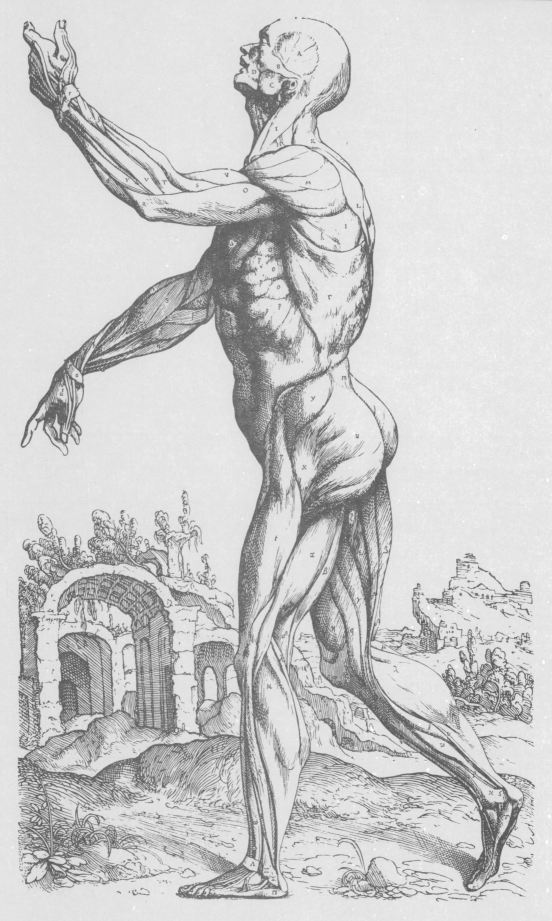

# CLEMENTE · ANATOMY

CLEMENTE · ANATOMY

# ANATOMY

## *A Regional Atlas of the Human Body*

Carmine D. Clemente Ph. D.

Professor of Anatomy and Director of the Brain Research Institute
University of California at Los Angeles School of Medicine
and
Professor of Surgery (Anatomy)
Charles R. Drew Postgraduate Medical School
Los Angeles, California

*Second Edition*

Urban & Schwarzenberg · Baltimore–Munich 1981

The pictures on the end leaves of the present volume show reproductions of the work of "Andreas Vesalii de corporis humani fabrica libri septem", which appeared in Basel in 1542. Andreas Vesalius (* Brussels 1514, † 1564) urged and practiced the dissection of human bodies and may be considered to be the founder of Modern Anatomy.

Editor's address:

Carmine D. Clemente, Ph. D., Professor of Anatomy and Director, Brain Research Institute UCLA School of Medicine, Los Angeles, California 90024 USA

Publisher's addresses:

Urban & Schwarzenberg, Inc.
7 East Redwood Street
Baltimore, Maryland 21202
USA

Urban & Schwarzenberg
Pettenkoferstraße 18
D-8000 München 2
Germany


The illustrations of this atlas were originally published in
      Sobotta/Becher, Atlas der Anatomie des Menschen, edited by H. Ferner and J. Staubesand,
      Urban & Schwarzenberg
with the exception of figures: 13, 15, 151, 152, 270, 286, 288, 316, 335, 352, 354, 439, 450, 517, 526, 527, 538, 542, 547, 548, 652, 662, 665, 693, 695, 705, 714 (from Benninghoff/Goerttler, Lehrbuch der Anatomie des Menschen, edited by H. Ferner and J. Staubesand, Urban & Schwarzenberg); 33, 165, 179, 232, 259, 263, 293, 347, 348 (from Lothar Wicke, Atlas of Radiologic Anatomy, 2nd Ed., Urban & Schwarzenberg); 11, 54, 55, 100, 115, 155, 157, 173, 174, 177, 180, 184, 185, 193, 205−207, 214, 218, 219, 257, 336, 337, 346, 419−424, 448, 449, 454, 507, 520, 524, 546, 568, 570, 596, 604, 630−639, 641−643, 653, 655, 692, 700, 702 (from Eduard Pernkopf, Atlas of Topographical and Applied Human Anatomy, 2nd Ed., edited by H. Ferner, Urban & Schwarzenberg).
Figures 14, 105, 195, 201, 435, 437 were drawn for this atlas by Jill Penkhus.

The first edition of this atlas was published in 1975 by Urban & Schwarzenberg (ISBN 3-541-07141-9) and copublished in North America by Lea & Febiger, Philadelphia (ISBN 0-8121-0496-X).

**Library of Congress Cataloging in Publication Data**

Clemente, Carmine D.
   Anatomy, a regional atlas of the human body.

   Includes index.
   1. Anatomy, Surgical and topographical--Atlases. I. Title. [DNLM: 1. Anatomy, Regional--Atlases. QS 17 C626a]
   QM531.C57   1981      611'.0022'2      80-28394
   ISBN 0-8067-0322-9

Fourth Printing 1984

© Urban & Schwarzenberg 1981

Printed in Germany by Kastner & Callwey, Fotosatz, Offsetdruck, München.

ISBN 0-8067-0322-9 Baltimore

ISBN 3-541-70322-9 München

# PREFACE TO THE SECOND EDITION

Seldom does a professor experience more gratification than when students at home and throughout the world express kind words regarding a teaching resource which he had offered tentatively and, initially, with some trepidation. After publication of the first edition of this atlas, I received nearly two hundred letters from medical and dental students, students of kinesiology, physical therapy and nursing as well as residents in the surgical specialties. Not one failed to comment in some manner on the beauty of the reproduced Sobotta figures (for which the publishers should be commended), and most letters made excellent suggestions of items to be included in future editions, while others uncovered typographical errors or mistaken facts. I am most grateful because this feedback information allowed me to alter labels and correct misspellings in time for the subsequent reprintings of the first edition and to add important transition figures in this edition.

The wide distribution and adoption of this atlas has allowed an opportunity for its revision. I have observed the use of the first edition in the classroom and in the gross anatomy laboratory setting for over five years, and this has given me further direction in assembling this revision. The addition of 130 figures and the elimination of only 10 published in the first edition represents an increase of 120 figures, or slightly over 20 percent. These have not been distributed equally among the seven parts of the atlas. Nearly one-third of the new figures were added to the section on neck and head, another one-third to the sections on thorax and abdomen, and the remaining one-third to the extremities, the pelvis and the back. I was fortunate to have the opportunity of selecting figures from the famous atlas published by Professor Eduard Pernkopf, *Atlas of Topographical and Applied Human Anatomy,* as well as having access to certain radiographs from the elegant *Atlas of Radiologic Anatomy* published by Dr. Lothar Wicke from Vienna. These new sources account for one-half of the additional figures selected, while the remainder come from the Sobotta and Benninghoff-Goerttler collections, used almost exclusively in the first edition. My appreciation is extended to Professor Helmut Ferner of Vienna and Professor Jochen Staubesand of Freiburg, who individually or together currently edit the German editions of the Sobotta and Pernkopf atlases and the Benninghoff-Goerttler text.

Some special emphasis has been placed in this edition on the inclusion of figures illustrating radiographic views of different regions, lymphatic drainage, the anatomy of the newborn, more material on the oral cavity, as well as additional cross sections of the limbs. Many of the recommendations received from students and faculty could be adopted, and my colleague here at UCLA, Dr. David S. Maxwell, offered a number of constructive suggestions which were incorporated. To all of these friends I express my gratitude. I wish to thank the publishers, Urban & Schwarzenberg, for their generosity in allowing a significant enlargement of this edition, without an inordinant increase in the cost of the book to students.

There are others, as well, to whom I am most grateful. Dr. Caroline Belz contributed superb editorial assistance in the preparation of the text for this edition and Mrs. Joyce Fried spent many hours helping to revise the index. From Urban & Schwarzenberg, I wish to thank Mr. Michael Urban, Dr. Richard Degkwitz and Mr. Klaus Gullath in Munich and Mr. Braxton Mitchell in Baltimore for their conceptual suggestions and for the practical solution of innumerable problems. And, as always, to my wife, Julie, I owe a continuing debt of gratitude for her selflessness and for her true understanding of the academic way of life.

Los Angeles, California, January 1981
CARMINE D. CLEMENTE

# FROM THE PREFACE TO THE FIRST EDITION

Twenty-five years ago, while a student at the University of Pennsylvania, I marvelled at the clarity, completeness, and boldness of the anatomical illustrations of the original German editions of Professor Johannes Sobotta's Atlas and their excellent three-volume, English counterparts, the recent editions of which were authored by the late Professor Frank H. J. Figge. It is a matter of record that before World War II these atlases were the most popular ones consulted by American medical students. In the United States, with the advent of other anatomical atlases, the shortening of courses of anatomy in the medical schools, and the increase in publishing costs, the excellent but larger editions of the Sobotta atlases have become virtually unknown to a full generation of students. During the past twenty years of teaching Gross Anatomy at the University of California at Los Angeles I have found only a handful of students who are familiar with the beautiful and still unexcelled Sobotta illustrations.

With this background I enthusiastically accepted the proposal of creating a single-volume atlas from the Sobotta plates and those subsequently drawn by Professor Erich Lepier of Vienna, with the objective of making this teaching resource material once again available to American students, this time at a relatively low cost.

This volume introduces several departures from the former Sobotta atlases. It is the first English edition that presents the Sobotta plates in a regional sequence – the pectoral region and upper extremity, the thorax, the abdomen, the pelvis and perineum, the lower extremity, the back, verterbral column and spinal cord, and finally the neck and head. This sequence is consistent with that followed in many courses presented in the United States and Canada and one which should be useful to students in other countries.

English instead of Latin labels have been used in all the figures. In most instances the terminology of the labels represents the English translation of the Nomina Anatomica designations. In rare instances in which the problem and discrepancies in nomenclature found among modern anatomical texts could not be resolved by consulting the Nomina Anatomica, I have elected to be consistent with the terminology presented in the Twenty-ninth American Edition of Gray's Anatomy. The text consists simply of notes intended to amplify the illustrations but not to exclude the need for an anatomy textbook.

Several illustrations never before published are presented in this Atlas. These have been drawn by Jill Penkhus, who for a number of years has been the resident medical artist in the Anatomy Department at the UCLA School of Medicine.

Many have contributed to bringing this Atlas to fruition. I wish to thank Dr. David S. Maxwell, Professor and Vice Chairman for Gross Anatomy and my colleague at UCLA, for his encouragement and suggestions. I also wish to express my appreciation to my friends Mr. John Febiger Spahr and Mr. George Mundorff, of Lea & Febiger in Philadelphia, and Mr. Michael Urban, of Urban and Schwarzenberg in Munich, for proposing this work and for assistance in seeing it to completion. I am indebted to Klaus Gullath and Sabine Rheineck, of Urban and Schwarzenberg, who have contributed much to the editing and format of this Atlas, and to Caroline Belz and Louise Campbell, who spent many hours proofreading and typing the original text. I especially wish to thank Mary Mansor, of Lea & Febiger, for constructing the index – a most laborious task. I am grateful to Barbara Robins for her assistance in typing some of the early parts of the manuscript, and above all, to her sister Julie, who is my wife and who makes all of my efforts worthwhile through her encouragement and devotion.

Los Angeles, California, January 1975

CARMINE D. CLEMENTE

# CONTENTS

# PART I: PECTORAL REGION AND UPPER EXTREMITY

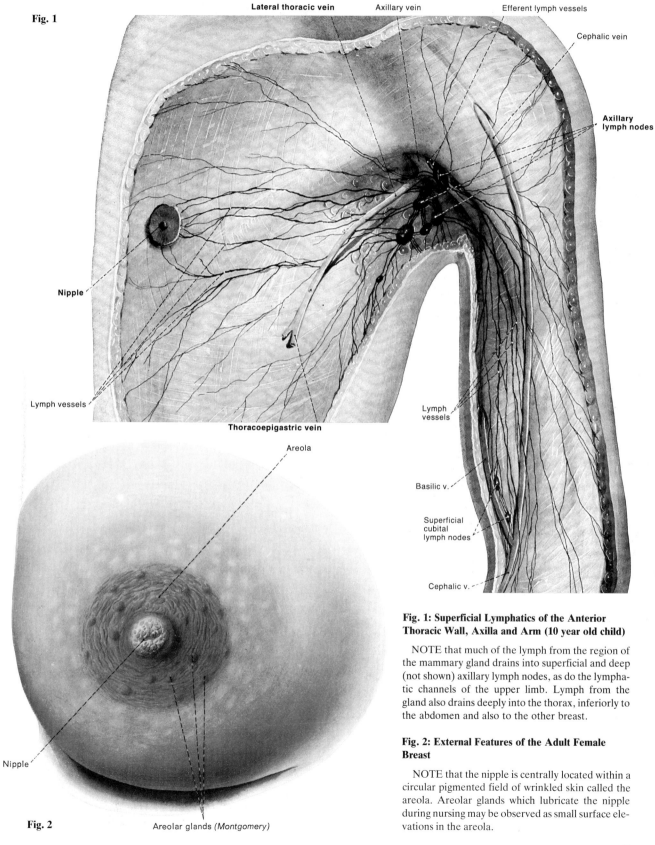

**Fig. 1**

Lateral thoracic vein

Axillary vein

Efferent lymph vessels

Cephalic vein

**Axillary lymph nodes**

**Nipple**

Lymph vessels

**Thoracoepigastric vein**

Lymph vessels

Basilic v.

Superficial cubital lymph nodes

Cephalic v.

Areola

Nipple

**Fig. 2**

Areolar glands (*Montgomery*)

### Fig. 1: Superficial Lymphatics of the Anterior Thoracic Wall, Axilla and Arm (10 year old child)

NOTE that much of the lymph from the region of the mammary gland drains into superficial and deep (not shown) axillary lymph nodes, as do the lymphatic channels of the upper limb. Lymph from the gland also drains deeply into the thorax, inferiorly to the abdomen and also to the other breast.

### Fig. 2: External Features of the Adult Female Breast

NOTE that the nipple is centrally located within a circular pigmented field of wrinkled skin called the areola. Areolar glands which lubricate the nipple during nursing may be observed as small surface elevations in the areola.

Figs. 1, 2    **I**

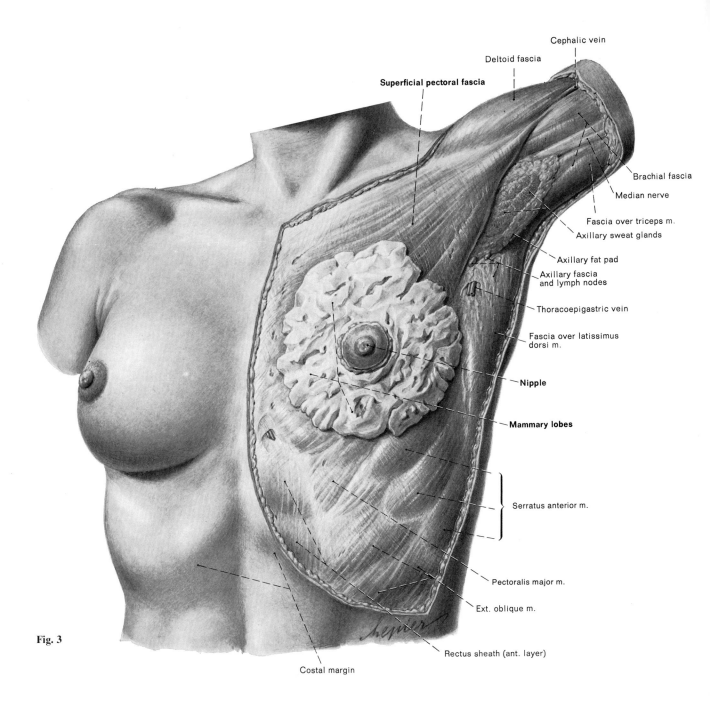

Cephalic vein

Deltoid fascia

**Superficial pectoral fascia**

Brachial fascia

Median nerve

Fascia over triceps m.

Axillary sweat glands

Axillary fat pad

Axillary fascia and lymph nodes

Thoracoepigastric vein

Fascia over latissimus dorsi m.

**Nipple**

**Mammary lobes**

Serratus anterior m.

Pectoralis major m.

Ext. oblique m.

**Fig. 3**

Rectus sheath (ant. layer)

Costal margin

**Fig. 3: Anterior Pectoral Dissection (Adult Female)**
   NOTE: 1) the lobular nature of the mammary gland extending toward the axilla and its location anterior to the pectoralis major muscle.
   2) the superficial axillary lymph and sudoriferous (sweat) glands.

**Fig. 4: Sagittal Section through Mammary Gland of Gravid Female**
   NOTE: 1) the radial arrangement of the lobes of glandular tissue. These lobes are comprised of smaller lobules and are separated from one another by fat and the supporting connective tissue.
   2) the lactiferous duct system. Each of the 15 to 20 lobes has its own duct which opens by means of a small orifice onto the nipple.
   3) that the mammary gland is separated from the pectoralis major muscle by the pectoral fascia and that connective tissue strands (suspensory ligaments of Cooper) within the gland extend toward this fascia.

**Fig. 5: Right Mammary Gland: Dissection of the Nipple**
   A circular piece of skin has been removed in this dissection. With the incised margin of the skin around the nipple retracted, the lactiferous ducts can be observed perforating onto the surface and arranged circumferentially around the nipple.

**Fig. 6: Two Typical Spinal Nerves: Their Origin, Branches and Connections to the Sympathetic Trunk**
   NOTE: 1) each spinal nerve attaches to the spinal cord by two roots: an afferent or sensory dorsal root and an efferent or motor ventral root. Each dorsal root contains a spinal ganglion comprised of afferent neuron cell bodies.
   2) the two spinal roots join to form the spinal nerve, which in turn divides into a dorsal ramus coursing posteriorly and a ventral ramus coursing anteriorly. During their course, these rami divide further to innervate the body segment with both sensory and motor fibers.
   3) the spinal nerve communicates with the sympathetic trunk carrying preganglionic sympathetic fibers to the trunk (white ramus) and postganglionic fibers from the trunk (gray ramus).

Fig. 3

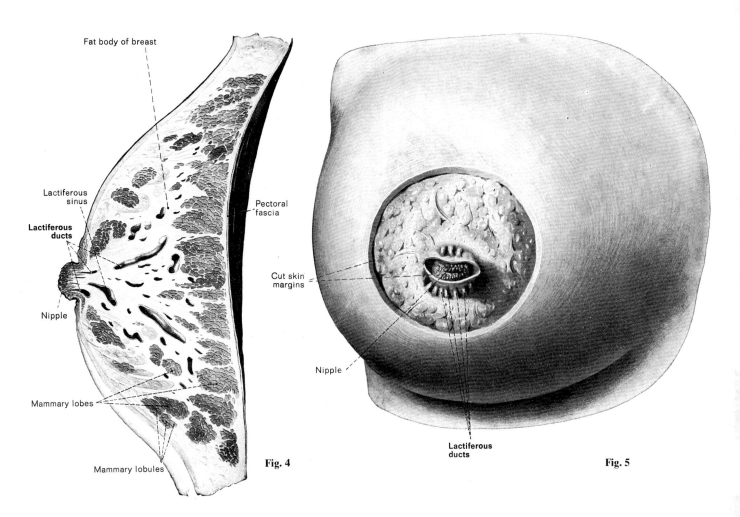

Fig. 4

Fat body of breast

Lactiferous sinus

**Lactiferous ducts**

Nipple

Mammary lobes

Mammary lobules

Pectoral fascia

Fig. 5

Cut skin margins

Nipple

Lactiferous ducts

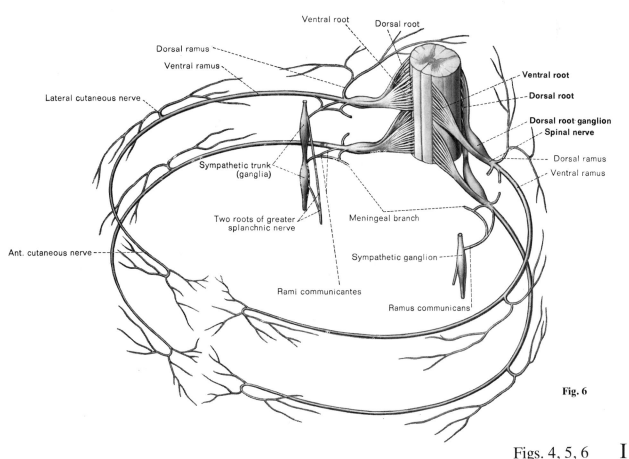

Ventral root

Dorsal root

Dorsal ramus

Ventral ramus

Lateral cutaneous nerve

**Ventral root**

**Dorsal root**

**Dorsal root ganglion**
**Spinal nerve**

Dorsal ramus

Ventral ramus

Sympathetic trunk (ganglia)

Two roots of greater splanchnic nerve

Meningeal branch

Ant. cutaneous nerve

Sympathetic ganglion

Rami communicantes

Ramus communicans

Fig. 6

Figs. 4, 5, 6   I

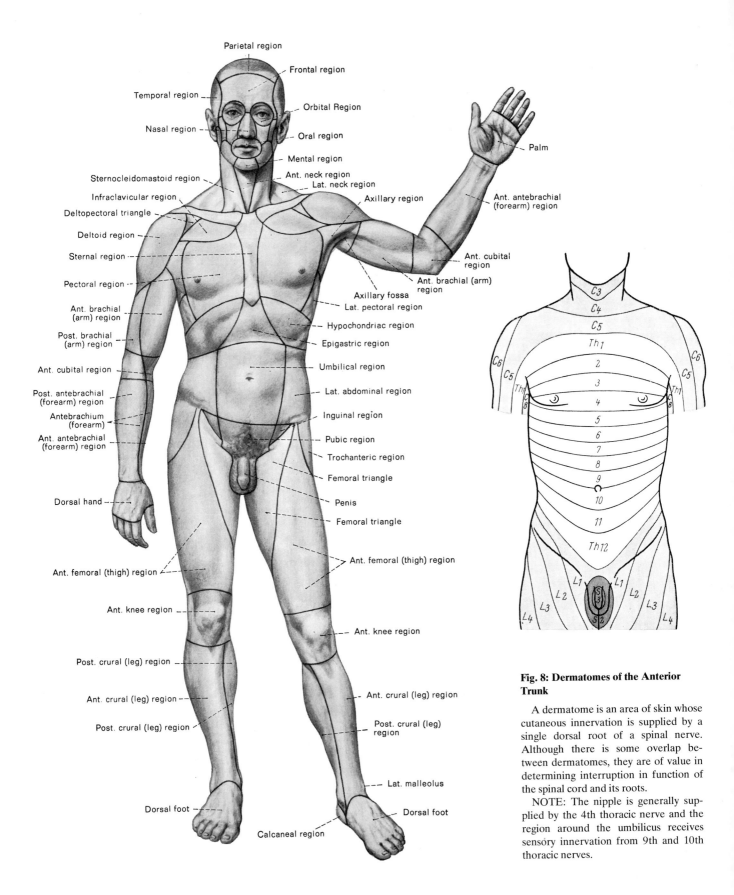

Parietal region
Frontal region
Temporal region
Orbital Region
Nasal region
Oral region
Mental region
Sternocleidomastoid region
Ant. neck region
Lat. neck region
Infraclavicular region
Axillary region
Deltopectoral triangle
Deltoid region
Sternal region
Pectoral region
Ant. brachial (arm) region
Post. brachial (arm) region
Ant. cubital region
Post. antebrachial (forearm) region
Antebrachium (forearm)
Ant. antebrachial (forearm) region
Dorsal hand

Palm
Ant. antebrachial (forearm) region
Ant. cubital region
Ant. brachial (arm) region
Axillary fossa
Lat. pectoral region
Hypochondriac region
Epigastric region
Umbilical region
Lat. abdominal region
Inguinal region
Pubic region
Trochanteric region
Femoral triangle
Penis
Femoral triangle

Ant. femoral (thigh) region
Ant. knee region
Post. crural (leg) region
Ant. crural (leg) region
Post. crural (leg) region
Dorsal foot
Calcaneal region

Ant. femoral (thigh) region
Ant. knee region
Ant. crural (leg) region
Post. crural (leg) region
Lat. malleolus
Dorsal foot

*(Fig. 8 dermatome labels: C3, C4, C5, Th1, 2, 3, 4, 5, 6, 7, 8, 9, 10, 11, Th12, C6, C5, Th1, C8, L1, L2, L3, L4, S3, S4)*

**Fig. 8: Dermatomes of the Anterior Trunk**

A dermatome is an area of skin whose cutaneous innervation is supplied by a single dorsal root of a spinal nerve. Although there is some overlap between dermatomes, they are of value in determining interruption in function of the spinal cord and its roots.

NOTE: The nipple is generally supplied by the 4th thoracic nerve and the region around the umbilicus receives sensory innervation from 9th and 10th thoracic nerves.

**Fig 7: The Regions of the Body: Anterior View**

Every surface area and region of the body has been identified by a specific name in order to describe more precisely the location of anatomical structures. Note that regions are named after underlying or adjacent bones (sternal, parietal, frontal, temporal, infraclavicular, femoral) while other regions are named for underlying muscles (sternocleidomastoid, deltoid, pectoral). Still other regions are named after specialized anatomical structures (umbilical, oral, nasal).

Figs. 7, 8

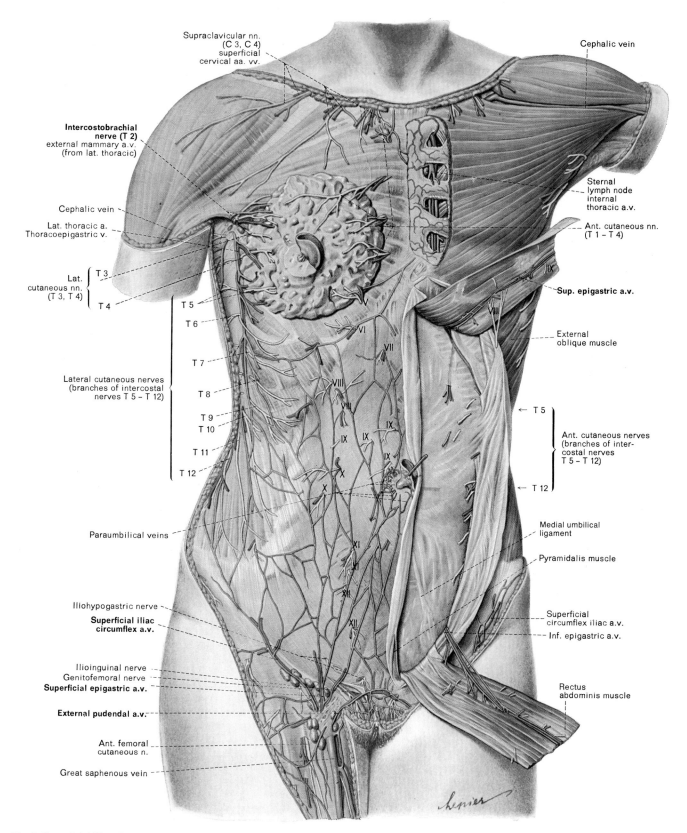

**Fig. 9: Superficial Vessels and Nerves of the Ventral Trunk: Pectoral Region and Anterior Abdominal Wall**

OBSERVE: 1) the cutaneous innervation of the anterior trunk which is derived from a) the supraclavicular nerves ($C_3$, $C_4$);
b) the intercostal nerves (anterior cutaneous T 1 – T 12; lateral cutaneous T 2 – T 12); c) iliohypogastric and ilioinguinal nerves (L 1).

2) the thoracoepigastric venous anastomosis between the thoracoepigastric and lateral thoracic veins superiorly and the superficial circumflex iliac and superficial epigastric veins inferiorly.

3) the mammary gland: its innervation (T2–T6) and its blood supply (branches of internal thoracic artery, lateral thoracic artery). Additionally, the mammary gland may receive small branches from the intercostal arteries which may enter the deep surface of the gland.

4) the nipple at the level of T 4 and the umbilicus at the level of T 10.

Fig. 9    I

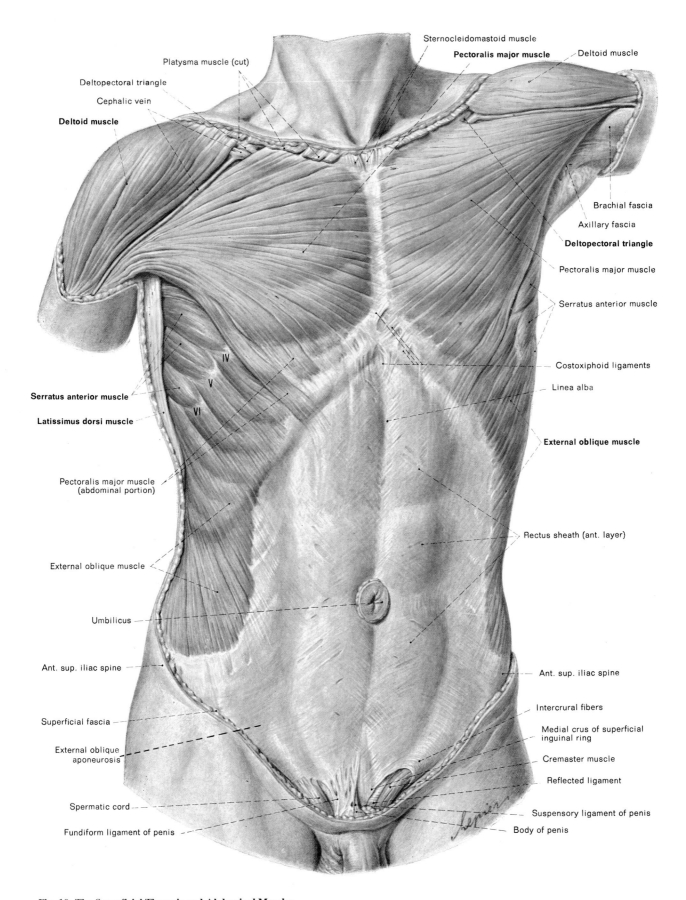

**Fig. 10: The Superficial Thoracic and Abdominal Muscles**

   OBSERVE that the pectoralis major arises from the medial half of the clavicle, the costal margin of the sternum, the 2nd to 6th ribs and the upper part of the aponeurosis of the external oblique. Also note the deltopectoral triangle and the course of the cephalic vein as it empties into the axillary vein.

Fig. 10

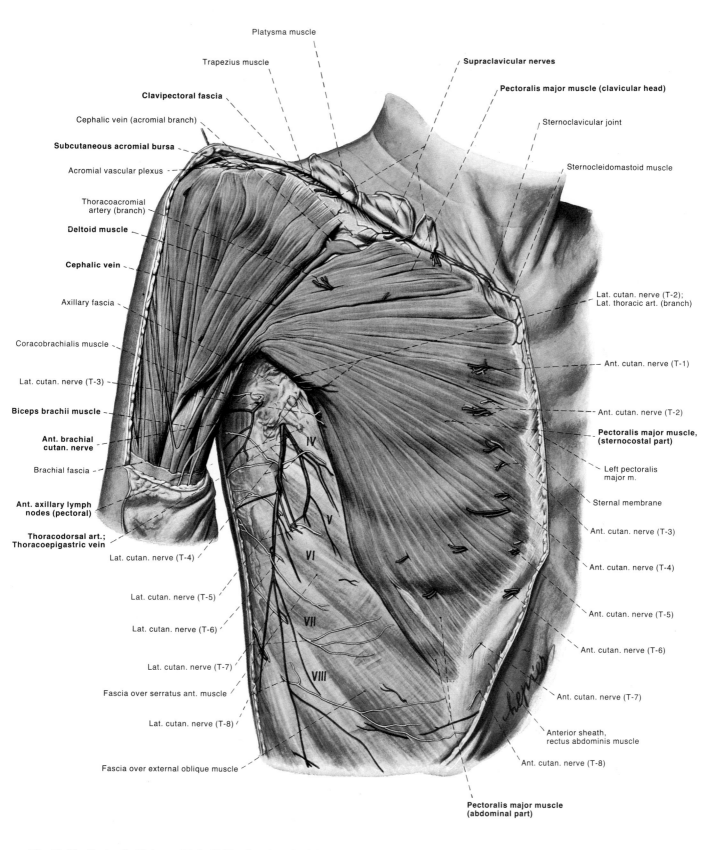

Platysma muscle

Trapezius muscle

**Clavipectoral fascia**

Cephalic vein (acromial branch)

**Subcutaneous acromial bursa**

Acromial vascular plexus

Thoracoacromial artery (branch)

**Deltoid muscle**

**Cephalic vein**

Axillary fascia

Coracobrachialis muscle

Lat. cutan. nerve (T-3)

**Biceps brachii muscle**

**Ant. brachial cutan. nerve**

Brachial fascia

**Ant. axillary lymph nodes (pectoral)**

**Thoracodorsal art.; Thoracoepigastric vein**

Lat. cutan. nerve (T-4)

Lat. cutan. nerve (T-5)

Lat. cutan. nerve (T-6)

Lat. cutan. nerve (T-7)

Fascia over serratus ant. muscle

Lat. cutan. nerve (T-8)

Fascia over external oblique muscle

**Supraclavicular nerves**

**Pectoralis major muscle (clavicular head)**

Sternoclavicular joint

Sternocleidomastoid muscle

Lat. cutan. nerve (T-2); Lat. thoracic art. (branch)

Ant. cutan. nerve (T-1)

Ant. cutan. nerve (T-2)

**Pectoralis major muscle, (sternocostal part)**

Left pectoralis major m.

Sternal membrane

Ant. cutan. nerve (T-3)

Ant. cutan. nerve (T-4)

Ant. cutan. nerve (T-5)

Ant. cutan. nerve (T-6)

Ant. cutan. nerve (T-7)

Anterior sheath, rectus abdominis muscle

Ant. cutan. nerve (T-8)

**Pectoralis major muscle (abdominal part)**

**Fig. 11: The Pectoralis Major and Deltoid Muscles, Anterior View**

NOTE: 1) segmentally arranged lateral and anterior cutaneous nerves which branch from the intercostal nerves. These penetrate through the intercostal spaces approximately in the mid-axillary line (lateral cutaneous nerves) and, more anteriorly, along the lateral border of the sternum through the substance of the pectoralis major muscle (anterior cutaneous nerves).

2) the 4th to the 8th ribs are numbered sequentially with Roman numerals.

3) the thoracoepigastric vein and the thoracodorsal artery piercing the deep fascia and coursing along the mid-axillary line.

Fig. 11   I

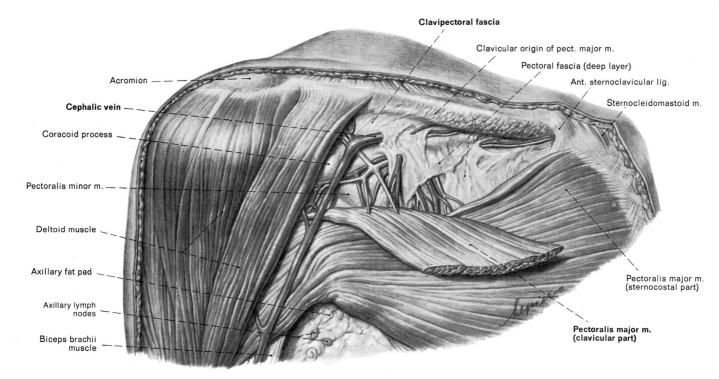

Acromion

**Cephalic vein**

Coracoid process

Pectoralis minor m.

Deltoid muscle

Axillary fat pad

Axillary lymph nodes

Biceps brachii muscle

**Clavipectoral fascia**

Clavicular origin of pect. major m.

Pectoral fascia (deep layer)

Ant. sternoclavicular lig.

Sternocleidomastoid m.

Pectoralis major m. (sternocostal part)

**Pectoralis major m. (clavicular part)**

**Fig. 12: The Deltopectoral Triangle (Right)**

With the clavicular head of the pectoralis major muscle severed,
    OBSERVE: 1) the internal investing layer of fascia deep to the pectoralis major;
2) the clavipectoral fascia which lies between the pectoralis major and the thoracic wall;
3) the course of the cephalic vein as it pierces the clavipectoral fascia to join the axillary vein.

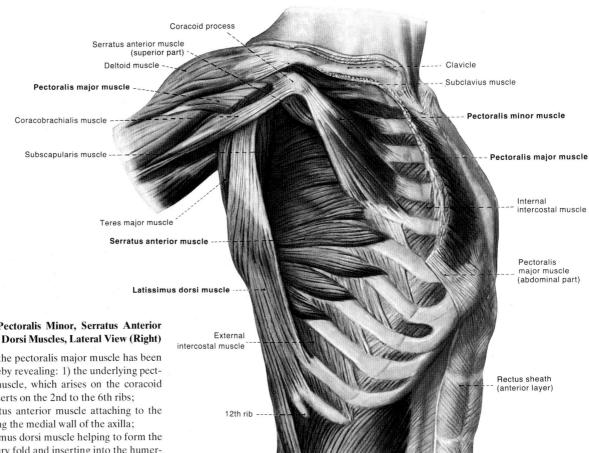

Coracoid process

Serratus anterior muscle (superior part)

Deltoid muscle

**Pectoralis major muscle**

Coracobrachialis muscle

Subscapularis muscle

Teres major muscle

**Serratus anterior muscle**

**Latissimus dorsi muscle**

Clavicle

Subclavius muscle

**Pectoralis minor muscle**

**Pectoralis major muscle**

Internal intercostal muscle

Pectoralis major muscle (abdominal part)

External intercostal muscle

12th rib

Rectus sheath (anterior layer)

**Fig. 13: The Pectoralis Minor, Serratus Anterior and Latissimus Dorsi Muscles, Lateral View (Right)**

NOTE that the pectoralis major muscle has been reflected, thereby revealing: 1) the underlying pectoralis minor muscle, which arises on the coracoid process and inserts on the 2nd to 6th ribs;

2) the serratus anterior muscle attaching to the ribs and forming the medial wall of the axilla;

3) the latissimus dorsi muscle helping to form the posterior axillary fold and inserting into the humerus.

Figs. 12, 13

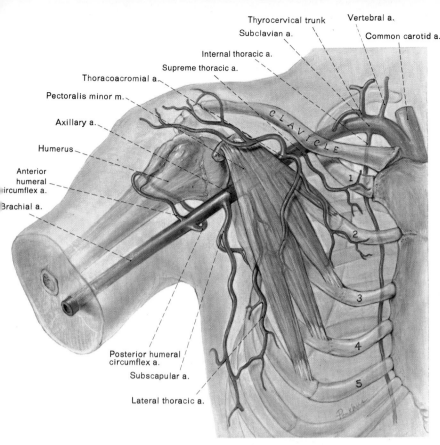

Thyrocervical trunk
Subclavian a.
Internal thoracic a.
Supreme thoracic a.
Thoracoacromial a.
Pectoralis minor m.
Axillary a.
Humerus
Anterior humeral circumflex a.
Brachial a.

Vertebral a.
Common carotid a.

CLAVICLE

Posterior humeral circumflex a.
Subscapular a.
Lateral thoracic a.

## Fig. 14: The Branches of the Axillary Artery

NOTE: 1) as the subclavian artery passes beneath the clavicle, it becomes the axillary artery. The axillary artery becomes the brachial artery in the upper arm (at the level of the tendon of the teres major muscle). In the axilla the pectoralis minor muscle crosses anterior to the axillary artery, thereby, for descriptive purposes, dividing the vessel into three parts.

2) from the 1st part of the axillary artery (medial to the pectoralis minor and lateral to the clavicle) branches one vessel, the supreme thoracic artery. From the 2nd part (beneath the muscle) branch two vessels, the thoracoacromial artery and the lateral thoracic. From the 3rd part of the axillary (lateral to the pectoralis minor muscle) are derived three branches, the subscapular artery and the anterior and posterior humeral circumflex arteries.

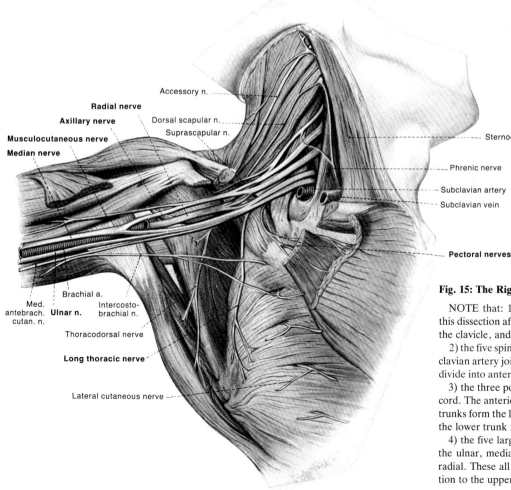

Radial nerve
Axillary nerve
Musculocutaneous nerve
Median nerve

Accessory n.
Dorsal scapular n.
Suprascapular n.

Sternocleidomastoid muscle
Phrenic nerve
Subclavian artery
Subclavian vein

Pectoral nerves

Med. antebrach. cutan. n.
Ulnar n.
Brachial a.
Intercosto-brachial n.
Thoracodorsal nerve
Long thoracic nerve
Lateral cutaneous nerve

## Fig. 15: The Right Brachial Plexus

NOTE that: 1) the brachial plexus is exposed in this dissection after removal of the pectoral muscles, the clavicle, and the axillary vessels;

2) the five spinal roots immediately above the subclavian artery join to form three trunks, which then divide into anterior and posterior divisions;

3) the three posterior divisions form the posterior cord. The anterior divisions of the upper and middle trunks form the lateral cord. The anterior division of the lower trunk forms the medial cord;

4) the five large terminal nerves of the plexus are the ulnar, median, musculocutaneous, axillary and radial. These all supply motor and sensory innervation to the upper limb.

Figs. 14, 15    I

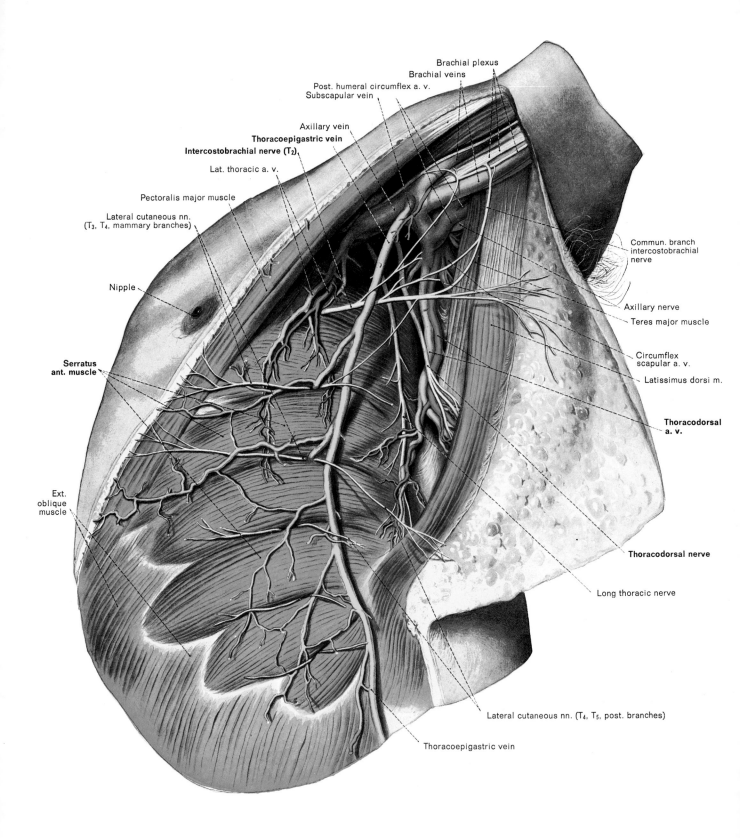

**Brachial plexus**

**Brachial veins**

**Post. humeral circumflex a. v.**

**Subscapular vein**

**Axillary vein**

**Thoracoepigastric vein**

**Intercostobrachial nerve (T₂)**

Lat. thoracic a. v.

Pectoralis major muscle

Lateral cutaneous nn.
(T₃, T₄, mammary branches)

Nipple

**Serratus
ant. muscle**

Ext.
oblique
muscle

Commun. branch
intercostobrachial
nerve

Axillary nerve

Teres major muscle

Circumflex
scapular a. v.

Latissimus dorsi m.

**Thoracodorsal
a. v.**

**Thoracodorsal nerve**

Long thoracic nerve

Lateral cutaneous nn. (T₄, T₅, post. branches)

Thoracoepigastric vein

**Fig. 16: The Axilla: Superficial Vessels and Nerves (left)**

OBSERVE: 1) that the boundaries of the axilla are, a) anteriorly, the pectoralis major muscle; b) posteriorly, the subscapularis, teres major and latissimus dorsi muscles; c) medially, the serratus anterior muscle covering the ribs, and; d) laterally, the bicipital groove of the humerus.

2) that the inferior portion of the serratus anterior muscle arises from the lower ribs as fleshy interdigitations with the external oblique muscle.

3) the serratus anterior is innervated by the long thoracic nerve (C 5, 6, 7) and the latissimus dorsi is innervated by the thoracodorsal nerve (C 5, 6, 7).

4) the axillary vein lies medial to the axillary artery and the cords of the brachial plexus.

5) the descending course of the thoracoepigastric vein and the lateral thoracic artery and vein.

Fig. 16

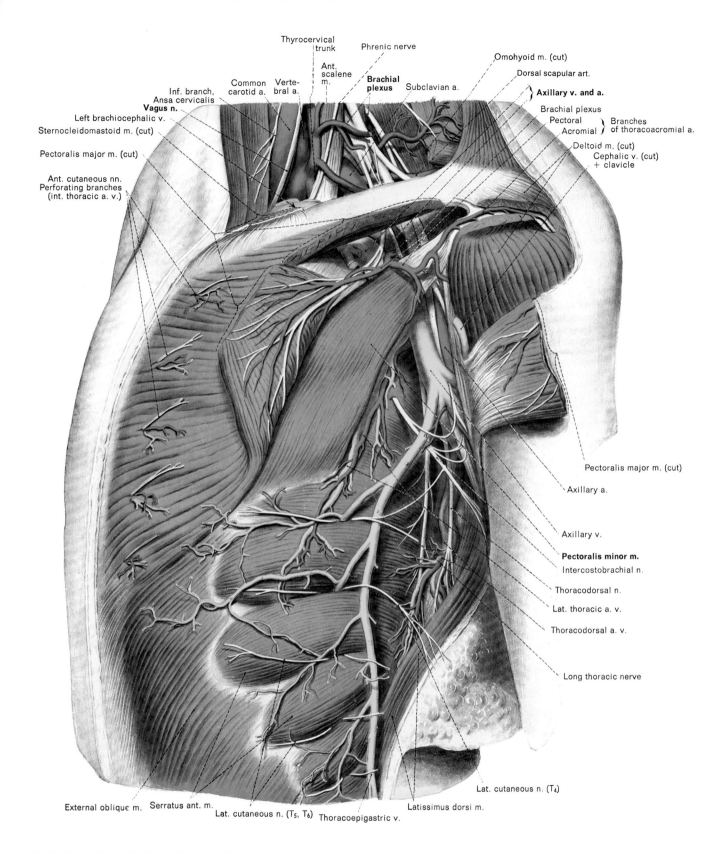

Thyrocervical trunk
Phrenic nerve
Ant. scalene m.
Brachial plexus
Subclavian a.
Common carotid a.
Verte-bral a.
Omohyoid m. (cut)
Dorsal scapular art.
**Axillary v. and a.**
Inf. branch, Ansa cervicalis
**Vagus n.**
Brachial plexus
Pectoral
Acromial } Branches of thoracoacromial a.
Left brachiocephalic v.
Sternocleidomastoid m. (cut)
Deltoid m. (cut)
Cephalic v. (cut) + clavicle
Pectoralis major m. (cut)
Ant. cutaneous nn. Perforating branches (int. thoracic a. v.)

Pectoralis major m. (cut)

Axillary a.

Axillary v.

**Pectoralis minor m.**
Intercostobrachial n.
Thoracodorsal n.
Lat. thoracic a. v.
Thoracodorsal a. v.

Long thoracic nerve

Lat. cutaneous n. (T₄)
External oblique m.   Serratus ant. m.
Lat. cutaneous n. (T₅, T₆)   Thoracoepigastric v.
Latissimus dorsi m.

**Fig. 17: The Axilla (left): Deep Vessels and Nerves**

OBSERVE: 1) that the subclavian artery becomes the axillary artery as it passes beneath the clavicle;

2) that the pectoralis minor muscle is helpful in describing the underlying axillary artery in its course through the axilla, since the three parts of the axillary artery are medial, beneath and lateral to the pectoralis minor;

3) that the axillary vein courses medial to the axillary artery and it receives tributaries not only from the upper extremity but from the thorax as well;

4) that the axillary artery is surrounded by the three cords of the brachial plexus;

5) that the thoracoacromial artery divides into pectoral, acromial, deltoid and small clavicular branches (the latter are not shown in the figure);

6) that the intercostobrachial (T₂) nerve pierces the thoracic cage through the 2nd intercostal space in its course toward the axilla and arm.

Fig. 17   I

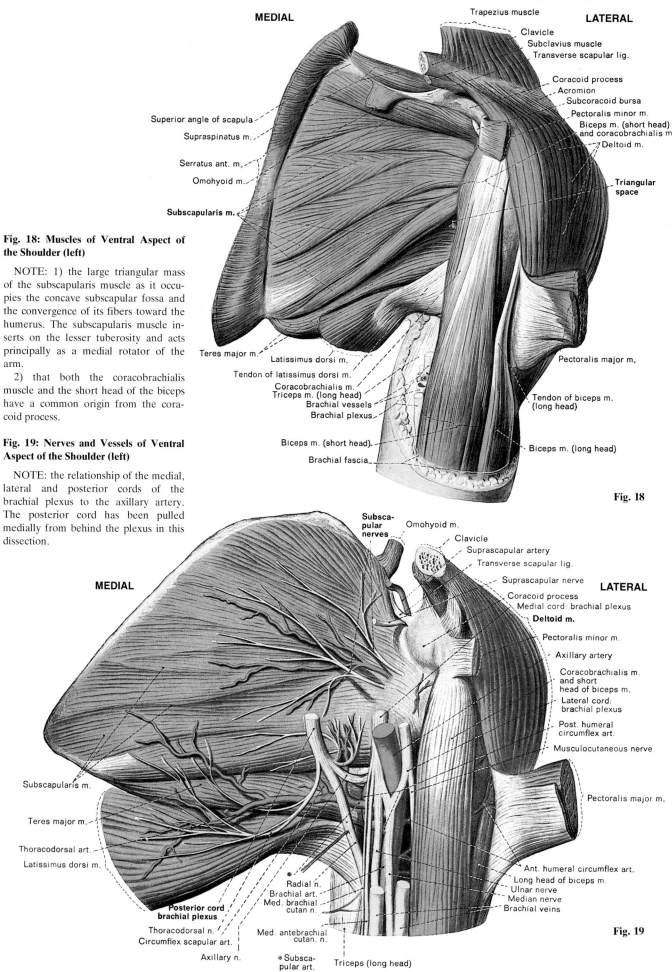

MEDIAL

Trapezius muscle

LATERAL

Clavicle
Subclavius muscle
Transverse scapular lig.

Coracoid process
Acromion
Subcoracoid bursa
Pectoralis minor m.
Biceps m. (short head)
and coracobrachialis m.
Deltoid m.

Superior angle of scapula

Supraspinatus m.

Serratus ant. m.

Omohyoid m.

Subscapularis m.

**Triangular space**

### Fig. 18: Muscles of Ventral Aspect of the Shoulder (left)

NOTE: 1) the large triangular mass of the subscapularis muscle as it occupies the concave subscapular fossa and the convergence of its fibers toward the humerus. The subscapularis muscle inserts on the lesser tuberosity and acts principally as a medial rotator of the arm.

2) that both the coracobrachialis muscle and the short head of the biceps have a common origin from the coracoid process.

### Fig. 19: Nerves and Vessels of Ventral Aspect of the Shoulder (left)

NOTE: the relationship of the medial, lateral and posterior cords of the brachial plexus to the axillary artery. The posterior cord has been pulled medially from behind the plexus in this dissection.

Teres major m.
Latissimus dorsi m.
Tendon of latissimus dorsi m.
Coracobrachialis m.
Triceps m. (long head)
Brachial vessels
Brachial plexus

Biceps m. (short head)

Brachial fascia

Pectoralis major m.

Tendon of biceps m. (long head)

Biceps m. (long head)

Fig. 18

Subscapular nerves
Omohyoid m.
Clavicle
Suprascapular artery
Transverse scapular lig.
Suprascapular nerve

MEDIAL

LATERAL

Coracoid process
Medial cord: brachial plexus
**Deltoid m.**

Pectoralis minor m.

Axillary artery

Coracobrachialis m. and short head of biceps m.

Lateral cord: brachial plexus

Post. humeral circumflex art.

Musculocutaneous nerve

Subscapularis m.

Teres major m.

Thoracodorsal art.
Latissimus dorsi m.

Pectoralis major m.

Ant. humeral circumflex art.
Long head of biceps m.
Ulnar nerve
Median nerve
Brachial veins

**Posterior cord brachial plexus**

Thoracodorsal n.
Circumflex scapular art.

Axillary n.

Radial n.
Brachial art.
Med. brachial cutan n.

Med. antebrachial cutan. n.

*Subscapular art.

Triceps (long head)

Fig. 19

Figs. 18, 19

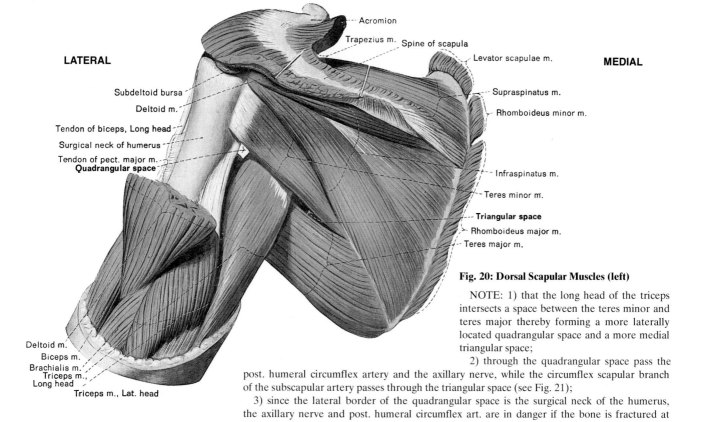

LATERAL                    MEDIAL

- Acromion
- Trapezius m.
- Spine of scapula
- Levator scapulae m.
- Subdeltoid bursa
- Deltoid m.
- Tendon of biceps, Long head
- Surgical neck of humerus
- Tendon of pect. major m.
- **Quadrangular space**
- Supraspinatus m.
- Rhomboideus minor m.
- Infraspinatus m.
- Teres minor m.
- **Triangular space**
- Rhomboideus major m.
- Teres major m.
- Deltoid m.
- Biceps m.
- Brachialis m.
- Triceps m.
- Long head
- **Triceps m., Lat. head**

**Fig. 20: Dorsal Scapular Muscles (left)**

NOTE: 1) that the long head of the triceps intersects a space between the teres minor and teres major thereby forming a more laterally located quadrangular space and a more medial triangular space;

2) through the quadrangular space pass the post. humeral circumflex artery and the axillary nerve, while the circumflex scapular branch of the subscapular artery passes through the triangular space (see Fig. 21);

3) since the lateral border of the quadrangular space is the surgical neck of the humerus, the axillary nerve and post. humeral circumflex art. are in danger if the bone is fractured at this site.

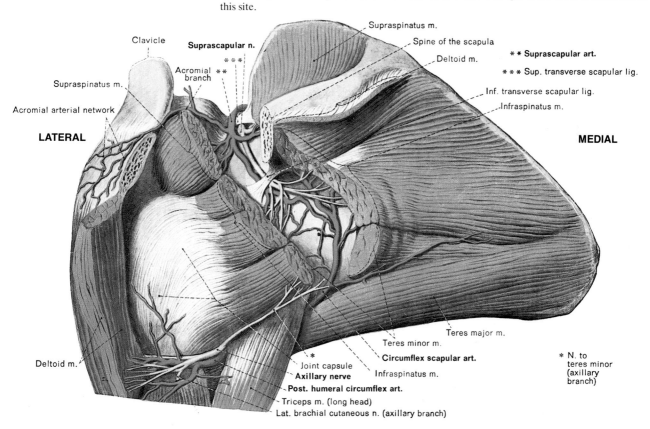

- Supraspinatus m.
- Spine of the scapula
- Clavicle
- **Suprascapular n.**
- * * *
- Deltoid m.
- **✱✱ Suprascapular art.**
- Acromial branch ✱✱
- Supraspinatus m.
- Acromial arterial network
- ✱✱✱ Sup. transverse scapular lig.
- Inf. transverse scapular lig.
- Infraspinatus m.
- LATERAL                    MEDIAL
- Teres major m.
- Teres minor m.
- **Circumflex scapular art.**
- Deltoid m.
- *
- Joint capsule
- **Axillary nerve**
- Infraspinatus m.
- **Post. humeral circumflex art.**
- Triceps m. (long head)
- Lat. brachial cutaneous n. (axillary branch)
- ✱ N. to teres minor (axillary branch)

**Fig. 21: Nerves and Vessels of Dorsal Scapular Region (left)**

NOTE: 1) that the sup. transverse scapular lig. bridges across the scapular notch and the suprascapular nerve passes beneath the ligament while the suprascapular artery usually passes above it;

2) that the axillary nerve supplies four structures: the deltoid muscle, the teres minor muscle, the capsule of the shoulder joint and the skin over the shoulder joint;

3) that the axillary nerve and post. humeral circumflex artery achieve the dorsal aspect of the shoulder through the quadrangular space while the circumflex scapular artery reaches the infraspinatus fossa through the triangular space.

Figs. 20, 21    **I**

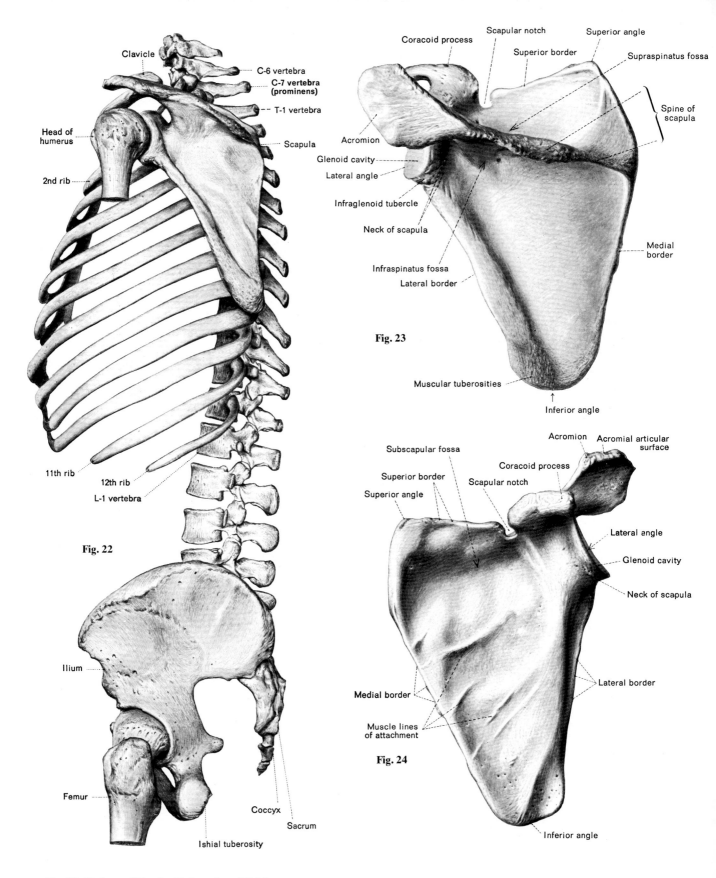

**Fig. 22: Skeleton of Trunk with Scapula and Pelvis**

NOTE that the flat triangular shaped scapula articulates with the head of the humerus and the clavicle. It is also attached to the rib cage by muscles.

**Fig. 23: The Left Scapula (Dorsal Surface)**

NOTE that the socket for the head of the humerus is formed by the glenoid cavity and is further enlarged by the coracoid and acromial processes along with their related ligaments. The spine of the scapula separates the dorsal surface into supraspinatus and infraspinatus fossae.

**Fig. 24: The Left Scapula (Ventral Surface)**

NOTE that much of the ventral surface is a concave fossa within which lies the subscapularis muscle.

Figs. 22, 23, 24

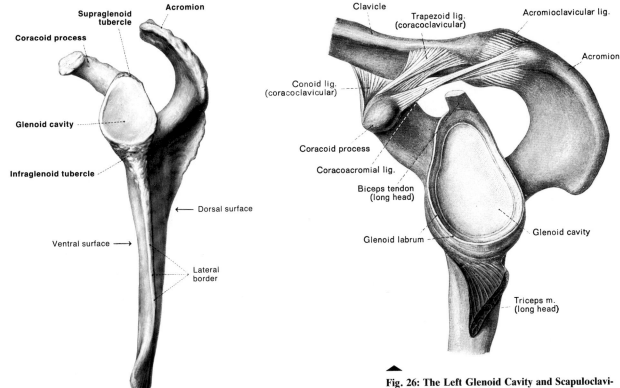

**Fig. 25: The Left Scapula, Lateral View**

NOTE: 1) the supraglenoid and infraglenoid tubercles from which arise the long heads of the biceps and triceps muscles, respectively;

2) the anteriorly projecting coracoid process to which are attached the pectoralis minor, short head of the biceps, and the coracobrachialis muscles.

**Fig. 26: The Left Glenoid Cavity and Scapuloclavicular Joint (Lateral View)**

NOTE: 1) exposure of the glenoid cavity was achieved by removal of the articular capsule at the glenoid labrum;

2) the attachment of the tendon of the long head of the biceps muscle at the supraglenoid tubercle and that of the long head of the triceps at the infraglenoid tubercle have been left intact;

3) the shallowness of the glenoid cavity is slightly deepened (4 to 6 mm.) by the glenoid labrum;

4) the protection afforded to the shoulder joint superiorly by the acromion, coracoid process and clavicle and their ligamentous attachments and by the tendon of the long head of the biceps.

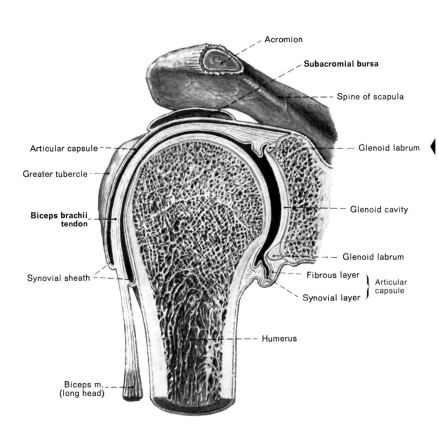

**Fig. 27: Frontal Section through Right Shoulder Joint**

NOTE: 1) that the tendon of the long head of the biceps arises from the supraglenoid tuberosity and is at once enclosed by a reflection of the synovial sheath. Thus, although the tendon passes through the joint, it is not contained within the synovial cavity of the joint;

2) the capsule of the joint is composed of a dense fibrous outer layer and a thin synovial inner layer. It is this thin inner layer which reflects itself around the biceps tendon in its course through the joint;

3) a bursa is a sac lined with a synovial-like membrane containing a small amount of fluid. Bursae are found at sites subjected to friction and normally do not communicate with the joint capsule. In the shoulder, separate bursae are found between the capsule and the subscapularis, infraspinatus and deltoid tendons as well as other muscles, and between the capsule and the coracoid and acromial processes (subacromial bursa).

Figs. 25, 26, 27    I

## Fig. 28: Left Shoulder Joint and Acromioclavicular Joint (Anterior View)

NOTE: 1) that the clavicle is attached by ligaments to both the acromion (acromioclavicular lig) and the coracoid process (coracoclavicular lig.) of the scapula. The acromion and coracoid process are themselves connected by the coracoacromial ligament;

2) neither the acromion nor the clavicle articulates directly with the humerus, whereas the coracoid process and the glenoid labrum afford attachment of the scapula to the humerus;

3) the acromion, coracoid process and clavicle assist in the protection of the shoulder joint from above. Thus, the joint is weakest inferiorly and anteriorly, the directions in which most dislocations occur;

4) the glenohumeral ligaments are thickened bands which tend to strenghten somewhat the capsule of the joint anteriorly;

5) the position of the long tendon of the biceps traversing the articular cavity to its point of attachment on the supraglenoid tubercle.

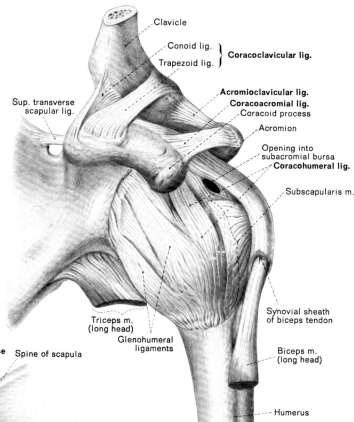

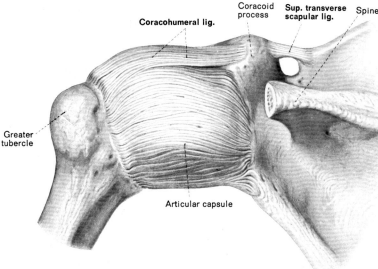

## Fig. 29: Capsule of Left Shoulder Joint (Posterior View)

NOTE: 1) the articular capsule completely surrounds the joint, being attached beyond the glenoid cavity on the scapula above and to the anatomical neck of the humerus below;

2) the superior part of the capsule is further strengthened by the coracohumeral ligament.

## Fig. 30: Left Shoulder Joint (Posterior View)

NOTE: 1) the shoulder joint is a freely moving ball and socket joint. The capsule of the joint is not drawn tightly between the humeral head and scapula but attached loosely over these bony structures;

2) the tendons of the supraspinatus, infraspinatus and teres minor blend superiorly and posteriorly with the capsule of the joint. These muscles along with the subscapularis anteriorly form a muscular encasement lending some support in the maintenance of the head of the humerus in its socket;

3) the close relationship of the long head of the triceps to the capsule of joint. When the arm is abducted the triceps is drawn even closer to the capsule to help prevent dislocation.

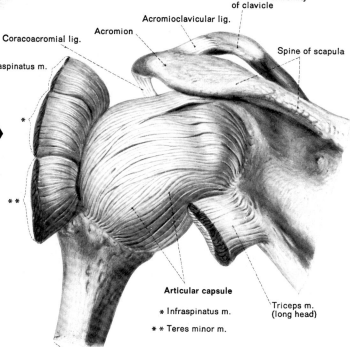

Figs. 28, 29, 30

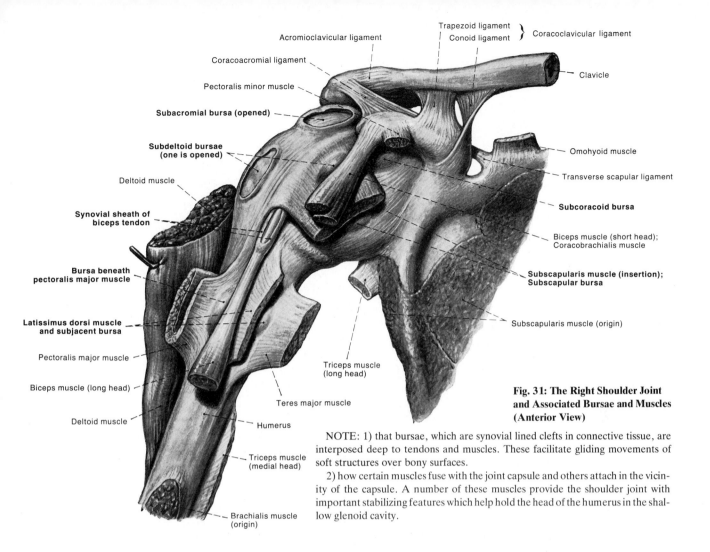

Acromioclavicular ligament

Trapezoid ligament
Conoid ligament } Coracoclavicular ligament

Coracoacromial ligament

Clavicle

Pectoralis minor muscle

**Subacromial bursa (opened)**

**Subdeltoid bursae
(one is opened)**

Omohyoid muscle

Deltoid muscle

Transverse scapular ligament

**Synovial sheath of
biceps tendon**

**Subcoracoid bursa**

Biceps muscle (short head);
Coracobrachialis muscle

**Bursa beneath
pectoralis major muscle**

**Subscapularis muscle (insertion);
Subscapular bursa**

**Latissimus dorsi muscle
and subjacent bursa**

Subscapularis muscle (origin)

Pectoralis major muscle

Biceps muscle (long head)

Triceps muscle
(long head)

Deltoid muscle

**Fig. 31: The Right Shoulder Joint
and Associated Bursae and Muscles
(Anterior View)**

Teres major muscle

Humerus

Triceps muscle
(medial head)

NOTE: 1) that bursae, which are synovial lined clefts in connective tissue, are interposed deep to tendons and muscles. These facilitate gliding movements of soft structures over bony surfaces.

2) how certain muscles fuse with the joint capsule and others attach in the vicinity of the capsule. A number of these muscles provide the shoulder joint with important stabilizing features which help hold the head of the humerus in the shallow glenoid cavity.

Brachialis muscle
(origin)

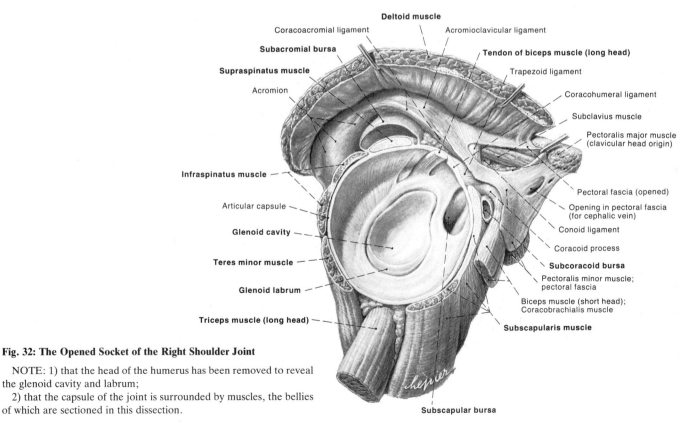

Deltoid muscle

Coracoacromial ligament

Acromioclavicular ligament

**Subacromial bursa**

**Tendon of biceps muscle (long head)**

**Supraspinatus muscle**

Trapezoid ligament

Acromion

Coracohumeral ligament

Subclavius muscle

Pectoralis major muscle
(clavicular head origin)

**Infraspinatus muscle**

Articular capsule

Pectoral fascia (opened)

Opening in pectoral fascia
(for cephalic vein)

**Glenoid cavity**

Conoid ligament

Coracoid process

**Teres minor muscle**

**Subcoracoid bursa**

Glenoid labrum

Pectoralis minor muscle;
pectoral fascia

Biceps muscle (short head);
Coracobrachialis muscle

**Triceps muscle (long head)**

**Subscapularis muscle**

**Subscapular bursa**

**Fig. 32: The Opened Socket of the Right Shoulder Joint**

NOTE: 1) that the head of the humerus has been removed to reveal the glenoid cavity and labrum;

2) that the capsule of the joint is surrounded by muscles, the bellies of which are sectioned in this dissection.

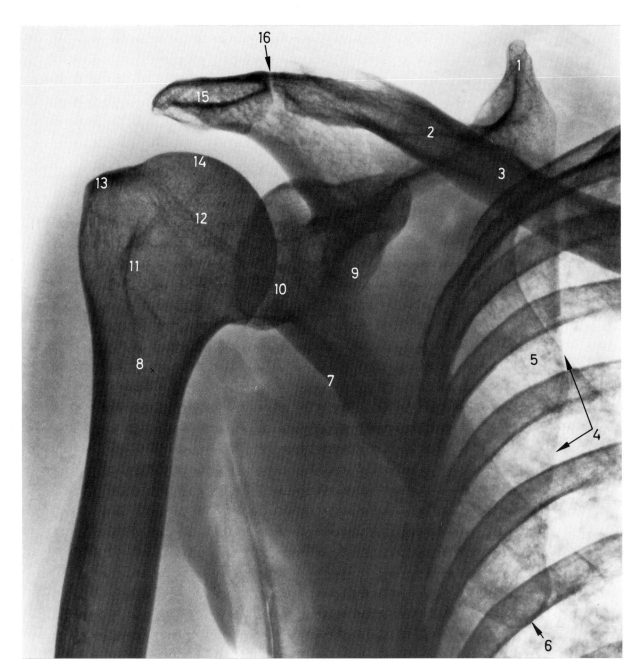

**Fig. 33: Radiograph of the Right Shoulder Region**

1. Superior angle of scapula
2. Spine of scapula
3. Clavicle
4. Medial margin of scapula
5. Second rib
6. Inferior angle of scapula
7. Lateral margin of scapula
8. Surgical neck of humerus
9. Coracoid process
10. Glenoid cavity
11. Lesser tubercle
12. Anatomical neck of humerus
13. Greater tubercle
14. Head of humerus
15. Acromion
16. Acromioclavicular joint

NOTE: 1) the clavicle, scapula and humerus are importantly involved in the radiographic anatomy of the shoulder region. The acromioclavicular joint is a planar joint formed by the apposition of the lateral end of the clavicle and the medial border of the acromion.

2) the glenohumeral joint, more commonly called the shoulder joint, is remarkably loose and provides a free range of movement. Observe the wide separation between the humeral head and glenoid cavity, and that only a small part of the humeral head is in contact with the cavity at any time.

3) that inferior *dislocations* of the head of the humerus are common because of minimal protection to this part of the joint. A *shoulder separation* results from the dislocation of the acromion beneath the lateral end of the clavicle, usually because of a strong blow to the lateral aspect of the joint.

**Fig. 34: Arm; Superficial Veins and Cutaneous Nerves of Left Upper Limb (Anterior Surface)**

NOTE: 1) the basilic vein ascends on the medial (ulnar) aspect of the arm, pierces the deep fascia and at the lower border of the teres major and joins the brachial vein to form the axillary vein. The cephalic vein ascends laterally in the arm in its course toward the axillary vein.

2) the principal sensory nerves of the anterior arm are the medial and lateral brachial cutaneous nerves and the intercostobrachial nerve.

Fig. 33

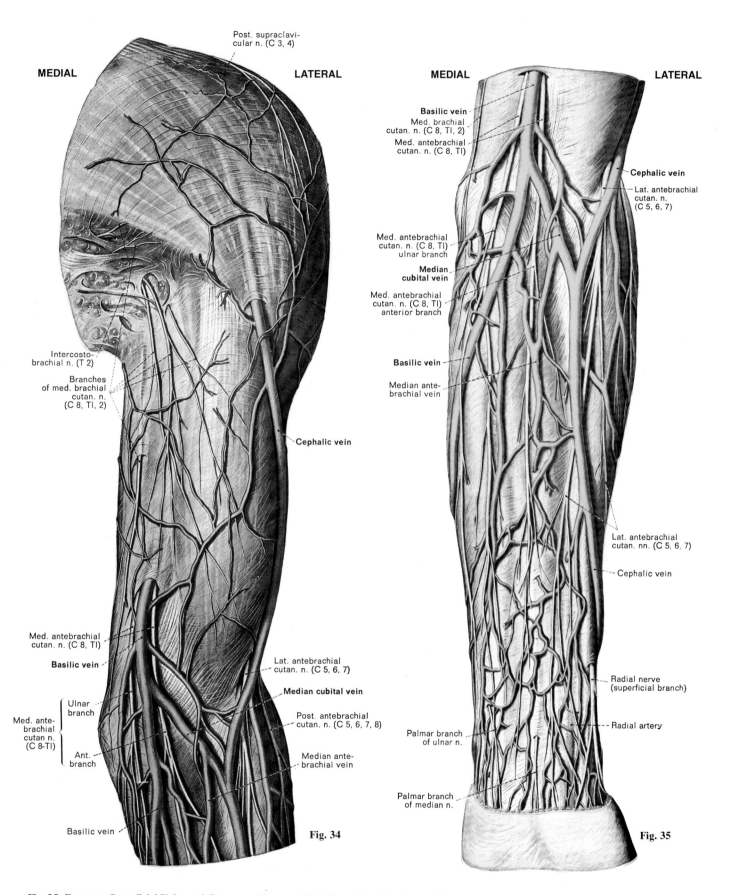

MEDIAL

Post. supraclavi-
cular n. (C 3, 4)

LATERAL

MEDIAL

LATERAL

Basilic vein
Med. brachial
cutan. n. (C 8, Tl, 2)
Med. antebrachial
cutan. n. (C 8, Tl)

Cephalic vein
Lat. antebrachial
cutan. n.
(C 5, 6, 7)

Med. antebrachial
cutan. n. (C 8, Tl)
ulnar branch

Median
cubital vein

Med. antebrachial
cutan. n. (C 8, Tl)
anterior branch

Basilic vein

Median ante-
brachial vein

Intercosto-
brachial n. (T 2)

Branches
of med. brachial
cutan. n.
(C 8, Tl, 2)

Cephalic vein

Lat. antebrachial
cutan. nn. (C 5, 6, 7)

Cephalic vein

Med. antebrachial
cutan. n. (C 8, Tl)

Basilic vein

Ulnar
branch

Med. ante-
brachial
cutan n.
(C 8-Tl)

Ant.
branch

Lat. antebrachial
cutan. n. (C 5, 6, 7)

Median cubital vein

Post. antebrachial
cutan. n. (C 5, 6, 7, 8)

Median ante-
brachial vein

Radial nerve
(superficial branch)

Radial artery

Palmar branch
of ulnar n.

Palmar branch
of median n.

Basilic vein

Fig. 34

Fig. 35

**Fig. 35: Forearm; Superficial Veins and Cutaneous Nerves of Left Upper Limb (Anterior Surface)**

NOTE: 1) the median cubital vein, interconnecting the cephalic and the basilic veins in the cubital fossa.

2) the main sensory nerves of the anterior forearm are the medial antebrachial cutaneous nerve (derived from the medial cord of the brachial plexus) and the lateral antebrachial cutaneous nerve, which is the continuation of the musculocutaneous nerve.

Figs. 34, 35     I

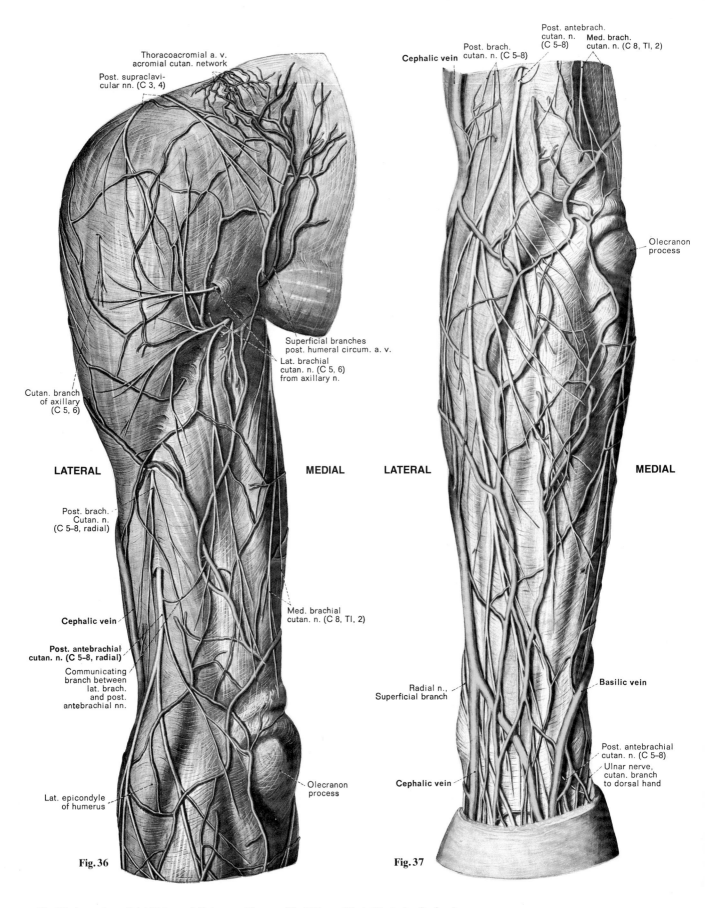

Thoracoacromial a. v.
acromial cutan. network

Post. supraclavi-
cular nn. (C 3, 4)

Post. brach.
cutan. n. (C 5-8)

Cephalic vein

Post. antebrach.
cutan. n.
(C 5-8)

Med. brach.
cutan. n. (C 8, Tl, 2)

Olecranon
process

Superficial branches
post. humeral circum. a. v.

Lat. brachial
cutan. n. (C 5, 6)
from axillary n.

Cutan. branch
of axillary
(C 5, 6)

**LATERAL**

**MEDIAL**

**LATERAL**

**MEDIAL**

Post. brach.
Cutan. n.
(C 5-8, radial)

**Cephalic vein**

**Post. antebrachial**
**cutan. n. (C 5-8, radial)**

Communicating
branch between
lat. brach.
and post.
antebrachial nn.

Med. brachial
cutan. n. (C 8, Tl, 2)

Radial n.,
Superficial branch

**Basilic vein**

**Cephalic vein**

Post. antebrachial
cutan. n. (C 5-8)

Ulnar nerve,
cutan. branch
to dorsal hand

Lat. epicondyle
of humerus

Olecranon
process

**Fig. 36**

**Fig. 37**

**Fig. 36: Arm: Superficial Veins and Cutaneous Nerves of Left Upper Limb (Posterior Surface)**

NOTE: the posterior surface of the arm receives cutaneous innervation from branches of the radial (post. brachial cutan. n) and axillary (lat. brachial cutan. n) nerves, both of which are derived from the posterior cord of the brachial plexus.

Figs. 36, 37

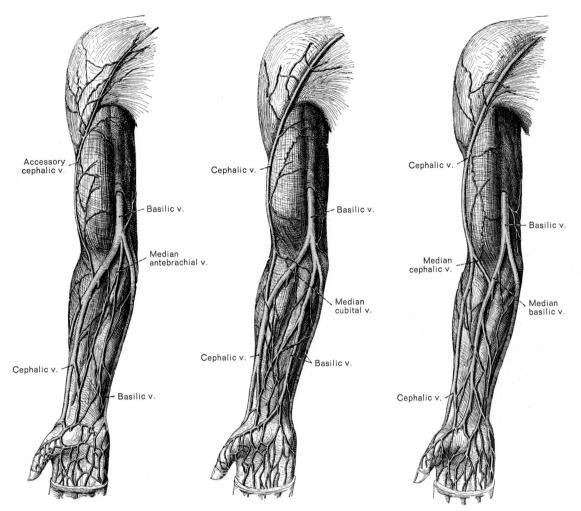

**Fig. 38: Variations in the Venous Pattern of the Upper Extremity**

NOTE that the superficial veins of the upper extremity are quite variable and yet are of significance clinically. The median cubital vein in the cubital fossa is especially used for the withdrawal of blood and for procedures necessitating the injection of fluids into the vascular system. In this regard, care must be taken not to injure the median nerve nor puncture the brachial artery, which both lie deep to the median cubital vein and the subjacent bicipital aponeurosis on which the vein rests.

**Fig. 39: Dermatomes of the Upper Limb**

NOTE: the dermatomes of the upper limb are supplied by the 5th cervical to the 1st thoracic segments of the spinal cord. The boundary between the 5th cervical and the 1st thoracic dermatomes ventrally is called the ventral axial line of the upper limb. The 4th cervical dermatome lies in the neck. Commencing with the 5th cervical dermatome and proceeding radially around the upper limb the dermatomes can be followed sequentially to the 1st thoracic and thus, the ventral axial line.

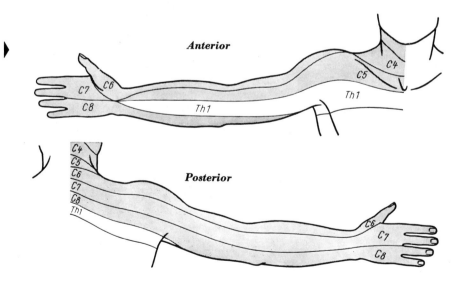

**Fig. 37: Forearm; Superficial Veins and Cutaneous Nerves of the Left Upper Limb (Posterior Surface)**

NOTE: 1) branches of the radial n. (post. antebrach. cutan. and superficial radial) supply the principal cutaneous innervation to the posterior forearm.

2) the basilic (ulnar side) and cephalic (radial side) veins commence on the dorsum of the hand in their ascent up the forearm.

Figs. 38, 39    I

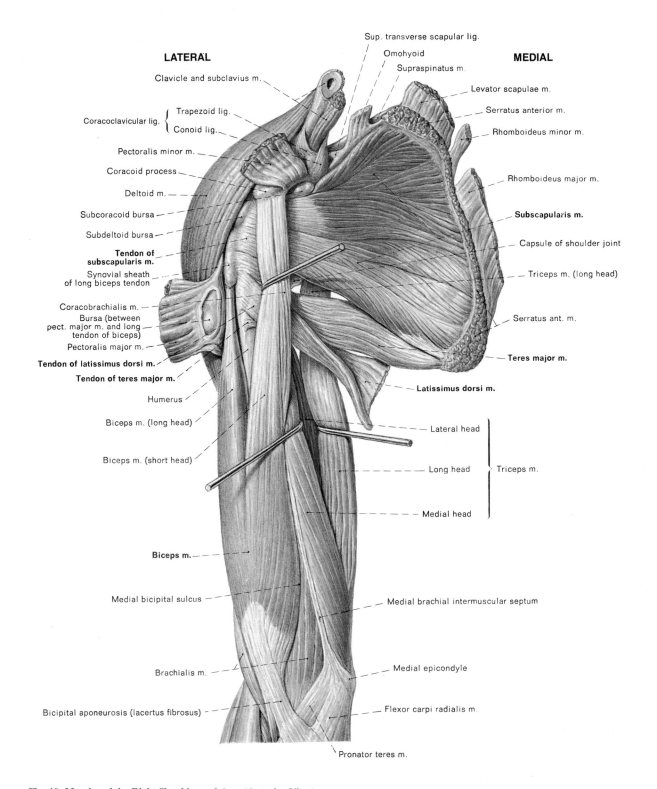

LATERAL

MEDIAL

Sup. transverse scapular lig.

Omohyoid

Supraspinatus m.

Clavicle and subclavius m.

Levator scapulae m.

Serratus anterior m.

Trapezoid lig.

Coracoclavicular lig.

Conoid lig.

Rhomboideus minor m.

Pectoralis minor m.

Rhomboideus major m.

Coracoid process

Deltoid m.

**Subscapularis m.**

Subcoracoid bursa

Capsule of shoulder joint

Subdeltoid bursa

**Tendon of subscapularis m.**

Triceps m. (long head)

Synovial sheath of long biceps tendon

Coracobrachialis m.

Serratus ant. m.

Bursa (between pect. major m. and long tendon of biceps)

Pectoralis major m.

**Teres major m.**

**Tendon of latissimus dorsi m.**

**Latissimus dorsi m.**

**Tendon of teres major m.**

Humerus

Biceps m. (long head)

Lateral head

Biceps m. (short head)

Long head

Triceps m.

Medial head

**Biceps m.**

Medial bicipital sulcus

Medial brachial intermuscular septum

Brachialis m.

Medial epicondyle

Bicipital aponeurosis (lacertus fibrosus)

Flexor carpi radialis m.

Pronator teres m.

**Fig. 40: Muscles of the Right Shoulder and Arm (Anterior View)**

NOTE: 1) the insertion of the subscapularis muscle on the lesser tubercle of the humerus. Distal to this, from medial to lateral, insert the teres major, latissimus dorsi and pectoralis major muscles.

2) attaching to the coracoid process are the pectoralis minor m., coracobrachialis m. and the short head of the biceps m.

3) the insertion of the pectoralis major m. and the long tendon of the biceps muscle are frequently separated by a bursa.

4) in the arm, the flexor compartment (biceps, coracobrachialis and brachialis) is separated from the extensor compartment (triceps) by an intermuscular septum of deep fascia.

Fig. 40

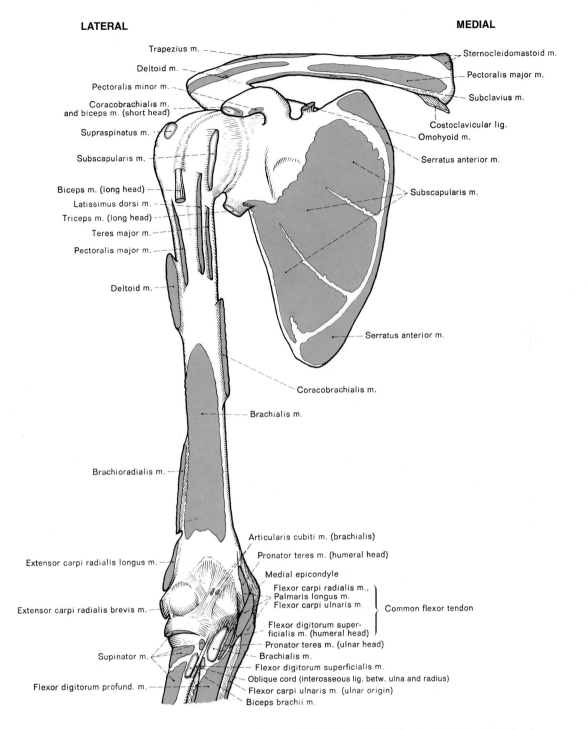

**LATERAL**        **MEDIAL**

Trapezius m.

Deltoid m.

Pectoralis minor m.

Coracobrachialis m.
and biceps m. (short head)

Supraspinatus m.

Subscapularis m.

Biceps m. (long head)

Latissimus dorsi m.

Triceps m. (long head)

Teres major m.

Pectoralis major m.

Deltoid m.

Brachioradialis m.

Sternocleidomastoid m.

Pectoralis major m.

Subclavius m.

Costoclavicular lig.

Omohyoid m.

Serratus anterior m.

Subscapularis m.

Serratus anterior m.

Coracobrachialis m.

Brachialis m.

Articularis cubiti m. (brachialis)

Pronator teres m. (humeral head)

Extensor carpi radialis longus m.

Medial epicondyle

Flexor carpi radialis m.,
Palmaris longus m.
Flexor carpi ulnaris m.

Common flexor tendon

Extensor carpi radialis brevis m.

Flexor digitorum super-
ficialis m. (humeral head)

Pronator teres m. (ulnar head)

Brachialis m.

Supinator m.

Flexor digitorum superficialis m.

Oblique cord (interosseous lig. betw. ulna and radius)

Flexor digitorum profund. m.

Flexor carpi ulnaris m. (ulnar origin)

Biceps brachii m.

**Fig. 41: Anterior View of Bones of the Upper Limb (Including Proximal End of Radius and Ulna) Showing Attachments of Muscles**

NOTE: 1) the broad *origin* of the subscapularis in the subscapular fossa of the scapula and its *insertion* on the lesser tubercle of the humerus proximal to the insertions of the latissimus dorsi and teres major muscles. The subscapularis is an adductor and medial rotator of the arm.

2) the brachialis muscle *arises* from the distal three-fifths of the anterior surface of the humerus and *inserts* on the coronoid process of the ulna. This muscle is the strongest flexor of the forearm.

3) the short head of the biceps m. *arises* with the coracobrachialis m. from the coracoid process, while the long head *arises* from the supraglenoid tubercle of the scapula.

4) the coracobrachialis *inserts* onto the shaft of the humerus near its middle, while the biceps inserts onto the tuberosity of the radius and onto the deep fascia of the forearm by way of the bicipital aponeurosis.

5) the coracobrachialis flexes and adducts the arm at the shoulder joint, while the biceps flexes and supinates the forearm, with the long head assisting in flexion of the arm at the shoulder joint.

Fig. 41    **I**

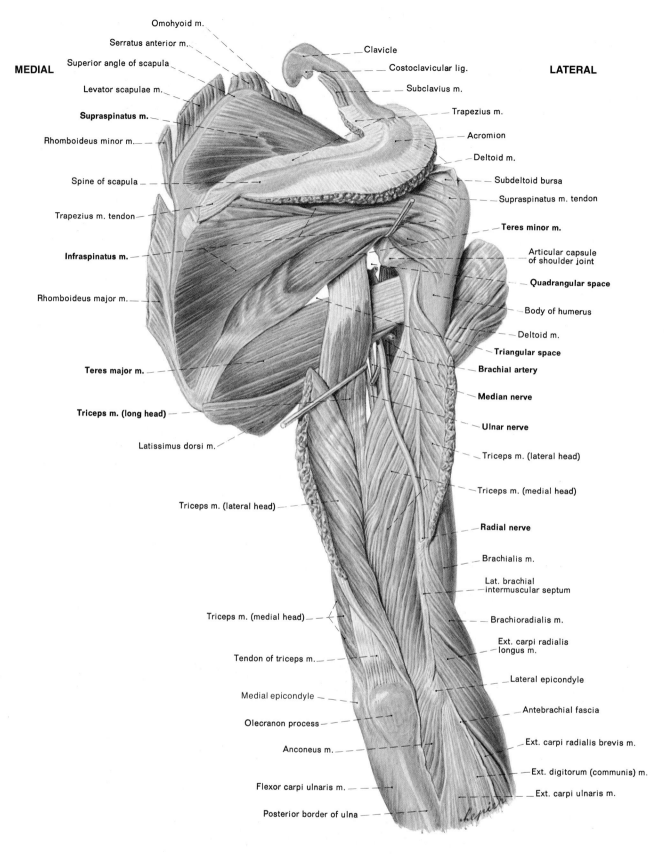

Omohyoid m.

Serratus anterior m.

Superior angle of scapula

**MEDIAL**

Levator scapulae m.

**Supraspinatus m.**

Rhomboideus minor m.

Spine of scapula

Trapezius m. tendon

**Infraspinatus m.**

Rhomboideus major m.

**Teres major m.**

**Triceps m. (long head)**

Latissimus dorsi m.

Triceps m. (lateral head)

Triceps m. (medial head)

Tendon of triceps m.

Medial epicondyle

Olecranon process

Anconeus m.

Flexor carpi ulnaris m.

Posterior border of ulna

Clavicle

Costoclavicular lig.

Subclavius m.

**LATERAL**

Trapezius m.

Acromion

Deltoid m.

Subdeltoid bursa

Supraspinatus m. tendon

**Teres minor m.**

Articular capsule of shoulder joint

**Quadrangular space**

Body of humerus

Deltoid m.

**Triangular space**

**Brachial artery**

**Median nerve**

**Ulnar nerve**

Triceps m. (lateral head)

Triceps m. (medial head)

**Radial nerve**

Brachialis m.

Lat. brachial intermuscular septum

Brachioradialis m.

Ext. carpi radialis longus m.

Lateral epicondyle

Antebrachial fascia

Ext. carpi radialis brevis m.

Ext. digitorum (communis) m.

Ext. carpi ulnaris m.

**Fig. 42: Muscles of the Shoulder and Deep Arm (Posterior View)**

NOTE: 1) that with the deltoid muscle and the lateral head of the triceps muscle severed, the course of the radial nerve in the upper arm is revealed.

2) the sequential insertions of the supraspinatus, infraspinatus and teres minor muscles on the greater tubercle of the humerus.

3) the boundaries of the quadrangular and triangular spaces.

Fig. 42

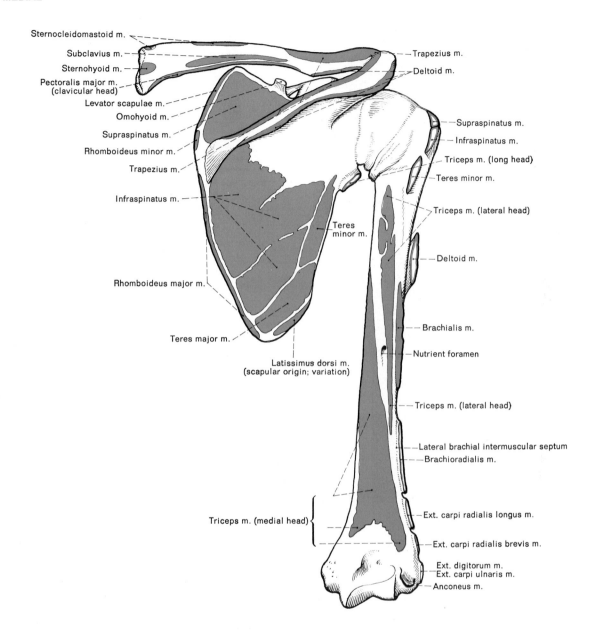

**Fig. 43: Posterior View of the Clavicle, Scapula and Humerus Showing Muscle Attachments**

NOTE: 1) that dorsally the vertebral border of the scapula is attached to the trunk by the levator scapulae and the rhomboideus major and minor muscles, whereas on the ventral scapular surface (see Fig. 41) the serratus anterior attaches along the vertebral border.

2) the supraspinatus muscle arising from the medial two-thirds of the supraspinatus fossa.

3) the origins of the teres major and teres minor muscles along the axillary border of the scapula, and the broad origin of the infraspinatus muscle from the infraspinatus fossa.

4) that onto the spine of the scapula and extending to the lateral third of the clavicle are attached the trapezius and deltoid muscles.

5) most of the posterior surface of the humerus affords origin to the medial and lateral heads of the triceps muscle, while the long head arises from the infraglenoid tubercle of the scapula.

6) the alignment of the tendinous insertions of the supraspinatus, infraspinatus, and teres minor muscles which, along with the tendon of the subscapularis (see Figs. 40 and 41), form the so-called "rotator cuff" of the shoulder joint. This musculotendinous cuff significantly strengthens the joint, but is also the site of inflammatory reactions resulting in pain brought on by trauma or aging.

Fig. 43   I

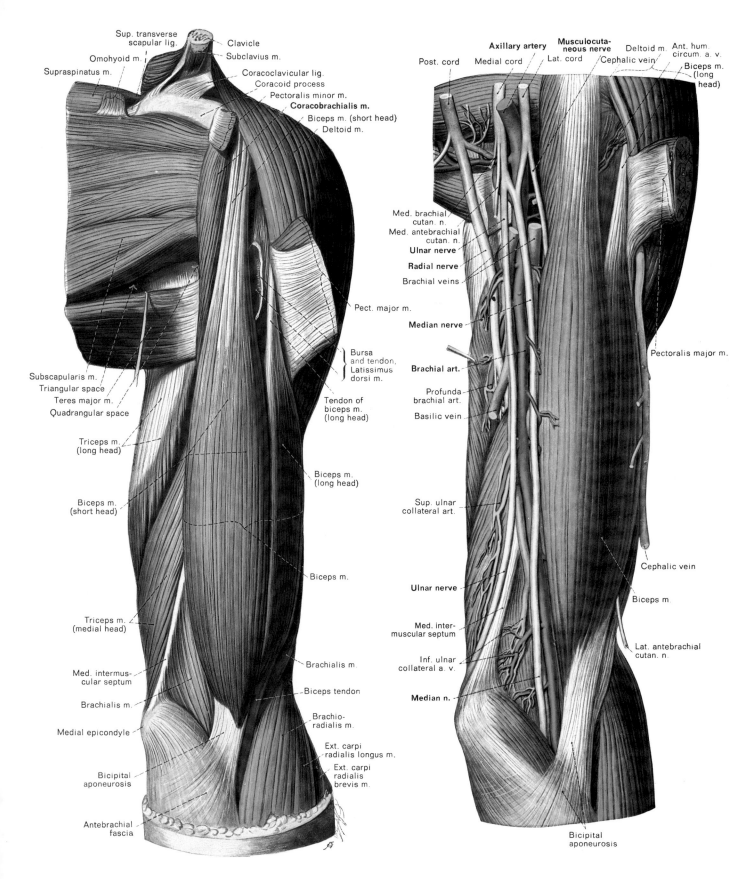

**Fig. 44:** Superficial View of Muscles on the Anterior Aspect of the Left Arm

NOTE: that the biceps muscle extends across both the shoulder and elbow joints, but that the coracobrachialis muscle extends only across the shoulder joint.

**Fig. 45:** Vessels and Nerves of the Anterior Arm (left)

NOTE: 1) the median nerve crosses the brachial artery anteriorly from lateral to medial just above the cubital fossa.
2) neither the ulnar nor median nerve gives off branches in the arm.

Figs. 44, 45

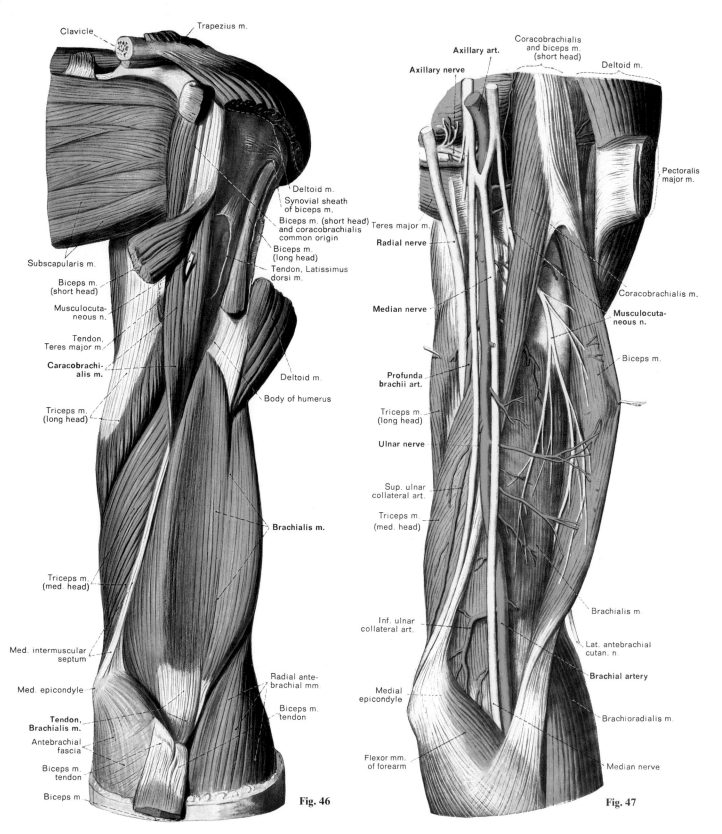

Fig. 46 labels:
- Clavicle
- Trapezius m.
- Deltoid m.
- Synovial sheath of biceps m.
- Biceps m. (short head) and coracobrachialis common origin
- Biceps m. (long head)
- Tendon, Latissimus dorsi m.
- Subscapularis m.
- Biceps m. (short head)
- Musculocutaneous n.
- Tendon, Teres major m.
- Caracobrachialis m.
- Triceps m. (long head)
- Deltoid m.
- Body of humerus
- Brachialis m.
- Triceps m. (med. head)
- Med. intermuscular septum
- Med. epicondyle
- Tendon, Brachialis m.
- Antebrachial fascia
- Biceps m. tendon
- Biceps m
- Radial antebrachial mm.
- Biceps m. tendon

**Fig. 46**

Fig. 47 labels:
- Axillary art.
- Axillary nerve
- Coracobrachialis and biceps m. (short head)
- Deltoid m.
- Pectoralis major m.
- Teres major m.
- Radial nerve
- Median nerve
- Coracobrachialis m.
- Musculocutaneous n.
- Biceps m.
- Profunda brachii art.
- Triceps m. (long head)
- Ulnar nerve
- Sup. ulnar collateral art.
- Triceps m. (med. head)
- Brachialis m.
- Lat. antebrachial cutan. n.
- Brachial artery
- Inf. ulnar collateral art.
- Medial epicondyle
- Brachioradialis m.
- Median nerve
- Flexor mm. of forearm

**Fig. 47**

**Fig. 46: Deep View of Muscles on the Anterior Aspect of the Left Arm**

NOTE: In this dissection both the long head and short head of the biceps brachii muscle have been severed and reflected in order to reveal the underlying brachialis muscle. The coracobrachialis muscle has been left intact.

**Fig. 47: The Nerves and Arteries of the Anterior Arm (left)**

NOTE: 1) the short head of the biceps muscle has been pulled aside to reveal the musculocutaneous nerve which supplies the coracobrachialis, biceps and brachialis muscles. This nerve continues into the forearm as the lateral antebrachial cutaneous nerve.

2) the superficial course of the brachial artery in the arm. Its branches include the profunda brachii artery and the superior and inferior ulnar collateral arteries in addition to its muscular branches.

Figs. 46, 47    I

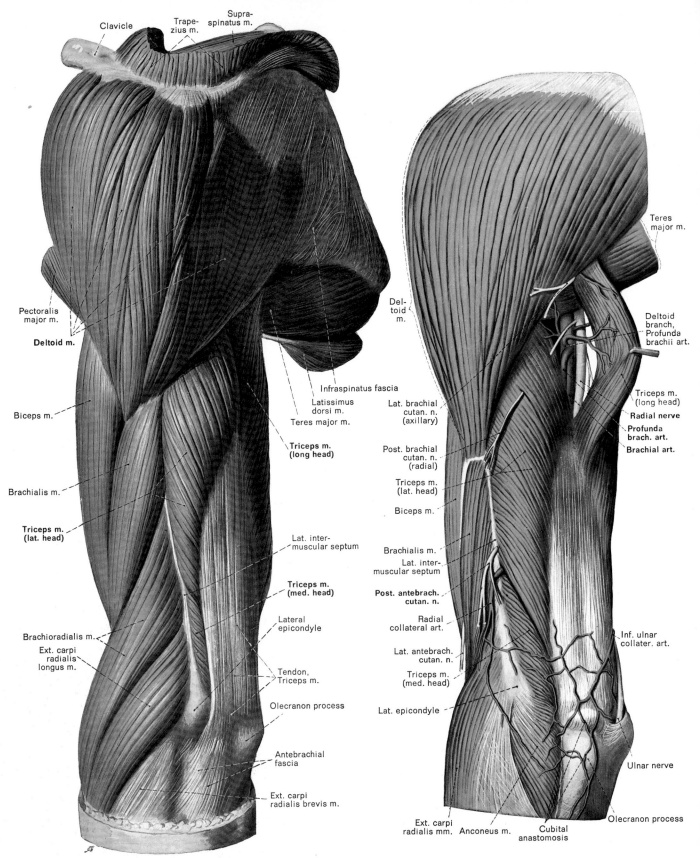

**Fig. 48: The Muscles of the Arm (Lateral View)**

NOTE: 1) the deltoid muscle acting as a whole abducts the arm. The clavicular portion flexes and medially rotates the arm, while the scapular portion extends and laterally rotates the arm.

2) the lateral intermuscular septum separates the anterior muscular compartment from the posterior muscular compartment.

**Fig. 49: Nerves and Arteries of the Left Posterior Arm (Superficial Branches)**

NOTE: 1) the origin of the profunda brachii artery from the brachial artery and its relationship to the radial nerve. The long head of the triceps has been pulled medially.

2) the relationship of the ulnar nerve to the olecranon process and the vascular anastomosis around the elbow.

Figs. 48, 49

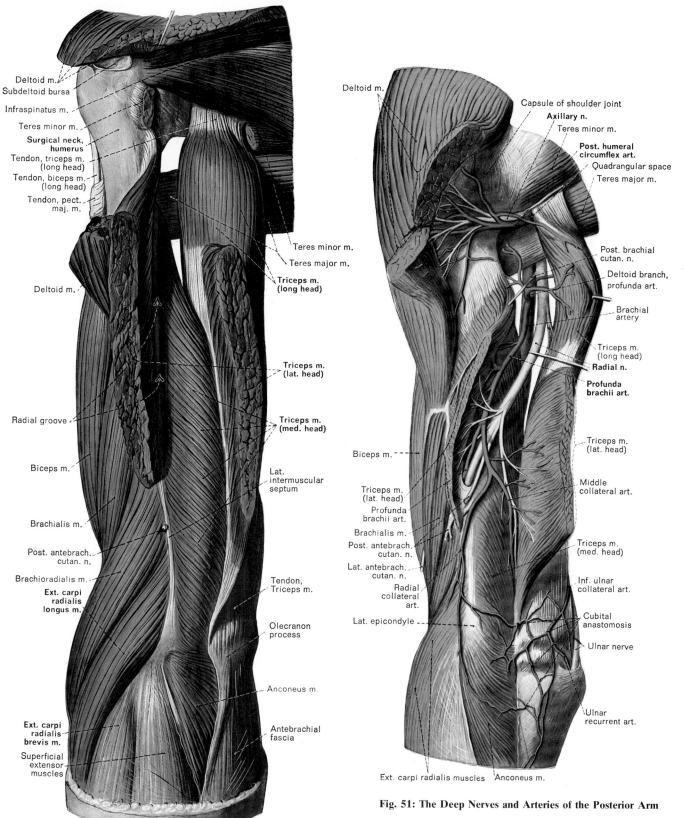

Deltoid m.
Subdeltoid bursa
Infraspinatus m.
Teres minor m.
**Surgical neck, humerus**
Tendon, triceps m. (long head)
Tendon, biceps m. (long head)
Tendon, pect. maj. m.

Deltoid m.

Radial groove

Biceps m.

Brachialis m.

Post. antebrach. cutan. n.

Brachioradialis m.

**Ext. carpi radialis longus m.**

**Ext. carpi radialis brevis m.**

Superficial extensor muscles

Teres minor m.
Teres major m.
**Triceps m. (long head)**

**Triceps m. (lat. head)**

**Triceps m. (med. head)**

Lat. intermuscular septum

Tendon, Triceps m.

Olecranon process

Anconeus m.

Antebrachial fascia

Deltoid m.

Capsule of shoulder joint
**Axillary n.**
Teres minor m.
**Post. humeral circumflex art.**
Quadrangular space
Teres major m.

Post. brachial cutan. n.
Deltoid branch, profunda art.
Brachial artery

Triceps m. (long head)
**Radial n.**
**Profunda brachii art.**

Triceps m. (lat. head)

Middle collateral art.

Biceps m.

Triceps m. (lat. head)
Profunda brachii art.
Brachialis m.
Post. antebrach. cutan. n.
Lat. antebrach. cutan. n.
Radial collateral art.
Lat. epicondyle

Triceps m. (med. head)

Inf. ulnar collateral art.

Cubital anastomosis

Ulnar nerve

Ulnar recurrent art.

Ext. carpi radialis muscles    Anconeus m.

**Fig. 50: Deep Muscles of the Arm and Shoulder (Posterolateral View)**

NOTE: in this dissection much of the deltoid and teres minor muscles was removed, and the lateral head of the triceps muscle was transected and reflected. Observe the radial groove between the medial and lateral heads of the triceps.

**Fig. 51: The Deep Nerves and Arteries of the Posterior Arm**

NOTE: 1) the course of the axillary nerve and posterior humeral circumflex artery through the quadrangular space to achieve the deltoid muscle and dorsal shoulder region.

2) the course of the radial nerve and profunda brachii artery along the musculospiral groove to the posterior brachial region. The groove lies along the body of the humerus between the origins of the lateral and medial heads of the triceps muscle.

3) the common insertion of the triceps muscle onto the olecranon process of the ulna.

Figs. 50, 51    I

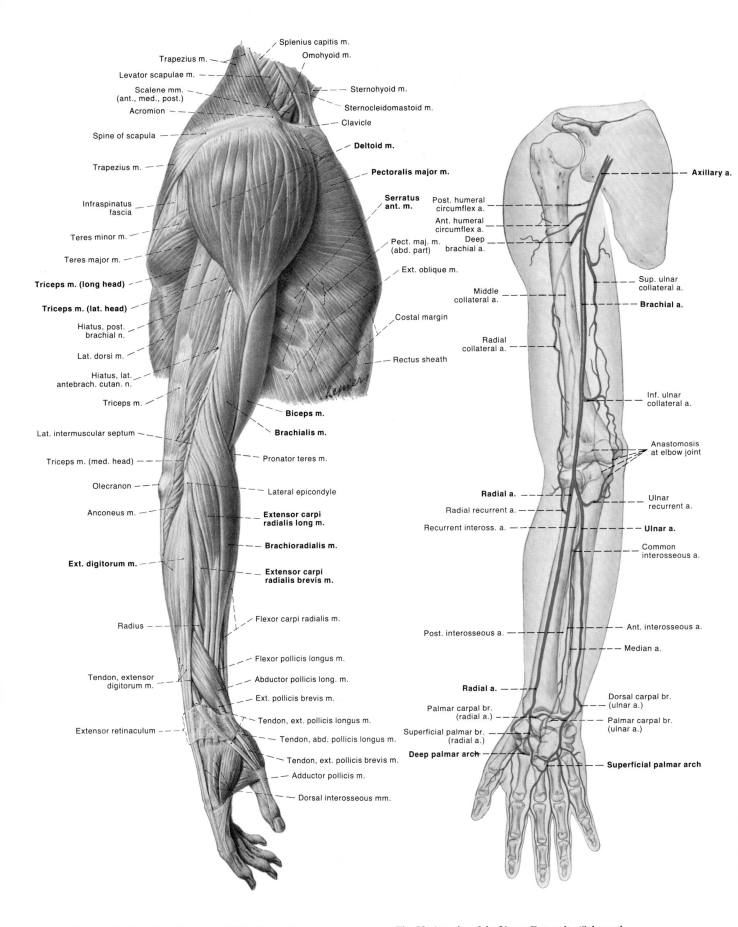

Splenius capitis m.

Trapezius m.

Levator scapulae m.

Scalene mm.
(ant., med., post.)

Acromion

Spine of scapula

Trapezius m.

Infraspinatus
fascia

Teres minor m.

Teres major m.

**Triceps m. (long head)**

**Triceps m. (lat. head)**

Hiatus, post.
brachial n.

Lat. dorsi m.

Hiatus, lat.
antebrach. cutan. n.

Triceps m.

Lat. intermuscular septum

Triceps m. (med. head)

Olecranon

Anconeus m.

**Ext. digitorum m.**

Radius

Tendon, extensor
digitorum m.

Extensor retinaculum

Omohyoid m.

Sternohyoid m.

Sternocleidomastoid m.

Clavicle

**Deltoid m.**

**Pectoralis major m.**

**Serratus
ant. m.**

Pect. maj. m.
(abd. part)

Ext. oblique m.

Costal margin

Rectus sheath

**Biceps m.**

**Brachialis m.**

Pronator teres m.

Lateral epicondyle

**Extensor carpi
radialis long m.**

**Brachioradialis m.**

**Extensor carpi
radialis brevis m.**

Flexor carpi radialis m.

Flexor pollicis longus m.

Abductor pollicis long. m.

Ext. pollicis brevis m.

Tendon, ext. pollicis longus m.

Tendon, abd. pollicis longus m.

Tendon, ext. pollicis brevis m.

Adductor pollicis m.

Dorsal interosseous mm.

**Axillary a.**

Post. humeral
circumflex a.

Ant. humeral
circumflex a.

Deep
brachial a.

Middle
collateral a.

Radial
collateral a.

Radial a.

Radial recurrent a.

Recurrent inteross. a.

Post. interosseous a.

**Radial a.**

Palmar carpal br.
(radial a.)

Superficial palmar br.
(radial a.)

**Deep palmar arch**

Sup. ulnar
collateral a.

**Brachial a.**

Inf. ulnar
collateral a.

Anastomosis
at elbow joint

Ulnar
recurrent a.

**Ulnar a.**

Common
interosseous a.

Ant. interosseous a.

Median a.

Dorsal carpal br.
(ulnar a.)

Palmar carpal br.
(ulnar a.)

**Superficial palmar arch**

**Fig. 52: Muscles of the Thorax and Right Upper Extremity,
Lateral View**

**Fig. 53: Arteries of the Upper Extremity (Schematic
Representation)**

Figs. 52, 53

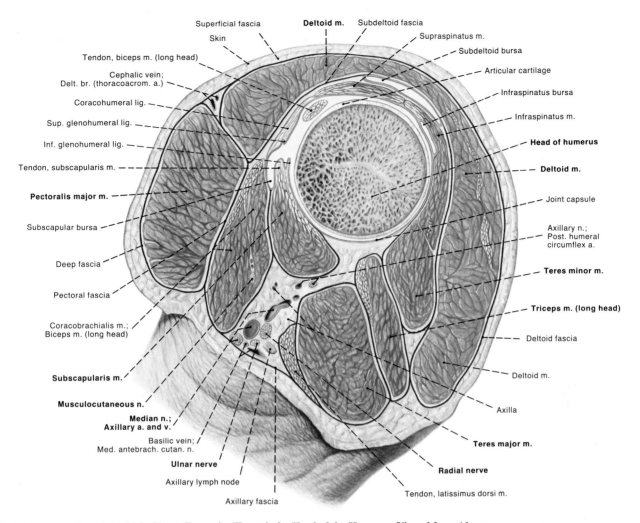

**Fig. 54: Cross Section of the Right Upper Extremity Through the Head of the Humerus, Viewed from Above**

Superficial fascia
Skin
Deltoid m.
Subdeltoid fascia
Supraspinatus m.
Tendon, biceps m. (long head)
Subdeltoid bursa
Cephalic vein;
Delt. br. (thoracoacrom. a.)
Articular cartilage
Coracohumeral lig.
Infraspinatus bursa
Sup. glenohumeral lig.
Infraspinatus m.
Inf. glenohumeral lig.
Head of humerus
Tendon, subscapularis m.
Deltoid m.
Pectoralis major m.
Joint capsule
Subscapular bursa
Axillary n.;
Post. humeral
circumflex a.
Deep fascia
Teres minor m.
Pectoral fascia
Triceps m. (long head)
Coracobrachialis m.;
Biceps m. (long head)
Deltoid fascia
Subscapularis m.
Deltoid m.
Musculocutaneous n.
Axilla
Median n.;
Axillary a. and v.
Basilic vein;
Med. antebrach. cutan. n.
Teres major m.
Ulnar nerve
Axillary lymph node
Radial nerve
Axillary fascia
Tendon, latissimus dorsi m.

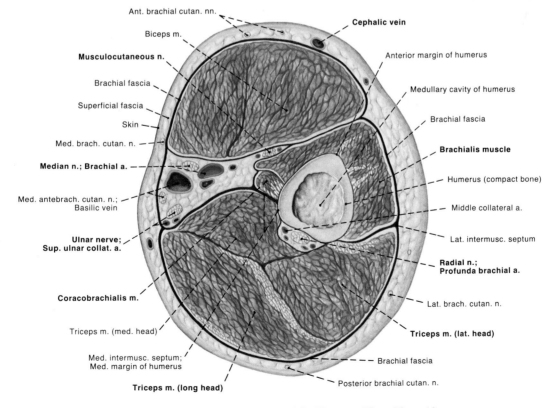

**Fig. 55: Cross Section of the Right Upper Extremity Through the Middle of the Humerus, Viewed from Above**

Ant. brachial cutan. nn.
Cephalic vein
Biceps m.
Anterior margin of humerus
Musculocutaneous n.
Medullary cavity of humerus
Brachial fascia
Superficial fascia
Brachial fascia
Skin
Brachialis muscle
Med. brach. cutan. n.
Median n.; Brachial a.
Humerus (compact bone)
Med. antebrach. cutan. n.;
Basilic vein
Middle collateral a.
Lat. intermusc. septum
Ulnar nerve;
Sup. ulnar collat. a.
Radial n.;
Profunda brachial a.
Coracobrachialis m.
Lat. brach. cutan. n.
Triceps m. (med. head)
Triceps m. (lat. head)
Med. intermusc. septum;
Med. margin of humerus
Brachial fascia
Triceps m. (long head)
Posterior brachial cutan. n.

Figs. 54, 55    **I**

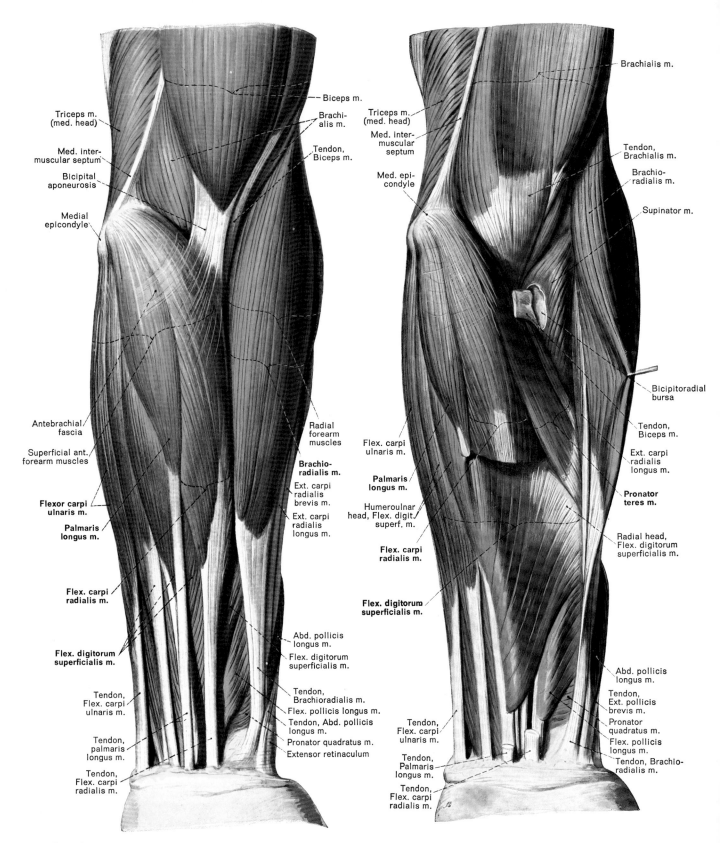

Triceps m.
(med. head)

Med. inter-
muscular septum

Bicipital
aponeurosis

Medial
epicondyle

Biceps m.

Brachi-
alis m.

Tendon,
Biceps m.

Antebrachial
fascia

Superficial ant.
forearm muscles

**Flexor carpi
ulnaris m.**

**Palmaris
longus m.**

Flex. carpi
radialis m.

**Flex. digitorum
superficialis m.**

Tendon,
Flex. carpi
ulnaris m.

Tendon,
palmaris
longus m.

Tendon,
Flex. carpi
radialis m.

Radial
forearm
muscles

**Brachio-
radialis m.**

Ext. carpi
radialis
brevis m.

Ext. carpi
radialis
longus m.

Abd. pollicis
longus m.

Flex. digitorum
superficialis m.

Tendon,
Brachioradialis m.

Flex. pollicis longus m.

Tendon, Abd. pollicis
longus m.

Pronator quadratus m.

Extensor retinaculum

Triceps m.
(med. head)

Med. inter-
muscular
septum

Med. epi-
condyle

Flex. carpi
ulnaris m.

**Palmaris
longus m.**

Humeroulnar
head, Flex. digit.
superf. m.

**Flex. carpi
radialis m.**

**Flex. digitorum
superficialis m.**

Tendon,
Flex. carpi
ulnaris m.

Tendon,
Palmaris
longus m.

Tendon,
Flex. carpi
radialis m.

Brachialis m.

Tendon,
Brachialis m.

Brachio-
radialis m.

Supinator m.

Bicipitoradial
bursa

Tendon,
Biceps m.

Ext. carpi
radialis
longus m.

**Pronator
teres m.**

Radial head,
Flex. digitorum
superficialis m.

Abd. pollicis
longus m.

Tendon,
Ext. pollicis
brevis m.

Pronator
quadratus m.

Flex. pollicis
longus m.

Tendon, Brachio-
radialis m.

**Fig. 56: The Left Anterior Forearm Muscles, Superficial Group**

NOTE: 1) that the brachioradialis m. is studied with the posterior forearm muscles instead of the anterior muscles.

2) that the anterior forearm muscles arise from the medial epicondyle of the humerus and include the pronator teres (not labelled), flexor carpi radialis, palmaris longus and flexor carpi ulnaris. Beneath these is the flexor digitorum superficialis.

**Fig. 57: The Flexor Digitorum Superficialis Muscle and Related Muscles (left)**

NOTE: 1) the palmaris longus, flexor carpi radialis and tendon of the biceps have been cut to reveal the flexor digitorum superficialis and pronator teres.

2) the triangular cubital fossa is bounded medially by the superficial flexors and laterally by the extensors. Its floor is the brachialis muscle.

Figs. 56, 57

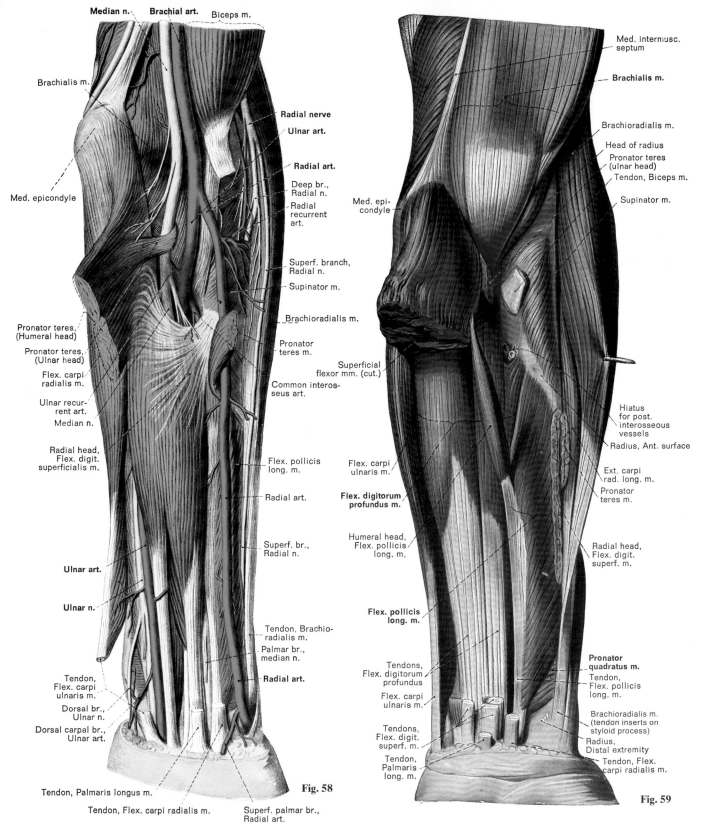

**Median n.**  **Brachial art.**  Biceps m.

Brachialis m.

Med. epicondyle

Pronator teres, (Humeral head)

Pronator teres, (Ulnar head)

Flex. carpi radialis m.

Ulnar recurrent art.

Median n.

Radial head, Flex. digit. superficialis m.

**Ulnar art.**

**Ulnar n.**

Tendon, Flex. carpi ulnaris m.

Dorsal br., Ulnar n.

Dorsal carpal br., Ulnar art.

Tendon, Palmaris longus m.

Tendon, Flex. carpi radialis m.

**Radial nerve**

**Ulnar art.**

**Radial art.**

Deep br., Radial n.

Radial recurrent art.

Superf. branch, Radial n.

Supinator m.

Brachioradialis m.

Pronator teres m.

Common interosseus art.

Flex. pollicis long. m.

Radial art.

Superf. br., Radial n.

Tendon, Brachioradialis m.

Palmar br., median n.

**Radial art.**

Superf. palmar br., Radial art.

**Fig. 58**

Med. epicondyle

Flex. carpi ulnaris m.

**Flex. digitorum profundus m.**

Humeral head, Flex. pollicis long. m.

**Flex. pollicis long. m.**

Tendons, Flex. digitorum profundus

Flex. carpi ulnaris m.

Tendons, Flex. digit. superf. m.

Tendon, Palmaris long. m.

Med. intermusc. septum

**Brachialis m.**

Brachioradialis m.

Head of radius
Pronator teres (ulnar head)
Tendon, Biceps m.

Supinator m.

Superficial flexor mm. (cut.)

Hiatus for post. interosseous vessels

Radius, Ant. surface

Ext. carpi rad. long. m.
Pronator teres m.

Radial head, Flex. digit. superf. m.

**Pronator quadratus m.**
Tendon, Flex. pollicis long. m.

Brachioradialis m. (tendon inserts on styloid process)
Radius, Distal extremity
Tendon, Flex. carpi radialis m.

**Fig. 59**

**Fig. 58: Nerves and Arteries, Anterior Aspect of Left Forearm**

NOTE: 1) the pronator teres and flexor carpi radialis muscles are reflected just below the cubital fossa to reveal the origins of the ulnar and radial arteries.

2) at the wrist, the flexor carpi ulnaris muscle is severed to expose the ulnar nerve and artery.

**Fig. 59: The Left Anterior Forearm Muscles, Deep Group**

NOTE: 1) the superficial anterior forearm muscles have been removed to reveal the three muscles of the deep group. These include the flexor digitorum profundus, the flexor pollicis longus and the pronator quadratus.

2) the pronator quadratus is a small quadrangular muscle situated at the distal end of the forearm beneath the tendons of the flexor digitorum profundus and flexor pollicis longus. It is only partially shown in this dissection and can better be seen in Fig. 97.

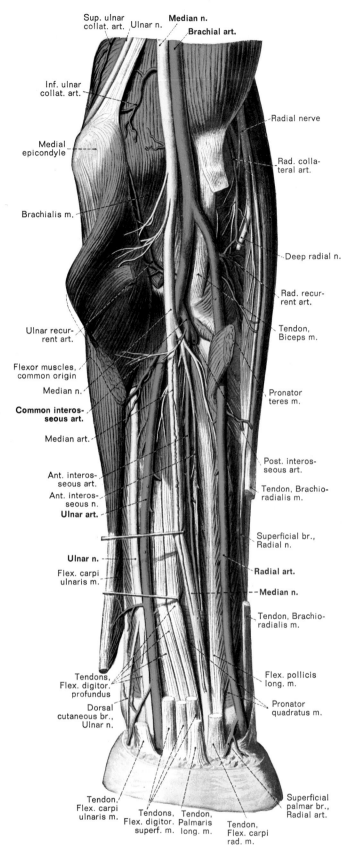

**Fig. 60: Nerves and Arteries of Left Anterior Forearm (Deep Dissection)**

NOTE the division of the brachial artery into the radial and ulnar. The common interosseous artery branches from the ulnar artery and divides immediately into anterior and posterior interosseous arteries. Observe the courses of the median and ulnar nerves.

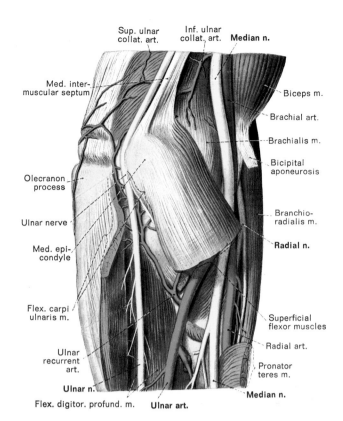

**Fig. 61: Nerves and Arteries at the Elbow (Medial View)**

NOTE: the ulnar nerve enters the forearm directly behind the medial epicondyle.

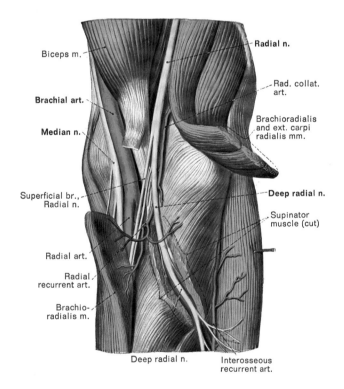

**Fig. 62: Nerves and Arteries at the Elbow (Lateral View)**

NOTE: the deep radial nerve passes into the forearm in front of the lateral part of the elbow joint. It then courses dorsally through the supinator muscle to supply the posterior forearm muscles.

Figs. 60, 61, 62

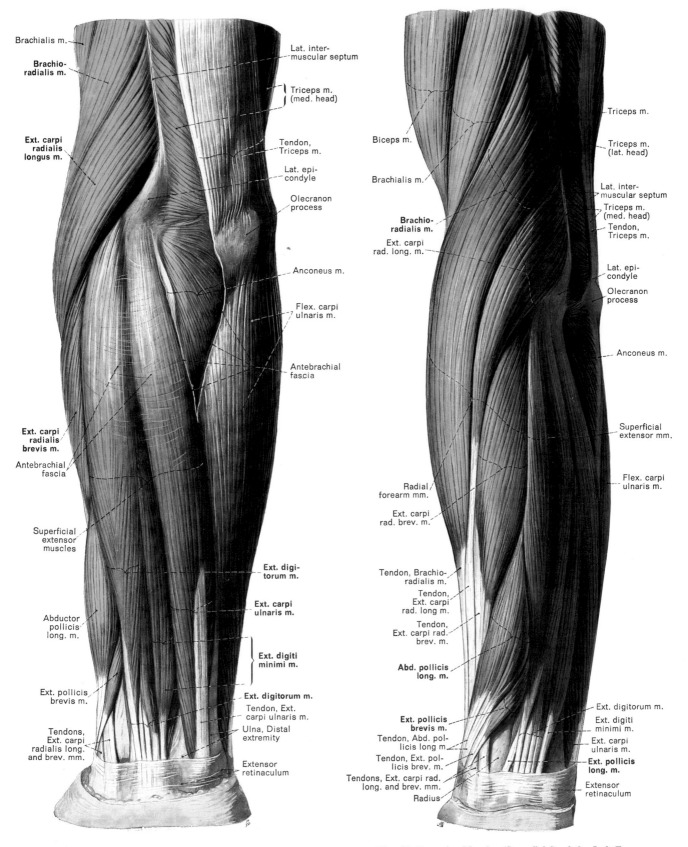

Brachialis m.

**Brachio-
radialis m.**

**Ext. carpi
radialis
longus m.**

**Ext. carpi
radialis
brevis m.**

Antebrachial
fascia

Superficial
extensor
muscles

Abductor
pollicis
long. m.

Ext. pollicis
brevis m.

Tendons,
Ext. carpi
radialis long.
and brev. mm.

Lat. inter-
muscular septum

Triceps m.
(med. head)

Tendon,
Triceps m.

Lat. epi-
condyle

Olecranon
process

Anconeus m.

Flex. carpi
ulnaris m.

Antebrachial
fascia

**Ext. digi-
torum m.**

**Ext. carpi
ulnaris m.**

**Ext. digiti
minimi m.**

**Ext. digitorum m.**

Tendon, Ext.
carpi ulnaris m.

Ulna, Distal
extremity

Extensor
retinaculum

Biceps m.

Brachialis m.

**Brachio-
radialis m.**

Ext. carpi
rad. long. m.

Radial
forearm mm.

Ext. carpi
rad. brev. m.

Tendon, Brachio-
radialis m.

Tendon,
Ext. carpi
rad. long m.

Tendon,
Ext. carpi rad.
brev. m.

**Abd. pollicis
long. m.**

**Ext. pollicis
brevis m.**

Tendon, Abd. pol-
licis long m.

Tendon, Ext. pol-
licis brev. m.

Tendons, Ext. carpi rad.
long. and brev. mm.

Radius

Triceps m.

Triceps m.
(lat. head)

Lat. inter-
muscular septum

Triceps m.
(med. head)

Tendon,
Triceps m.

Lat. epi-
condyle

Olecranon
process

Anconeus m.

Superficial
extensor mm.

Flex. carpi
ulnaris m.

Ext. digitorum m.

Ext. digiti
minimi m.

Ext. carpi
ulnaris m.

**Ext. pollicis
long. m.**

Extensor
retinaculum

**Fig. 63: Posterior Muscles of the Left Forearm, Superficial
Group**

NOTE that most of the superficial extensor muscles arise
from the lateral epicondyle of the humerus. These are the
extensor carpi radialis brevis, the extensor digitorum, the
extensor digiti minimi and the extensor carpi ulnaris. The
brachioradialis and extensor carpi radialis longus arise from
the supracondylar ridge.

**Fig. 64: Posterior Muscles (Superficial) of the Left Forearm,
Lateral View**

NOTE: 1) the superficial location of the brachioradialis
muscle.

2) three muscles of the thumb: extensor pollicis longus,
extensor pollicis brevis and abductor pollicis longus.

3) the closely investing extensor retinaculum under which
the extensor tendons pass into the dorsum of the hand.

Figs. 63, 64    **I**

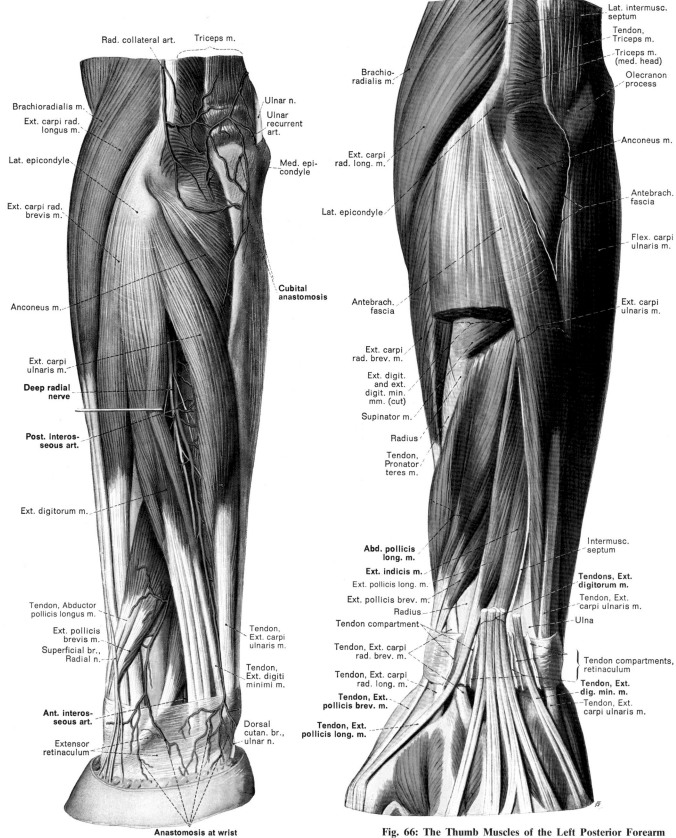

**Fig. 65:** Labels — Rad. collateral art. · Triceps m. · Brachioradialis m. · Ext. carpi rad. longus m. · Lat. epicondyle · Ext. carpi rad. brevis m. · Anconeus m. · Ext. carpi ulnaris m. · **Deep radial nerve** · **Post. interosseous art.** · Ext. digitorum m. · Tendon, Abductor pollicis longus m. · Ext. pollicis brevis m. · Superficial br., Radial n. · **Ant. interosseous art.** · Extensor retinaculum · Ulnar n. · Ulnar recurrent art. · Med. epicondyle · **Cubital anastomosis** · Tendon, Ext. carpi ulnaris m. · Tendon, Ext. digiti minimi m. · Dorsal cutan. br., ulnar n. · **Anastomosis at wrist**

**Fig. 66:** Labels — Lat. intermusc. septum · Tendon, Triceps m. · Triceps m. (med. head) · Olecranon process · Anconeus m. · Antebrach. fascia · Flex. carpi ulnaris m. · Ext. carpi ulnaris m. · Brachioradialis m. · Ext. carpi rad. long. m. · Lat. epicondyle · Antebrach. fascia · Ext. carpi rad. brev. m. · Ext. digit. and ext. digit. min. mm. (cut) · Supinator m. · Radius · Tendon, Pronator teres m. · **Abd. pollicis long. m.** · **Ext. indicis m.** · Ext. pollicis long. m. · Ext. pollicis brev. m. · Radius · Tendon compartment · Tendon, Ext. carpi rad. brev. m. · Tendon, Ext. carpi rad. long. m. · **Tendon, Ext. pollicis brev. m.** · **Tendon, Ext. pollicis long. m.** · Intermusc. septum · **Tendons, Ext. digitorum m.** · Tendon, Ext. carpi ulnaris m. · Ulna · Tendon compartments, retinaculum · **Tendon, Ext. dig. min. m.** · Tendon, Ext. carpi ulnaris m.

**Fig. 65: Nerves and Arteries of the Left Posterior Forearm**

NOTE: 1) the extensor digiti minimi and extensor digitorum have been separated from the extensor carpi ulnaris to expose the deep radial nerve and posterior interosseous artery coursing inferiorly in the posterior forearm.

2) the anastomoses at the elbow and wrist.

**Fig. 66: The Thumb Muscles of the Left Posterior Forearm**

NOTE: 1) that the three thumb muscles (abductor pollicis longus and extensors pollicis brevis and longus) are exposed when the extensor digitorum and extensor digiti minimi muscles are partially removed. Observe also the extensor indicis muscle coursing to the index finger.

2) the tendon compartments formed by the extensor retinaculum at the wrist.

Figs. 65, 66

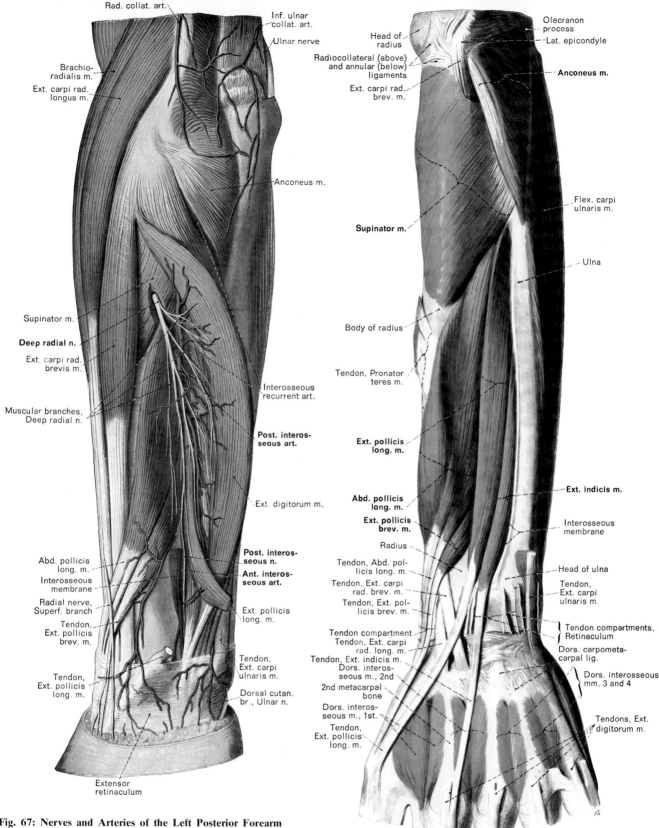

**Fig. 67: Nerves and Arteries of the Left Posterior Forearm (Deep Dissection)**

NOTE: 1) the extensor digitorum muscle is separated from the extensor carpi radialis brevis and pulled medially to reveal the posterior interosseous artery and deep radial nerve.

2) the emergence of the deep radial nerve to the posterior forearm through the supinator muscle.

3) the posterior interosseous nerve is a continuation inferiorly of the deep radial nerve and may be seen coursing deep to the extensor pollicis longus muscle. This muscle has been cut at the wrist in this dissection.

**Fig. 68: The Left Posterior Forearm Muscles, Deep Group**

NOTE: 1) all of the superficial posterior forearm muscles have been removed except the anconeus. The five deep muscles are the supinator, abductor pollicis longus, extensors pollicis brevis and longus and extensor indicis.

2) the supinator is a broad muscle, arising from the lateral epicondyle of the humerus and from the ridge of the ulna. It courses obliquely to insert around the upper third of the radius.

Figs. 67, 68    I

## Figs. 69 and 70: The Left Humerus

NOTE: 1) the humerus consists of a body and two extremities. The head of the humerus is shaped as a hemisphere and articulates with the scapula at the glenoid cavity.

2) the anatomical neck is a constricted zone just distal to the head of the humerus, and the surgical neck, where fractures frequently occur, lies just below the two tubercles.

3) the greater and lesser tubercles are roughened prominences which allow the insertion of muscles: the supraspinatus, infraspinatus, and the teres minor on the greater tubercle and the subscapularis on the lesser.

4) within the tubercular sulcus passes the tendon of the long head of the biceps.

5) adjacent to the radial groove courses the radial nerve, which is therefore endangered by fractures of the humerus. If the radial nerve does become injured by a fracture, a clinical condition called *wrist drop* develops because this nerve supplies all the extensors of the wrist and fingers.

6) the distal extremity affords articulation with the radius and ulna; the rounded capitulum (Fig. 70) articulates with the head of the radius, while the grooved trochlea fits into the trochlear notch of the ulna.

7) the radial fossa above the capitulum (Fig. 70) within which the radial head is received upon flexion of the forearm. Additionally, note the coronoid fossa which receives the coronoid process of the ulna.

8) the olecranon fossa (Fig. 69) for the olecranon process of the ulna. Finally, observe the medial and lateral epicondyles which allow attachment of muscles.

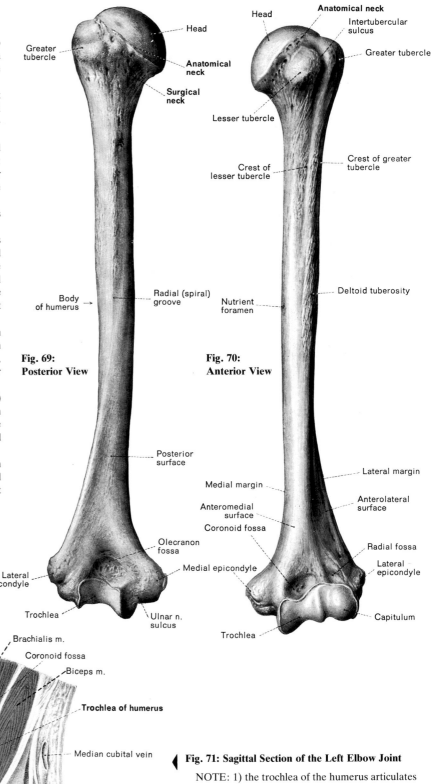

**Fig. 69: Posterior View**

**Fig. 70: Anterior View**

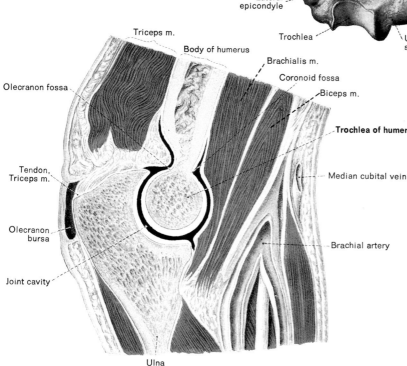

## Fig. 71: Sagittal Section of the Left Elbow Joint

NOTE: 1) the trochlea of the humerus articulates with the trochlear notch of the ulna to form a ginglymus or hinge joint. The adaptation of these two articular surfaces is such that only flexion and extension can take place and not lateral displacement.

2) the posterior aspect of the olecranon process is separated from the skin by a subcutaneous bursa, and the insertion of the triceps on the olecranon.

3) that the brachialis muscle lies immediately adjacent to the joint capsule anteriorly, and courses to insert on the roughened depression on the anterior surface of the coronoid process and onto the tuberosity of the ulna.

Figs. 69, 70, 71

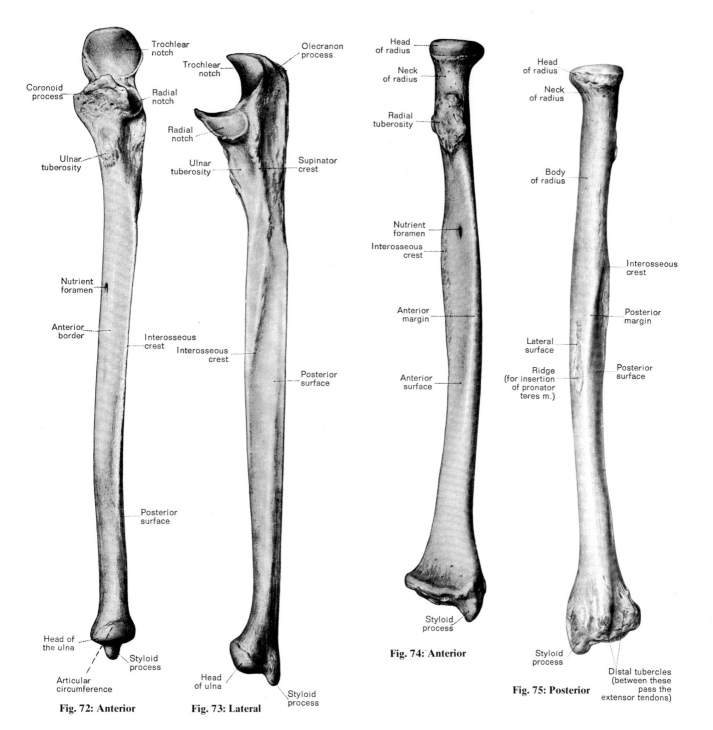

Trochlear notch

Trochlear notch

Olecranon process

Coronoid process

Radial notch

Radial notch

Ulnar tuberosity

Ulnar tuberosity

Supinator crest

Nutrient foramen

Anterior border

Interosseous crest

Interosseous crest

Posterior surface

Posterior surface

Head of the ulna

Styloid process

Head of ulna

Articular circumference

Styloid process

Styloid process

**Fig. 72: Anterior**

**Fig. 73: Lateral**

Head of radius

Neck of radius

Radial tuberosity

Nutrient foramen

Interosseous crest

Anterior margin

Anterior surface

Styloid process

**Fig. 74: Anterior**

Head of radius

Neck of radius

Body of radius

Interosseous crest

Posterior margin

Lateral surface

Ridge (for insertion of pronator teres m.)

Posterior surface

Styloid process

Distal tubercles (between these pass the extensor tendons)

**Fig. 75: Posterior**

### The Left Ulna (Figs. 72 and 73)

NOTE: 1) the ulna is the medial bone of the forearm. It presents a superior extremity, a body or shaft and an inferior extremity.

2) the superior extremity is marked by two processes, the olecranon and coronoid processes and two concave cavities, the radial notch for articulation with the radius, and the trochlear notch which serves for articulation with the trochlea of the humerus. The brachialis muscle inserts on the tuberosity of the ulna.

3) the tapering body of the ulna affords attachment of the interosseous membrane. The distal extremity is marked by the ulnar head laterally, and the styloid process postero-medially. The head of the ulna is attached to an articular disc which, in turn, articulates with the triquetral bone. Onto the styloid process of the ulna is attached the ulnar collateral ligament of the wrist joint.

### The Left Radius (Figs. 74 and 75)

NOTE: 1) the radius is situated lateral to the ulna in the forearm. It has a body and two extremities. The proximal extremity articulates with both the humerus and ulna. The larger distal extremity articulates inferiorly with the carpal bones (scaphoid, lunate and triquetrum) and medially with the ulna.

2) the proximal extremity is marked by a cylindrical head which articulates with both the capitulum of the humerus and the radial notch of the ulna. Just beneath the neck on the anteromedial aspect is found the radial tuberosity on which is inserted the biceps tendon.

3) the interosseous membrane is attached along the inter-osseous crest of the shaft.

4) the styloid process distally gives attachment to the brachioradialis muscle and the radial collateral ligament of the radiocarpal joint.

## Fig. 76: The Left Elbow Joint, Anterior View

NOTE: 1) the elbow joint is a hinge (ginglymus) joint in which the trochlear notch of the ulna receives the trochlea of the humerus, and the shallow fovea on the head of radius articulates with the capitulum of the humerus.

2) the entire joint is encased by an articular capsule which tends to be loose to allow flexion and extension of the forearm. The capsule is thickened medially by the ulnar collateral ligament and laterally by the radial collateral ligament.

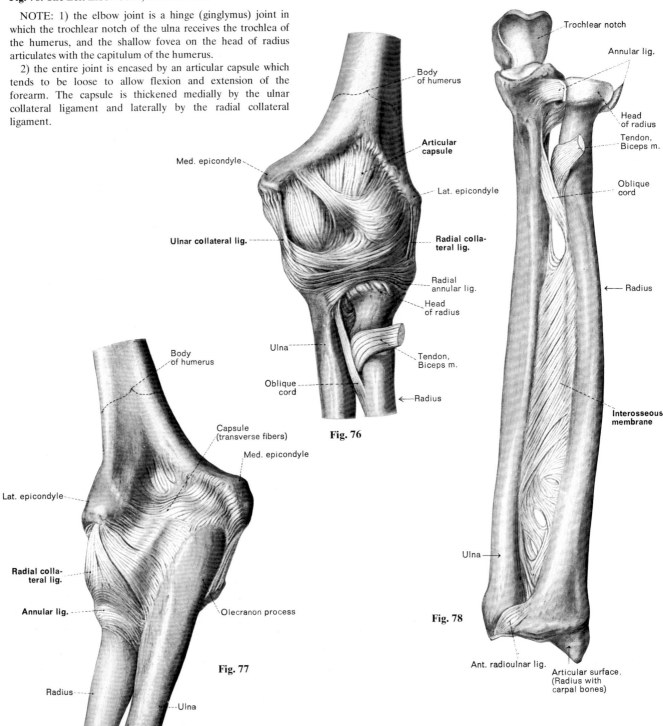

Fig. 76

Fig. 77

Fig. 78

## Fig. 77: The Left Elbow Joint, Posterolateral View

NOTE: 1) the fan-shaped form of the radial collateral ligament. It attaches superiorly to the lateral epicondyle and blends inferiorly with the capsule of the joint.

2) the superior portion of the radial annular ligament also blends with the articular capsule.

3) the transverse fibers of the articular capsule forming a band between the medial and lateral epicondyles and bridging the olecranon fossa.

## Fig. 78: Radioulnar Joints, Anterior View (left)

NOTE: 1) articulations between the radius and ulna occur proximally, along the shafts of the two bones and distally.

2) the proximal joint is a pivot (trochoid) type joint and consists of the head of the radius which rotates within the radial notch of the ulna. This joint is protected by the lower part of the capsule of the elbow joint and by an underlying annular ligament attached at both ends to the ulna and forming a circular band around the head of the radius.

3) the broad, fibrous interosseous membrane extends obliquely between the bones while distally the head of the ulna articulates with the ulnar notch of the radius.

Figs. 76, 77, 78

## Fig. 79: Roentgenogram of the Elbow Joint of 5½ Year Old Boy

NOTE: 1) the shaft of a long bone is called the *diaphysis* while a center of ossification, distinct from the shaft and usually at the extremity of a long bone, is known as an *epiphysis*.

2) the epihysis of the head of the radius is as yet not formed in the 5½-year old, while ossification has commenced in the humeral capitulum.

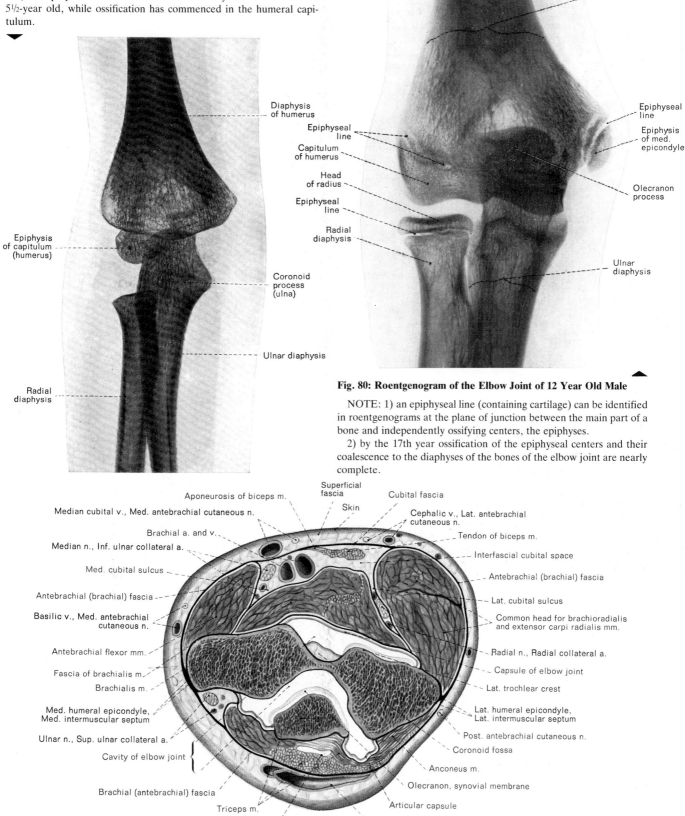

Fig. 79 labels:
- Diaphysis of humerus
- Epiphysis of capitulum (humerus)
- Ulnar diaphysis
- Radial diaphysis
- Coronoid process (ulna)

Fig. 80 labels:
- Diaphysis of humerus
- Epiphyseal line
- Capitulum of humerus
- Head of radius
- Epiphyseal line
- Radial diaphysis
- Epiphyseal line
- Epiphysis of med. epicondyle
- Olecranon process
- Ulnar diaphysis

## Fig. 80: Roentgenogram of the Elbow Joint of 12 Year Old Male

NOTE: 1) an epiphyseal line (containing cartilage) can be identified in roentgenograms at the plane of junction between the main part of a bone and independently ossifying centers, the epiphyses.

2) by the 17th year ossification of the epiphyseal centers and their coalescence to the diaphyses of the bones of the elbow joint are nearly complete.

Fig. 81 labels:
- Aponeurosis of biceps m.
- Superficial fascia
- Skin
- Cubital fascia
- Median cubital v., Med. antebrachial cutaneous n.
- Cephalic v., Lat. antebrachial cutaneous n.
- Brachial a. and v.
- Tendon of biceps m.
- Median n., Inf. ulnar collateral a.
- Interfascial cubital space
- Med. cubital sulcus
- Antebrachial (brachial) fascia
- Antebrachial (brachial) fascia
- Lat. cubital sulcus
- Basilic v., Med. antebrachial cutaneous n.
- Common head for brachioradialis and extensor carpi radialis mm.
- Antebrachial flexor mm.
- Radial n., Radial collateral a.
- Fascia of brachialis m.
- Capsule of elbow joint
- Brachialis m.
- Lat. trochlear crest
- Med. humeral epicondyle, Med. intermuscular septum
- Lat. humeral epicondyle, Lat. intermuscular septum
- Ulnar n., Sup. ulnar collateral a.
- Post. antebrachial cutaneous n.
- Cavity of elbow joint
- Coronoid fossa
- Anconeus m.
- Brachial (antebrachial) fascia
- Olecranon, synovial membrane
- Triceps m.
- Articular capsule
- Subtendinous bursa of triceps brachii m.
- Subcutaneous bursa of olecranon

## Fig. 81: Cross Section Through the Right Upper Extremity at the Level of the Elbow Joint

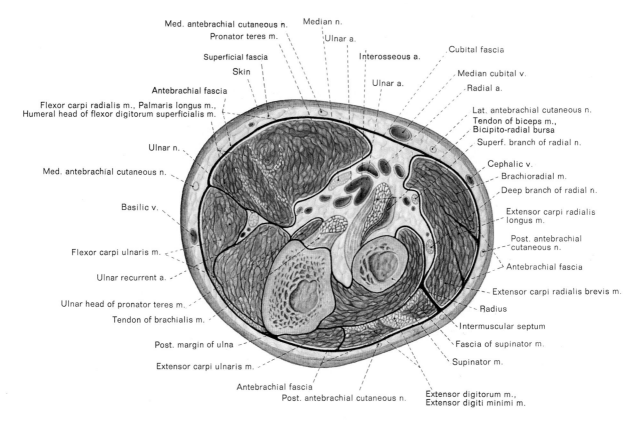

Med. antebrachial cutaneous n.
Pronator teres m.
Superficial fascia
Skin
Antebrachial fascia
Flexor carpi radialis m., Palmaris longus m.,
Humeral head of flexor digitorum superficialis m.
Ulnar n.
Med. antebrachial cutaneous n.
Basilic v.
Flexor carpi ulnaris m.
Ulnar recurrent a.
Ulnar head of pronator teres m.
Tendon of brachialis m.
Post. margin of ulna
Extensor carpi ulnaris m.
Antebrachial fascia
Post. antebrachial cutaneous n.

Median n.
Ulnar a.
Interosseous a.
Ulnar a.
Cubital fascia
Median cubital v.
Radial a.
Lat. antebrachial cutaneous n.
Tendon of biceps m.,
Bicipito-radial bursa
Superf. branch of radial n.
Cephalic v.
Brachioradial m.
Deep branch of radial n.
Extensor carpi radialis longus m.
Post. antebrachial cutaneous n.
Antebrachial fascia
Extensor carpi radialis brevis m.
Radius
Intermuscular septum
Fascia of supinator m.
Supinator m.
Extensor digitorum m.,
Extensor digiti minimi m.

**Fig. 82: Cross Section Through the Proximal Third of the Right Forearm**

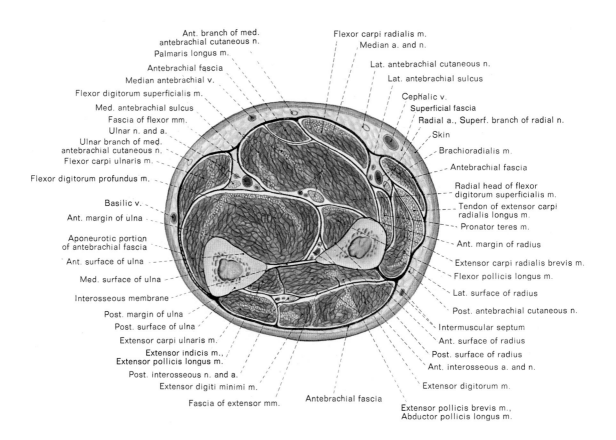

Ant. branch of med. antebrachial cutaneous n.
Palmaris longus m.
Antebrachial fascia
Median antebrachial v.
Flexor digitorum superficialis m.
Med. antebrachial sulcus
Fascia of flexor mm.
Ulnar n. and a.
Ulnar branch of med. antebrachial cutaneous n.
Flexor carpi ulnaris m.
Flexor digitorum profundus m.
Basilic v.
Ant. margin of ulna
Aponeurotic portion of antebrachial fascia
Ant. surface of ulna
Med. surface of ulna
Interosseous membrane
Post. margin of ulna
Post. surface of ulna
Extensor carpi ulnaris m.
Extensor indicis m.,
Extensor pollicis longus m.
Post. interosseous n. and a.
Extensor digiti minimi m.
Fascia of extensor mm.

Flexor carpi radialis m.
Median a. and n.
Lat. antebrachial cutaneous n.
Lat. antebrachial sulcus
Cephalic v.
Superficial fascia
Radial a., Superf. branch of radial n.
Skin
Brachioradialis m.
Antebrachial fascia
Radial head of flexor digitorum superficialis m.
Tendon of extensor carpi radialis longus m.
Pronator teres m.
Ant. margin of radius
Extensor carpi radialis brevis m.
Flexor pollicis longus m.
Lat. surface of radius
Post. antebrachial cutaneous n.
Intermuscular septum
Ant. surface of radius
Post. surface of radius
Ant. interosseous a. and n.
Extensor digitorum m.
Extensor pollicis brevis m.,
Abductor pollicis longus m.
Antebrachial fascia

**Fig. 83: Cross Section Through the Middle Third of the Right Forearm**

Figs. 82, 83

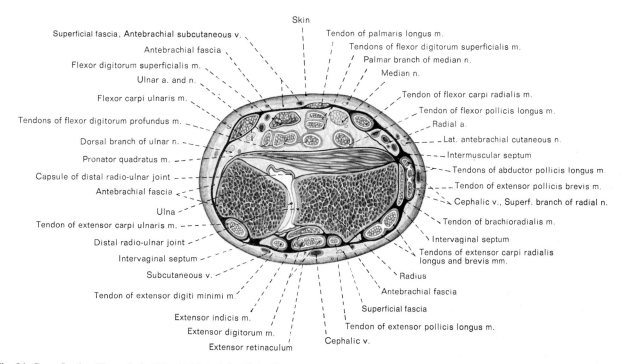

Skin
Superficial fascia, Antebrachial subcutaneous v.
Antebrachial fascia
Flexor digitorum superficialis m.
Ulnar a. and n.
Flexor carpi ulnaris m.
Tendons of flexor digitorum profundus m.
Dorsal branch of ulnar n.
Pronator quadratus m.
Capsule of distal radio-ulnar joint
Antebrachial fascia
Ulna
Tendon of extensor carpi ulnaris m.
Distal radio-ulnar joint
Intervaginal septum
Subcutaneous v.
Tendon of extensor digiti minimi m.
Extensor indicis m.
Extensor digitorum m.
Extensor retinaculum

Tendon of palmaris longus m.
Tendons of flexor digitorum superficialis m.
Palmar branch of median n.
Median n.
Tendon of flexor carpi radialis m.
Tendon of flexor pollicis longus m.
Radial a.
Lat. antebrachial cutaneous n.
Intermuscular septum
Tendons of abductor pollicis longus m.
Tendon of extensor pollicis brevis m.
Cephalic v., Superf. branch of radial n.
Tendon of brachioradialis m.
Intervaginal septum
Tendons of extensor carpi radialis longus and brevis mm.
Radius
Antebrachial fascia
Superficial fascia
Tendon of extensor pollicis longus m.
Cephalic v.

**Fig. 84: Cross Section Through the Distal Third of the Right Forearm**

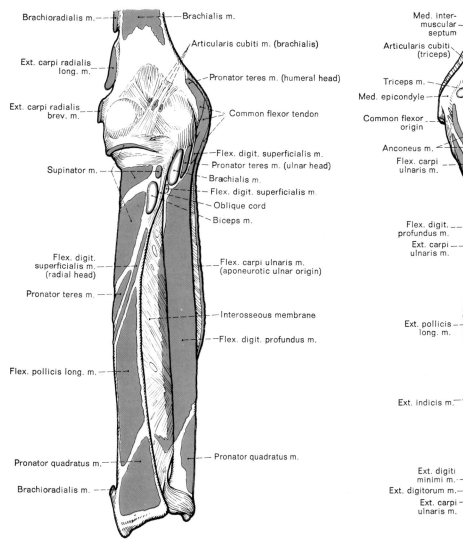

Brachioradialis m.
Brachialis m.
Articularis cubiti m. (brachialis)
Ext. carpi radialis long. m.
Pronator teres m. (humeral head)
Ext. carpi radialis brev. m.
Common flexor tendon
Flex. digit. superficialis m.
Pronator teres m. (ulnar head)
Supinator m.
Brachialis m.
Flex. digit. superficialis m.
Oblique cord
Biceps m.
Flex. digit. superficialis m. (radial head)
Flex. carpi ulnaris m. (aponeurotic ulnar origin)
Pronator teres m.
Interosseous membrane
Flex. digit. profundus m.
Flex. pollicis long. m.
Pronator quadratus m.
Pronator quadratus m.
Brachioradialis m.

**Fig. 85: Bones of the Right Forearm Showing Attachments of Muscles (Anterior View)**

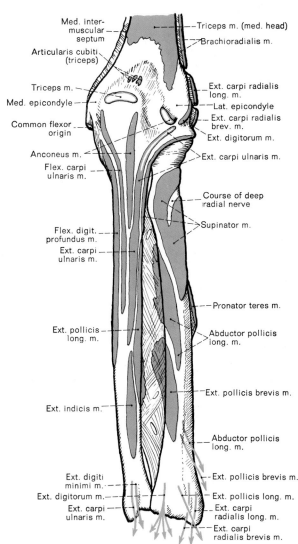

Med. intermuscular septum
Triceps m. (med. head)
Brachioradialis m.
Articularis cubiti (triceps)
Triceps m.
Med. epicondyle
Common flexor origin
Ext. carpi radialis long. m.
Lat. epicondyle
Ext. carpi radialis brev. m.
Ext. digitorum m.
Anconeus m.
Flex. carpi ulnaris m.
Ext. carpi ulnaris m.
Course of deep radial nerve
Supinator m.
Flex. digit. profundus m.
Ext. carpi ulnaris m.
Pronator teres m.
Abductor pollicis long. m.
Ext. pollicis long. m.
Ext. pollicis brevis m.
Ext. indicis m.
Abductor pollicis long. m.
Ext. digiti minimi m.
Ext. pollicis brevis m.
Ext. digitorum m.
Ext. pollicis long. m.
Ext. carpi ulnaris m.
Ext. carpi radialis long. m.
Ext. carpi radialis brevis m.

**Fig. 86: Bones of the Right Forearm Showing the Attachments of Muscles (Posterior View)**

Figs. 84, 85, 86   I

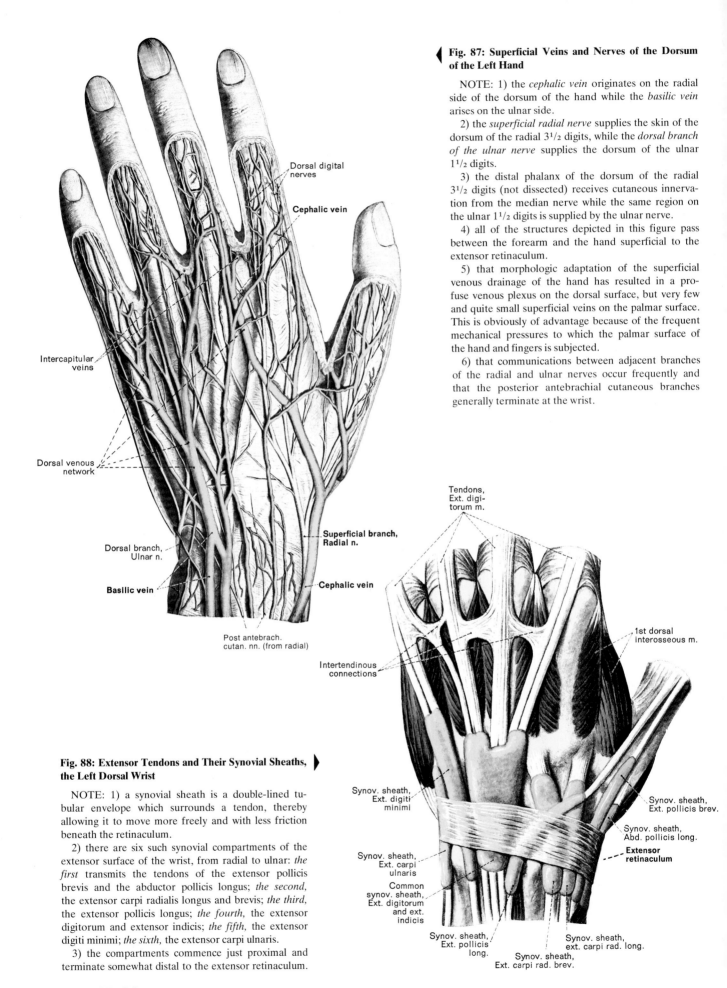

**Dorsal digital nerves**

**Cephalic vein**

Intercapitular veins

Dorsal venous network

Dorsal branch, Ulnar n.

**Basilic vein**

**Superficial branch, Radial n.**

**Cephalic vein**

Post antebrach. cutan. nn. (from radial)

Tendons, Ext. digitorum m.

1st dorsal interosseous m.

Intertendinous connections

Synov. sheath, Ext. digiti minimi

Synov. sheath, Ext. pollicis brev.

Synov. sheath, Abd. pollicis long.

**Extensor retinaculum**

Synov. sheath, Ext. carpi ulnaris

Common synov. sheath, Ext. digitorum and ext. indicis

Synov. sheath, Ext. pollicis long.

Synov. sheath, Ext. carpi rad. brev.

Synov. sheath, ext. carpi rad. long.

◀ **Fig. 87: Superficial Veins and Nerves of the Dorsum of the Left Hand**

NOTE: 1) the *cephalic vein* originates on the radial side of the dorsum of the hand while the *basilic vein* arises on the ulnar side.

2) the *superficial radial nerve* supplies the skin of the dorsum of the radial 3½ digits, while the *dorsal branch of the ulnar nerve* supplies the dorsum of the ulnar 1½ digits.

3) the distal phalanx of the dorsum of the radial 3½ digits (not dissected) receives cutaneous innervation from the median nerve while the same region on the ulnar 1½ digits is supplied by the ulnar nerve.

4) all of the structures depicted in this figure pass between the forearm and the hand superficial to the extensor retinaculum.

5) that morphologic adaptation of the superficial venous drainage of the hand has resulted in a profuse venous plexus on the dorsal surface, but very few and quite small superficial veins on the palmar surface. This is obviously of advantage because of the frequent mechanical pressures to which the palmar surface of the hand and fingers is subjected.

6) that communications between adjacent branches of the radial and ulnar nerves occur frequently and that the posterior antebrachial cutaneous branches generally terminate at the wrist.

**Fig. 88: Extensor Tendons and Their Synovial Sheaths,** ▶ **the Left Dorsal Wrist**

NOTE: 1) a synovial sheath is a double-lined tubular envelope which surrounds a tendon, thereby allowing it to move more freely and with less friction beneath the retinaculum.

2) there are six such synovial compartments of the extensor surface of the wrist, from radial to ulnar: *the first* transmits the tendons of the extensor pollicis brevis and the abductor pollicis longus; *the second*, the extensor carpi radialis longus and brevis; *the third*, the extensor pollicis longus; *the fourth*, the extensor digitorum and extensor indicis; *the fifth*, the extensor digiti minimi; *the sixth*, the extensor carpi ulnaris.

3) the compartments commence just proximal and terminate somewhat distal to the extensor retinaculum.

Figs. 87, 88

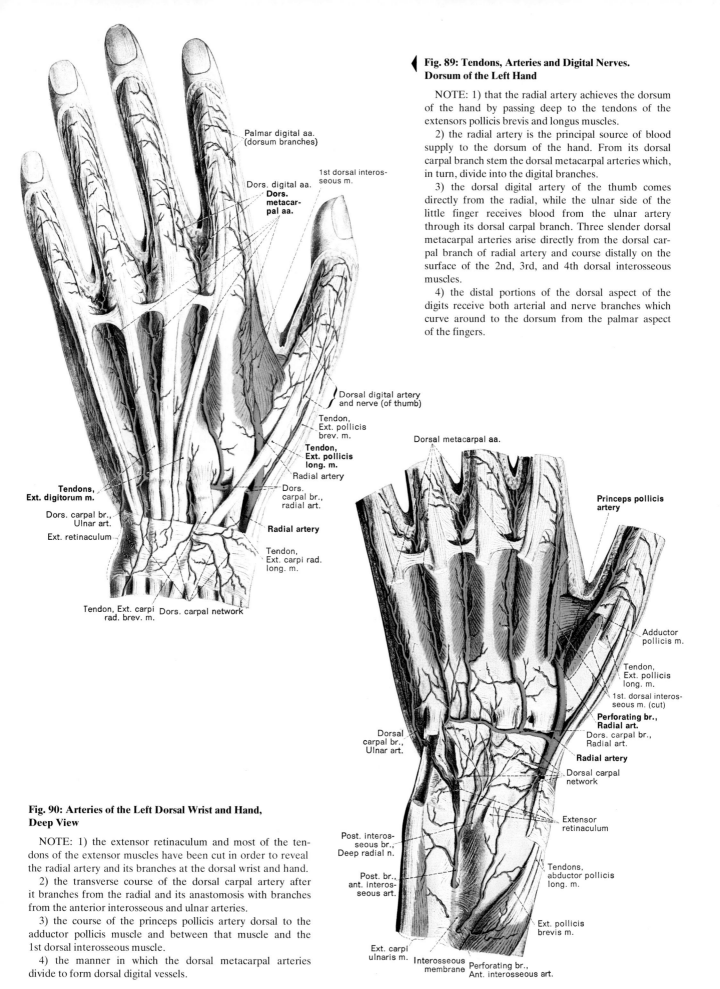

Palmar digital aa.
(dorsum branches)

Dors. digital aa.
**Dors.
metacar-
pal aa.**

1st dorsal interos-
seous m.

Dorsal digital artery
and nerve (of thumb)

Tendon,
Ext. pollicis
brev. m.

**Tendon,
Ext. pollicis
long. m.**

Radial artery

Dors.
carpal br.,
radial art.

**Radial artery**

Tendon,
Ext. carpi rad.
long. m.

**Tendons,
Ext. digitorum m.**

Dors. carpal br.,
Ulnar art.

Ext. retinaculum

Tendon, Ext. carpi
rad. brev. m.

Dors. carpal network

### Fig. 89: Tendons, Arteries and Digital Nerves. Dorsum of the Left Hand

NOTE: 1) that the radial artery achieves the dorsum of the hand by passing deep to the tendons of the extensors pollicis brevis and longus muscles.

2) the radial artery is the principal source of blood supply to the dorsum of the hand. From its dorsal carpal branch stem the dorsal metacarpal arteries which, in turn, divide into the digital branches.

3) the dorsal digital artery of the thumb comes directly from the radial, while the ulnar side of the little finger receives blood from the ulnar artery through its dorsal carpal branch. Three slender dorsal metacarpal arteries arise directly from the dorsal carpal branch of radial artery and course distally on the surface of the 2nd, 3rd, and 4th dorsal interosseous muscles.

4) the distal portions of the dorsal aspect of the digits receive both arterial and nerve branches which curve around to the dorsum from the palmar aspect of the fingers.

Dorsal metacarpal aa.

**Princeps pollicis
artery**

Adductor
pollicis m.

Tendon,
Ext. pollicis
long. m.

1st. dorsal interos-
seous m. (cut)

**Perforating br.,
Radial art.**

Dors. carpal br.,
Radial art.

**Radial artery**

Dorsal carpal
network

Extensor
retinaculum

Tendons,
abductor pollicis
long. m.

Ext. pollicis
brevis m.

Dorsal
carpal br.,
Ulnar art.

Post. interos-
seous br.,
Deep radial n.

Post. br.,
ant. interos-
seous art.

Ext. carpi
ulnaris m.

Interosseous
membrane

Perforating br.,
Ant. interosseous art.

### Fig. 90: Arteries of the Left Dorsal Wrist and Hand, Deep View

NOTE: 1) the extensor retinaculum and most of the tendons of the extensor muscles have been cut in order to reveal the radial artery and its branches at the dorsal wrist and hand.

2) the transverse course of the dorsal carpal artery after it branches from the radial and its anastomosis with branches from the anterior interosseous and ulnar arteries.

3) the course of the princeps pollicis artery dorsal to the adductor pollicis muscle and between that muscle and the 1st dorsal interosseous muscle.

4) the manner in which the dorsal metacarpal arteries divide to form dorsal digital vessels.

Figs. 89, 90    I

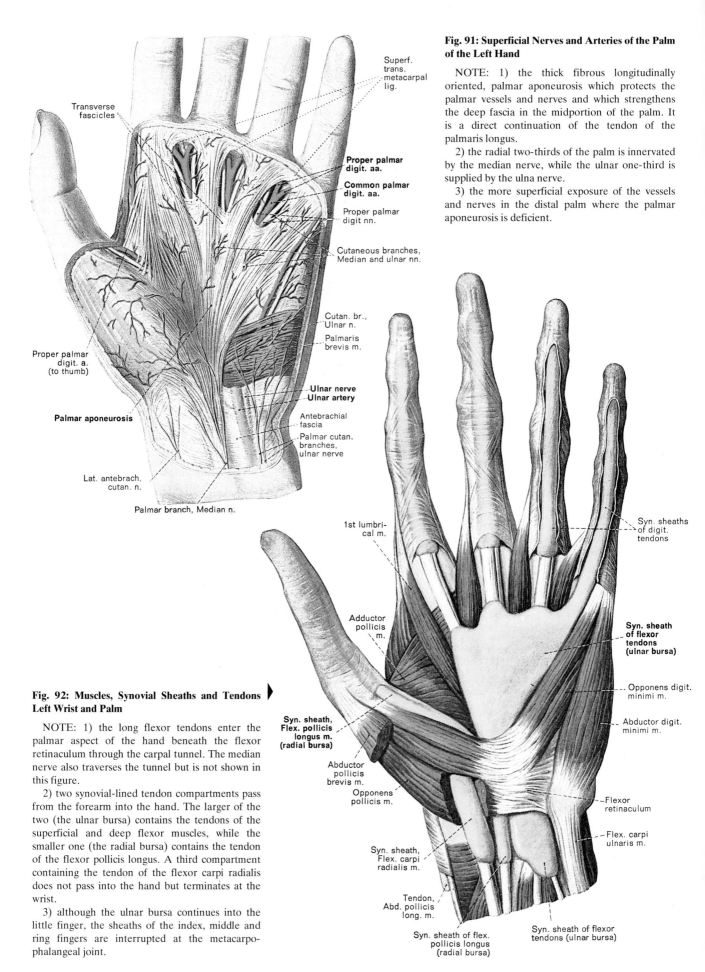

Transverse fascicles

Superf. trans. metacarpal lig.

**Proper palmar digit. aa.**

**Common palmar digit. aa.**

Proper palmar digit nn.

Cutaneous branches, Median and ulnar nn.

Proper palmar digit. a. (to thumb)

Cutan. br., Ulnar n.

Palmaris brevis m.

**Palmar aponeurosis**

**Ulnar nerve**
**Ulnar artery**

Antebrachial fascia

Palmar cutan. branches, ulnar nerve

Lat. antebrach. cutan. n.

Palmar branch, Median n.

### Fig. 91: Superficial Nerves and Arteries of the Palm of the Left Hand

NOTE: 1) the thick fibrous longitudinally oriented, palmar aponeurosis which protects the palmar vessels and nerves and which strengthens the deep fascia in the midportion of the palm. It is a direct continuation of the tendon of the palmaris longus.

2) the radial two-thirds of the palm is innervated by the median nerve, while the ulnar one-third is supplied by the ulna nerve.

3) the more superficial exposure of the vessels and nerves in the distal palm where the palmar aponeurosis is deficient.

1st lumbrical m.

Syn. sheaths of digit. tendons

Adductor pollicis m.

**Syn. sheath of flexor tendons (ulnar bursa)**

Opponens digit. minimi m.

Abductor digit. minimi m.

**Syn. sheath, Flex. pollicis longus m. (radial bursa)**

Abductor pollicis brevis m.

Opponens pollicis m.

Flexor retinaculum

Flex. carpi ulnaris m.

Syn. sheath, Flex. carpi radialis m.

Tendon, Abd. pollicis long. m.

Syn. sheath of flex. pollicis longus (radial bursa)

Syn. sheath of flexor tendons (ulnar bursa)

### Fig. 92: Muscles, Synovial Sheaths and Tendons Left Wrist and Palm

NOTE: 1) the long flexor tendons enter the palmar aspect of the hand beneath the flexor retinaculum through the carpal tunnel. The median nerve also traverses the tunnel but is not shown in this figure.

2) two synovial-lined tendon compartments pass from the forearm into the hand. The larger of the two (the ulnar bursa) contains the tendons of the superficial and deep flexor muscles, while the smaller one (the radial bursa) contains the tendon of the flexor pollicis longus. A third compartment containing the tendon of the flexor carpi radialis does not pass into the hand but terminates at the wrist.

3) although the ulnar bursa continues into the little finger, the sheaths of the index, middle and ring fingers are interrupted at the metacarpophalangeal joint.

Figs. 91, 92

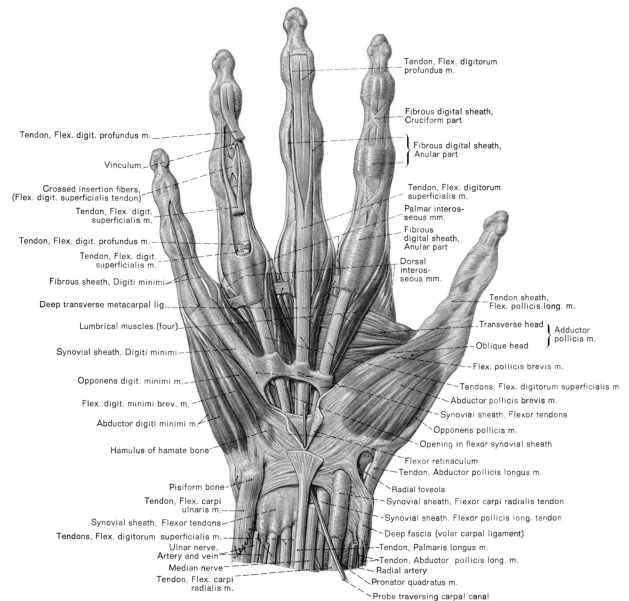

Tendon, Flex. digitorum profundus m.

Fibrous digital sheath, Cruciform part

Fibrous digital sheath, Anular part

Tendon, Flex. digit. profundus m.

Vinculum

Crossed insertion fibers, (Flex. digit. superficialis tendon)

Tendon, Flex. digit. superficialis m.

Tendon, Flex. digit. profundus m.

Tendon, Flex. digit. superficialis m.

Fibrous sheath, Digiti minimi

Deep transverse metacarpal lig.

Lumbrical muscles (four)

Synovial sheath, Digiti minimi

Opponens digit. minimi m.

Flex. digit. minimi brev. m.

Abductor digiti minimi m.

Hamulus of hamate bone

Pisiform bone

Tendon, Flex. carpi ulnaris m.

Synovial sheath, Flexor tendons

Tendons, Flex. digitorum superficialis m.

Ulnar nerve, Artery and vein

Median nerve

Tendon, Flex. carpi radialis m.

Tendon, Flex. digitorum superficialis m.

Palmar interosseous mm.

Fibrous digital sheath, Anular part

Dorsal interosseous mm.

Tendon sheath, Flex. pollicis long. m.

Transverse head } Adductor pollicis m.

Oblique head

Flex. pollicis brevis m.

Tendons, Flex. digitorum superficialis m.

Abductor pollicis brevis m.

Synovial sheath, Flexor tendons

Opponens pollicis m.

Opening in flexor synovial sheath

Flexor retinaculum

Tendon, Abductor pollicis longus m.

Radial foveola

Synovial sheath, Flexor carpi radialis tendon

Synovial sheath, Flexor pollicis long. tendon

Deep fascia (volar carpal ligament)

Tendon, Palmaris longus m.

Tendon, Abductor pollicis long. m.

Radial artery

Pronator quadratus m.

Probe traversing carpal canal

**Fig. 93: Muscles of the Right Hand**

NOTE: 1) how the flexor digit. profundus achieves its insertion on the distal phalanx. The tendon of the flexor digit. superficialis divides into two slips, allowing the corresponding deep flexor tendon to pass.

2) that along the fingers, the tendons are encased in a synovial sheath and then they are bound by both crossed and transverse (cruciate and annular) fibrous sheaths.

3) the muscles of the thenar eminence: abductor pollicis brevis, flexor pollicis brevis and the underlying opponens pollicis muscle.

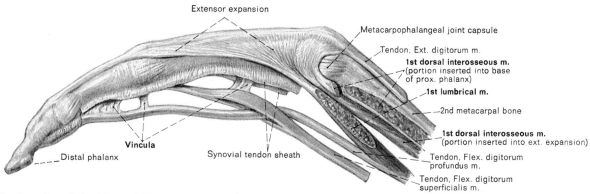

Extensor expansion

Metacarpophalangeal joint capsule

Tendon, Ext. digitorum m.

**1st dorsal interosseous m.** (portion inserted into base of prox. phalanx)

**1st lumbrical m.**

2nd metacarpal bone

**1st dorsal interosseous m.** (portion inserted into ext. expansion)

Tendon, Flex. digitorum profundus m.

Tendon, Flex. digitorum superficialis m.

**Vincula**

Distal phalanx

Synovial tendon sheath

**Fig. 94: Tendon Insertions, Index Finger of Right Hand (Radial Side)**

NOTE: 1) the flexor digit. superficialis inserts on the middle phalanx while the flexor digit. profundus inserts on the distal phalanx.

2) the dorsal interosseous and lumbrical muscles join the diverging extensor fibers in the formation of the extensor expansion on the dorsum of the finger.

3) the vincula are remnants of mesotendons and attach both superficial and deep flexor tendons to the digital sheath.

Figs. 93, 94    I

## Fig. 95: Nerves and Arteries of the Left Palm, Superficial Palmar Arch

NOTE: 1) the median nerve enters the palm beneath the flexor retinaculum and supplies the muscles of the thenar eminence: abductor pollicis brevis, opponens pollicis and flexor pollicis brevis (superficial head). Additionally, it supplies the two most lateral lumbrical muscles and the palmar surface of the lateral three and one-half fingers.

2) the superficial location of the small but important "recurrent" branch of the median nerve which supplies several of the thenar muscles. Its location, just below the deep fascia on the thenar eminence, makes it vulnerable to injury.

3) the ulnar nerve enters the palm superficial to the flexor retinaculum, supplies the medial one and one-half fingers and all the remaining musculature of the hand: three hypothenar muscles, seven interosseous muscles, two medial lumbrical muscles, the adductor pollicis and the flexor pollicis brevis (deep head).

4) the superficial palmar arch is derived principally from the ulnar artery. It crosses the palm to the radial side superficial to the nerves and tendons and is joined by a palmar branch of the radial artery. Three or four common palmar digital arteries arise from the arch, proceed distally and divide into proper palmar digital arteries which course along the fingers with corresponding digital nerves.

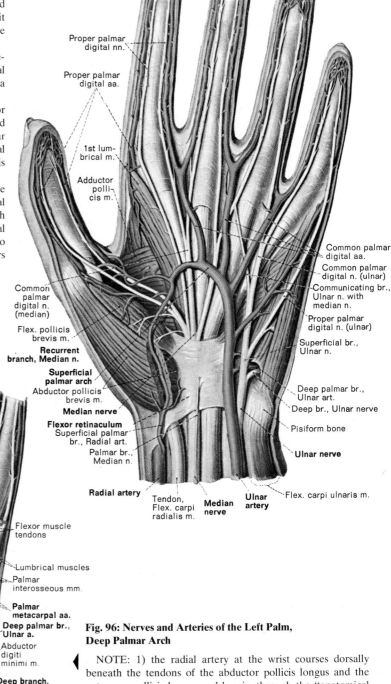

## Fig. 96: Nerves and Arteries of the Left Palm, Deep Palmar Arch

NOTE: 1) the radial artery at the wrist courses dorsally beneath the tendons of the abductor pollicis longus and the extensors pollicis longus and brevis, through the "anatomical snuff box" (see figures 89 and 90), then passes distally to perforate to the palm of the hand through the two heads of the 1st dorsal interosseous muscle. In the palm it forms the deep palmar arch which crosses the palm to the ulnar side to unite with the deep palmar branch of the ulnar artery.

2) palmar metacarpal arteries stem from the deep arch as does the princeps pollicis artery. There is rich anastomosis between the superficial and deep palmar arches.

3) the deep branch of the ulnar nerve coursing with the deep palmar arch to supply all of the muscles in the deep palm.

4) the palmar carpal anastomosis between the ulnar and radial arteries.

Figs. 95, 96

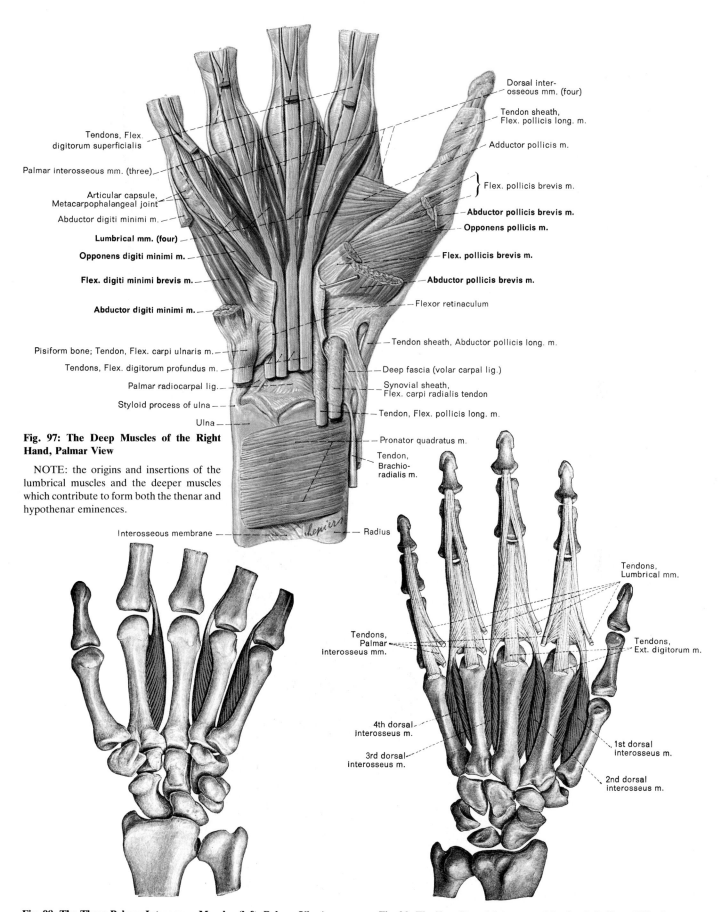

Tendons, Flex. digitorum superficialis

Palmar interosseous mm. (three)

Articular capsule, Metacarpophalangeal joint

Abductor digiti minimi m.

**Lumbrical mm. (four)**

**Opponens digiti minimi m.**

**Flex. digiti minimi brevis m.**

**Abductor digiti minimi m.**

Pisiform bone; Tendon, Flex. carpi ulnaris m.

Tendons, Flex. digitorum profundus m.

Palmar radiocarpal lig.

Styloid process of ulna

Ulna

Dorsal interosseous mm. (four)

Tendon sheath, Flex. pollicis long. m.

Adductor pollicis m.

Flex. pollicis brevis m.

**Abductor pollicis brevis m.**

**Opponens pollicis m.**

**Flex. pollicis brevis m.**

**Abductor pollicis brevis m.**

Flexor retinaculum

Tendon sheath, Abductor pollicis long. m.

Deep fascia (volar carpal lig.)

Synovial sheath, Flex. carpi radialis tendon

Tendon, Flex. pollicis long. m.

Pronator quadratus m.

Tendon, Brachio-radialis m.

**Fig. 97: The Deep Muscles of the Right Hand, Palmar View**

NOTE: the origins and insertions of the lumbrical muscles and the deeper muscles which contribute to form both the thenar and hypothenar eminences.

Interosseous membrane

Radius

Tendons, Lumbrical mm.

Tendons, Palmar interosseus mm.

Tendons, Ext. digitorum m.

4th dorsal interosseus m.

3rd dorsal interosseus m.

1st dorsal interosseus m.

2nd dorsal interosseus m.

**Fig. 98: The Three Palmar Interosseus Muscles (left, Palmar View)**

**Fig. 99: The Four Dorsal Interosseus Muscles (left, Dorsal View)**

NOTE: whereas the three palmar interosseus muscles (figure 98) are adductors of the fingers, the four dorsal interosseus muscles (figure 99) are abductors. All of the interossei flex the metacarpophalangeal joint and extend the interphalangeal joints, and they are all supplied by the ulnar nerve.

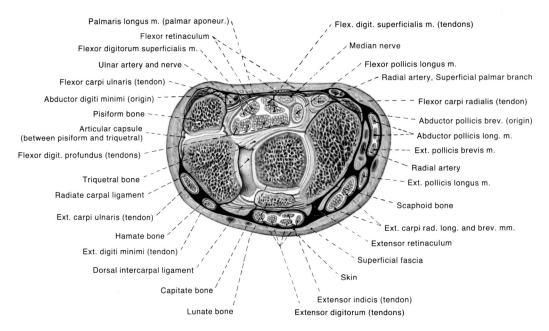

Palmaris longus m. (palmar aponeur.)
Flexor retinaculum
Flexor digitorum superficialis m.
Ulnar artery and nerve
Flexor carpi ulnaris (tendon)
Abductor digiti minimi (origin)
Pisiform bone
Articular capsule
(between pisiform and triquetral)
Flexor digit. profundus (tendons)
Triquetral bone
Radiate carpal ligament
Ext. carpi ulnaris (tendon)
Hamate bone
Ext. digiti minimi (tendon)
Dorsal intercarpal ligament
Capitate bone
Lunate bone

Flex. digit. superficialis m. (tendons)
Median nerve
Flexor pollicis longus m.
Radial artery, Superficial palmar branch
Flexor carpi radialis (tendon)
Abductor pollicis brev. (origin)
Abductor pollicis long. m.
Ext. pollicis brevis m.
Radial artery
Ext. pollicis longus m.
Scaphoid bone
Ext. carpi rad. long. and brev. mm.
Extensor retinaculum
Superficial fascia
Skin
Extensor indicis (tendon)
Extensor digitorum (tendons)

**Fig. 100: Cross Section Through the Hand at the Level of the First Row of Carpal Bones**

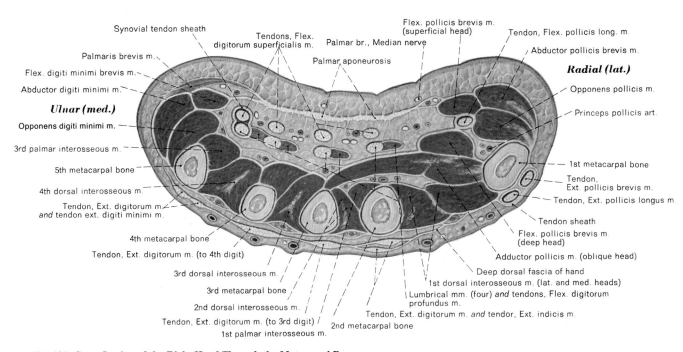

Synovial tendon sheath
Palmaris brevis m.
Flex. digiti minimi brevis m.
Abductor digiti minimi m.
*Ulnar (med.)*
Opponens digiti minimi m.
3rd palmar interosseous m.
5th metacarpal bone
4th dorsal interosseous m.
Tendon, Ext. digitorum m.
*and* tendon ext. digiti minimi m.
4th metacarpal bone
Tendon, Ext. digitorum m. (to 4th digit)
3rd dorsal interosseous m.
3rd metacarpal bone
2nd dorsal interosseous m.
Tendon, Ext. digitorum m. (to 3rd digit)
1st palmar interosseous m.

Tendons, Flex.
digitorum superficialis m.
Palmar aponeurosis

Flex. pollicis brevis m.
(superficial head)
Palmar br., Median nerve

Tendon, Flex. pollicis long. m.
Abductor pollicis brevis m.
*Radial (lat.)*
Opponens pollicis m.
Princeps pollicis art.
1st metacarpal bone
Tendon,
Ext. pollicis brevis m.
Tendon, Ext. pollicis longus m.
Tendon sheath
Flex. pollicis brevis m.
(deep head)
Adductor pollicis m. (oblique head)
Deep dorsal fascia of hand
1st dorsal interosseous m. (lat. and med. heads)
Lumbrical mm. (four) *and* tendons, Flex. digitorum
profundus m.
Tendon, Ext. digitorum m. *and* tendor, Ext. indicis m.
2nd metacarpal bone

**Fig. 101: Cross Section of the Right Hand Through the Metacarpal Bones**

IDENTIFY a) the four dorsal interossei which act as abductors of the fingers and which fill the intervals between the metacarpal bones, b) the three palmar interossei which act as adductors of the fingers, c) the thenar and hypothenar muscles and d) the tendons and lumbrical muscles in the palmar compartment.

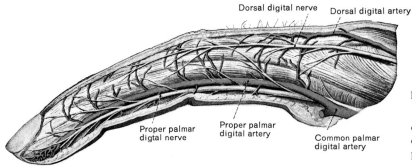

Dorsal digital nerve    Dorsal digital artery

Proper palmar
digtal nerve
Proper palmar
digital artery
Common palmar
digital artery

**Fig. 102: Nerves and Arteries of the Index Finger**

NOTE: the dorsal digital nerve and artery extend only two-thirds the length of the finger. The palmar digital nerve and artery supply not only the entire palmar surface but also the distal one-third of the dorsal surface.

Figs. 100, 101, 102

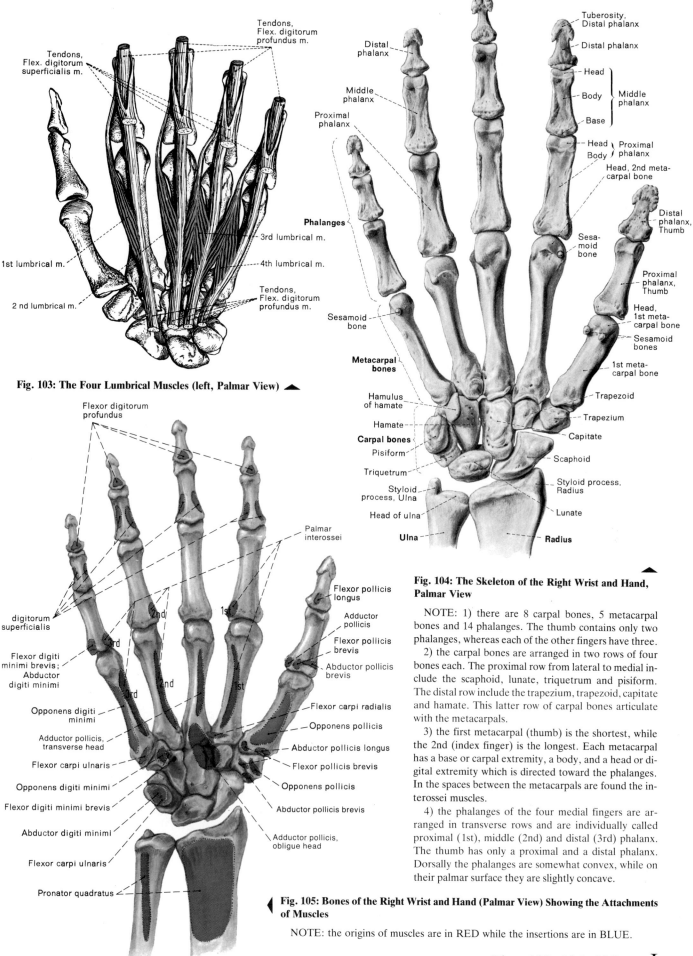

Tendons, Flex. digitorum superficialis m.

Tendons, Flex. digitorum profundus m.

1st lumbrical m.

2 nd lumbrical m.

**Phalanges**

3rd lumbrical m.

4th lumbrical m.

Tendons, Flex. digitorum profundus m.

**Fig. 103: The Four Lumbrical Muscles (left, Palmar View)** ▲

Distal phalanx

Middle phalanx

Proximal phalanx

Tuberosity, Distal phalanx

Distal phalanx

Head

Body } Middle phalanx

Base

Head } Proximal phalanx
Body /

Head, 2nd metacarpal bone

Distal phalanx, Thumb

Proximal phalanx, Thumb

Head, 1st metacarpal bone

Sesamoid bones

1st metacarpal bone

Trapezoid

Trapezium

Capitate

Scaphoid

Styloid process, Radius

Lunate

**Radius**

Sesamoid bone

**Metacarpal bones**

Hamulus of hamate

Hamate

**Carpal bones**

Pisiform

Triquetrum

Styloid process, Ulna

Head of ulna

**Ulna**

**Fig. 104: The Skeleton of the Right Wrist and Hand, Palmar View**

NOTE: 1) there are 8 carpal bones, 5 metacarpal bones and 14 phalanges. The thumb contains only two phalanges, whereas each of the other fingers have three.

2) the carpal bones are arranged in two rows of four bones each. The proximal row from lateral to medial include the scaphoid, lunate, triquetrum and pisiform. The distal row include the trapezium, trapezoid, capitate and hamate. This latter row of carpal bones articulate with the metacarpals.

3) the first metacarpal (thumb) is the shortest, while the 2nd (index finger) is the longest. Each metacarpal has a base or carpal extremity, a body, and a head or digital extremity which is directed toward the phalanges. In the spaces between the metacarpals are found the interossei muscles.

4) the phalanges of the four medial fingers are arranged in transverse rows and are individually called proximal (1st), middle (2nd) and distal (3rd) phalanx. The thumb has only a proximal and a distal phalanx. Dorsally the phalanges are somewhat convex, while on their palmar surface they are slightly concave.

Flexor digitorum profundus

Palmar interossei

digitorum superficialis

Flexor digiti minimi brevis; Abductor digiti minimi

Opponens digiti minimi

Adductor pollicis, transverse head

Flexor carpi ulnaris

Opponens digiti minimi

Flexor digiti minimi brevis

Abductor digiti minimi

Flexor carpi ulnaris

Pronator quadratus

Flexor pollicis longus

Adductor pollicis

Flexor pollicis brevis

Abductor pollicis brevis

Flexor carpi radialis

Opponens pollicis

Abductor pollicis longus

Flexor pollicis brevis

Opponens pollicis

Abductor pollicis brevis

Adductor pollicis, obligue head

**Fig. 105: Bones of the Right Wrist and Hand (Palmar View) Showing the Attachments of Muscles**

NOTE: the origins of muscles are in RED while the insertions are in BLUE.

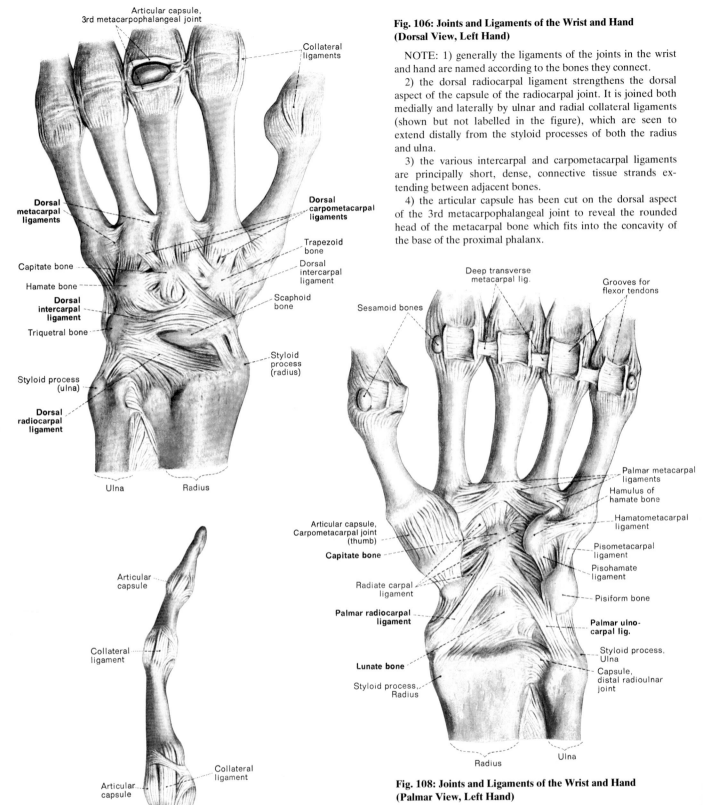

**Fig. 106: Joints and Ligaments of the Wrist and Hand (Dorsal View, Left Hand)**

NOTE: 1) generally the ligaments of the joints in the wrist and hand are named according to the bones they connect.

2) the dorsal radiocarpal ligament strengthens the dorsal aspect of the capsule of the radiocarpal joint. It is joined both medially and laterally by ulnar and radial collateral ligaments (shown but not labelled in the figure), which are seen to extend distally from the styloid processes of both the radius and ulna.

3) the various intercarpal and carpometacarpal ligaments are principally short, dense, connective tissue strands extending between adjacent bones.

4) the articular capsule has been cut on the dorsal aspect of the 3rd metacarpophalangeal joint to reveal the rounded head of the metacarpal bone which fits into the concavity of the base of the proximal phalanx.

**Fig.107: Joints and Ligaments of the Middle Finger**

NOTE: the articular capsules of the metacarpophalangeal and interphalangeal joints are strengthened by longitudinally oriented collateral ligaments.

**Fig. 108: Joints and Ligaments of the Wrist and Hand (Palmar View, Left Hand)**

NOTE: 1) the radiocarpal and ulnocarpal ligamentous bands strengthening the palmar aspect of the radiocarpal joint.

2) identify several strong ligaments in the palmar hand including the pisohamate, pisometacarpal and the radiate ligament surrounding the capitate bone.

3) the bases of the metacarpal bones are joined by the palmar metacarpal ligaments, while the more distal heads of these bones are interconnected by the deep transverse metacarpal ligament.

Figs. 106, 107, 108

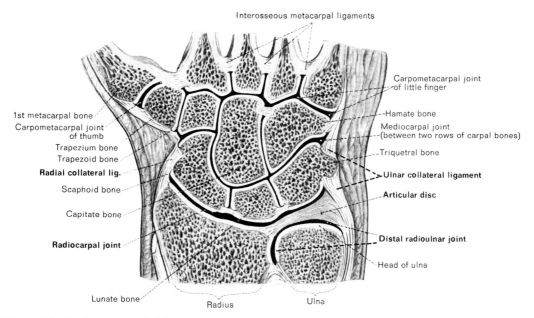

Interosseous metacarpal ligaments

Carpometacarpal joint of little finger
Hamate bone
Mediocarpal joint (between two rows of carpal bones)
Triquetral bone
Ulnar collateral ligament
Articular disc
Distal radioulnar joint
Head of ulna

1st metacarpal bone
Carpometacarpal joint of thumb
Trapezium bone
Trapezoid bone
Radial collateral lig.
Scaphoid bone
Capitate bone
Radiocarpal joint

Lunate bone
Radius
Ulna

**Fig. 109: Coronal (Frontal) Section Through the Left Wrist Joints**

NOTE: 1) the articular disc situated at the distal end of the ulna. Thus, the radiocarpal joint consists of the radius and articular disc proximally and the scaphoid, lunate and triquetrum distally.

2) the ulnar and radial collateral ligaments which provide the wrist joints with strong longitudinally oriented fibrous bands both laterally and medially.

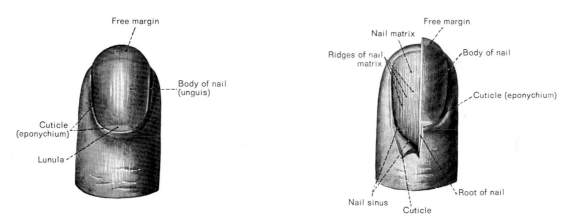

Free margin
Body of nail (unguis)
Cuticle (eponychium)
Lunula

**Fig. 110: Finger Nail, Normal Position (Dorsal View)**

Free margin
Nail matrix
Ridges of nail matrix
Body of nail
Cuticle (eponychium)
Nail sinus
Cuticle
Root of nail

**Fig. 111: Left Half of Finger Nail Bed Exposed**

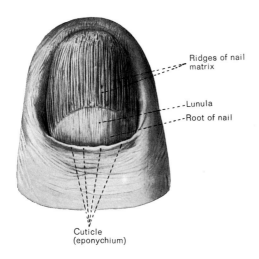

Ridges of nail matrix
Lunula
Root of nail
Cuticle (eponychium)

**Fig. 112: Nail Bed of Thumb after Removal of Nail**

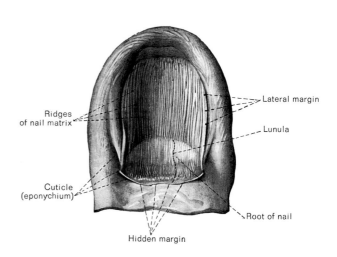

Ridges of nail matrix
Lateral margin
Lunula
Cuticle (eponychium)
Root of nail
Hidden margin

**Fig. 113: Nail Bed of Thumb and Reflection of Cuticle**

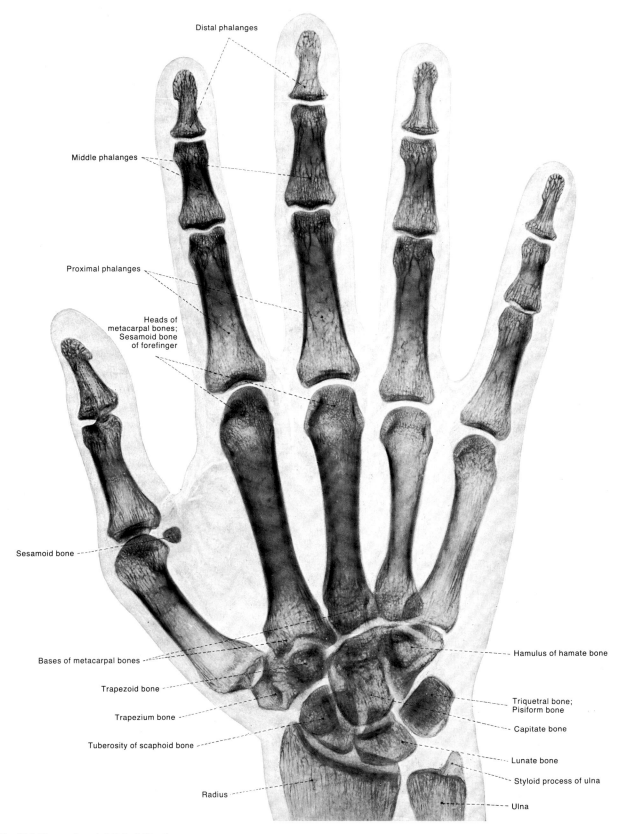

Distal phalanges

Middle phalanges

Proximal phalanges

Heads of
metacarpal bones;
Sesamoid bone
of forefinger

Sesamoid bone

Bases of metacarpal bones

Trapezoid bone

Trapezium bone

Tuberosity of scaphoid bone

Radius

Hamulus of hamate bone

Triquetral bone;
Pisiform bone

Capitate bone

Lunate bone

Styloid process of ulna

Ulna

**Fig. 114: X-ray of on Adult Left Hand**

NOTE: 1) the expanded distal surface of the radius and its articulation inferolaterally with the scaphoid bone and inferomedially with the lunate. The distal extremity of the ulna is lengthened by the styloid process and has an interposed fibrocartilaginous articular disc between it, the radius, and the triquetral bone;

2) the shadow of the pisiform overlies that of the triquetrum. Thus, the proximal row of carpal bones includes the scaphoid, lunate, and triquetrum (with its superimposed pisiform);

3) the articulation of the scaphoid with the trapezium and trapezoid distally and the lunate and capitate laterally;

4) the size and central location of the capitate bone within the wrist. In addition to the capitate, the distal row of carpal bones includes the trapezium, trapezoid, and hamate.

Fig. 114

# PART II: THE THORAX

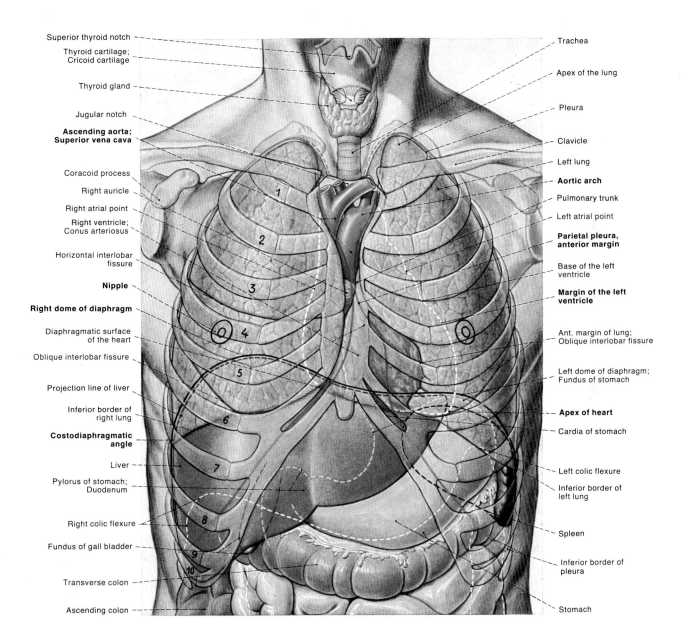

Superior thyroid notch
Thyroid cartilage; Cricoid cartilage
Thyroid gland
Jugular notch
**Ascending aorta; Superior vena cava**
Coracoid process
Right auricle
Right atrial point
Right ventricle; Conus arteriosus
Horizontal interlobar fissure
**Nipple**
**Right dome of diaphragm**
Diaphragmatic surface of the heart
Oblique interlobar fissure
Projection line of liver
Inferior border of right lung
**Costodiaphragmatic angle**
Liver
Pylorus of stomach; Duodenum
Right colic flexure
Fundus of gall bladder
Transverse colon
Ascending colon

Trachea
Apex of the lung
Pleura
Clavicle
Left lung
**Aortic arch**
Pulmonary trunk
Left atrial point
**Parietal pleura, anterior margin**
Base of the left ventricle
**Margin of the left ventricle**
Ant. margin of lung; Oblique interlobar fissure
Left dome of diaphragm; Fundus of stomach
**Apex of heart**
Cardia of stomach
Left colic flexure
Inferior border of left lung
Spleen
Inferior border of pleura
Stomach

**Fig. 115: Thoracic and Upper Abdominal Viscera Viewed from the Anterior Aspect**

NOTE: 1) the outline of the heart and great vessels (white broken line) deep to the anteromedial portion of the lungs;

2) that the liver, lying below the diaphragm, extends superiorly as high as the fourth interspace on the right and to the fifth interspace on the left (red broken line);

3) the superficial position of the superior vena cava and ascending aorta just deep to the manubrium of the sternum in the superior mediastinum;

4) that an upper triangular region containing the great vessels and a lower triangular region overlying the heart (area of superficial cardiac dullness) are not covered by pleura.

Fig. 115    II

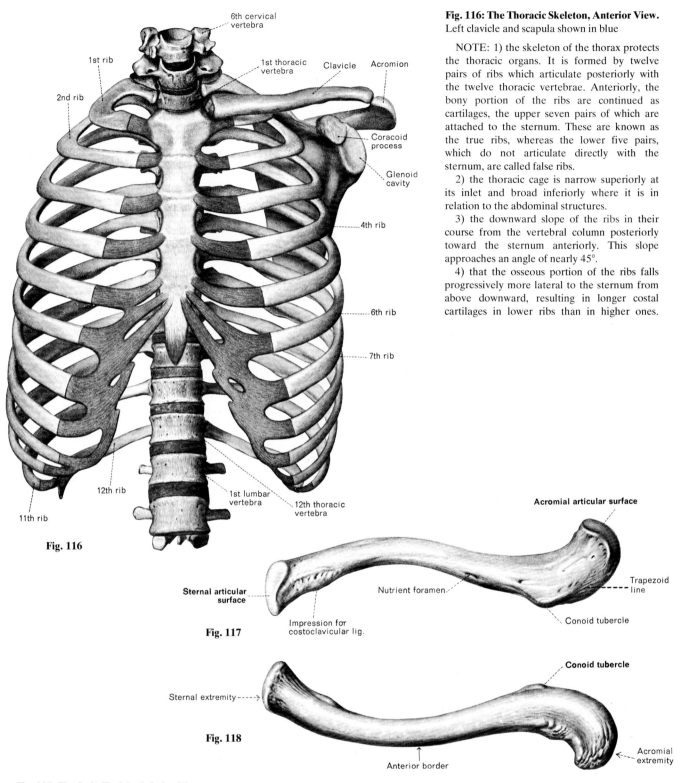

**Fig. 116: The Thoracic Skeleton, Anterior View.**
Left clavicle and scapula shown in blue

NOTE: 1) the skeleton of the thorax protects the thoracic organs. It is formed by twelve pairs of ribs which articulate posteriorly with the twelve thoracic vertebrae. Anteriorly, the bony portion of the ribs are continued as cartilages, the upper seven pairs of which are attached to the sternum. These are known as the true ribs, whereas the lower five pairs, which do not articulate directly with the sternum, are called false ribs.

2) the thoracic cage is narrow superiorly at its inlet and broad inferiorly where it is in relation to the abdominal structures.

3) the downward slope of the ribs in their course from the vertebral column posteriorly toward the sternum anteriorly. This slope approaches an angle of nearly 45°.

4) that the osseous portion of the ribs falls progressively more lateral to the sternum from above downward, resulting in longer costal cartilages in lower ribs than in higher ones.

6th cervical vertebra
1st rib
2nd rib
1st thoracic vertebra
Clavicle
Acromion
Coracoid process
Glenoid cavity
4th rib
6th rib
7th rib
12th rib
1st lumbar vertebra
12th thoracic vertebra
11th rib

**Fig. 116**

Acromial articular surface
Sternal articular surface
Nutrient foramen
Trapezoid line
Conoid tubercle
Impression for costoclavicular lig.

**Fig. 117**

Conoid tubercle
Sternal extremity
Acromial extremity
Anterior border

**Fig. 118**

**Fig. 117: The Left Clavicle, Inferior View**

NOTE: 1) the clavicle is a double-curved bone which articulates medially with the sternum just above the first rib and laterally with the acromion of the scapula.

2) the inferior surface has roughened areas for the attachment of the costoclavicular ligament medially and the conoid and trapezoid fascicles of the coracoclavicular ligament laterally. The subclavius muscle attaches along the middle third of the inferior surface.

**Fig. 118: The Left Clavicle, Superior View**

NOTE: 1) the superior surface of the clavicle affords attachment of the pectoralis major and sternocleidomastoid muscles medially and the deltoid and trapezius muscles laterally.

2) the claviculoacromial articulation associates the clavicle with all the movements of the scapula, while the sternal articulation of the clavicle is a more secure and less movable joint.

Figs. 116, 117, 118

### Fig. 119: The Sternum, Anterior View

NOTE: 1) the sternum consists of three parts: the manubrium, the body and the xiphoid process and forms the middle portion of the anterior wall of the thorax.

2) the manubrium articulates with the body of the sternum at somewhat of an angle called the sternal angle. The xiphoid process is thin and usually cartilaginous.

3) the concave jugular notch which marks the superior border of the manubrium. Lateral to this are the two clavicular notches, each of which receives the medial end of the respective clavicle.

4) the entire sternum measures between 15 and 20 cm (6 to 7 inches). Its anterior surface is roughened and affords attachment to the sternocleidomastoid and pectoralis major muscles.

### Fig. 120: The Sternum, Lateral View

NOTE: 1) the clavicle and the 1st rib articulate with the manubrium. The 2nd rib articulates at the sternal angle where the sternal manubrium and body join. The 3rd to the 6th ribs articulate with the body of the sternum, while the 7th joins the sternum inferiorly at the junction of the xiphoid process.

2) A line projected posteriorly through the sternal angle would meet the vertebral column at the 4th thoracic vertebral level, while the xiphisternal junction lies at vertebral level T-9.

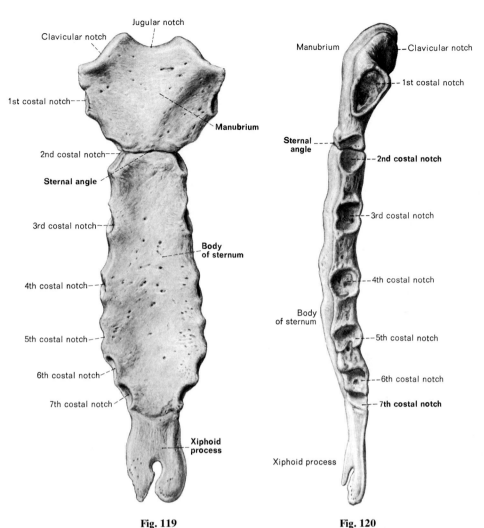

Fig. 119

Fig. 120

### Fig. 121: The Sternoclavicular and the First Two Sternocostal Joints

NOTE: 1) the sternoclavicular joint is formed by the junction of the clavicle with a) the upper lateral aspect of the manubrium and b) the cartilage of the first rib. A flat articular disc is interposed between the clavicle and the sternum. An articular capsule and fibrous ligamentous bands protect the joint.

2) the cartilages of the 2nd through the 7th ribs articulate with the sternum by means of movable diarthrodial joints, whereas the cartilage of the 1st rib is directly joined to the sternum and, without a joint cavity, forms an immovable articulation (synarthrosis).

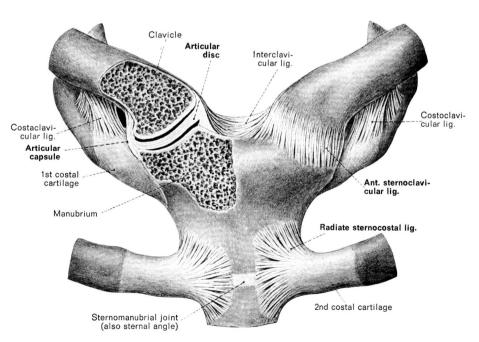

Figs. 119, 120, 121    II

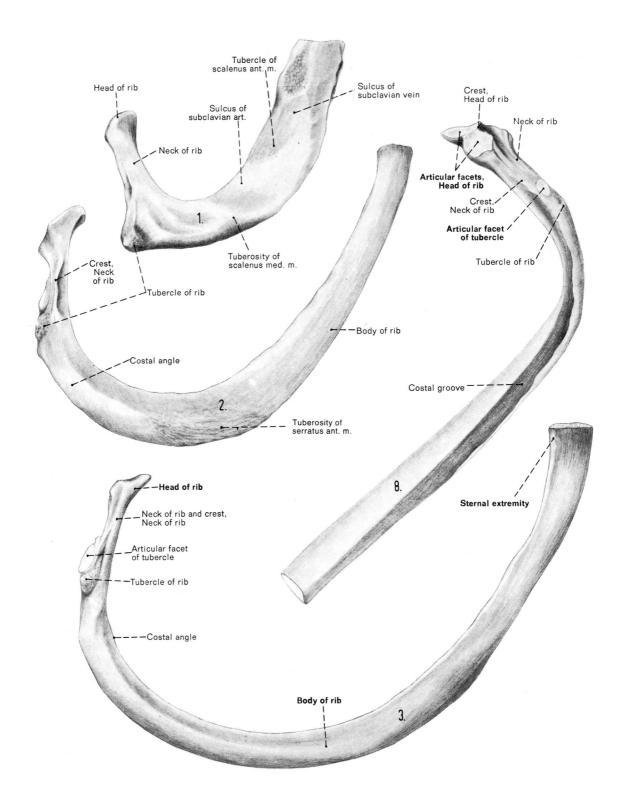

**Fig. 122: The 1st, 2nd, 3rd and 8th Right Ribs**

NOTE: 1) the superior surfaces of the first, second and third ribs are illustrated in this figure, while the inferior surface of the eighth rib is shown.

2) each rib has a vertebral extremity directed posteriorly, and a sternal extremity directed anteriorly. The body of the rib is the shaft which stretches between these two extremities.

3) the vertebral extremity is marked by a head, a neck and a tubercle. The head contains two facets for articulation with the bodies of the thoracic vertebrae, while the tubercle consists of a non-articular roughened elevation and an articular facet for connection with the transverse process of the thoracic vertebrae.

4) the 1st, 2nd, 10th, 11th and 12th ribs present somewhat different structural characteristics from the 3rd through the 9th ribs. The 1st rib is the most curved of all the ribs and has only a single articular facet on the head of the rib. The 10th, 11th and 12th ribs also have only a single facet on the rib head. The 2nd rib is shaped similar to the 1st rib but is longer.

Fig. 122

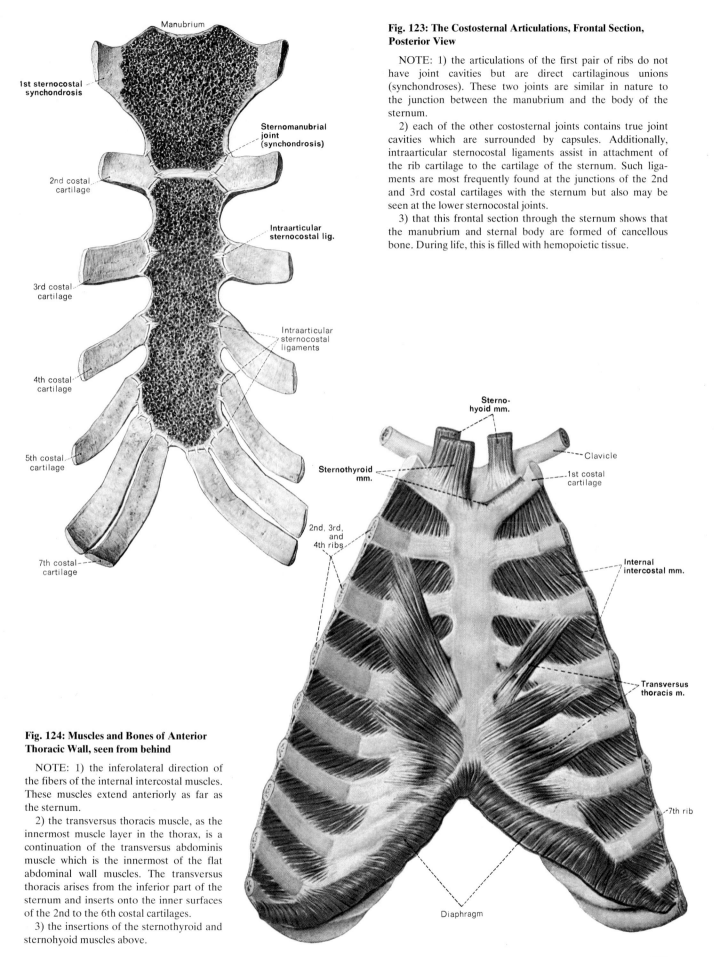

Manubrium

1st sternocostal
synchondrosis

Sternomanubrial
joint
(synchondrosis)

2nd costal
cartilage

Intraarticular
sternocostal lig.

3rd costal
cartilage

Intraarticular
sternocostal
ligaments

4th costal
cartilage

5th costal
cartilage

7th costal
cartilage

**Fig. 123: The Costosternal Articulations, Frontal Section, Posterior View**

NOTE: 1) the articulations of the first pair of ribs do not have joint cavities but are direct cartilaginous unions (synchondroses). These two joints are similar in nature to the junction between the manubrium and the body of the sternum.

2) each of the other costosternal joints contains true joint cavities which are surrounded by capsules. Additionally, intraarticular sternocostal ligaments assist in attachment of the rib cartilage to the cartilage of the sternum. Such ligaments are most frequently found at the junctions of the 2nd and 3rd costal cartilages with the sternum but also may be seen at the lower sternocostal joints.

3) that this frontal section through the sternum shows that the manubrium and sternal body are formed of cancellous bone. During life, this is filled with hemopoietic tissue.

Sterno-
hyoid mm.

Clavicle

Sternothyroid
mm.

1st costal
cartilage

2nd, 3rd,
and
4th ribs

Internal
intercostal mm.

Transversus
thoracis m.

7th rib

Diaphragm

**Fig. 124: Muscles and Bones of Anterior Thoracic Wall, seen from behind**

NOTE: 1) the inferolateral direction of the fibers of the internal intercostal muscles. These muscles extend anteriorly as far as the sternum.

2) the transversus thoracis muscle, as the innermost muscle layer in the thorax, is a continuation of the transversus abdominis muscle which is the innermost of the flat abdominal wall muscles. The transversus thoracis arises from the inferior part of the sternum and inserts onto the inner surfaces of the 2nd to the 6th costal cartilages.

3) the insertions of the sternothyroid and sternohyoid muscles above.

Figs. 123, 124    II

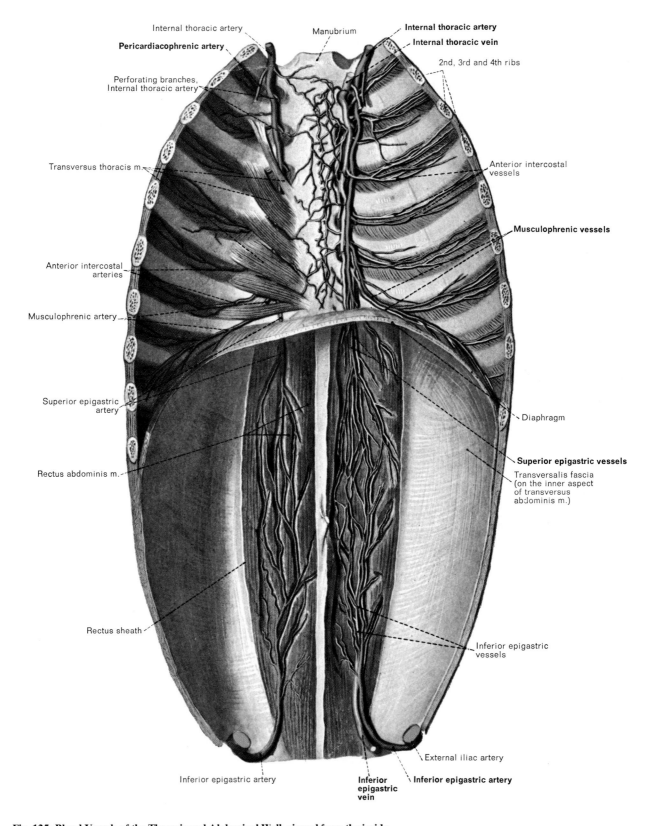

Internal thoracic artery
Pericardiacophrenic artery
Manubrium
**Internal thoracic artery**
**Internal thoracic vein**

Perforating branches,
Internal thoracic artery
2nd, 3rd and 4th ribs

Transversus thoracis m.
Anterior intercostal
vessels

**Musculophrenic vessels**

Anterior intercostal
arteries

Musculophrenic artery

Superior epigastric
artery

Diaphragm

**Superior epigastric vessels**

Rectus abdominis m.
Transversalis fascia
(on the inner aspect
of transversus
abdominis m.)

Rectus sheath

Inferior epigastric
vessels

External iliac artery

Inferior epigastric artery
**Inferior
epigastric
vein**
**Inferior epigastric artery**

**Fig. 125: Blood Vessels of the Thoracic and Abdominal Wall, viewed from the inside**

NOTE: 1) the principal vessels dissected include the internal thoracic and inferior epigastric arteries and veins and their terminal branches.

2) the internal thoracic artery branches from the subclavian artery and descends behind the costal cartilages on the inner aspect of the anterior thoracic wall parallel to the lateral margin of the sternum. In its course the internal thoracic artery gives rise to the pericardiacophrenic artery, small anterior mediastinal vessels to the thymus and bronchial structures, perforating branches to the chest wall, anterior intercostal branches which anastomose with the intercostal arteries, and finally it terminates as the musculophrenic and superior epigastric arteries.

3) the superior epigastric artery anastomoses with the inferior epigastric artery, which is a branch of the external iliac artery and which ascends in the abdominal wall from below. The anastomosis occurs in the substance of the rectus abdominis muscle.

Fig. 125

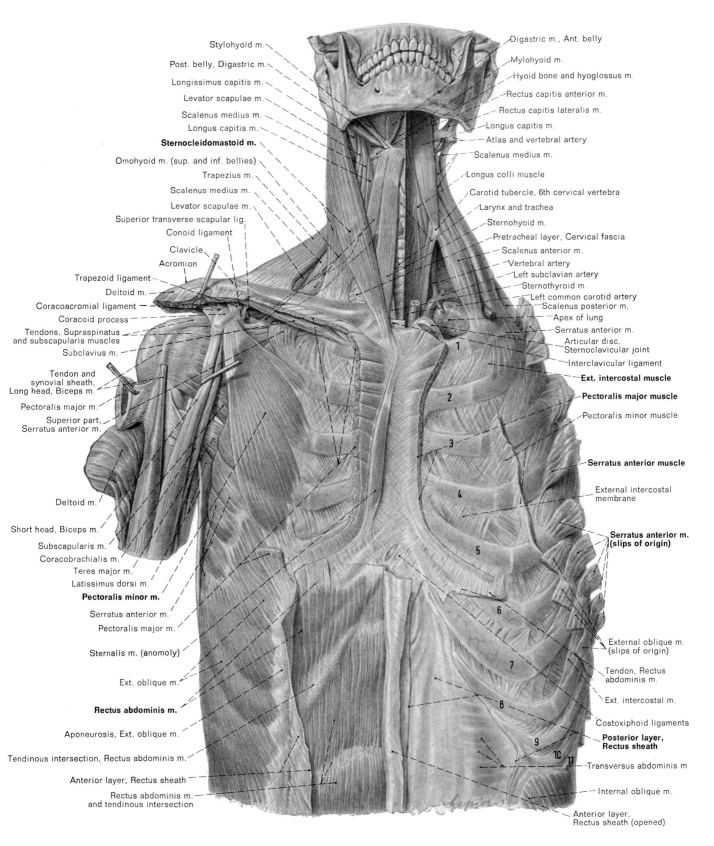

Stylohyoid m.
Post. belly, Digastric m.
Longissimus capitis m.
Levator scapulae m.
Scalenus medius m.
Longus capitis m.
**Sternocleidomastoid m.**
Omohyoid m. (sup. and inf. bellies)
Trapezius m.
Scalenus medius m.
Levator scapulae m.
Superior transverse scapular lig.
Conoid ligament
Clavicle
Acromion
Trapezoid ligament
Deltoid m.
Coracoacromial ligament
Coracoid process
Tendons, Supraspinatus
and subscapularis muscles
Subclavius m.
Tendon and
synovial sheath,
Long head, Biceps m.
Pectoralis major m.
Superior part,
Serratus anterior m.

Deltoid m.

Short head, Biceps m.
Subscapularis m.
Coracobrachialis m.
Teres major m.
Latissimus dorsi m.
**Pectoralis minor m.**
Serratus anterior m.
Pectoralis major m.
Sternalis m. (anomoly)
Ext. oblique m.
**Rectus abdominis m.**
Aponeurosis, Ext. oblique m.
Tendinous intersection, Rectus abdominis m.
Anterior layer, Rectus sheath
Rectus abdominis m.
and tendinous intersection

Digastric m., Ant. belly
Mylohyoid m.
Hyoid bone and hyoglossus m.
Rectus capitis anterior m.
Rectus capitis lateralis m.
Longus capitis m.
Atlas and vertebral artery
Scalenus medius m.
Longus colli muscle
Carotid tubercle, 6th cervical vertebra
Larynx and trachea
Sternohyoid m.
Pretracheal layer, Cervical fascia
Scalenus anterior m.
Vertebral artery
Left subclavian artery
Sternothyroid m.
Left common carotid artery
Scalenus posterior m.
Apex of lung
Serratus anterior m.
Articular disc,
Sternoclavicular joint
Interclavicular ligament
**Ext. intercostal muscle**
**Pectoralis major muscle**
Pectoralis minor muscle
**Serratus anterior muscle**
External intercostal
membrane
**Serratus anterior m.
(slips of origin)**
External oblique m.
(slips of origin)
Tendon, Rectus
abdominis m.
Ext. intercostal m.
Costoxiphoid ligaments
**Posterior layer,
Rectus sheath**
Transversus abdominis m
Internal oblique m.
Anterior layer,
Rectus sheath (opened)

**Fig. 126: Anterior Cervical, Thoracic and Abdominal Musculature**

NOTE: 1) on the right side the muscles of the shoulder and upper arm are demonstrated following the removal of the pectoralis major muscle. The anterior layer of the rectus sheath has been opened.

2) on the left side the upper limb has been removed, as have all of the more superficial trunk and cervical musculature, revealing the thoracic cage and the deeper soft tissues.

Fig. 126    **II**

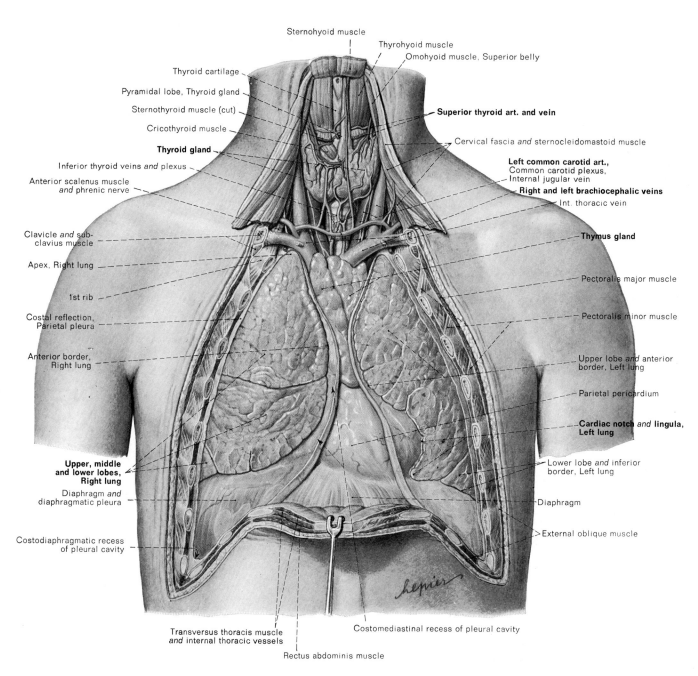

Sternohyoid muscle

Thyrohyoid muscle

Omohyoid muscle, Superior belly

Thyroid cartilage

Pyramidal lobe, Thyroid gland

Sternothyroid muscle (cut)

Cricothyroid muscle

**Thyroid gland**

Inferior thyroid veins *and* plexus

Anterior scalenus muscle *and* phrenic nerve

Clavicle *and* subclavius muscle

Apex, Right lung

1st rib

Costal reflection, Parietal pleura

Anterior border, Right lung

**Upper, middle and lower lobes, Right lung**

Diaphragm *and* diaphragmatic pleura

Costodiaphragmatic recess of pleural cavity

**Superior thyroid art. and vein**

Cervical fascia *and* sternocleidomastoid muscle

**Left common carotid art.,** Common carotid plexus, Internal jugular vein

**Right and left brachiocephalic veins**

Int. thoracic vein

**Thymus gland**

Pectoralis major muscle

Pectoralis minor muscle

Upper lobe *and* anterior border, Left lung

Parietal pericardium

**Cardiac notch** *and* **lingula, Left lung**

Lower lobe *and* inferior border, Left lung

Diaphragm

External oblique muscle

Transversus thoracis muscle *and* internal thoracic vessels

Costomediastinal recess of pleural cavity

Rectus abdominis muscle

**Fig. 127: The Thoracic Viscera and the Root of the Neck, Anterior Exposure**

NOTE: 1) the anterior thoracic wall has been removed along with the medial portion of both clavicles to reveal the normal position of the heart, lungs, thymus and thyroid gland. The great vessels at the superior aperture to the thorax are also exposed.

2) the parietal pleura, likewise, has been removed arteriorly. The thymus is situated between the two lungs superiorly, whereas inferiorly is found the bare area of the heart. With the heart's apex directed more toward the left, a deficiency can be observed along the border of the left lung. This is called the cardiac notch.

3) the basal surface of both lungs and the inferior aspect of the heart rest on the diaphragm. Superiorly, the apex of each lung extends slightly above the level of the first rib.

4) at the root of the neck, the common carotid artery and internal jugular vein lie lateral and somewhat posterior to the thyroid gland.

5) the rather transverse course in the superior mediastinum of the left brachiocephalic vein in contrast to the nearly vertical course of the right brachiocephalic vein. On either side each of these vessels is formed by a junction of the internal jugular and subclavian veins. The two brachiocephalic veins join (deep to the thymus) to form the superior vena cava.

Fig. 127

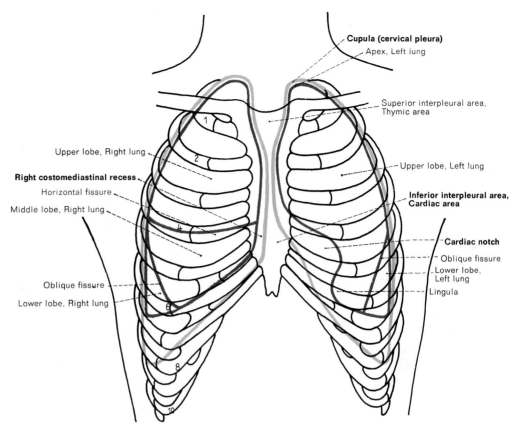

Cupula (cervical pleura)
Apex, Left lung
Superior interpleural area, Thymic area
Upper lobe, Right lung
Upper lobe, Left lung
**Right costomediastinal recess**
Horizontal fissure
**Inferior interpleural area, Cardiac area**
Middle lobe, Right lung
**Cardiac notch**
Oblique fissure
Lower lobe, Left lung
Lingula
Oblique fissure
Lower lobe, Right lung

**Figs. 128 and 129:**
**Pleural Reflections (blue) and Lungs (red)**
**Projected onto Thoracic Wall**

**Fig. 128: Anterior View**

NOTE: 1) each lung is invested by two layers of pleural membrane which are continuous with each other at the hilum of the lung, thereby forming an invaginated sac. The parietal layer of pleura (represented in blue) is the outermost of the two layers and lines the inner surface of the thoracic wall and the superior surface of the diaphragm. The visceral, innermost layer of pleura closely invests and adheres to the surfaces of the lungs (represented in red).

2) the potential space between the two pleural layers is called the pleural cavity and contains only a small amount of serous fluid in the healthy individual, but may contain considerable fluid and blood in pathological conditions.

3) although the parietal pleura is a continuous sheet for each lung, portions of it are described in relation to their adjacent surfaces. Thus, lining the inner surface of the ribs is the costal pleura, while the diaphragmatic and mediastinal pleurae are applied onto the surfaces of the diaphragm and mediastinal structures. Superiorly, the apex of each lung extends above the clavicle into the root of the neck. This is covered by the cupula, or cervical pleura.

4) because of the curvature of the diaphragm, a narrow recess is formed around its periphery into which the surface of the lung (visceral pleura) does not extend. This potential space, lying between reflections of the costal and diaphragmatic pleurae, is called the costodiaphragmatic recess and is of clinical importance, since it may be punctured and drained without damage to lung tissue.

5) similarly, the costomediastinal recess is another pleural space which is situated anterior to the heart, and which is formed at that site by the reflections of the costal and mediastinal pleurae.

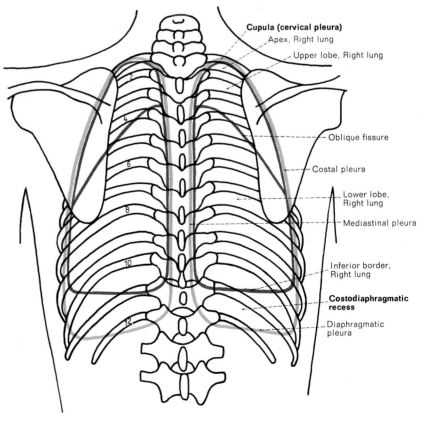

Cupula (cervical pleura)
Apex, Right lung
Upper lobe, Right lung
Oblique fissure
Costal pleura
Lower lobe, Right lung
Mediastinal pleura
Inferior border, Right lung
**Costodiaphragmatic recess**
Diaphragmatic pleura

**Fig. 129: Posterior View**

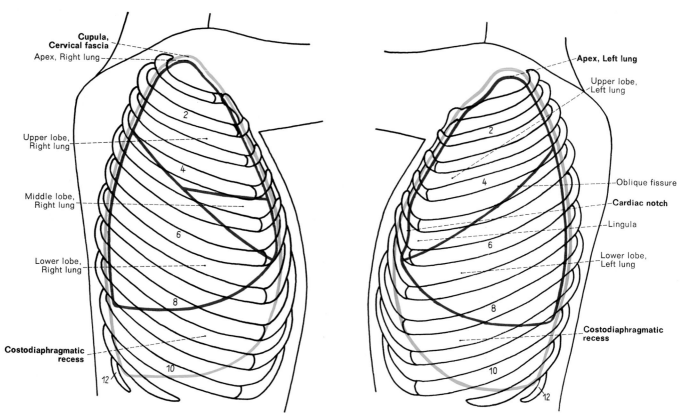

**Fig. 130: Right Lateral View**　　　　　　　　　　**Fig. 131: Left Lateral View**
**Pleural Reflections (blue) and Lungs (red) Projected onto Thoracic Wall**

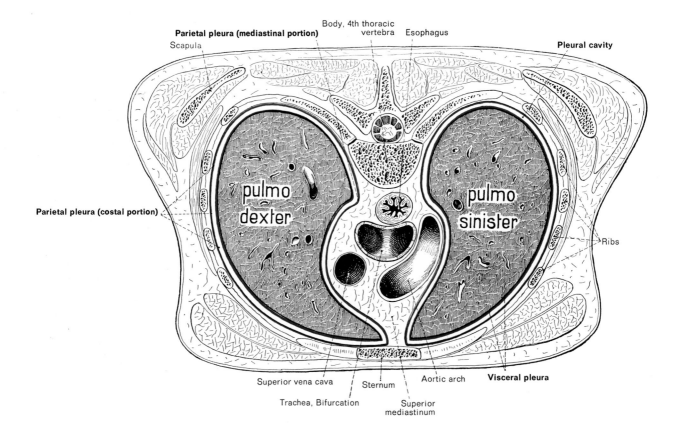

**Fig. 132: Cross Section of Thorax at the Level of the Tracheal Bifurcation and the 4th Thoracic Vertebra (Pleura is shown in red)**

Figs. 130, 131, 132

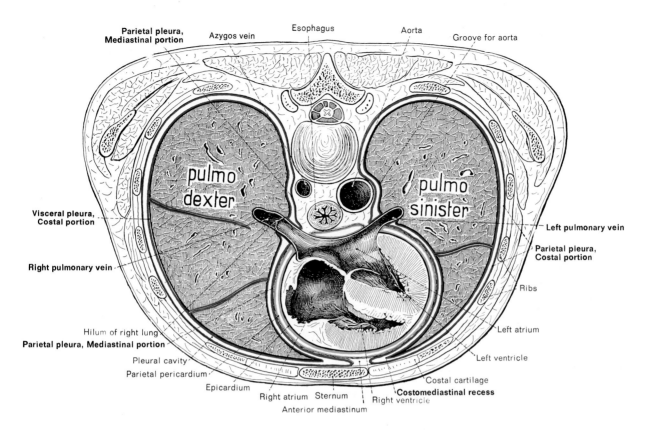

**Fig. 133: Cross Section of Thorax Through the Hilum of the Lung at the Level of the Pulmonary Vein (Pleura in red, Pericardium in blue)**

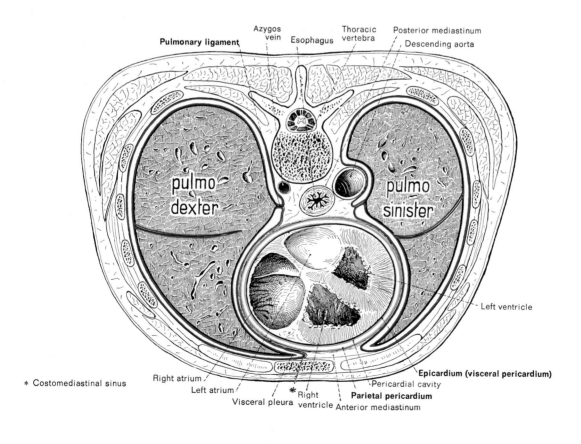

**Fig. 134: Cross Section of the Thorax Inferior to the Hilum at the Level of the Pulmonary Ligament (Pleura in red, Pericardium in blue)**

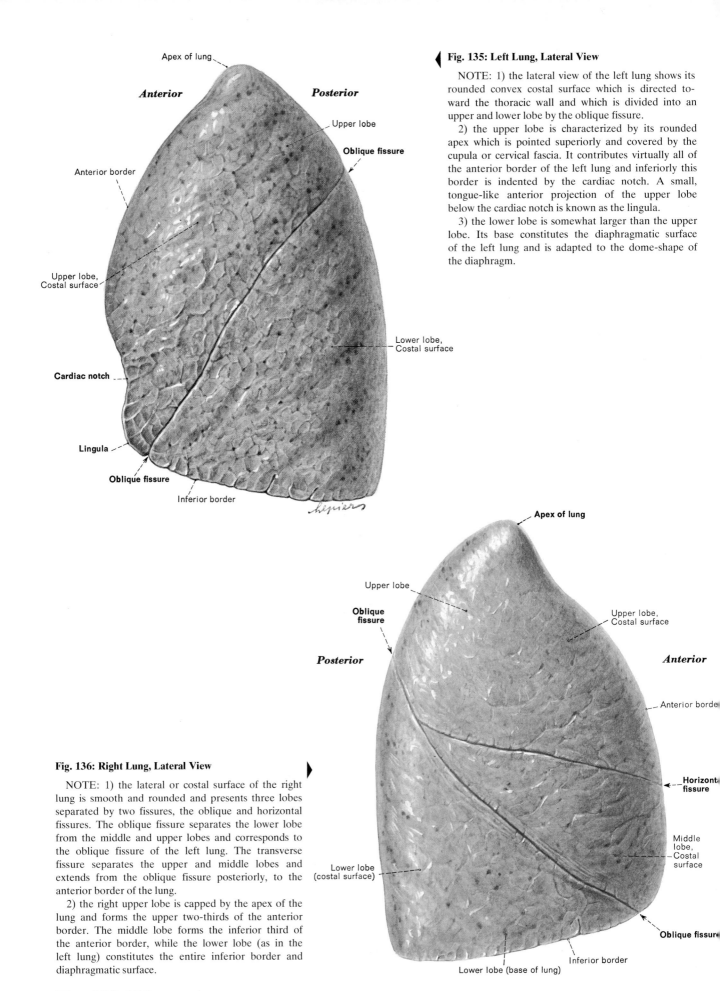

Apex of lung

**Anterior**    **Posterior**

Upper lobe

**Oblique fissure**

Anterior border

Upper lobe,
Costal surface

Lower lobe,
Costal surface

**Cardiac notch**

**Lingula**

**Oblique fissure**

Inferior border

### Fig. 135: Left Lung, Lateral View

NOTE: 1) the lateral view of the left lung shows its rounded convex costal surface which is directed toward the thoracic wall and which is divided into an upper and lower lobe by the oblique fissure.

2) the upper lobe is characterized by its rounded apex which is pointed superiorly and covered by the cupula or cervical fascia. It contributes virtually all of the anterior border of the left lung and inferiorly this border is indented by the cardiac notch. A small, tongue-like anterior projection of the upper lobe below the cardiac notch is known as the lingula.

3) the lower lobe is somewhat larger than the upper lobe. Its base constitutes the diaphragmatic surface of the left lung and is adapted to the dome-shape of the diaphragm.

Apex of lung

Upper lobe

Upper lobe,
Costal surface

**Oblique
fissure**

**Posterior**    **Anterior**

Anterior border

**Horizontal
fissure**

Middle
lobe,
Costal
surface

Lower lobe
(costal surface)

**Oblique fissure**

Inferior border

Lower lobe (base of lung)

### Fig. 136: Right Lung, Lateral View

NOTE: 1) the lateral or costal surface of the right lung is smooth and rounded and presents three lobes separated by two fissures, the oblique and horizontal fissures. The oblique fissure separates the lower lobe from the middle and upper lobes and corresponds to the oblique fissure of the left lung. The transverse fissure separates the upper and middle lobes and extends from the oblique fissure posteriorly, to the anterior border of the lung.

2) the right upper lobe is capped by the apex of the lung and forms the upper two-thirds of the anterior border. The middle lobe forms the inferior third of the anterior border, while the lower lobe (as in the left lung) constitutes the entire inferior border and diaphragmatic surface.

Figs. 135, 136

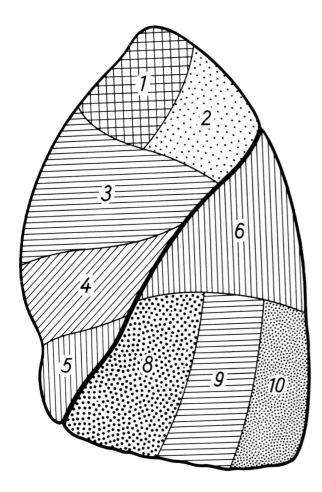

◀ **Fig. 137: Left Lung, Bronchopulmonary Segments, Lateral View**

NOTE: 1) bronchopulmonary segments are anatomical subdivisions of the lung, each of which is supplied by its own segmental tertiary bronchus and artery, and drained by intersegmental veins.

2) the trachea divides into two primary bronchi, each of which supplies an entire lung. Each primary bronchus divides into secondary or lobar bronchi. There are two lobar bronchi on the left and three on the right, each supplying a single lobe. The secondary bronchi divide into the segmental or tertiary bronchi, which are distributed to the bronchopulmonary segments. Usual descriptions of the bronchopulmonary segments enumerate 8 to 10 segments in the left lung.

3) the bronchopulmonary segments of the left lung are numbered and named as follows:

**Upper lobe**
1 Apical        ⎫
2 Posterior     ⎬ Frequently considered as a single segment
3 Anterior
4 Superior    ⎫
5 Inferior      ⎬ Lingular

**Lower lobe**
6 Superior
7 Medial basal    ⎫ Usually considered as a single segment;
8 Anterior basal   ⎬ Medial basal cannot be seen from lateral view.
9 Lateral basal
10 Posterior basal

4) in the left lower lobe the medial basal bronchus arises separate from the anterior basal in only about 13 % of humans studied. Thus, in most instances the medial basal and anterior basal segments combine as an anteromedial basal segment.

**Fig. 138: Right Lung, Bronchopulmonary Segments, Lateral View** ▶

NOTE: 1) the concept of subdividing the lungs into functional bronchopulmonary segments allows the surgeon to determine whether segments of lung might be resected in operations in preference to entire lobes.

2) although minor variations exist in the division of the bronchial tree, a significant consistency has become recognized in the bronchopulmonary segmentation. The nomenclature utilized here was offered by Jackson and Huber in 1943 (Dis. of Chest **9:** 319–326) and has now become generally accepted because it is the simplest and most straightforward of the many suggested.

3) the bronchopulmonary segments of the right lung are numbered and named as follows:

| Upper lobe | Middle lobe |
|---|---|
| 1 Apical | 4 Lateral |
| 2 Posterior | 5 Medial |
| 3 Anterior | |

**Lower lobe**
6 Superior
7 Medial basal (cannot be seen from lateral view)
8 Anterior basal
9 Lateral basal
10 Posterior basal

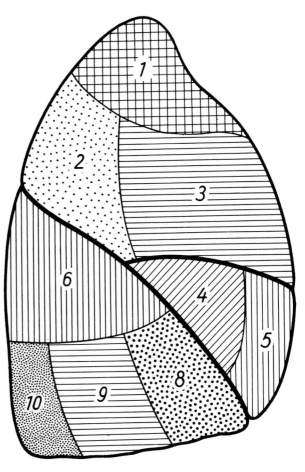

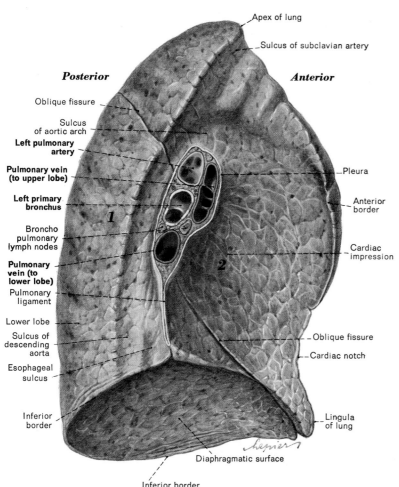

Apex of lung

Sulcus of subclavian artery

*Posterior*

*Anterior*

Oblique fissure

Sulcus of aortic arch

**Left pulmonary artery**

**Pulmonary vein (to upper lobe)**

**Left primary bronchus**

Broncho pulmonary lymph nodes

**Pulmonary vein (to lower lobe)**

Pulmonary ligament

Lower lobe

Sulcus of descending aorta

Esophageal sulcus

Inferior border

*1*

*2*

Pleura

Anterior border

Cardiac impression

Oblique fissure

Cardiac notch

Lingula of lung

Diaphragmatic surface

Inferior border

### Fig. 139: Left Lung, Mediastinal and Diaphragmatic surfaces

NOTE: 1) the pulmonary arteries are shown in blue since their blood contains less oxygen than that in the pulmonary veins which are shown in red.

2) the concave diaphragmatic surface of the left lung is shaped to cover most of the convex dome of the diaphragm which is completely covered by diaphragmatic pleura. However, the lung does not completely fill the peripheral rim of the diaphragm, thereby forming the costodiaphragmatic recess.

3) the mediastinal (or medial) surface of the left lung is also concave and presents the contours of the adjacent organs in the mediastinum. The large anterior concavity is the cardiac impression. Also found are grooves for the aortic arch and the descending aorta as well as the subclavian artery superiorly and the esophagus inferiorly.

4) the structures which form the root of the left lung at the hilum include the left pulmonary artery, found most superior and below which is found the left bronchus. The left pulmonary veins lie anterior and inferior to the artery and bronchus. The oblique fissure extends across the mediastinal surface from the costal surface to the diaphragm, completely dividing the lung into its two lobes.

### Fig. 140: Right Lung, Mediastinal and Diaphragmatic Surfaces

NOTE: 1) the diaphragmatic surface of the right lung, similar to that on the left, is shaped to the contour of the diaphragm, while the mediastinal surface superiorly shows grooves for the superior vena cava and subclavian artery. Just above the hilum of the right lung is the arched sulcus for the azygos vein, and this is continued inferiorly behind the root of the lung. The cardiac impression on the right lung is somewhat more shallow than on the left.

2) since the right bronchus frequently branches before the right pulmonary artery it is not unusual for the most superior structure at the root of the right lung to be the bronchus to the upper lobe (eparterial bronchus). The pulmonary artery lies anterior to the bronchus, while the pulmonary veins are located anterior and inferior to these structures.

3) the hilum of the lung is ensheathed by parietal pleura, the layers of which come into contact inferiorly to form the pulmonary ligament. It extends from the inferior border of the hilum to a point just above the diaphragm.

4) the numbers 1 and 2 on this figure and on Fig. 139 refer to the costal and mediastinal portions of the medial surface of the lung.

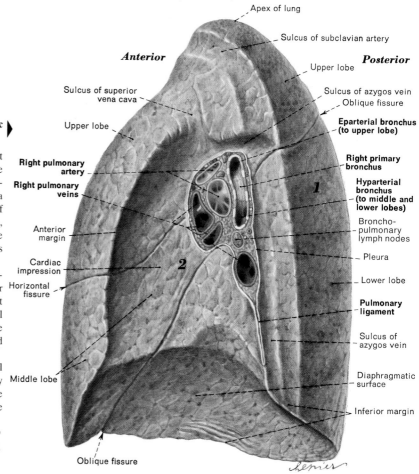

Apex of lung

Sulcus of subclavian artery

*Anterior*

*Posterior*

Upper lobe

Sulcus of azygos vein

Oblique fissure

**Eparterial bronchus (to upper lobe)**

**Right primary bronchus**

**Hyparterial bronchus (to middle and lower lobes)**

Bronchopulmonary lymph nodes

Pleura

Lower lobe

**Pulmonary ligament**

Sulcus of azygos vein

Diaphragmatic surface

Inferior margin

Sulcus of superior vena cava

Upper lobe

**Right pulmonary artery**

**Right pulmonary veins**

Anterior margin

Cardiac impression

Horizontal fissure

Middle lobe

*1*

*2*

Oblique fissure

Figs. 139, 140

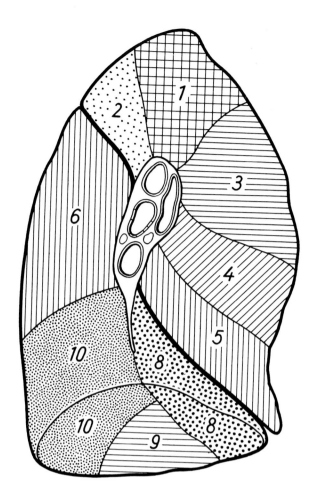

## Fig. 141: Left Lung, Bronchopulmonary Segments, Medial View

NOTE: the bronchopulmonary segments of the left lung have been identified as follows:

**Upper lobe**
1 Apical ⎫ Frequently
2 Posterior ⎬ considered as one segment
3 Anterior
4 Superior ⎫ Lingular
5 Inferior ⎭

**Lower lobe**
6 Superior
7 Medial basal *
8 Anterior basal *
9 Lateral basal
10 Posterior basal

\* the medial basal and anterior basal segments were at one time frequently considered as a single bronchopulmonary segment. Today, however, they have been recognized as separate segments in a majority of left lungs. Therefore, on this figure that portion of segment 8 just inferior to the oblique fissure should be marked 7 and identified as medial basal.

## Fig. 142: Right Lung, Bronchopulmonary Segments, Medial View

NOTE: the bronchopulmonary segments of the right lung have been identified as follows:

**Upper lobe**
1 Apical
2 Posterior
3 Anterior

**Middle lobe**
4 Lateral (not seen from this view)
5 Medial

**Lower lobe**
6 Superior
7 Medial basal
8 Anterior basal
9 Lateral basal
10 Posterior basal

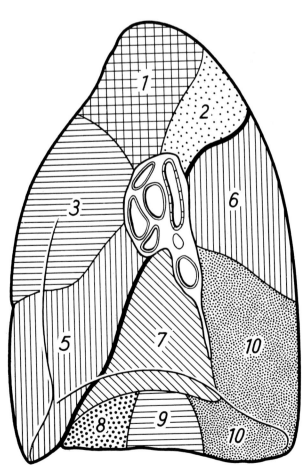

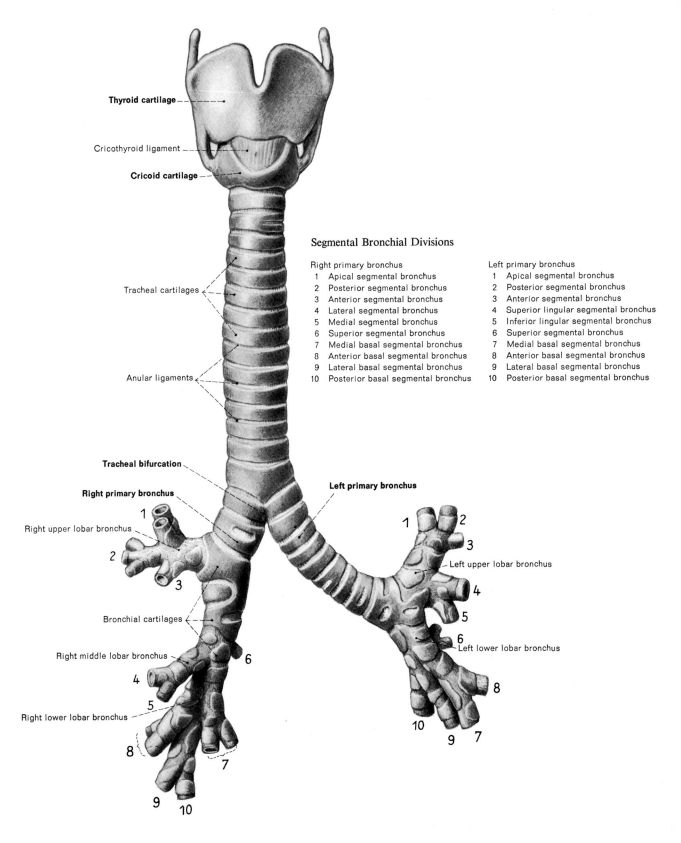

Thyroid cartilage

Cricothyroid ligament

Cricoid cartilage

Tracheal cartilages

Anular ligaments

Tracheal bifurcation

Right primary bronchus

Right upper lobar bronchus

Bronchial cartilages

Right middle lobar bronchus

Right lower lobar bronchus

Left primary bronchus

Left upper lobar bronchus

Left lower lobar bronchus

## Segmental Bronchial Divisions

| Right primary bronchus | | Left primary bronchus | |
|---|---|---|---|
| 1 | Apical segmental bronchus | 1 | Apical segmental bronchus |
| 2 | Posterior segmental bronchus | 2 | Posterior segmental bronchus |
| 3 | Anterior segmental bronchus | 3 | Anterior segmental bronchus |
| 4 | Lateral segmental bronchus | 4 | Superior lingular segmental bronchus |
| 5 | Medial segmental bronchus | 5 | Inferior lingular segmental bronchus |
| 6 | Superior segmental bronchus | 6 | Superior segmental bronchus |
| 7 | Medial basal segmental bronchus | 7 | Medial basal segmental bronchus |
| 8 | Anterior basal segmental bronchus | 8 | Anterior basal segmental bronchus |
| 9 | Lateral basal segmental bronchus | 9 | Lateral basal segmental bronchus |
| 10 | Posterior basal segmental bronchus | 10 | Posterior basal segmental bronchus |

**Fig. 143: Anterior Aspect of Larynx, Trachea, and Bronchi**

NOTE: 1) the trachea bifurcates into two principal (primary) bronchi. These then divide into lobar (secondary) bronchi which in turn give rise to segmental (tertiary) bronchi.

2) the larynx is located in the anterior aspect of the neck, and its thyroid and cricoid cartilages can be felt through the skin.

3) the thyroid cartilage, projected posteriorly, lies at the level of the 4th and 5th cervical vertebrae, while the cricoid cartilage is at the 6th cervical level. The trachea commences at the lower end of the cricoid and extends slightly more than four inches before bifurcating into the two primary bronchi at the level of T-4. Two inches of trachea lie above the suprasternal notch in the neck, while about two inches of trachea are intrathoracic above its bifurcation.

Fig. 143

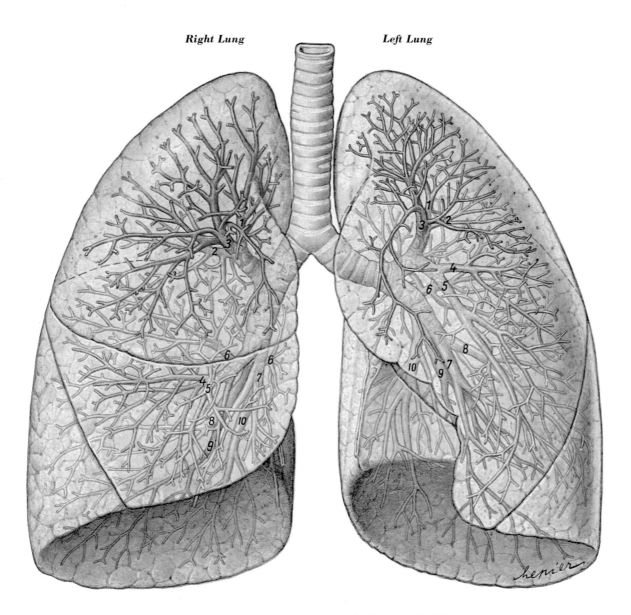

**Right Lung**          **Left Lung**

**Fig. 144: Diagram of the Bronchial Tree and its Lobar and Bronchopulmonary Divisions, Anterior View**

NOTE: 1) as the trachea divides, the left primary bronchus diverges at a more abrupt angle than the right primary bronchus to reach their respective lungs. Thus, the left bronchus is directed more transversely and the right bronchus more inferiorly.

2) on the right side the upper lobar bronchus branches from the primary bronchus almost immediately, even above the pulmonary artery (eparterial), while the bronchus directed toward the middle and lower lobes branches below the position of the main stem of the pulmonary artery (hyparterial).

3) on the left side the initial lobar bronchus, branching from the primary bronchus, is directed upward and lateralward to the upper lobe segments and its lingular segments. The remaining lobar bronchus is directed inferiorly and soon divides into the segmental bronchi of the lower lobe.

4) the segmental bronchi numbered above are as follows:

**Right lung:**

| | | | |
|---|---|---|---|
| 1 | Apical | 6 | Superior |
| 2 | Posterior | 7 | Medial basal |
| 3 | Anterior | 8 | Anterior basal |
| 4 | Lateral | 9 | Lateral basal |
| 5 | Medial | 10 | Posterior basal |

**Left lung:**

| | | | |
|---|---|---|---|
| 1 | Apical | 6 | Superior |
| 2 | Posterior | 7 | Medial basal |
| 3 | Anterior | 8 | Anterior basal |
| 4 | Superior lingular | 9 | Lateral basal |
| 5 | Inferior lingular | 10 | Posterior basal |

Fig. 144      **II**

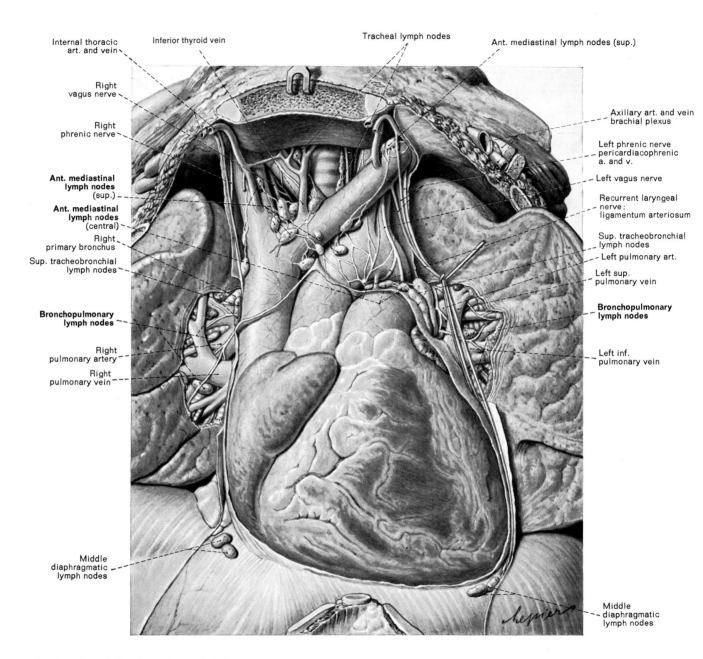

Internal thoracic art. and vein

Inferior thyroid vein

Tracheal lymph nodes

Ant. mediastinal lymph nodes (sup.)

Right vagus nerve

Right phrenic nerve

Axillary art. and vein brachial plexus

Left phrenic nerve pericardiacophrenic a. and v.

Left vagus nerve

**Ant. mediastinal lymph nodes (sup.)**

**Ant. mediastinal lymph nodes (central)**

Recurrent laryngeal nerve; ligamentum arteriosum

Right primary bronchus

Sup. tracheobronchial lymph nodes

Sup. tracheobronchial lymph nodes

Left pulmonary art.

Left sup. pulmonary vein

**Bronchopulmonary lymph nodes**

**Bronchopulmonary lymph nodes**

Right pulmonary artery

Left inf. pulmonary vein

Right pulmonary vein

Middle diaphragmatic lymph nodes

Middle diaphragmatic lymph nodes

## Fig. 145: Lymphatics of the Thorax, Anterior Aspect

NOTE: 1) in this dissection the anterior thoracic wall was removed along with the ventral portion of the pericardium. Further, the anterior borders of the lungs have been pulled laterally to reveal the lymphatic channels at the roots of the lungs. The thymus has also been removed and the manubrium reflected superiorly to expose the organs at the thoracic inlet and their associated lymphatics.

2) the lymph nodes in the anterior aspect of the thoracic cavity might be divided into those associated with the thoracic cage (parietal) and those associated with the organs (visceral). Probably all of the nodes indicated in this figure are visceral nodes.

3) situated ventrally are the *anterior mediastinal nodes* which include a superior group lying ventral to the brachiocephalic veins along their course in the superior mediastinum and at their junction to form the superior vena cava. A more centrally located group lies ventral to the arch of the aorta. Inferiorly, anterior diaphragmatic nodes are sometimes also classified as part of the anterior mediastinal nodes.

4) large numbers of lymph nodes are associated with the trachea, the bronchi and the other structures at the root of the lung. These nodes have been aptly named tracheal, tracheobronchial, bronchopulmonary and pulmonary.

Fig. 145

## Fig. 146: Projection of the Heart and its Valves onto Anterior Thoracic Wall

NOTE: 1) the broken lines indicate the limits of the area of deep cardiac dullness from which a dull resonance can be obtained by percussion. Lung tissue covers the area of deep cardiac dullness but does not cover the area limited by the dotted lines from which a less resonant superficial cardiac dullness can be obtained by percussion.

2) the apex of the normal heart is usually found in the 5th interspace about 9 centimeters to the left of the midline.

3) that the *pulmonary valve* lies behind the sternal end of the third left costal cartilage. The *aortic valve* is behind the sternum at the level of the 3rd intercostal space. The *bicuspid valve* lies behind the 4th left sternocostal joint, and the *tricuspid valve* lies posterior to the middle of the sternum at the level of the 4th intercostal space.

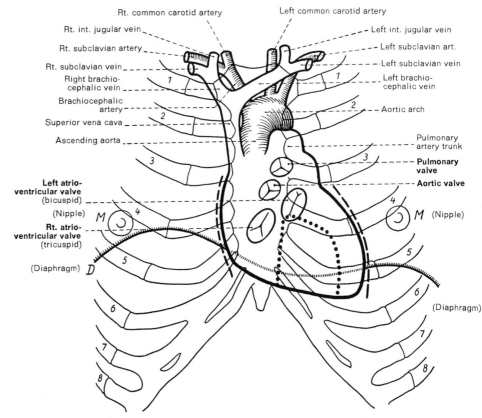

## Fig. 147: Thoracic Viscera of a Young Boy, Anterior View

NOTE: 1) the thymus gland consists of two lobulated lateral lobes and is situated anterior to the roots of the great vessels. It achieves its largest weight at puberty and then commences gradually to involute.

2) the arterial supply to the thymus is derived from the internal thoracic and superior and inferior thyroid arteries. Its veins drain into the left brachiocephalic and the thyroid veins.

3) the anterior borders of the lungs have been pulled laterally to reveal the pericardial sac encasing the heart.

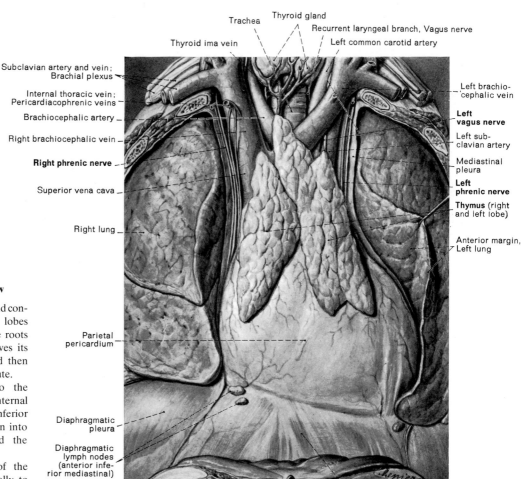

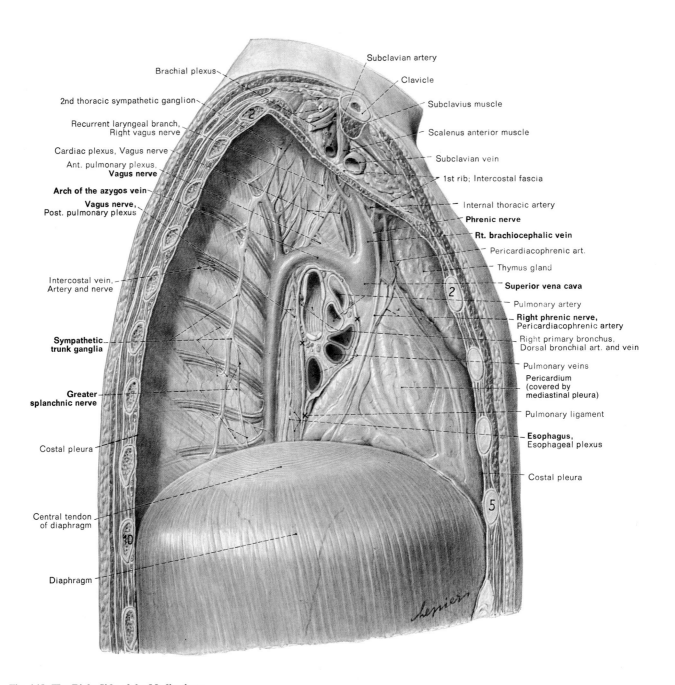

**Fig. 148: The Right Side of the Mediastinum**

NOTE: 1) with the right lung removed and the structures at its hilum transected, the organs of the mediastinum are exposed and their right lateral surface viewed.

2) the right side of the heart covered by the pericardium and the course of the phrenic nerve and pericardiacophrenic vessels.

3) the ascending course of the azygos vein, its arch and its junction with the superior vena cava.

4) that the right vagus nerve descends in the thorax behind the root of the right lung to form the posterior pulmonary plexus. It then helps form the esophageal plexus and leaves the thorax on the posterior aspect of the esophagus.

5) the dome of the diaphragm on the right side, taking the rounded form of the underlying liver. The inferior (diaphragmatic) surface of the heart rests on the diaphragm.

6) the position of the thoracic sympathetic chain of ganglia coursing longitudinally along the inner surface of the thoracic wall. Observe the greater splanchnic nerve.

Fig. 148

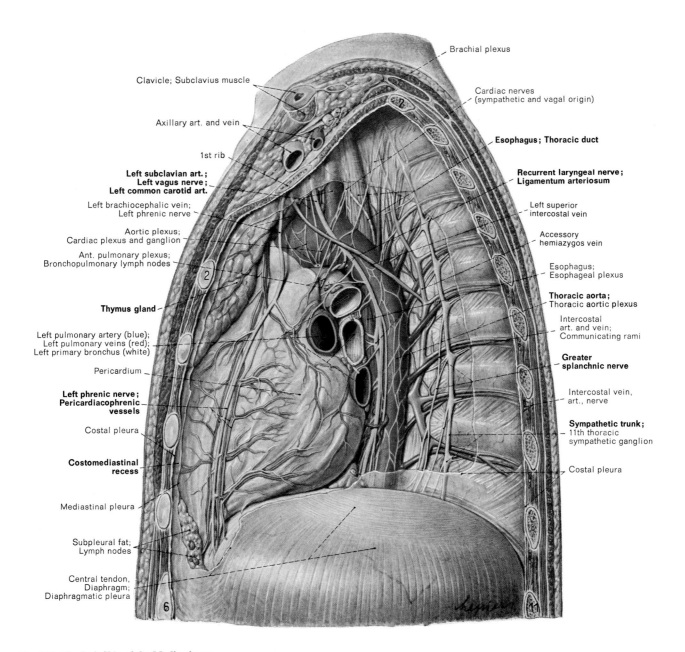

Brachial plexus

Clavicle; Subclavius muscle

Cardiac nerves
(sympathetic and vagal origin)

Axillary art. and vein

**Esophagus; Thoracic duct**

1st rib

**Recurrent laryngeal nerve;
Ligamentum arteriosum**

**Left subclavian art.;
Left vagus nerve;
Left common carotid art.**

Left superior
intercostal vein

Left brachiocephalic vein;
Left phrenic nerve

Accessory
hemiazygos vein

Aortic plexus;
Cardiac plexus and ganglion

Esophagus;
Esophageal plexus

Ant. pulmonary plexus;
Bronchopulmonary lymph nodes

**Thoracic aorta;
Thoracic aortic plexus**

Intercostal
art. and vein;
Communicating rami

**Thymus gland**

**Greater
splanchnic nerve**

Left pulmonary artery (blue);
Left pulmonary veins (red);
Left primary bronchus (white)

Pericardium

Intercostal vein,
art., nerve

**Left phrenic nerve;
Pericardiacophrenic
vessels**

**Sympathetic trunk;
11th thoracic
sympathetic ganglion**

Costal pleura

Costal pleura

**Costomediastinal
recess**

Mediastinal pleura

Subpleural fat;
Lymph nodes

Central tendon,
Diaphragm;
Diaphragmatic pleura

## Fig. 149: The Left Side of the Mediastinum

NOTE: 1) with the left lung removed along with most of the mediastinal pleura, the structures of the mediastinum are observed from their left side.

2) the left phrenic nerve and pericardiacophrenic vessels coursing to the diaphragm along the pericardium covering the left side of the heart.

3) the aorta ascends about two inches before it arches posteriorly and to the left of the vertebral column. The descending thoracic aorta commences at about the level of the 4th thoracic vertebra and as it descends, it comes to lie directly anterior to the vertebral column. The intercostal arteries branch directly from the thoracic aorta.

4) the left vagus nerve lies lateral to the aortic arch and gives off its recurrent laryngeal branch which passes inferior to the ligamentum arteriosum. The left vagus then continues to descend, contributes to the esophageal plexus, and enters the abdomen on the anterior aspect of the esophagus.

5) the position of the thymus gland anterior to the root of the great vessels at their attachments to the heart.

6) that the typical intercostal artery and vein course along the inferior border of their respective rib. Because the superior border of the ribs is free of vessels and nerves, it is a safer site for injection or drainage of the thorax.

Fig. 149    II

## Fig. 150: Diagram of Main Arteries: Systemic Circulation

NOTE that the heart is outlined in red dots. The black dots are sites along the course of main arteries which may be used as pressure points to interrupt blood flow in the pelvis and limbs during surgery.

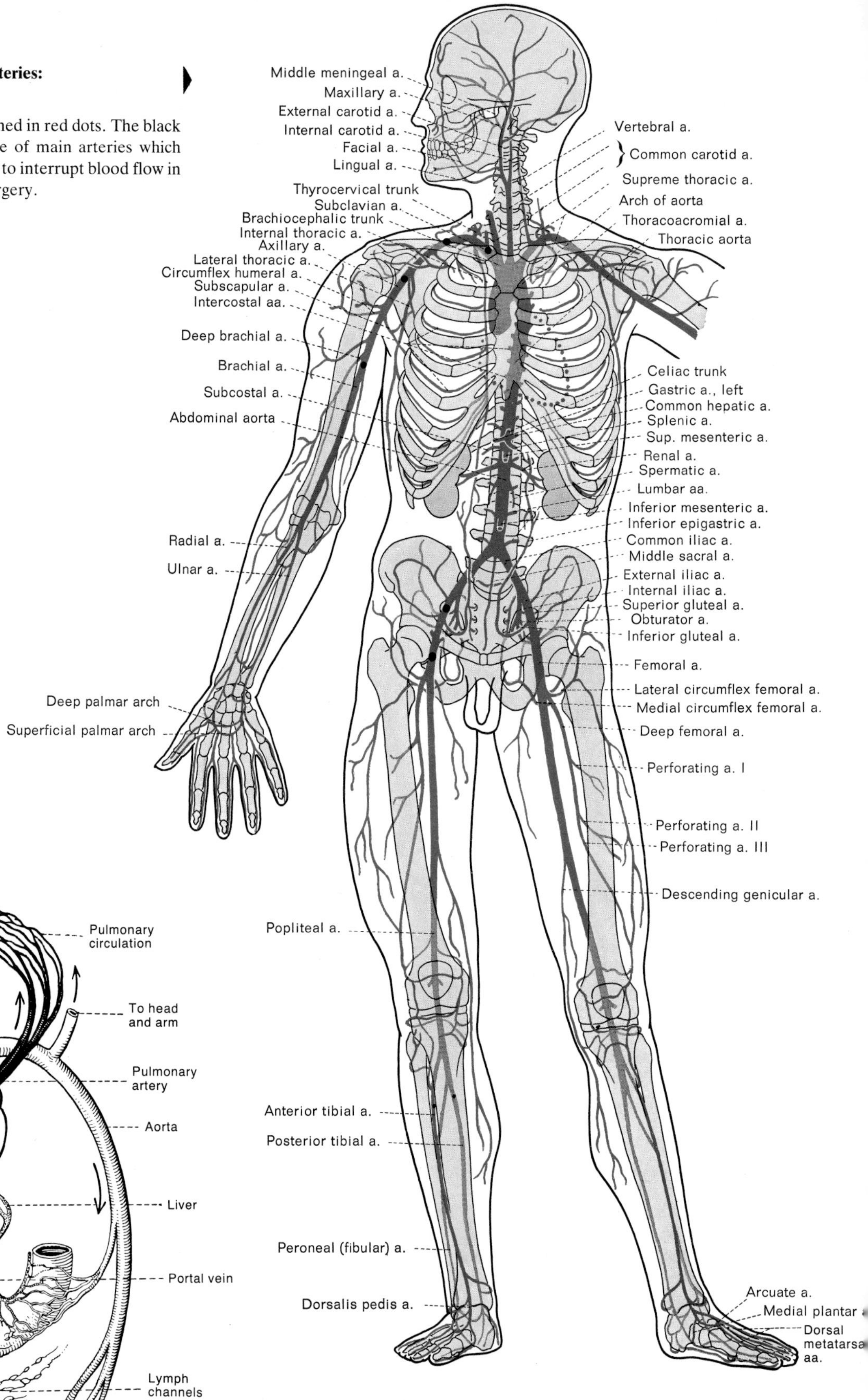

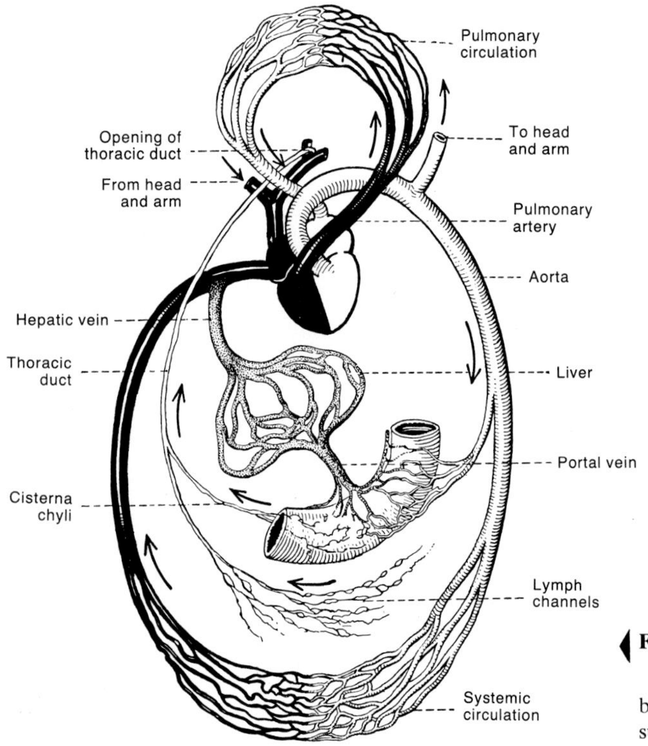

Middle meningeal a.
Maxillary a.
External carotid a.
Internal carotid a.
Facial a.
Lingual a.
Vertebral a.
Common carotid a.
Supreme thoracic a.
Arch of aorta
Thoracoacromial a.
Thoracic aorta
Thyrocervical trunk
Subclavian a.
Brachiocephalic trunk
Internal thoracic a.
Axillary a.
Lateral thoracic a.
Circumflex humeral a.
Subscapular a.
Intercostal aa.
Deep brachial a.
Brachial a.
Celiac trunk
Gastric a., left
Common hepatic a.
Splenic a.
Sup. mesenteric a.
Subcostal a.
Abdominal aorta
Renal a.
Spermatic a.
Lumbar aa.
Inferior mesenteric a.
Inferior epigastric a.
Common iliac a.
Middle sacral a.
External iliac a.
Internal iliac a.
Superior gluteal a.
Obturator a.
Inferior gluteal a.
Radial a.
Ulnar a.
Femoral a.
Lateral circumflex femoral a.
Medial circumflex femoral a.
Deep femoral a.
Perforating a. I
Deep palmar arch
Superficial palmar arch
Perforating a. II
Perforating a. III
Descending genicular a.
Popliteal a.
Anterior tibial a.
Posterior tibial a.
Peroneal (fibular) a.
Dorsalis pedis a.
Arcuate a.
Medial plantar
Dorsal metatarsal aa.

Pulmonary circulation
Opening of thoracic duct
From head and arm
To head and arm
Pulmonary artery
Aorta
Hepatic vein
Thoracic duct
Liver
Portal vein
Cisterna chyli
Lymph channels
Systemic circulation

### Fig. 151: Schema of Normal Blood Flow

NOTE: 1) that lymph from the abdomen and much of the lower region of the body flows through the thoracic duct. This duct has its origin at the cisterna chyli and subsequently opens into the left subclavian vein close to its junction (with the internal jugular vein) into the left brachiocephalic vein. In this manner circulating lymph in the tissues is returned to the general circulation.

2) the systemic, pulmonary and portal circulatory channels.

Figs. 150, 151

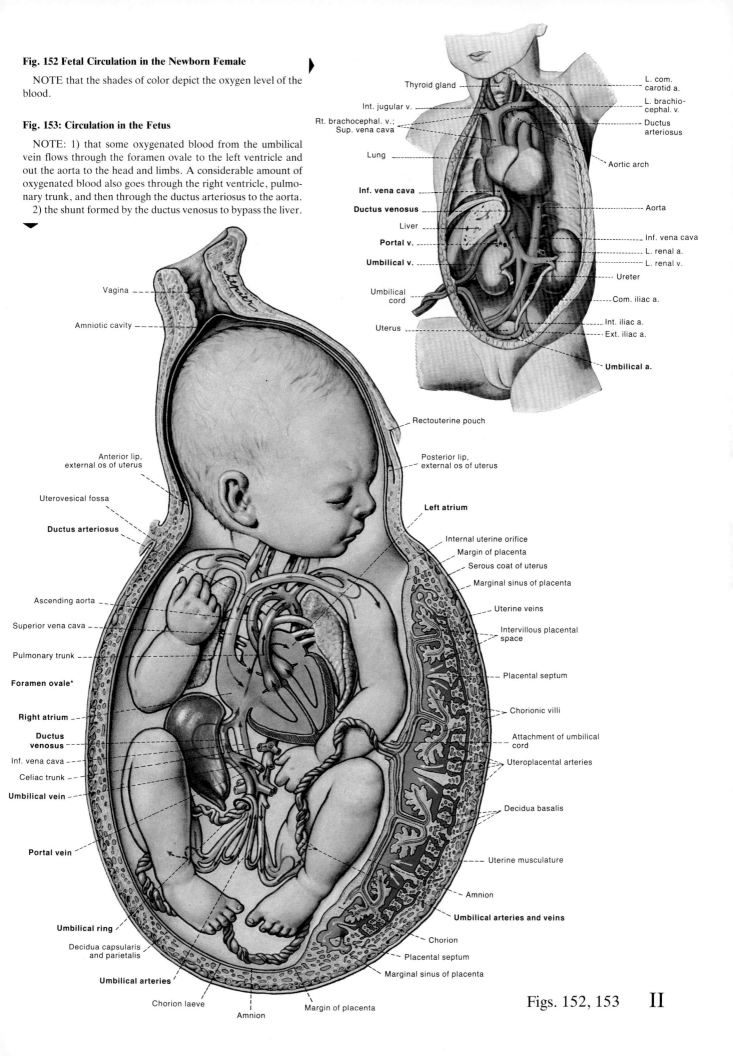

**Fig. 152 Fetal Circulation in the Newborn Female**

NOTE that the shades of color depict the oxygen level of the blood.

**Fig. 153: Circulation in the Fetus**

NOTE: 1) that some oxygenated blood from the umbilical vein flows through the foramen ovale to the left ventricle and out the aorta to the head and limbs. A considerable amount of oxygenated blood also goes through the right ventricle, pulmonary trunk, and then through the ductus arteriosus to the aorta.

2) the shunt formed by the ductus venosus to bypass the liver.

Thyroid gland
L. com. carotid a.
Int. jugular v.
L. brachio-cephal. v.
Rt. brachocephal. v.; Sup. vena cava
Ductus arteriosus
Lung
Aortic arch
**Inf. vena cava**
**Ductus venosus**
Aorta
Liver
Inf. vena cava
**Portal v.**
L. renal a.
**Umbilical v.**
L. renal v.
Ureter
Umbilical cord
Com. iliac a.
Int. iliac a.
Uterus
Ext. iliac a.
**Umbilical a.**

Vagina
Amniotic cavity

Rectouterine pouch

Anterior lip, external os of uterus
Posterior lip, external os of uterus

Uterovesical fossa
**Left atrium**

**Ductus arteriosus**
Internal uterine orifice
Margin of placenta
Serous coat of uterus
Marginal sinus of placenta

Ascending aorta
Superior vena cava
Uterine veins
Pulmonary trunk
Intervillous placental space
**Foramen ovale***
Placental septum
**Right atrium**
Chorionic villi
**Ductus venosus**
Attachment of umbilical cord
Inf. vena cava
Celiac trunk
Uteroplacental arteries
**Umbilical vein**
Decidua basalis
**Portal vein**
Uterine musculature
Amnion
**Umbilical arteries and veins**
**Umbilical ring**
Chorion
Decidua capsularis and parietalis
Placental septum
Marginal sinus of placenta
**Umbilical arteries**
Chorion laeve
Margin of placenta
Amnion

Figs. 152, 153   II

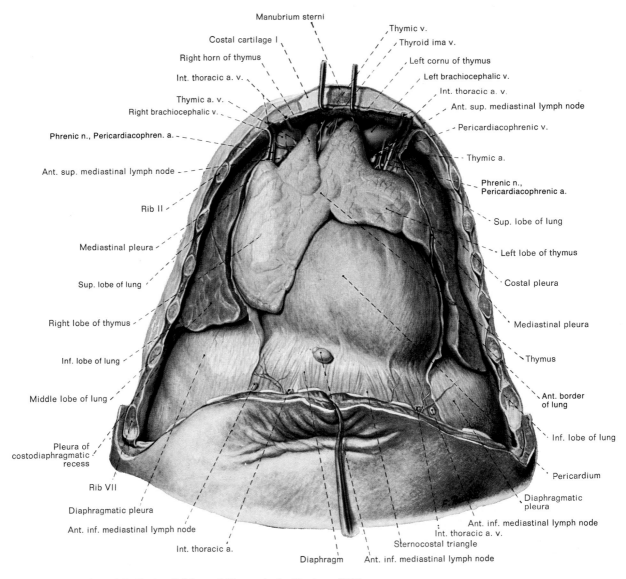

Manubrium sterni

Costal cartilage I

Right horn of thymus

Int. thoracic a. v.

Thymic a. v.

Right brachiocephalic v.

Phrenic n., Pericardiacophren. a.

Ant. sup. mediastinal lymph node

Rib II

Mediastinal pleura

Sup. lobe of lung

Right lobe of thymus

Inf. lobe of lung

Middle lobe of lung

Pleura of costodiaphragmatic recess

Rib VII

Diaphragmatic pleura

Ant. inf. mediastinal lymph node

Int. thoracic a.

Diaphragm

Ant. inf. mediastinal lymph node

Thymic v.

Thyroid ima v.

Left cornu of thymus

Left brachiocephalic v.

Int. thoracic a. v.

Ant. sup. mediastinal lymph node

Pericardiacophrenic v.

Thymic a.

Phrenic n., Pericardiacophrenic a.

Sup. lobe of lung

Left lobe of thymus

Costal pleura

Mediastinal pleura

Thymus

Ant. border of lung

Inf. lobe of lung

Pericardium

Diaphragmatic pleura

Ant. inf. mediastinal lymph node

Int. thoracic a. v.

Sternocostal triangle

**Fig. 154: Anterior View of the Pericardial Sac and Thymus in the Newborn Child**

NOTE that the great vessels of the superior mediastinum and the parietal pericardium over the base of the heart are covered by the thymus gland. The thymus also extends into the root of the neck in the newborn child.

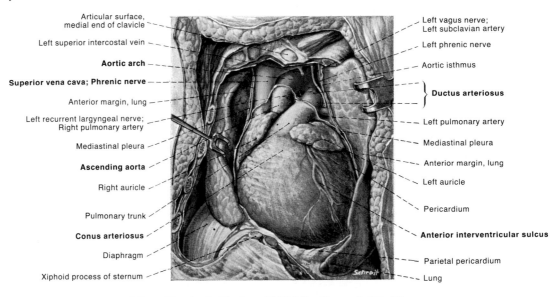

Articular surface, medial end of clavicle

Left superior intercostal vein

**Aortic arch**

**Superior vena cava; Phrenic nerve**

Anterior margin, lung

Left recurrent largyngeal nerve; Right pulmonary artery

Mediastinal pleura

**Ascending aorta**

Right auricle

Pulmonary trunk

**Conus arteriosus**

Diaphragm

Xiphoid process of sternum

Left vagus nerve; Left subclavian artery

Left phrenic nerve

Aortic isthmus

**Ductus arteriosus**

Left pulmonary artery

Mediastinal pleura

Anterior margin, lung

Left auricle

Pericardium

**Anterior interventricular sulcus**

Parietal pericardium

Lung

**Fig. 155: Anterior View of the Heart and Great Vessels of a Newborn Child After Removal of the Thymus**

NOTE that the ductus arteriosus is still an enlarged structure immediately after birth.

Figs. 154, 155

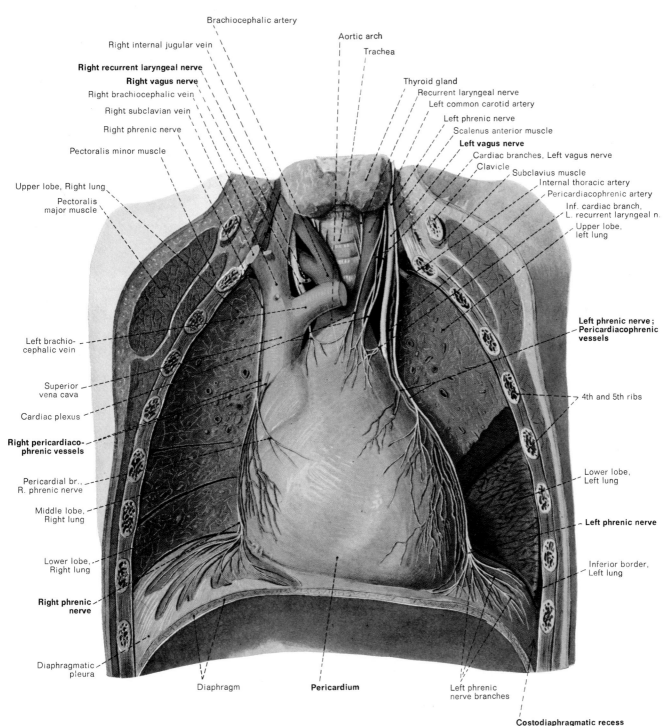

Brachiocephalic artery

Right internal jugular vein

**Right recurrent laryngeal nerve**

**Right vagus nerve**

Right brachiocephalic vein

Right subclavian vein

Right phrenic nerve

Pectoralis minor muscle

Upper lobe, Right lung

Pectoralis major muscle

Aortic arch

Trachea

Thyroid gland

Recurrent laryngeal nerve

Left common carotid artery

Left phrenic nerve

Scalenus anterior muscle

**Left vagus nerve**

Cardiac branches, Left vagus nerve

Clavicle

Subclavius muscle

Internal thoracic artery

Pericardiacophrenic artery

Inf. cardiac branch, L. recurrent laryngeal n.

Upper lobe, left lung

Left brachio-cephalic vein

Superior vena cava

Cardiac plexus

**Right pericardiaco-phrenic vessels**

Pericardial br., R. phrenic nerve

Middle lobe, Right lung

Lower lobe, Right lung

**Right phrenic nerve**

Diaphragmatic pleura

**Left phrenic nerve; Pericardiacophrenic vessels**

4th and 5th ribs

Lower lobe, Left lung

**Left phrenic nerve**

Inferior border, Left lung

Diaphragm

**Pericardium**

Left phrenic nerve branches

**Costodiaphragmatic recess**

**Fig. 156: The Adult Heart, Pericardium and Superior Mediastinal Structures, Anterior View**

NOTE: 1) in this frontal section through the thorax, the anterior thoracic wall and the anterior aspect of the lungs and diaphragm have been removed, leaving the pericardium, its contents and its associated vessels and nerves intact. The courses of the vagus nerves and their branches in the superior mediastinum are also demonstrated.

2) the phrenic nerves originate in the neck (C3, 4, 5) and descend almost vertically to innervate the diaphragm. In the superior mediastinum they join the pericardiacophrenic vessels, travel along the lateral surfaces of the pericardium and are distributed principally to the diaphragm, sending some sensory fibers to the pericardium as well.

3) the pericardium is formed by an outer fibrous layer which is lined by an inner serous sac. As the heart develops it invaginates into the inner serous sac, thereby being covered by a visceral layer of serous pericardium (epicardium) and a parietal layer of serous pericardium. The outer fibrous pericardium has only a parietal layer.

Fig. 156    II

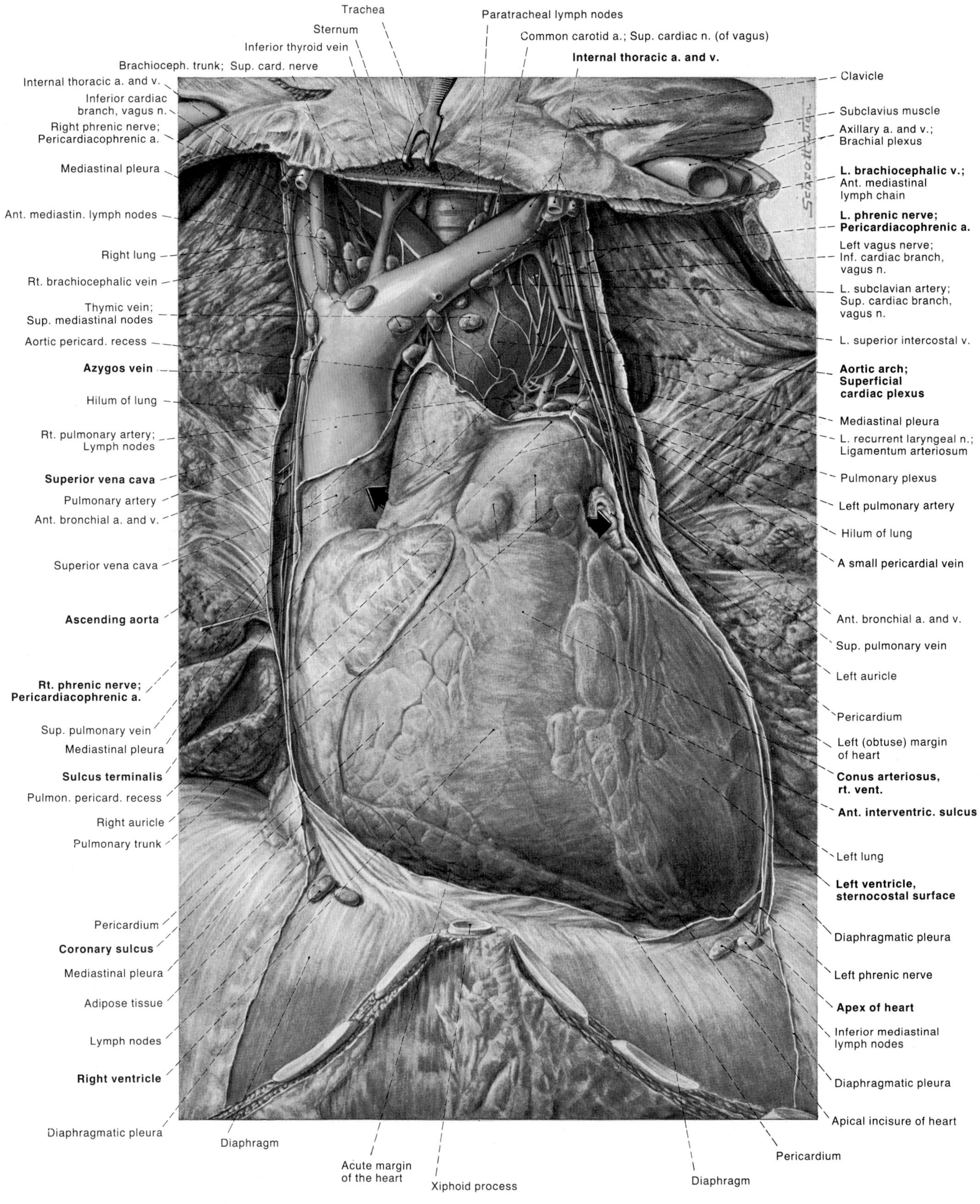

Trachea
Sternum
Inferior thyroid vein
Brachioceph. trunk; Sup. card. nerve
Paratracheal lymph nodes
Common carotid a.; Sup. cardiac n. (of vagus)
Internal thoracic a. and v.
Internal thoracic a. and v.
Inferior cardiac branch, vagus n.
Right phrenic nerve; Pericardiacophrenic a.
Mediastinal pleura
Ant. mediastin. lymph nodes
Right lung
Rt. brachiocephalic vein
Thymic vein; Sup. mediastinal nodes
Aortic pericard. recess
Azygos vein
Hilum of lung
Rt. pulmonary artery; Lymph nodes
Superior vena cava
Pulmonary artery
Ant. bronchial a. and v.
Superior vena cava
Ascending aorta
Rt. phrenic nerve; Pericardiacophrenic a.
Sup. pulmonary vein
Mediastinal pleura
Sulcus terminalis
Pulmon. pericard. recess
Right auricle
Pulmonary trunk
Pericardium
Coronary sulcus
Mediastinal pleura
Adipose tissue
Lymph nodes
Right ventricle
Diaphragmatic pleura
Diaphragm
Acute margin of the heart
Xiphoid process
Diaphragm
Pericardium
Clavicle
Subclavius muscle
Axillary a. and v.; Brachial plexus
L. brachiocephalic v.; Ant. mediastinal lymph chain
L. phrenic nerve; Pericardiacophrenic a.
Left vagus nerve; Inf. cardiac branch, vagus n.
L. subclavian artery; Sup. cardiac branch, vagus n.
L. superior intercostal v.
Aortic arch; Superficial cardiac plexus
Mediastinal pleura
L. recurrent laryngeal n.; Ligamentum arteriosum
Pulmonary plexus
Left pulmonary artery
Hilum of lung
A small pericardial vein
Ant. bronchial a. and v.
Sup. pulmonary vein
Left auricle
Pericardium
Left (obtuse) margin of heart
Conus arteriosus, rt. vent.
Ant. interventric. sulcus
Left lung
Left ventricle, sternocostal surface
Diaphragmatic pleura
Left phrenic nerve
Apex of heart
Inferior mediastinal lymph nodes
Diaphragmatic pleura
Apical incisure of heart


**Fig. 157: The Heart and Great Vessels, Anterior View**

NOTE that the anterior portion of the pericardium has been removed along with the remnants of the thymus to reveal the heart in its normal position within the middle mediastinum. The arrow is in the transverse pericardial sinus.

Fig. 157

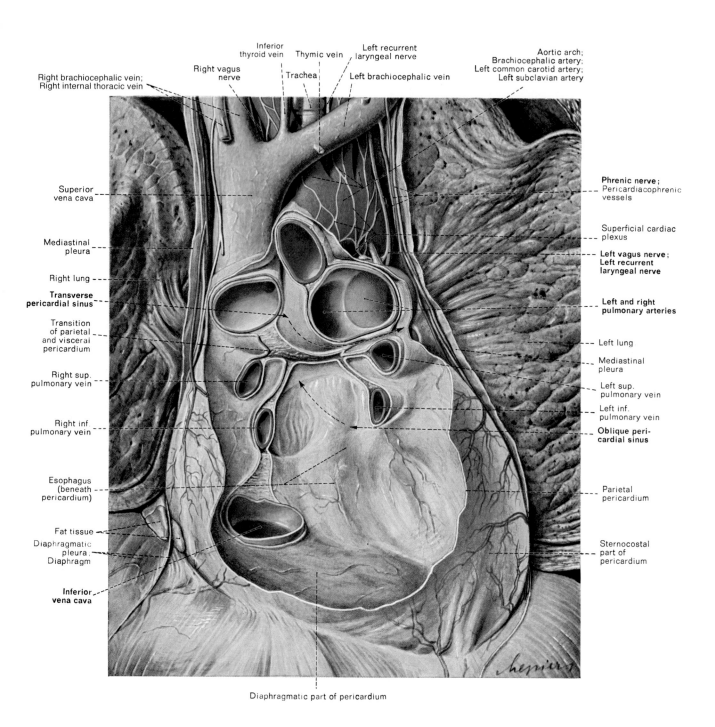

Right brachiocephalic vein;
Right internal thoracic vein

Inferior
thyroid vein

Right vagus
nerve

Thymic vein

Trachea

Left recurrent
laryngeal nerve

Left brachiocephalic vein

Aortic arch;
Brachiocephalic artery;
Left common carotid artery;
Left subclavian artery

Superior
vena cava

Mediastinal
pleura

Right lung

Transverse
pericardial sinus

Transition
of parietal
and visceral
pericardium

Right sup.
pulmonary vein

Right inf.
pulmonary vein

Esophagus
(beneath
pericardium)

Fat tissue
Diaphragmatic
pleura
Diaphragm

Inferior
vena cava

Phrenic nerve;
Pericardiacophrenic
vessels

Superficial cardiac
plexus

Left vagus nerve;
Left recurrent
laryngeal nerve

Left and right
pulmonary arteries

Left lung

Mediastinal
pleura

Left sup.
pulmonary vein

Left inf.
pulmonary vein

Oblique peri-
cardial sinus

Parietal
pericardium

Sternocostal
part of
pericardium

Diaphragmatic part of pericardium

## Fig. 158: Interior of the Pericardium, Anterior View

NOTE: 1) the pericardium has been opened anteriorly and the heart has been severed from the great vessels and removed. Eight vessels have been cut: the superior and inferior venae cavae, the four pulmonary veins, the pulmonary artery and the aorta.

2) the oblique pericardial sinus is located in the central portion of this posterior wall and is bounded by the pericardial reflections over the pulmonary veins and the venae cavae (venous mesocardium). With the heart in place, the oblique pericardial sinus may be palpated by inserting several fingers behind the heart and probing superiorly until the blind pouch of the sinus is felt.

3) the transverse pericardial sinus lies behind the pericardial reflection surrounding the aorta and pulmonary artery (arterial mesocardium). It may be located by probing from right to left with the index finger immediately posterior to the pulmonary trunk.

4) the site of bifurcation of the pulmonary trunk beneath the arch of the aorta and the course of the left recurrent laryngeal nerve beneath the ligamentum arteriosum (not labelled).

Fig. 158    II

## Fig. 159: The Coronary Vessels, Anterior View

NOTE: 1) both the left and right coronary arteries arise from the ascending aorta. The *left coronary* is directed toward the left and soon divides into a *descending anterior interventricular branch* which courses toward the apex and a circumflex branch which passes posteriorly as far as the posterior interventricular sulcus.

2) the right coronary artery is directed toward the right, passing to the posterior aspect of the heart within the coronary sulcus. In its course, branches from the right coronary supply the anterior surface of the right side (anterior cardiac artery). Its largest branch is the posterior interventricular artery which courses toward the apex on the posterior or diaphragmatic surface of the heart.

3) the principal veins of the heart drain into the coronary sinus which in turn flows into the right atrium. The distribution and course of the veins is generally similar to the arteries.

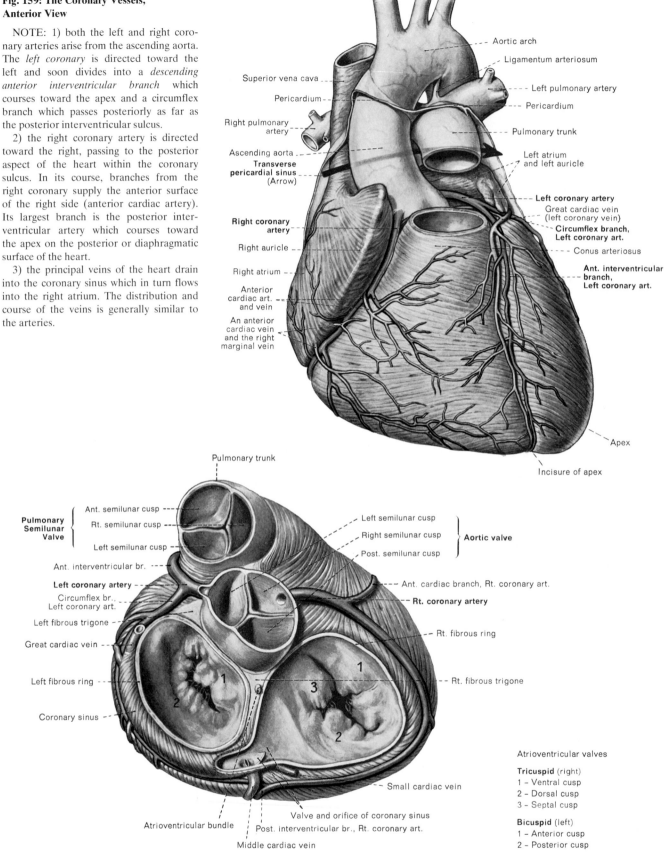

Aortic arch
Ligamentum arteriosum
Left pulmonary artery
Pericardium
Pulmonary trunk
Left atrium and left auricle
**Left coronary artery**
Great cardiac vein (left coronary vein)
**Circumflex branch, Left coronary art.**
Conus arteriosus
**Ant. interventricular branch, Left coronary art.**
Apex
Incisure of apex

Superior vena cava
Pericardium
Right pulmonary artery
Ascending aorta
**Transverse pericardial sinus (Arrow)**
**Right coronary artery**
Right auricle
Right atrium
Anterior cardiac art. and vein
An anterior cardiac vein and the right marginal vein

Pulmonary trunk

**Pulmonary Semilunar Valve**
Ant. semilunar cusp
Rt. semilunar cusp
Left semilunar cusp

Left semilunar cusp
Right semilunar cusp
Post. semilunar cusp
**Aortic valve**

Ant. interventricular br.
**Left coronary artery**
Circumflex br., Left coronary art.
Left fibrous trigone
Great cardiac vein
Left fibrous ring
Coronary sinus

Ant. cardiac branch, Rt. coronary art.
**Rt. coronary artery**
Rt. fibrous ring
Rt. fibrous trigone

Small cardiac vein

Atrioventricular bundle
Post. interventricular br., Rt. coronary art.
Valve and orifice of coronary sinus
Middle cardiac vein

Atrioventricular valves

**Tricuspid** (right)
1 – Ventral cusp
2 – Dorsal cusp
3 – Septal cusp

**Bicuspid** (left)
1 – Anterior cusp
2 – Posterior cusp

## Fig. 160: The Valves of the Heart and the Origin of the Coronary Vessels, Superior View

NOTE that the left coronary artery arises from the aortic sinus behind the left semilunar cusp and the right coronary artery stems from the aortic sinus behind the right semilunar cusp.

Figs. 159, 160

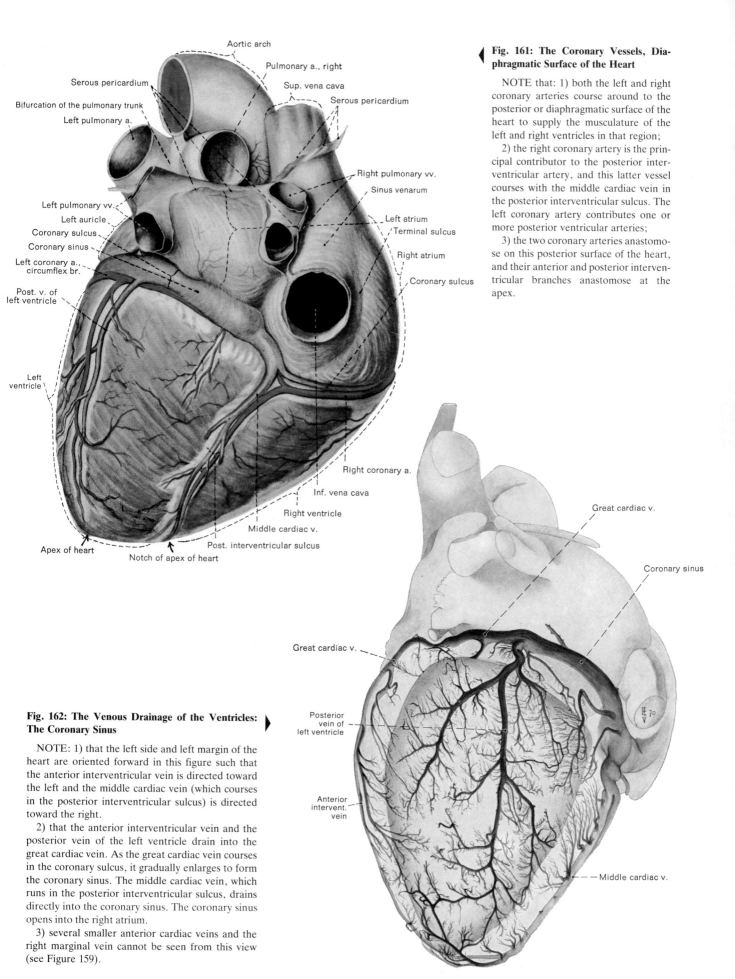

Aortic arch

Pulmonary a., right

Serous pericardium

Sup. vena cava

Bifurcation of the pulmonary trunk

Serous pericardium

Left pulmonary a.

Right pulmonary vv.

Sinus venarum

Left pulmonary vv.

Left auricle

Left atrium

Coronary sulcus

Terminal sulcus

Coronary sinus

Right atrium

Left coronary a., circumflex br.

Coronary sulcus

Post. v. of left ventricle

Left ventricle

Right coronary a.

Inf. vena cava

Right ventricle

Apex of heart

Middle cardiac v.

Notch of apex of heart

Post. interventricular sulcus

Great cardiac v.

Coronary sinus

Great cardiac v.

Posterior vein of left ventricle

Anterior intervent. vein

Middle cardiac v.

**Fig. 161: The Coronary Vessels, Diaphragmatic Surface of the Heart**

NOTE that: 1) both the left and right coronary arteries course around to the posterior or diaphragmatic surface of the heart to supply the musculature of the left and right ventricles in that region;

2) the right coronary artery is the principal contributor to the posterior interventricular artery, and this latter vessel courses with the middle cardiac vein in the posterior interventricular sulcus. The left coronary artery contributes one or more posterior ventricular arteries;

3) the two coronary arteries anastomose on this posterior surface of the heart, and their anterior and posterior interventricular branches anastomose at the apex.

**Fig. 162: The Venous Drainage of the Ventricles: The Coronary Sinus**

NOTE: 1) that the left side and left margin of the heart are oriented forward in this figure such that the anterior interventricular vein is directed toward the left and the middle cardiac vein (which courses in the posterior interventricular sulcus) is directed toward the right.

2) that the anterior interventricular vein and the posterior vein of the left ventricle drain into the great cardiac vein. As the great cardiac vein courses in the coronary sulcus, it gradually enlarges to form the coronary sinus. The middle cardiac vein, which runs in the posterior interventricular sulcus, drains directly into the coronary sinus. The coronary sinus opens into the right atrium.

3) several smaller anterior cardiac veins and the right marginal vein cannot be seen from this view (see Figure 159).

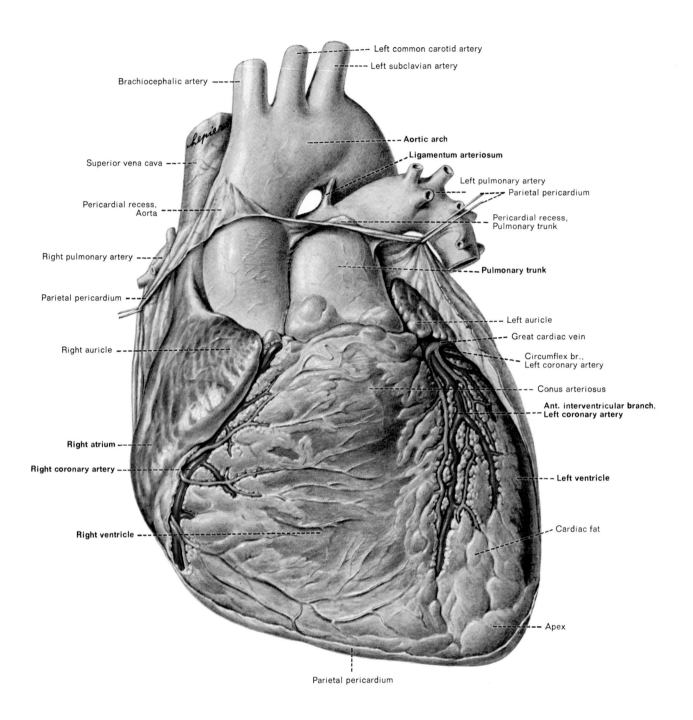

Left common carotid artery

Left subclavian artery

Brachiocephalic artery

**Aortic arch**

**Ligamentum arteriosum**

Superior vena cava

Left pulmonary artery

Parietal pericardium

Pericardial recess,
Aorta

Pericardial recess,
Pulmonary trunk

Right pulmonary artery

**Pulmonary trunk**

Parietal pericardium

Left auricle

Great cardiac vein

Right auricle

Circumflex br.,
Left coronary artery

Conus arteriosus

**Ant. interventricular branch,
Left coronary artery**

**Right atrium**

**Right coronary artery**

**Left ventricle**

Cardiac fat

**Right ventricle**

Apex

Parietal pericardium

**Fig. 163: Ventral View of the Heart and Great Vessels**

NOTE: 1) the heart is a muscular organ with its apex pointed inferiorly, toward the left and slightly anteriorly. The base of the heart is opposite to the apex and is, therefore, directed superiorly and toward the right. The great vessels attach to the heart at its base, and the pericardium is reflected over these vessels at their origin.

2) the anterior surface of the heart is its sternocostal surface. The auricular portion of the right atrium and especially the right ventricle is seen from this anterior view; also a small part of the left ventricle is visible on the left side.

3) the pulmonary trunk originates from the right ventricle. To its right and slightly behind can be seen the aorta which arises from the left ventricle. The superior vena cava can be seen opening into the upper aspect of the right atrium.

4) the ligamentum arteriosum. This fibrous structure, attaching the left pulmonary artery to the arch of the aorta, is the postnatal remnant of the fetal ductus arteriosus which, before birth, acted as a shunt diverting some of the blood directed for the lungs back into the aorta for general systemic distribution.

Fig. 163

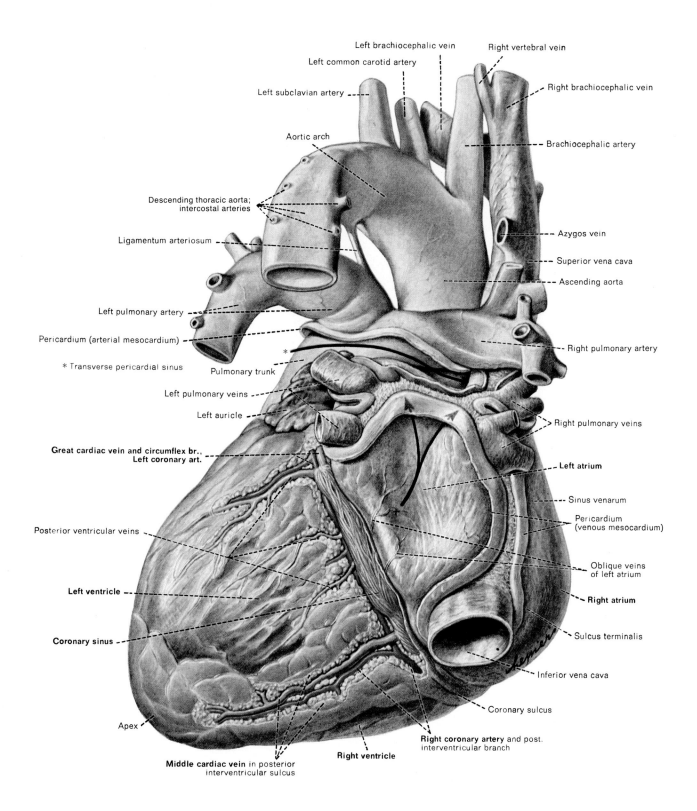

Left brachiocephalic vein
Left common carotid artery
Right vertebral vein
Left subclavian artery
Right brachiocephalic vein
Aortic arch
Brachiocephalic artery
Descending thoracic aorta; intercostal arteries
Azygos vein
Ligamentum arteriosum
Superior vena cava
Ascending aorta
Left pulmonary artery
Pericardium (arterial mesocardium)
Right pulmonary artery
* Transverse pericardial sinus
Pulmonary trunk
Left pulmonary veins
Right pulmonary veins
Left auricle
**Great cardiac vein and circumflex br., Left coronary art.**
**Left atrium**
Sinus venarum
Posterior ventricular veins
Pericardium (venous mesocardium)
Oblique veins of left atrium
**Left ventricle**
**Right atrium**
**Coronary sinus**
Sulcus terminalis
Inferior vena cava
Apex
Coronary sulcus
**Right coronary artery** and post. interventricular branch
**Middle cardiac vein** in posterior interventricular sulcus
**Right ventricle**

## Fig. 164: Posterior View of the Heart and Great Vessels

NOTE: 1) the two pericardial sinuses. The long transverse arrow indicates the *transverse pericardial sinus* which lies between the arterial mesocardium and the venous mesocardium. The double arrows lie in the *oblique pericardial sinus*, the boundaries of which are actually demarcated by the pericardial reflections around the pulmonary veins.

2) the transverse sinus can be identified by placing your index finger behind the pulmonary artery and aorta with the heart *in situ*. The oblique sinus is open inferiorly, while superiorly it forms a closed sac. This sinus can also be felt by cupping your fingers behind the heart and pushing superiorly.

3) the coronary sinus separates the posterior surface regions of the atria (above and to the right) and the ventricles (below and to the left). The posterior atrial surface principally consists of the left atrium, into which flow the pulmonary veins, although below and to the right can be seen the right atrium and its inferior vena cava. The posterior atrial surface lies anterior to the vertebral column. The posterior ventricular surface is formed principally by the left ventricle and this surface lies over the diaphragm.

Fig. 164    II

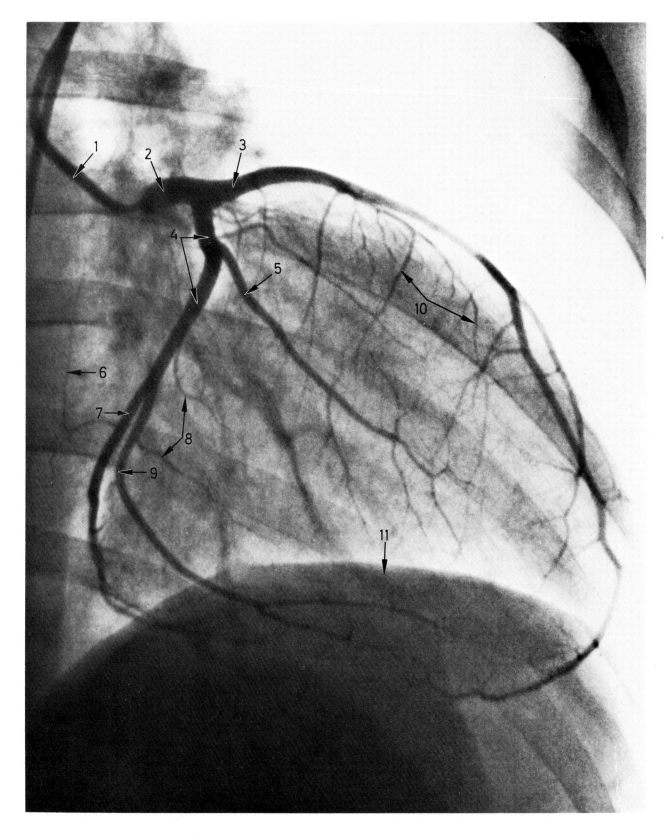

**Fig. 165: Left Coronary Arteriogram**

NOTE that this arteriogram of the left coronary artery is viewed from a right antero-oblique direction.

1. Catheter
2. Left coronary artery
3. Anterior interventricular branch
4. Circumflex branch
5. Left marginal branch of circumflex
6. Posterior atrial branch
7. Left posterolateral branch of circumflex
8. Posterior ventricular branches
9. Posterior interventricular branch
10. Septal branches
11. Diaphragm

Fig. 165

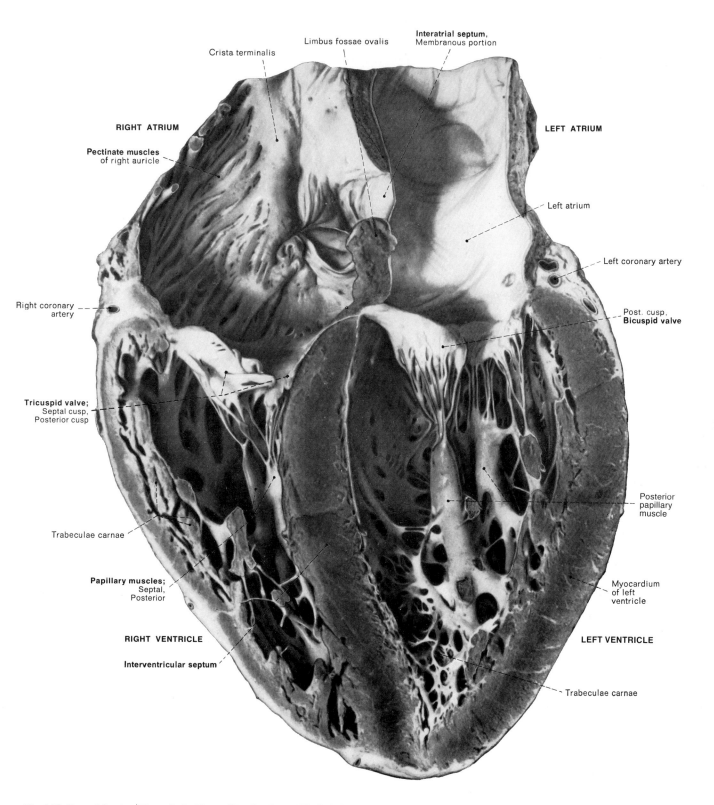

Crista terminalis

Limbus fossae ovalis

**Interatrial septum,** Membranous portion

RIGHT ATRIUM

LEFT ATRIUM

**Pectinate muscles** of right auricle

Left atrium

Left coronary artery

Right coronary artery

Post. cusp, **Bicuspid valve**

**Tricuspid valve;** Septal cusp, Posterior cusp

Posterior papillary muscle

Trabeculae carnae

**Papillary muscles;** Septal, Posterior

Myocardium of left ventricle

RIGHT VENTRICLE

LEFT VENTRICLE

Interventricular septum

Trabeculae carnae

**Fig. 166: Frontal Section Through the Heart, Showing Dorsal Half of Heart**

NOTE: 1) the human heart is a four-chambered muscular organ consisting of an atrium and a ventricle on each side. The walls of the ventricles are thicker than those of the atria. The atrial chambers are separated by an interatrial septum, and this is continuous with the interventricular septum dividing the two ventricles. Blood passes simultaneously from the two atria into their respective ventricles through the atrioventricular valves.

2) on the right side the atrioventricular valve (AV valve) consists of three cusps and is called the tricuspid valve. On the left side the AV valve has two cusps and is called the bicuspid or mitral valve.

3) the inner surfaces of the atria are relatively smooth, whereas muscular projections, the papillary muscles, protrude from the inner walls of the ventricles to attach to the cusps of the AV valves by way of fibrous, thin cords, the chordae tendineae. (These cords are shown but not labelled.)

4) other elevated muscular bundles on the inner heart wall to not attach to the valves. In the ventricles these are called the trabeculae carnae, while in the right auricle they are named the pectinate muscles.

Fig. 166  II

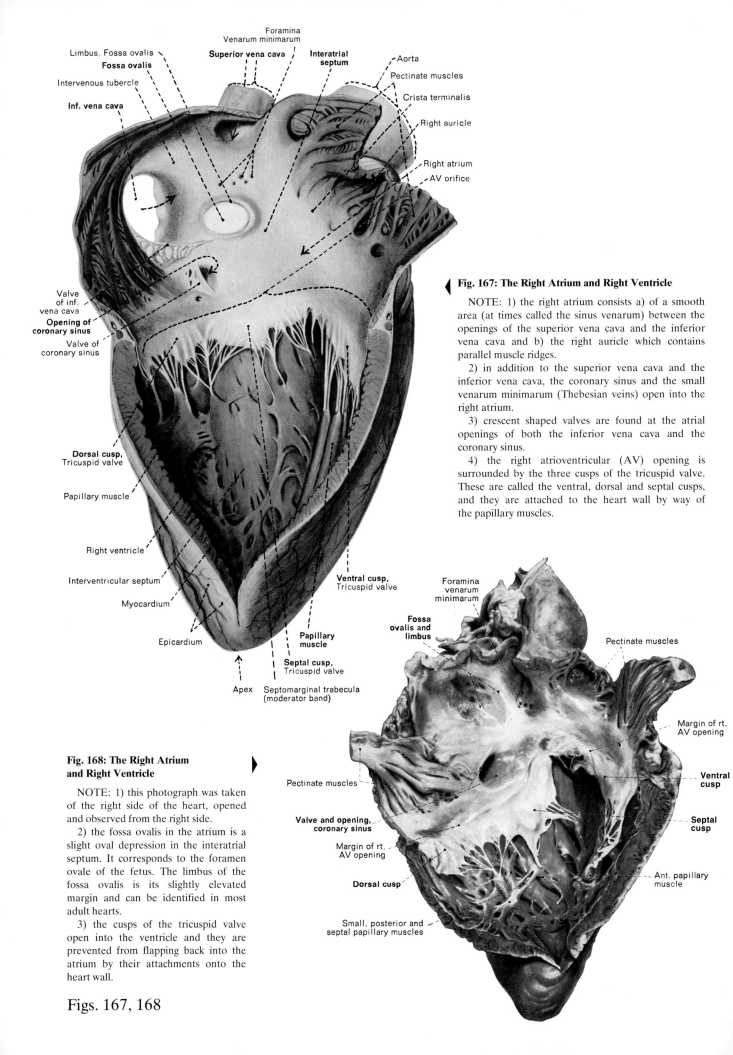

Foramina
Venarum minimarum
Limbus, Fossa ovalis
**Fossa ovalis**
Intervenous tubercle
**Inf. vena cava**
**Superior vena cava**
**Interatrial septum**
Aorta
Pectinate muscles
Crista terminalis
Right auricle
Right atrium
AV orifice

Valve
of inf.
vena cava
**Opening of
coronary sinus**
Valve of
coronary sinus

**Dorsal cusp,**
Tricuspid valve

Papillary muscle

Right ventricle

Interventricular septum

Myocardium

Epicardium

Apex

**Ventral cusp,**
Tricuspid valve

**Papillary
muscle**

**Septal cusp,**
Tricuspid valve

Septomarginal trabecula
(moderator band)

### Fig. 167: The Right Atrium and Right Ventricle

NOTE: 1) the right atrium consists a) of a smooth area (at times called the sinus venarum) between the openings of the superior vena cava and the inferior vena cava and b) the right auricle which contains parallel muscle ridges.

2) in addition to the superior vena cava and the inferior vena cava, the coronary sinus and the small venarum minimarum (Thebesian veins) open into the right atrium.

3) crescent shaped valves are found at the atrial openings of both the inferior vena cava and the coronary sinus.

4) the right atrioventricular (AV) opening is surrounded by the three cusps of the tricuspid valve. These are called the ventral, dorsal and septal cusps, and they are attached to the heart wall by way of the papillary muscles.

### Fig. 168: The Right Atrium and Right Ventricle

NOTE: 1) this photograph was taken of the right side of the heart, opened and observed from the right side.

2) the fossa ovalis in the atrium is a slight oval depression in the interatrial septum. It corresponds to the foramen ovale of the fetus. The limbus of the fossa ovalis is its slightly elevated margin and can be identified in most adult hearts.

3) the cusps of the tricuspid valve open into the ventricle and they are prevented from flapping back into the atrium by their attachments onto the heart wall.

Foramina
venarum
minimarum

**Fossa
ovalis and
limbus**

Pectinate muscles

Margin of rt.
AV opening

**Ventral
cusp**

**Septal
cusp**

Pectinate muscles

**Valve and opening,
coronary sinus**

Margin of rt.
AV opening

**Dorsal cusp**

Ant. papillary
muscle

Small, posterior and
septal papillary muscles

Figs. 167, 168

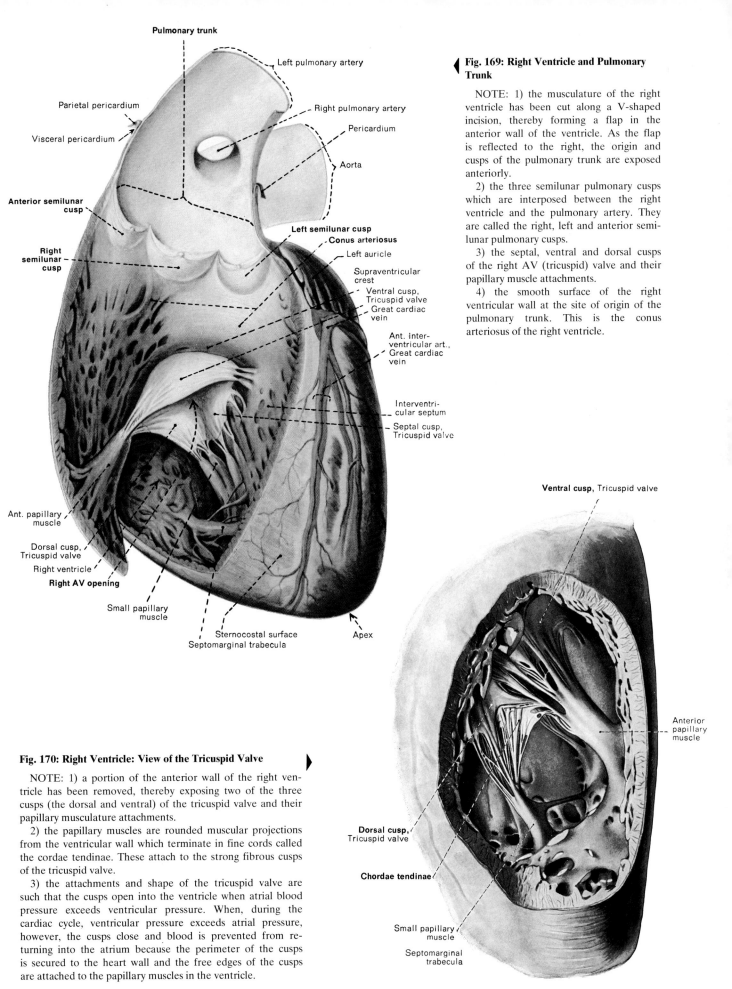

Pulmonary trunk

Left pulmonary artery

Right pulmonary artery

Parietal pericardium

Pericardium

Visceral pericardium

Aorta

**Anterior semilunar cusp**

**Left semilunar cusp**

**Conus arteriosus**

**Right semilunar cusp**

Left auricle

Supraventricular crest

Ventral cusp, Tricuspid valve

Great cardiac vein

Ant. interventricular art., Great cardiac vein

Interventricular septum

Septal cusp, Tricuspid valve

Ant. papillary muscle

Dorsal cusp, Tricuspid valve

Right ventricle

**Right AV opening**

Small papillary muscle

Sternocostal surface
Septomarginal trabecula

Apex

### Fig. 169: Right Ventricle and Pulmonary Trunk

NOTE: 1) the musculature of the right ventricle has been cut along a V-shaped incision, thereby forming a flap in the anterior wall of the ventricle. As the flap is reflected to the right, the origin and cusps of the pulmonary trunk are exposed anteriorly.

2) the three semilunar pulmonary cusps which are interposed between the right ventricle and the pulmonary artery. They are called the right, left and anterior semilunar pulmonary cusps.

3) the septal, ventral and dorsal cusps of the right AV (tricuspid) valve and their papillary muscle attachments.

4) the smooth surface of the right ventricular wall at the site of origin of the pulmonary trunk. This is the conus arteriosus of the right ventricle.

Ventral cusp, Tricuspid valve

Anterior papillary muscle

**Dorsal cusp,** Tricuspid valve

**Chordae tendinae**

Small papillary muscle

Septomarginal trabecula

### Fig. 170: Right Ventricle: View of the Tricuspid Valve

NOTE: 1) a portion of the anterior wall of the right ventricle has been removed, thereby exposing two of the three cusps (the dorsal and ventral) of the tricuspid valve and their papillary musculature attachments.

2) the papillary muscles are rounded muscular projections from the ventricular wall which terminate in fine cords called the cordae tendinae. These attach to the strong fibrous cusps of the tricuspid valve.

3) the attachments and shape of the tricuspid valve are such that the cusps open into the ventricle when atrial blood pressure exceeds ventricular pressure. When, during the cardiac cycle, ventricular pressure exceeds atrial pressure, however, the cusps close and blood is prevented from returning into the atrium because the perimeter of the cusps is secured to the heart wall and the free edges of the cusps are attached to the papillary muscles in the ventricle.

Figs. 169, 170    II

## Fig. 171: The Left Atrium and Left Ventricle

NOTE: 1) in this specimen a longitudinal section has been made through the left side of the heart, thereby exposing the smooth-walled left atrium above and the thickened, muscular-walled left ventricle below. The left atrium opens into the left ventricle through the left atrioventricular (AV) orifice at which is located the left AV valve. This valve is also called the mitral or bicuspid valve.

2) the mitral valve consists of two cusps, an anterior cusp and a posterior cusp, and these are attached to the left ventricular wall by means of papillary muscles in a manner similar to that seen on the right side of the heart. Observe the chordae tendineae interposed between the cusps and the papillary muscles.

3) the interatrial septum is marked by the valve of the foramen ovale (falx septi), which represents the remnant of the septum primum during the development of the interatrial septum.

4) the left atrium receives the four pulmonary veins (two from each lung) while the left ventricle leads into (indicated by arrow) the aorta.

5) the thick muscular layer of the heart, called the myocardium, is lined on its inner surface by a layer of endothelium, consistent and continuous with the inner lining of blood vessels that enter and leave the heart. The outer covering, called the epicardium, is a serous membrane which serves as the visceral layer of pericardium.

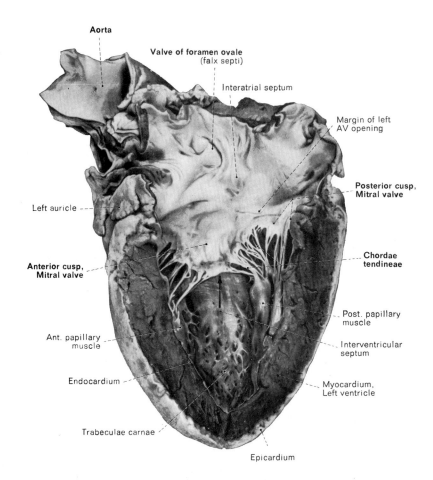

Aorta

Valve of foramen ovale (falx septi)

Interatrial septum

Margin of left AV opening

Left auricle

Posterior cusp, Mitral valve

Chordae tendineae

Anterior cusp, Mitral valve

Post. papillary muscle

Ant. papillary muscle

Interventricular septum

Endocardium

Myocardium, Left ventricle

Trabeculae carnae

Epicardium

## Fig. 172: The Left Ventricle and Ascending Aorta

NOTE: 1) the heart has been cut longitudinally in such a manner that the left ventricular cavity is exposed along with the origin of the ascending aorta.

2) the aortic opening is guarded by three semilunar cusps. These are named the posterior, left and right semilunar aortic cusps. Behind each cusp a small *cul de sac* is formed by the cusp and the wall of the aorta. These small dilated pockets are called the aortic sinuses (sinuses of Valsalva) and from the aortic sinuses behind the left and right semilunar aortic cusps, the left and right coronary arteries arise.

3) during ventricular contraction the blood pressure in the left ventricle is elevated over that in the aorta, thereby causing the aortic valve to open and blood to pass into the aorta. Soon, however, the aortic pressure exceeds ventricular pressure and blood then tends to rush back into the ventricle. In the normal heart, the aortic sinuses trap the regurgitating blood and thereby force the aortic cusps to close.

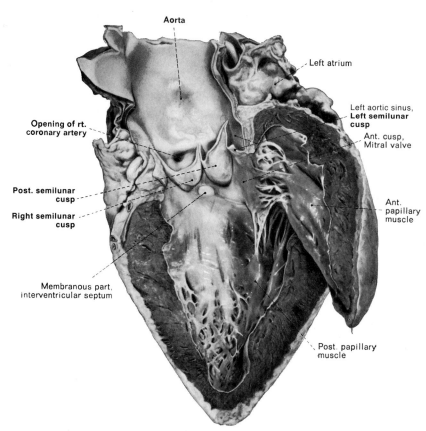

Aorta

Left atrium

Left aortic sinus, Left semilunar cusp

Ant. cusp, Mitral valve

Opening of rt. coronary artery

Post. semilunar cusp

Right semilunar cusp

Ant. papillary muscle

Membranous part, interventricular septum

Post. papillary muscle

Figs. 171, 172

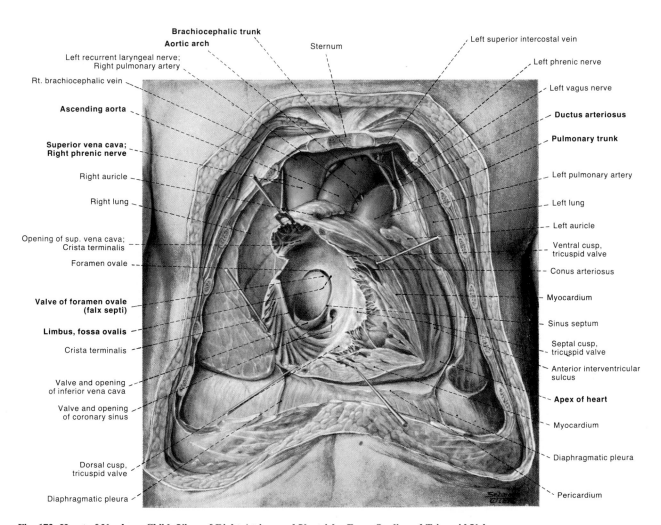

**Fig. 173: Heart of Newborn Child: View of Right Atrium and Ventricle, Fossa Ovalis and Tricuspid Valve**

Brachiocephalic trunk
Aortic arch
Left recurrent laryngeal nerve;
Right pulmonary artery
Sternum
Left superior intercostal vein
Left phrenic nerve
Rt. brachiocephalic vein
Left vagus nerve
Ascending aorta
Ductus arteriosus
Superior vena cava;
Right phrenic nerve
Pulmonary trunk
Right auricle
Left pulmonary artery
Right lung
Left lung
Left auricle
Opening of sup. vena cava;
Crista terminalis
Ventral cusp, tricuspid valve
Foramen ovale
Conus arteriosus
Myocardium
Valve of foramen ovale (falx septi)
Sinus septum
Limbus, fossa ovalis
Septal cusp, tricuspid valve
Crista terminalis
Anterior interventricular sulcus
Valve and opening of inferior vena cava
Apex of heart
Valve and opening of coronary sinus
Myocardium
Diaphragmatic pleura
Dorsal cusp, tricuspid valve
Pericardium
Diaphragmatic pleura

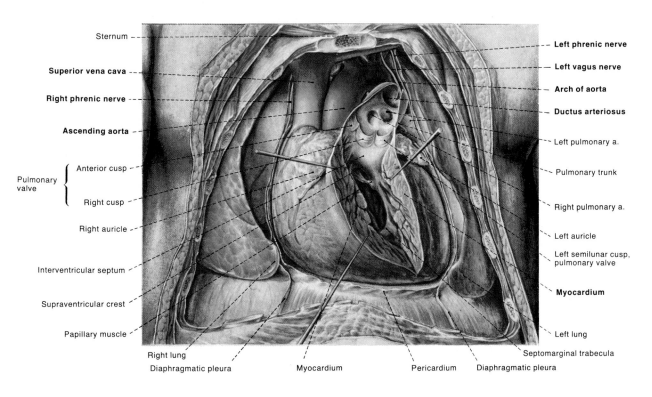

**Fig. 174: Heart of Newborn Child: View of Pulmonary Trunk and Opened Right Ventricle**

Sternum
Left phrenic nerve
Superior vena cava
Left vagus nerve
Right phrenic nerve
Arch of aorta
Ascending aorta
Ductus arteriosus
Anterior cusp
Left pulmonary a.
Pulmonary valve
Pulmonary trunk
Right cusp
Right pulmonary a.
Right auricle
Left auricle
Left semilunar cusp, pulmonary valve
Interventricular septum
Supraventricular crest
Myocardium
Papillary muscle
Left lung
Right lung
Septomarginal trabecula
Diaphragmatic pleura
Myocardium
Pericardium
Diaphragmatic pleura

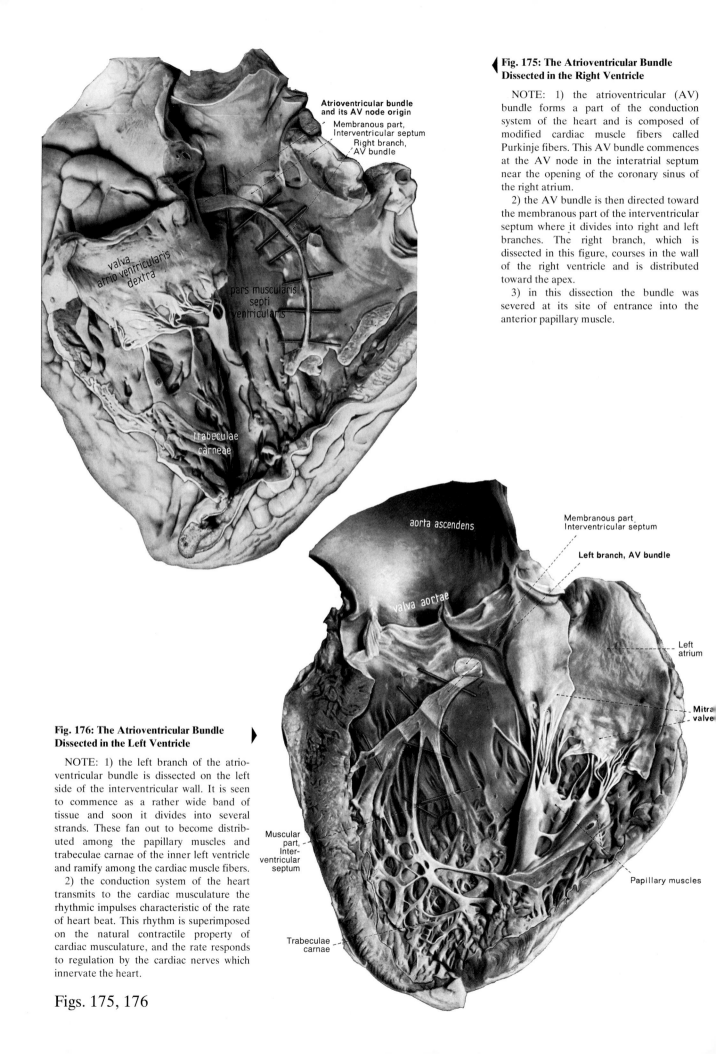

**Atrioventricular bundle and its AV node origin**

Membranous part, Interventricular septum

Right branch, AV bundle

valva atrio ventricularis dextra

pars muscularis septi ventricularis

trabeculae carneae

## Fig. 175: The Atrioventricular Bundle Dissected in the Right Ventricle

NOTE: 1) the atrioventricular (AV) bundle forms a part of the conduction system of the heart and is composed of modified cardiac muscle fibers called Purkinje fibers. This AV bundle commences at the AV node in the interatrial septum near the opening of the coronary sinus of the right atrium.

2) the AV bundle is then directed toward the membranous part of the interventricular septum where it divides into right and left branches. The right branch, which is dissected in this figure, courses in the wall of the right ventricle and is distributed toward the apex.

3) in this dissection the bundle was severed at its site of entrance into the anterior papillary muscle.

aorta ascendens

valva aortae

Membranous part, Interventricular septum

**Left branch, AV bundle**

Left atrium

Mitral valve

Papillary muscles

Muscular part, Interventricular septum

Trabeculae carneae

## Fig. 176: The Atrioventricular Bundle Dissected in the Left Ventricle

NOTE: 1) the left branch of the atrioventricular bundle is dissected on the left side of the interventricular wall. It is seen to commence as a rather wide band of tissue and soon it divides into several strands. These fan out to become distributed among the papillary muscles and trabeculae carnae of the inner left ventricle and ramify among the cardiac muscle fibers.

2) the conduction system of the heart transmits to the cardiac musculature the rhythmic impulses characteristic of the rate of heart beat. This rhythm is superimposed on the natural contractile property of cardiac musculature, and the rate responds to regulation by the cardiac nerves which innervate the heart.

Figs. 175, 176

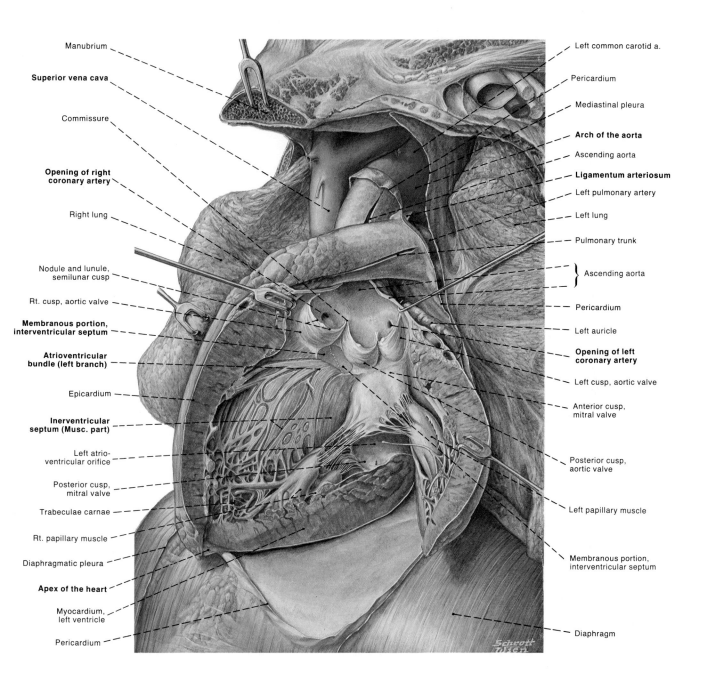

Manubrium

Superior vena cava

Commissure

Opening of right
coronary artery

Right lung

Nodule and lunule,
semilunar cusp

Rt. cusp, aortic valve

Membranous portion,
interventricular septum

Atrioventricular
bundle (left branch)

Epicardium

Inerventricular
septum (Musc. part)

Left atrio-
ventricular orifice

Posterior cusp,
mitral valve

Trabeculae carnae

Rt. papillary muscle

Diaphragmatic pleura

Apex of the heart

Myocardium,
left ventricle

Pericardium

Left common carotid a.

Pericardium

Mediastinal pleura

Arch of the aorta

Ascending aorta

Ligamentum arteriosum

Left pulmonary artery

Left lung

Pulmonary trunk

Ascending aorta

Pericardium

Left auricle

Opening of left
coronary artery

Left cusp, aortic valve

Anterior cusp,
mitral valve

Posterior cusp,
aortic valve

Left papillary muscle

Membranous portion,
interventricular septum

Diaphragm

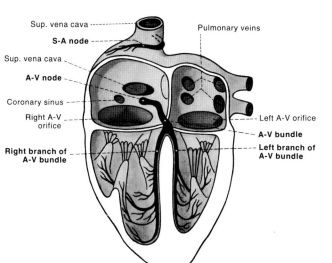

Sup. vena cava

S-A node

Sup. vena cava

A-V node

Coronary sinus

Right A-V
orifice

Right branch of
A-V bundle

Pulmonary veins

Left A-V orifice

A-V bundle

Left branch of
A-V bundle

**Fig. 177: Lateral View of the Atrioventricular Bundle (Left Branch)**

NOTE: 1) that in this dissection the left branch of the A-V bundle
has been dissected (and shown in yellow) in its course along the left side
of the interventricular septum. It is observed from within the opened
left ventricle;

2) the anterior and posterior cusps and the associated papillary muscles of the mitral valve, and the right, posterior and left cusps of the aortic valve.

**Fig. 178: Diagram of the Conduction System of the Heart**

NOTE that the sinoatrial node (S-A node) is located in the wall of
the right atrium at the junction of the superior vena cava with the right
atrium. The atrioventricular node (A-V node) lies in the septal wall of
the right atrium near the opening of the coronary sinus.

Figs. 177, 178    II

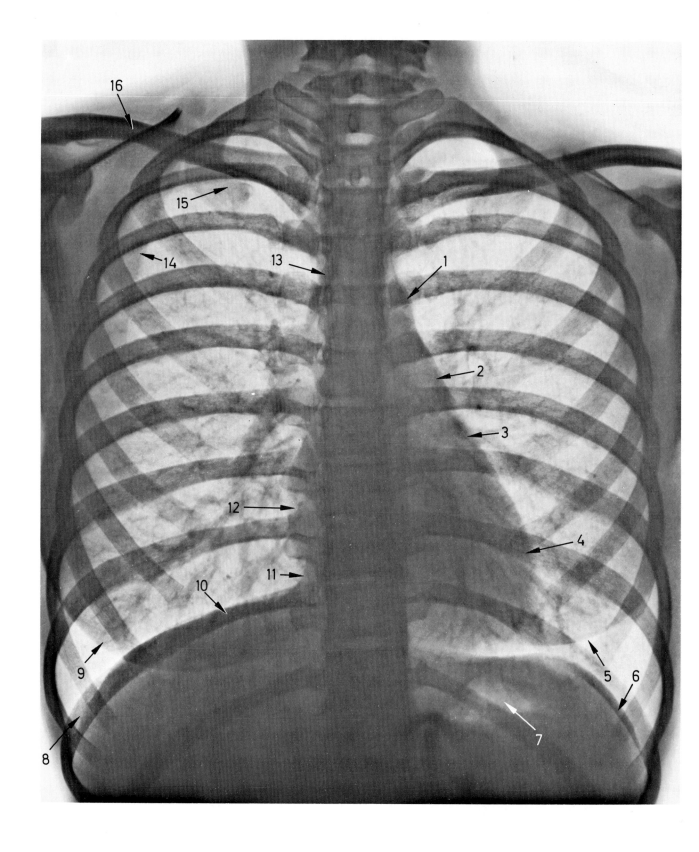

**Fig. 179: Posterior-Anterior Radiograph of the Thorax Showing the Heart and Lungs**

NOTE that this radiograph was contrast-enhanced and converted to a positive print to bring out greater detail of anatomical structures. The labelled structures are:

1. Arch of aorta
2. Pulmonary trunk
3. Left auricle
4. Left ventricle
5. Contour of left breast
6. Diaphragm
7. Air in fundus of stomach
8. Costodiaphragmatic recess
9. Contour of right breast
10. Diaphragm
11. Inferior vena cava
12. Right atrium
13. Superior vena cava
14. Medial border of scapula
15. First rib
16. Right clavicle

Fig. 179

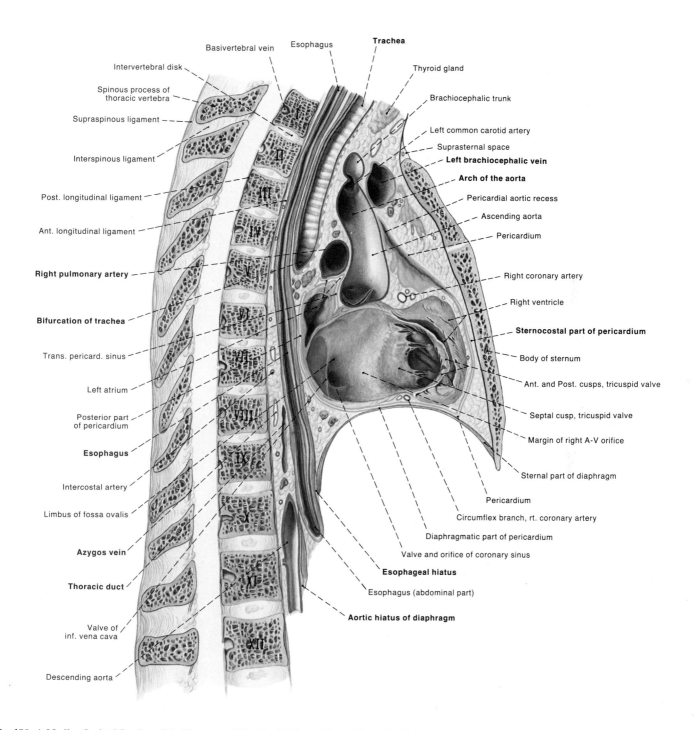

**Fig. 180: A Median Sagittal Section of the Thorax and Vertebral Column Viewed from the Right Side**

NOTE that:  1) the bodies of the thoracic vertebrae have been numbered from I to XII;

2)  a line drawn directly back from the manubriosternal joint (not labelled) to the spinal column crosses the lower end of the body of the 4th thoracic vertebra, whereas the superior border of the sternum projects back to the 2nd thoracic vertebra, and the lowest point of the xiphoid process lies at the level of the 9th thoracic vertebra;

3)  the trachea bifurcates at the level of the upper border of the 5th thoracic vertebra. The esophageal hiatus lies at the upper border of the 10th thoracic vertebra, while somewhat lower, the aortic hiatus is seen at the 11th or between the 11th and 12th thoracic vertebra;

4)  because the diaphragmatic opening for the inferior vena cava is to the right of the midline, it cannot be seen in this section; however, the vena caval foramen lies at a level between the 8th and 9th thoracic vertebrae.

Fig. 180    II

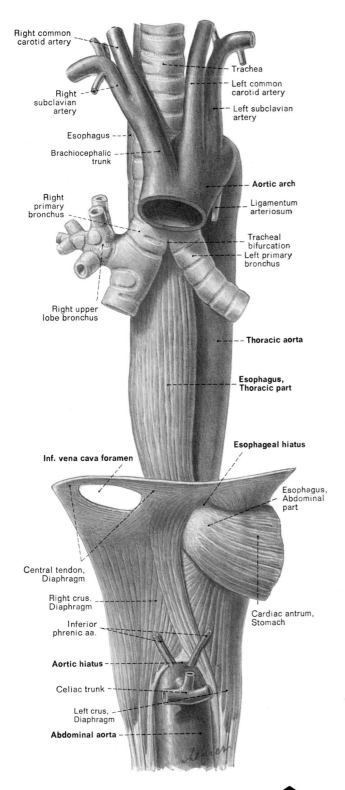

Right common
carotid artery

Right
subclavian
artery

Esophagus

Brachiocephalic
trunk

Right
primary
bronchus

Right upper
lobe bronchus

Trachea

Left common
carotid artery

Left subclavian
artery

**Aortic arch**

Ligamentum
arteriosum

Tracheal
bifurcation

Left primary
bronchus

**Thoracic aorta**

**Esophagus,
Thoracic part**

**Esophageal hiatus**

**Inf. vena cava foramen**

Esophagus,
Abdominal
part

Central tendon,
Diaphragm

Right crus,
Diaphragm

Inferior
phrenic aa.

Cardiac antrum,
Stomach

**Aortic hiatus**

Celiac trunk

Left crus,
Diaphragm

**Abdominal aorta**

## Fig. 181: The Aorta and Lower Esophagus at the Tracheal Bifurcation and Diaphragm

NOTE: 1) at the level of the bifurcation of the trachea (T-5), the esophagus lies between the trachea and the thoracic aorta. The esophagus then descends into the thorax with the aorta somewhat to its left. In the lower thorax the esophagus bends to the left and thus crosses over the aorta anteriorly from right to left.

2) the esophagus enters the abdomen through the esophageal hiatus of the diaphragm, while the aorta passes through the aortic hiatus.

Figs. 181, 182

## Fig. 182: The Relationship of the Esophagus to the Aorta and Trachea, Viewed from Right Side

NOTE: the esophagus commences above as an inferior extension of the pharynx. Superiorly, the esophagus is in relationship with the larynx and thyroid gland. Its middle third courses in relation to the trachea, bronchi and the arch of the aorta, while its lower third descends with the thoracic aorta.

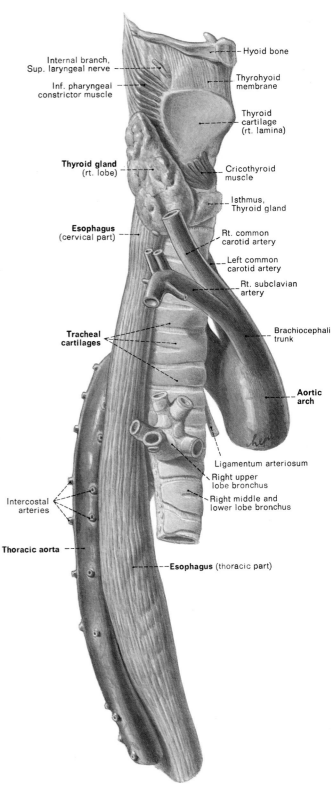

Internal branch,
Sup. laryngeal nerve

Inf. pharyngeal
constrictor muscle

Hyoid bone

Thyrohyoid
membrane

Thyroid
cartilage
(rt. lamina)

**Thyroid gland**
(rt. lobe)

Cricothyroid
muscle

Isthmus,
Thyroid gland

**Esophagus**
(cervical part)

Rt. common
carotid artery

Left common
carotid artery

Rt. subclavian
artery

**Tracheal
cartilages**

Brachiocephali
trunk

**Aortic
arch**

Ligamentum arteriosum

Right upper
lobe bronchus

Right middle and
lower lobe bronchus

Intercostal
arteries

**Thoracic aorta**

**Esophagus** (thoracic part)

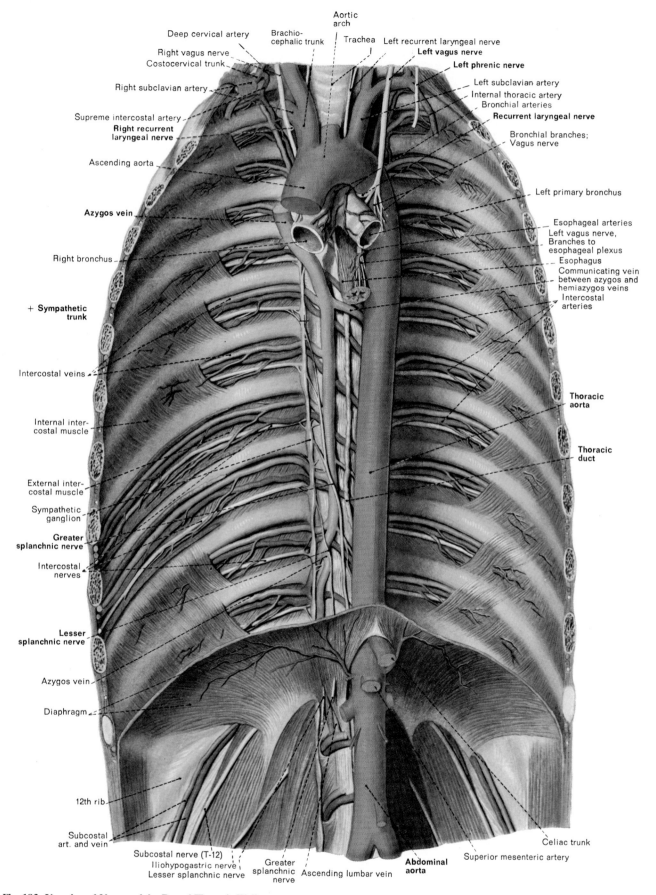

**Fig. 183: Vessels and Nerves of the Dorsal Thoracic Wall**

NOTE that the aorta ascends from the left ventricle, arches to the left behind the left pulmonary hilum, and descends through most of the thorax, just to the left side of the vertebral columm. In this course through the posterior mediastinum, the aorta gradually shifts toward the midline, which it achieves by the time it traverses the aortic hiatus to enter the abdomen.

Fig. 183    **II**

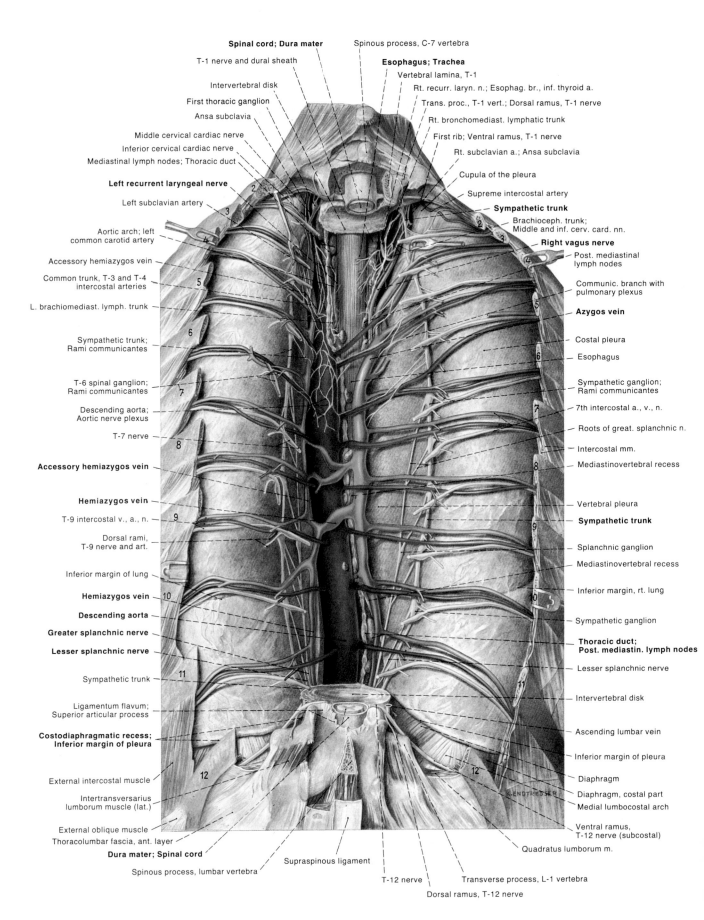

**Fig. 184: Dorsal View of the Mediastinum and Lungs with the Thoracic Vertebral Column Removed**

NOTE the azygos, hemiazygos and accessory azygos venous pattern that flows in the mediastinum but drains the intercostal spaces. Observe also the relationship of the thoracic sympathetic chain and its ganglia to the intercostal nerves.

Fig. 184

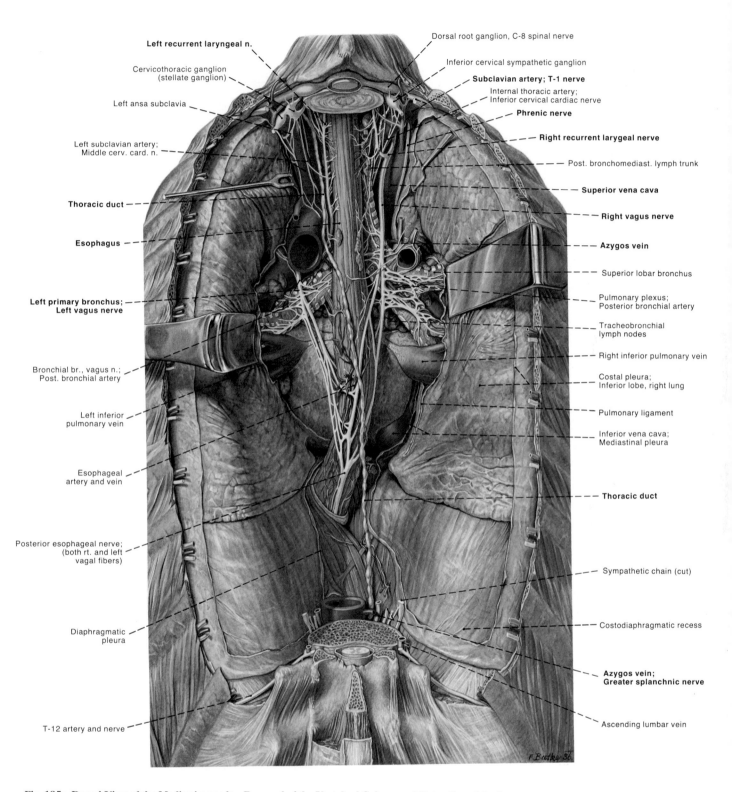

Left recurrent laryngeal n.

Cervicothoracic ganglion
(stellate ganglion)

Left ansa subclavia

Left subclavian artery;
Middle cerv. card. n.

Thoracic duct

Esophagus

Left primary bronchus;
Left vagus nerve

Bronchial br., vagus n.;
Post. bronchial artery

Left inferior
pulmonary vein

Esophageal
artery and vein

Posterior esophageal nerve;
(both rt. and left
vagal fibers)

Diaphragmatic
pleura

T-12 artery and nerve

Dorsal root ganglion, C-8 spinal nerve

Inferior cervical sympathetic ganglion

Subclavian artery; T-1 nerve

Internal thoracic artery;
Inferior cervical cardiac nerve

Phrenic nerve

Right recurrent larygeal nerve

Post. bronchomediast. lymph trunk

Superior vena cava

Right vagus nerve

Azygos vein

Superior lobar bronchus

Pulmonary plexus;
Posterior bronchial artery

Tracheobronchial
lymph nodes

Right inferior pulmonary vein

Costal pleura;
Inferior lobe, right lung

Pulmonary ligament

Inferior vena cava;
Mediastinal pleura

Thoracic duct

Sympathetic chain (cut)

Costodiaphragmatic recess

Azygos vein;
Greater splanchnic nerve

Ascending lumbar vein

**Fig. 185: Dorsal View of the Mediastinum after Removal of the Vertebral Column and Retraction of the Lungs**

NOTE: 1) that in addition to the vertebral column, the descending thoracic aorta has been removed in order to reveal the mediastinal course of the thoracic duct and esophagus. Observe the gradual right to left course of the thoracic duct as it ascends in the mediastinum;

2) that the esophagus descends behind the trachea in the superior mediastinum, but lies directly behind the pericardium below the bifurcation of the trachea;

3) the autonomic plexus of nerves, lymph nodes and bronchial vessels which characterize the hilum of each lung;

4) the course of the right vagus nerve, and observe that the right recurrent laryngeal nerve arches behind the right subclavian artery in order to achieve the neck in its ascent to the larynx.

Fig. 185    II

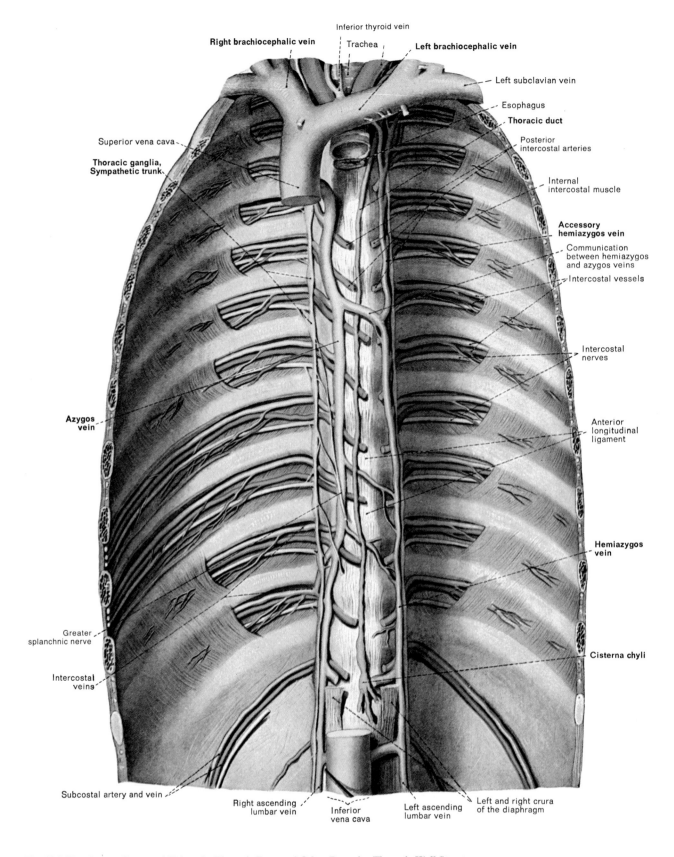

Inferior thyroid vein

**Right brachiocephalic vein**

Trachea

**Left brachiocephalic vein**

Left subclavian vein

Esophagus

**Thoracic duct**

Posterior intercostal arteries

Superior vena cava

**Thoracic ganglia, Sympathetic trunk**

Internal intercostal muscle

**Accessory hemiazygos vein**

Communication between hemiazygos and azygos veins

Intercostal vessels

Intercostal nerves

**Azygos vein**

Anterior longitudinal ligament

**Hemiazygos vein**

Cisterna chyli

Greater splanchnic nerve

Intercostal veins

Subcostal artery and vein

Right ascending lumbar vein

Inferior vena cava

Left ascending lumbar vein

Left and right crura of the diaphragm

**Fig. 186: The Azygos System of Veins, the Thoracic Duct and Other Posterior Thoracic Wall Structures**

NOTE: 1) with all the organs of the thorax and mediastinum removed or cut, the hemiazygos and accessory hemiazygos veins to the left of the vertebral column are seen communicating across the midline with the larger azygos vein. This latter vessel also ascends in the thorax to flow into the superior vena cava.

2) the thoracic duct as it arises from the cisterna chyli at the 1st lumbar level.

Fig. 186

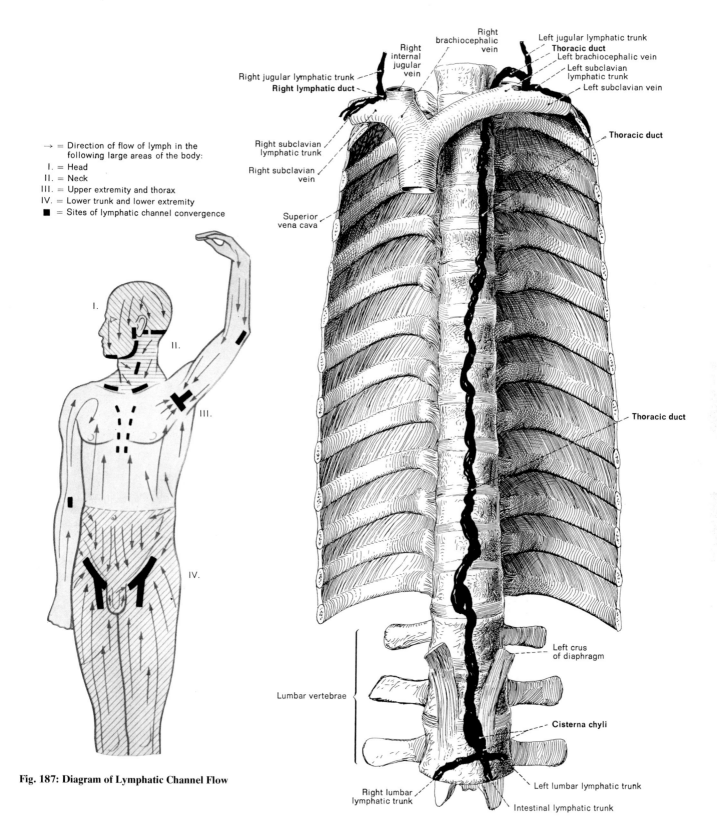

**Fig. 187: Diagram of Lymphatic Channel Flow**

→ = Direction of flow of lymph in the following large areas of the body:
I. = Head
II. = Neck
III. = Upper extremity and thorax
IV. = Lower trunk and lower extremity
■ = Sites of lymphatic channel convergence

Right internal jugular vein

Right brachiocephalic vein

Right jugular lymphatic trunk

**Right lymphatic duct**

Left jugular lymphatic trunk

**Thoracic duct**

Left brachiocephalic vein

Left subclavian lymphatic trunk

Left subclavian vein

Right subclavian lymphatic trunk

Right subclavian vein

Superior vena cava

**Thoracic duct**

**Thoracic duct**

Left crus of diaphragm

Lumbar vertebrae

**Cisterna chyli**

Right lumbar lymphatic trunk

Left lumbar lymphatic trunk

Intestinal lymphatic trunk

**Fig. 188: The Thoracic Duct: Its Origin and Course**

NOTE: 1) the thoracic duct collects the lymph from most of the body tissues and transmits it back into the blood stream. It originates in the abdomen anterior to the 2nd lumbar vertebra at the cisterna chyli. The duct then ascends into the thorax through the aortic hiatus of the diaphragm slightly to the right of the midline. Within the posterior mediastinum of the thorax and still coursing just ventral to the vertebral column, it gradually crosses the midline to the left. The duct then ascends into the root of the neck on the left side and opens into the left subclavian vein near the junction of the right internal jugular vein.

2) the right lymphatic duct receives lymph from the right side of the head, neck and trunk and from the right upper extremity. It empties into the right subclavian vein.

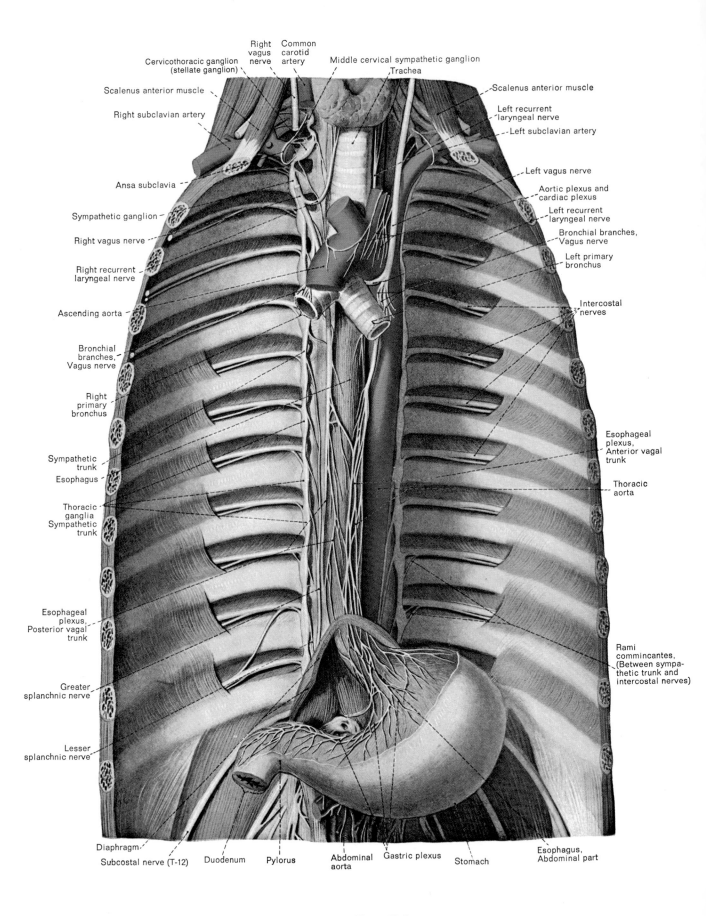

Right vagus nerve

Common carotid artery

Cervicothoracic ganglion (stellate ganglion)

Middle cervical sympathetic ganglion

Trachea

Scalenus anterior muscle

Scalenus anterior muscle

Right subclavian artery

Left recurrent laryngeal nerve

Left subclavian artery

Ansa subclavia

Left vagus nerve

Aortic plexus and cardiac plexus

Sympathetic ganglion

Left recurrent laryngeal nerve

Right vagus nerve

Bronchial branches, Vagus nerve

Right recurrent laryngeal nerve

Left primary bronchus

Ascending aorta

Intercostal nerves

Bronchial branches, Vagus nerve

Right primary bronchus

Sympathetic trunk

Esophagus

Esophageal plexus, Anterior vagal trunk

Thoracic ganglia Sympathetic trunk

Thoracic aorta

Esophageal plexus, Posterior vagal trunk

Rami commincantes, (Between sympathetic trunk and intercostal nerves)

Greater splanchnic nerve

Lesser splanchnic nerve

Diaphragm

Subcostal nerve (T-12)

Duodenum

Pylorus

Abdominal aorta

Gastric plexus

Stomach

Esophagus, Abdominal part

Fig. 189: The Sympathetic Trunks and Vagus Nerves in the Thorax and Upper Abdomen

Fig. 189

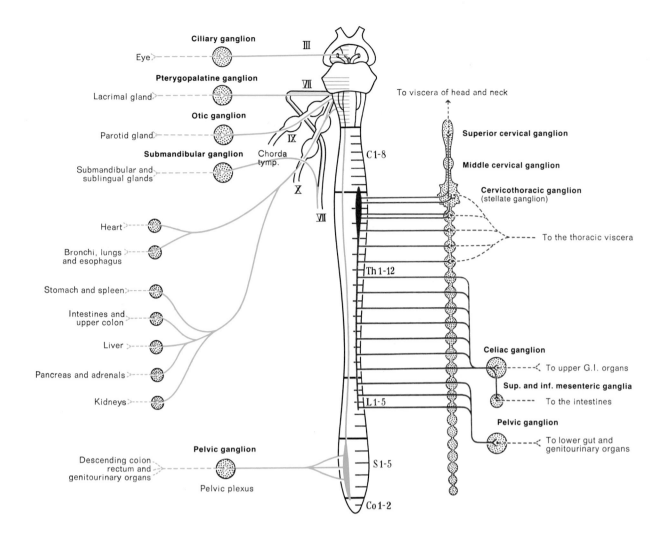

**Fig. 190: Diagram of the Autonomic Nervous System.** Blue = parasympathetic; red = sympathetic; solid lines = presynaptic neurons; broken lines = postsynaptic neurons.

NOTE: 1) the autonomic nervous system, by definition, is a two motor neuron system with the neuron cell bodies of the *presynaptic neurons* (solid lines) somewhere within the central nervous system, and the cell bodies of the *postsynaptic neurons* (broken lines) located in ganglia distributed peripherally in the body.

2) the autonomic nervous system is comprised of the nerve fibers which supply all the glands and blood vessels of the body including the heart. In so doing, all the smooth and cardiac muscle tissues (sometimes called involuntary muscles) are thereby innervated.

3) the autonomic nervous system is composed of two major divisions called the parasympathetic (in blue) and sympathetic (in red) divisions. The autonomic regulation of visceral function is, therefore, a dualistic control, i.e., most organs receive postganglionic fibers of both parasympathetic and sympathetic source.

4) the *parasympathetic division* is sometimes called a craniosacral outflow because the preganglionic cell bodies of this division lie in the brainstem and in the sacral segments of the spinal cord. Parasympathetic preganglionic fibers are found in four cranial nerves, III (oculomotor), VII (facial), IX (glossopharyngeal) and X (vagus) and in the 2nd, 3rd and 4th sacral nerves.

5) these *pre*ganglionic parasympathetic fibers then synapse with *post*ganglionic parasympathetic cell bodies in peripheral ganglia. From these ganglia the *post*ganglionic nerve fibers innervate the various organs.

6) the *sympathetic division* is sometimes called the thoracolumbar outflow because the *pre*ganglionic sympathetic neuron cell bodies are located in the lateral horn of the spinal cord between the 1st thoracic spinal segment and the 2nd or 3rd lumbar spinal segment, (i.e., from T-1 to L-3).

7) these *pre*ganglionic fibers emerge from the cord with their corresponding spinal roots and communicate with the sympathetic trunk and its ganglia where some *pre*synaptic sympathetic fibers synapse with *post*ganglionic sympathetic neurons. Other presynaptic fibers (especially those of the upper thoracic segments) ascend in the sympathetic chain and synapse with *post*ganglionic neurons in the cervicothoracic, middle and superior cervical ganglia. *Post*ganglionic fibers from these latter ganglia are then distributed to the viscera of the head and neck. Still other *pre*synaptic sympathetic fibers do not synapse in the sympathetic chain of ganglia at all, but collect to form the splanchnic nerves. These nerves course to the collateral sympathetic ganglia (celiac, superior and inferior mesenteric and pelvic ganglia) where synapse with the *post*ganglionic neuron occurs. The *post*ganglionic neurons of the sympathetic division then course to the viscera to supply sympathetic innervation.

8) the functions of the parasympathetic and sympathetic divisions of the autonomic nervous system are antagonistic to each other. The parasympathetic division constricts the pupil, decelerates the heart, lowers blood pressure, relaxes the sphincters of the gut and contracts the longitudinal musculature of the hollow organs. It is the division which is active during periods of calm and tranquility and aids in digestion and absorption. In contrast, the *sympathetic division* dilates the pupil, accelerates the heart, increases blood pressure, contracts the sphincters of the gut and relaxes the longitudinal musculature of hollow organs. It is active when the organism is challenged. It prepares for fight and flight and generally comes to the individual's defense during periods of stress and adversity.

Fig. 190    II

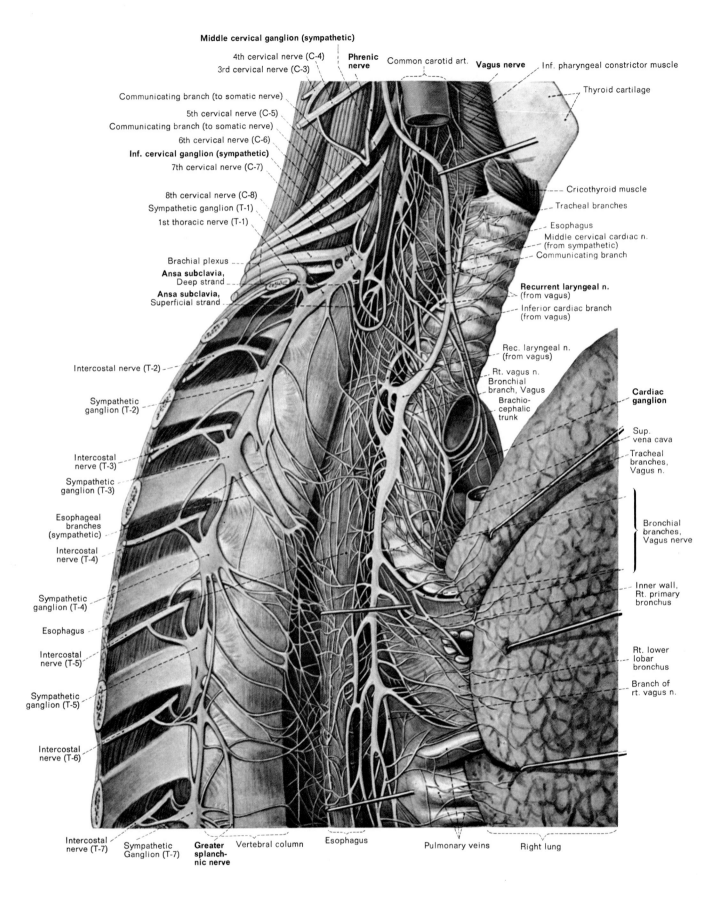

Middle cervical ganglion (sympathetic)

4th cervical nerve (C-4)

3rd cervical nerve (C-3)

**Phrenic nerve**

Common carotid art.

**Vagus nerve**

Inf. pharyngeal constrictor muscle

Thyroid cartilage

Communicating branch (to somatic nerve)

5th cervical nerve (C-5)

Communicating branch (to somatic nerve)

6th cervical nerve (C-6)

**Inf. cervical ganglion (sympathetic)**

7th cervical nerve (C-7)

8th cervical nerve (C-8)

Sympathetic ganglion (T-1)

1st thoracic nerve (T-1)

Brachial plexus

**Ansa subclavia,** Deep strand

**Ansa subclavia,** Superficial strand

Cricothyroid muscle

Tracheal branches

Esophagus

Middle cervical cardiac n. (from sympathetic)

Communicating branch

**Recurrent laryngeal n.** (from vagus)

Inferior cardiac branch (from vagus)

Rec. laryngeal n. (from vagus)

Rt. vagus n.

Bronchial branch, Vagus

Brachio-cephalic trunk

**Cardiac ganglion**

Sup. vena cava

Tracheal branches, Vagus n.

Intercostal nerve (T-2)

Sympathetic ganglion (T-2)

Intercostal nerve (T-3)

Sympathetic ganglion (T-3)

Esophageal branches (sympathetic)

Intercostal nerve (T-4)

Sympathetic ganglion (T-4)

Esophagus

Intercostal nerve (T-5)

Sympathetic ganglion (T-5)

Intercostal nerve (T-6)

Bronchial branches, Vagus nerve

Inner wall, Rt. primary bronchus

Rt. lower lobar bronchus

Branch of rt. vagus n.

Intercostal nerve (T-7)

Sympathetic Ganglion (T-7)

**Greater splanchnic nerve**

Vertebral column

Esophagus

Pulmonary veins

Right lung

**Fig. 191: The Cervical and Upper Thoracic Distribution of Autonomic Nerves**

NOTE: the organs of the posterior mediastinum are viewed from the right side by pulling the lungs forward and removing certain of the organs. Observe the two major descending nerve trunks and their associated complexes: the right vagus nerve situated more anteriorly and the right sympathetic trunk descending more posteriorly in the thorax adjacent to the costovertebral joints.

Fig. 191

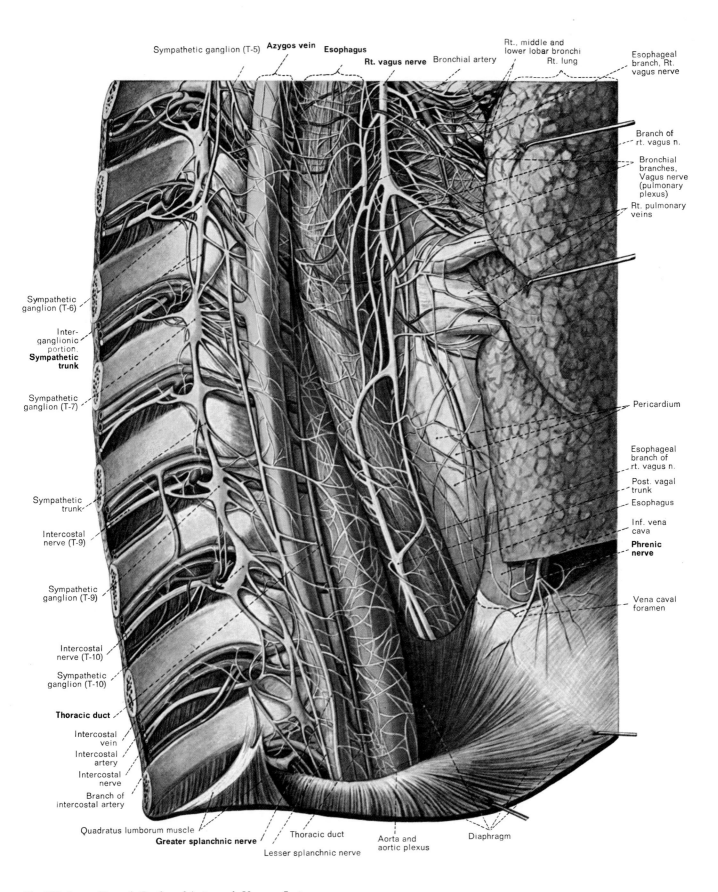

Sympathetic ganglion (T-5)  Azygos vein  Esophagus  Rt. vagus nerve  Bronchial artery  Rt., middle and lower lobar bronchi  Rt. lung  Esophageal branch, Rt. vagus nerve

Branch of rt. vagus n.

Bronchial branches, Vagus nerve (pulmonary plexus)

Rt. pulmonary veins

Sympathetic ganglion (T-6)

Inter-ganglionic portion, **Sympathetic trunk**

Sympathetic ganglion (T-7)

Pericardium

Esophageal branch of rt. vagus n.

Post. vagal trunk

Esophagus

Sympathetic trunk

Intercostal nerve (T-9)

Inf. vena cava

**Phrenic nerve**

Sympathetic ganglion (T-9)

Vena caval foramen

Intercostal nerve (T-10)

Sympathetic ganglion (T-10)

**Thoracic duct**

Intercostal vein

Intercostal artery

Intercostal nerve

Branch of intercostal artery

Quadratus lumborum muscle  **Greater splanchnic nerve**  Thoracic duct  Aorta and aortic plexus  Diaphragm

Lesser splanchnic nerve

**Fig. 192: Lower Thoracic Portion of Autonomic Nervous System**

NOTE: 1) the formation of the greater and lesser splanchnic nerves. The greater splanchnic nerve is derived from preganglionic sympathetic fibers which emerge from sympathetic ganglia T-6 to T-9 or T-10, whereas the lesser splanchnic nerve is derived from ganglia T-10 and T-11.

2) the right vagus nerve after contributing parasympathetic fibers to the esophageal plexus becomes the posterior vagal trunk dorsal to the esophagus as that organ passes through the diaphragm.

Fig. 192    II

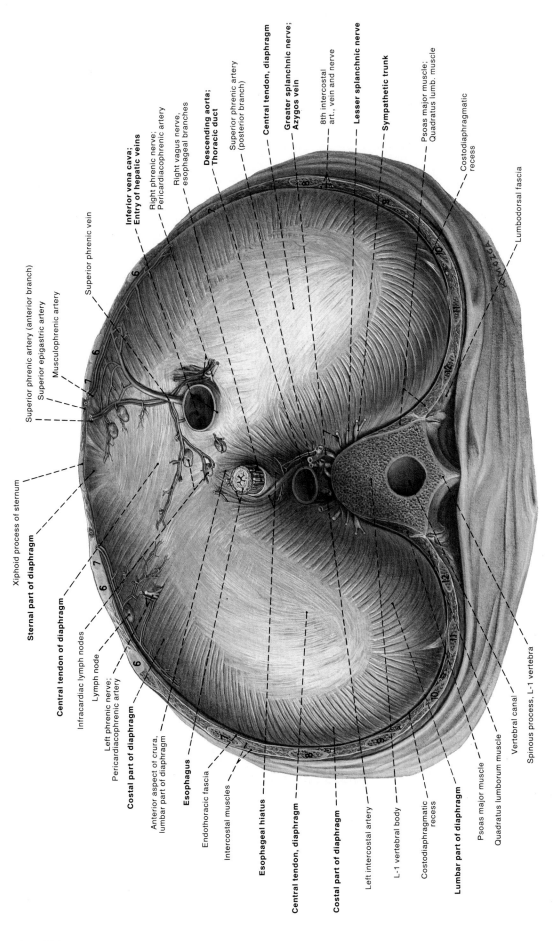

**Fig. 193: The Diaphragm: Its Openings, Blood Vessels and Nerves Viewed From Above**

NOTE: 1) that the thoracic cage has been severed transversely in a plane extending from the xiphoid process anteriorly and the body of the first lumbar vertebra posteriorly. The diaphragmatic pleurae and the pericardium have been stripped from the superior (thoracic) surface of the diaphragm;

2) the relative location of the vena caval orifice and the esophageal and aortic hiatuses. The *vena caval opening* lies to the right of the midline, is more anterior and higher (8th to 9th thoracic vertebra) than the other two. The *esophageal hiatus* lies in the midline and is the most posterior and the most inferior (L–1) of these large apertures. The *aortic hiatus*, also in the midline, lies anterior to the aortic hiatus at about the level of the 10th thoracic vertebra.

Fig. 193

Superior phrenic artery (anterior branch)

Superior epigastric artery

Musculophrenic artery

Superior phrenic vein

**Inferior vena cava;**
**Entry of hepatic veins**

Right phrenic nerve;
Pericardiacophrenic artery

Right vagus nerve,
esophageal branches

**Descending aorta;**
**Thoracic duct**

Superior phrenic artery
(posterior branch)

**Central tendon, diaphragm**

**Greater splanchnic nerve;**
**Azygos vein**

8th intercostal
art., vein and nerve

**Lesser splanchnic nerve**

**Sympathetic trunk**

Psoas major muscle;
Quadratus lumb. muscle

Costodiaphragmatic
recess

Lumbodorsal fascia

Xiphoid process of sternum

**Sternal part of diaphragm**

**Central tendon of diaphragm**

Infracardiac lymph nodes

Lymph node

**Costal part of diaphragm**

Left phrenic nerve;
Pericardiacophrenic artery

Anterior aspect of crura,
lumbar part of diaphragm

**Esophagus**

Endothoracic fascia

Intercostal muscles

**Esophageal hiatus**

**Central tendon, diaphragm**

**Costal part of diaphragm**

Left intercostal artery

L-1 vertebral body

Costodiaphragmatic
recess

**Lumbar part of diaphragm**

Psoas major muscle

Quadratus lumborum muscle

Vertebral canal

Spinous process, L-1 vertebra

# PART III: THE ABDOMEN

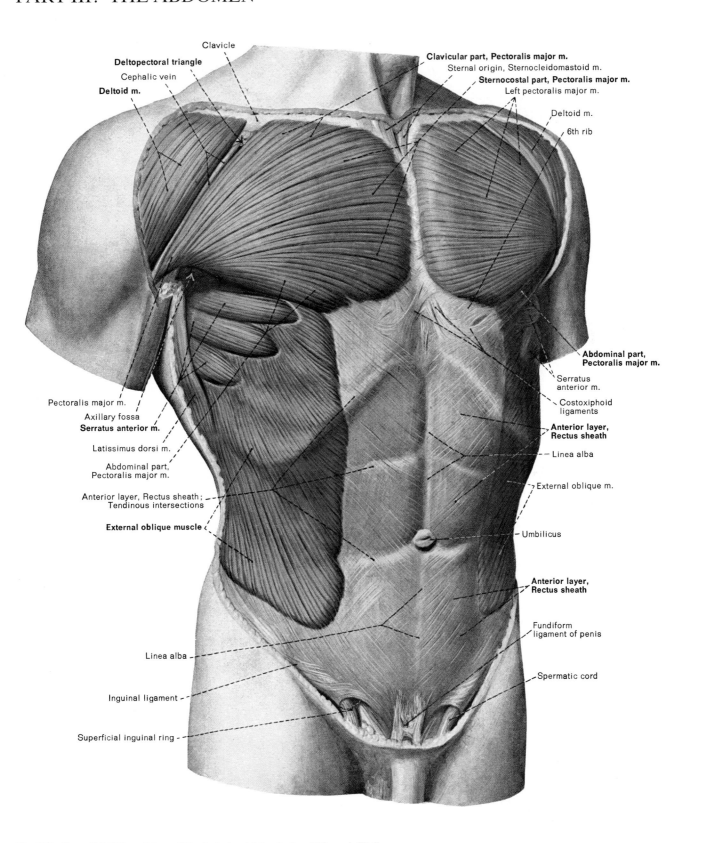

Clavicle

Deltopectoral triangle

Cephalic vein

Deltoid m.

Clavicular part, Pectoralis major m.

Sternal origin, Sternocleidomastoid m.

Sternocostal part, Pectoralis major m.

Left pectoralis major m.

Deltoid m.

6th rib

Abdominal part, Pectoralis major m.

Serratus anterior m.

Costoxiphoid ligaments

Anterior layer, Rectus sheath

Linea alba

External oblique m.

Umbilicus

Anterior layer, Rectus sheath

Fundiform ligament of penis

Spermatic cord

Pectoralis major m.

Axillary fossa

Serratus anterior m.

Latissimus dorsi m.

Abdominal part, Pectoralis major m.

Anterior layer, Rectus sheath; Tendinous intersections

External oblique muscle

Linea alba

Inguinal ligament

Superficial inguinal ring

**Fig. 194: Superficial Musculature of the Anterior Abdominal and Thoracic Wall**

NOTE:  1) the first layer of abdominal musculature consists principally of the external oblique muscle and its broad, flat aponeurosis which extends medially to the midline (forming the anterior layer of the sheath of the rectus abdominis muscle) and inferiorly as the inguinal ligament.

2)  the external oblique arises by means of 7 or 8 fleshy slips from the outer surfaces of the lower ribs (ribs 5 to 12), thereby interdigitating with the fleshy origin of the serratus anterior muscle.

Fig. 194    III

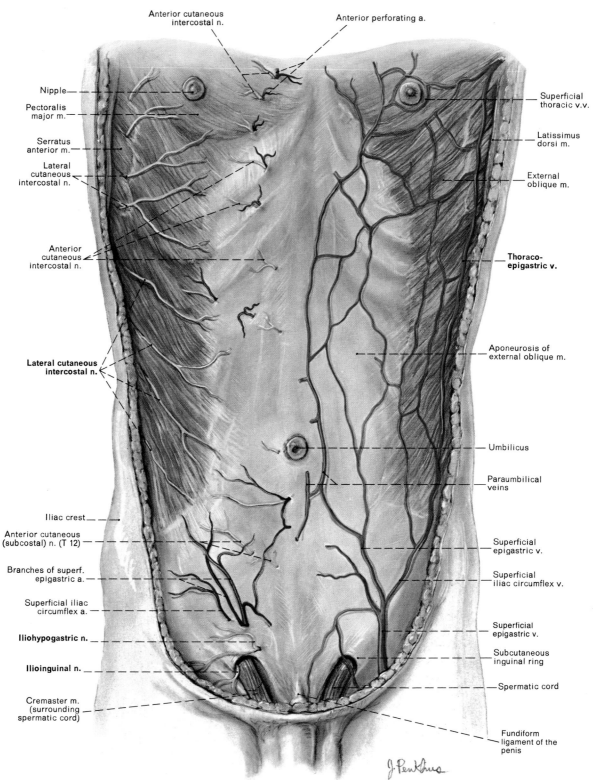

Anterior cutaneous intercostal n.

Anterior perforating a.

Nipple

Pectoralis major m.

Serratus anterior m.

Lateral cutaneous intercostal n.

Anterior cutaneous intercostal n.

**Lateral cutaneous intercostal n.**

Iliac crest

Anterior cutaneous (subcostal) n. (T 12)

Branches of superf. epigastric a.

Superficial iliac circumflex a.

**Iliohypogastric n.**

**Ilioinguinal n.**

Cremaster m. (surrounding spermatic cord)

Superficial thoracic v.v.

Latissimus dorsi m.

External oblique m.

**Thoraco-epigastric v.**

Aponeurosis of external oblique m.

Umbilicus

Paraumbilical veins

Superficial epigastric v.

Superficial iliac circumflex v.

Superficial epigastric v.

Subcutaneous inguinal ring

Spermatic cord

Fundiform ligament of the penis

**Fig. 195: Superficial Nerves and Vessels of the Anterior Abdominal Wall**

NOTE: 1) the distribution of the superficial vessels and cutaneous nerves is demonstrated upon the removal of the skin and superficial fatty layers over the lower thoracic and anterior abdominal wall.

2) the thoracic intercostal nerves supply the abdominal surface with lateral and anterior cutaneous branches.

3) in the inguinal region, the ilioinguinal and iliohypogastric branches of the 1st lumbar nerve become superficial in the region of the superficial inguinal ring.

4) the branches of superficial epigastric artery (which arises from the femoral artery) as they ascend in the inguinal region toward the umbilicus. Note also the superficial branches of the intercostal arteries.

5) the thoracoepigastric vein which serves as a means of communication between the femoral vein and the axillary vein. In cases of obstruction of the portal vein, these superficial veins become greatly enlarged forming varicose veins over the abdominal wall (sometimes this condition is called *caput medusae*).

Fig. 195

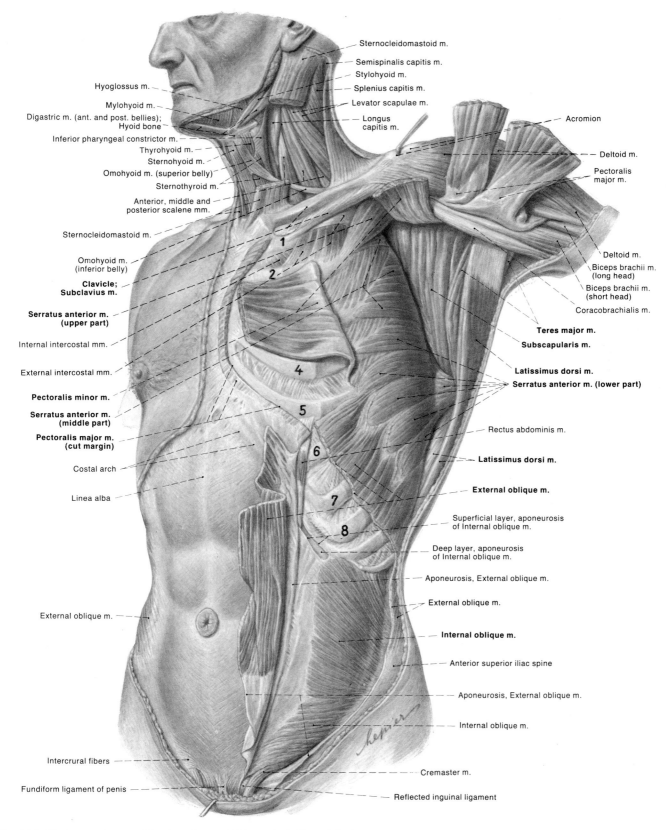

Sternocleidomastoid m.
Semispinalis capitis m.
Stylohyoid m.
Splenius capitis m.
Levator scapulae m.
Longus capitis m.

Hyoglossus m.
Mylohyoid m.
Digastric m. (ant. and post. bellies);
Hyoid bone
Inferior pharyngeal constrictor m.
Thyrohyoid m.
Sternohyoid m.
Omohyoid m. (superior belly)
Sternothyroid m.
Anterior, middle and posterior scalene mm.
Sternocleidomastoid m.
Omohyoid m. (inferior belly)
**Clavicle; Subclavius m.**
**Serratus anterior m. (upper part)**
Internal intercostal mm.
External intercostal mm.
**Pectoralis minor m.**
**Serratus anterior m. (middle part)**
**Pectoralis major m. (cut margin)**
Costal arch
Linea alba

External oblique m.

Intercrural fibers
Fundiform ligament of penis

Acromion
Deltoid m.
Pectoralis major m.
Deltoid m.
Biceps brachii m. (long head)
Biceps brachii m. (short head)
Coracobrachialis m.
**Teres major m.**
**Subscapularis m.**
**Latissimus dorsi m.**
**Serratus anterior m. (lower part)**
Rectus abdominis m.
**Latissimus dorsi m.**
**External oblique m.**
Superficial layer, aponeurosis of Internal oblique m.
Deep layer, aponeurosis of Internal oblique m.
Aponeurosis, External oblique m.
External oblique m.
**Internal oblique m.**
Anterior superior iliac spine
Aponeurosis, External oblique m.
Internal oblique m.
Cremaster m.
Reflected inguinal ligament

1
2
4
5
6
7
8

**Fig. 196: The Deeper Layers of the Musculature of the Trunk, Axilla and Neck**

NOTE that: 1) the pectoralis major and minor muscles have been reflected to reveal the underlying digitations of the serratus anterior muscle as these strands attach to the ribs forming the thoracic wall. Observe that the external oblique muscle covers a relatively large portion of the infero-lateral thoracic wall as well as stretching across the anterior abdominal wall as its external muscular layer.

2) the external oblique muscle and the lower lateral part of its aponeurosis have been severed in a semicircular manner near their origin in order to reveal the underlying internal oblique muscle. There are certain generalities about the attachments of the external and internal oblique muscles which also apply to the deepest of the anterior abdominal wall muscles, the transversus abdominis muscle: a) they all attach to the last six ribs (the external oblique frequently extending one or two ribs higher), b) they all are attached to both the iliac crest and the inguinal ligament, and c) they all insert into the linea alba.

Fig. 196    III

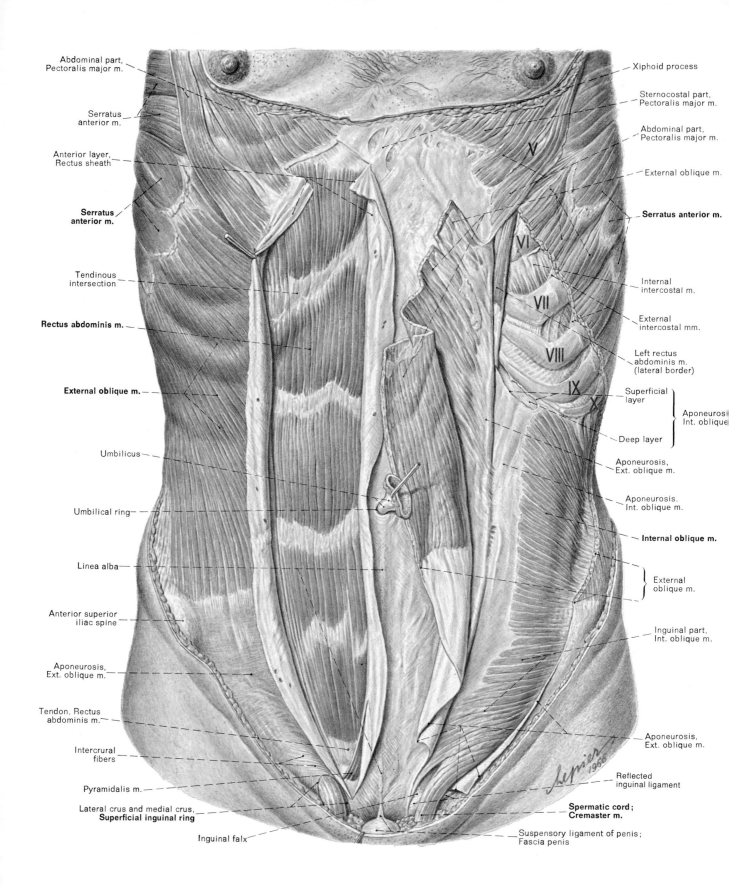

Abdominal part, Pectoralis major m.
Serratus anterior m.
Anterior layer, Rectus sheath
**Serratus anterior m.**
Tendinous intersection
**Rectus abdominis m.**
**External oblique m.**
Umbilicus
Umbilical ring
Linea alba
Anterior superior iliac spine
Aponeurosis, Ext. oblique m.
Tendon, Rectus abdominis m.
Intercrural fibers
Pyramidalis m.
Lateral crus and medial crus, **Superficial inguinal ring**
Inguinal falx

Xiphoid process
Sternocostal part, Pectoralis major m.
Abdominal part, Pectoralis major m.
External oblique m.
**Serratus anterior m.**
Internal intercostal m.
External intercostal mm.
Left rectus abdominis m. (lateral border)
Superficial layer
Deep layer
Aponeurosis, Int. oblique
Aponeurosis, Ext. oblique m.
Aponeurosis, Int. oblique m.
**Internal oblique m.**
External oblique m.
Inguinal part, Int. oblique m.
Aponeurosis, Ext. oblique m.
Reflected inguinal ligament
**Spermatic cord; Cremaster m.**
Suspensory ligament of penis; Fascia penis

V  VI  VII  VIII  IX  X

**Fig. 197: Anterior Abdominal Wall: Rectus Abdominis and Internal Oblique Muscles**

NOTE: 1) the specimen's right rectus sheath has been opened (reader's left) to reveal the right rectus abdominis muscle which is marked by transversely oriented tendinous intersections. On the specimen's left side, the external oblique muscle has been severed to reveal the second muscular layer, the internal oblique muscle. This also reveals ribs 6 through 10.

2) the muscle fibers of the external oblique course inferomedially (or in the same direction as you would put your hands in your side pockets), whereas most of the fibers of the internal oblique course in the opposite direction.

Fig. 197

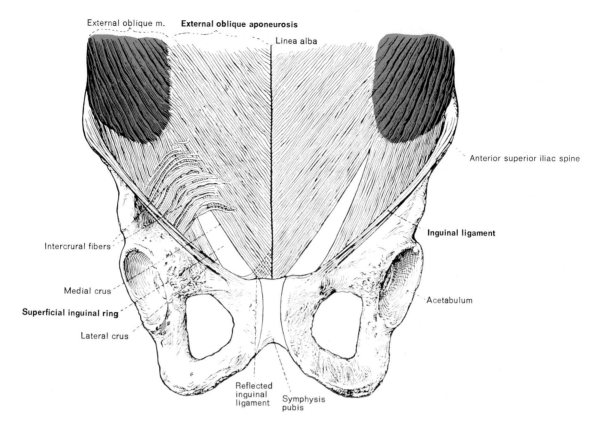

**Fig. 198: The Aponeurosis of the External Oblique Muscle**

NOTE: 1) the superficial inguinal ring is a triangular slit-like opening in the aponeurosis of the external oblique muscle. Observe how the intercrural fibers would strengthen the lateral aspect of the superficial ring by extending between the medial crus and lateral crus.

2) the inguinal ligament which extends between the anterior superior iliac spine and the pubic tubercle. This ligament is formed by the lowermost fibers of the external oblique aponeurosis and lends support to the inferior portion of the anterior abdominal wall.

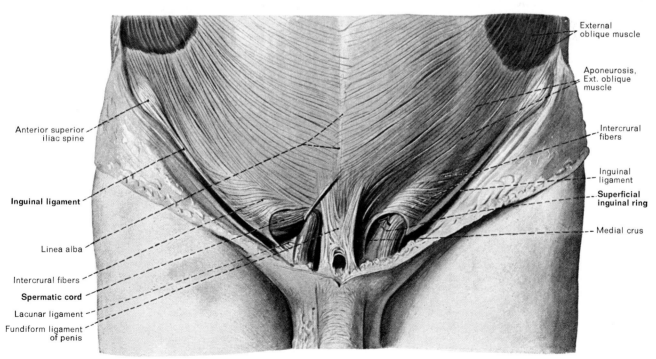

**Fig. 199: The Superficial Inguinal Ring and Spermatic Cord**

NOTE: 1) the superficial inguinal ring transmits the spermatic cord in the male and the round ligament of the uterus in the female. In this dissection, the right spermatic cord has been lifted in order to show the lateral crus of the inguinal ring.

2) the tendinous fibers of the aponeurosis are continuous with the fleshy fibers of the external oblique. They are directed inferiorly and medially and either decussate or insert into the linea alba.

Figs. 198, 199    **III**

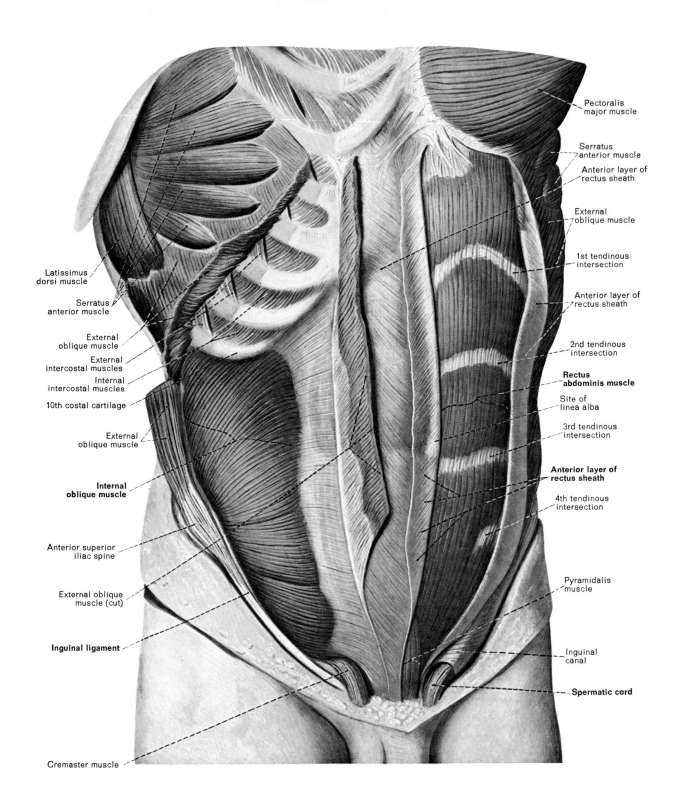

Pectoralis major muscle

Serratus anterior muscle

Anterior layer of rectus sheath

External oblique muscle

1st tendinous intersection

Anterior layer of rectus sheath

2nd tendinous intersection

**Rectus abdominis muscle**

Site of linea alba

3rd tendinous intersection

**Anterior layer of rectus sheath**

4th tendinous intersection

Pyramidalis muscle

Inguinal canal

**Spermatic cord**

Latissimus dorsi muscle

Serratus anterior muscle

External oblique muscle

External intercostal muscles

Internal intercostal muscles

10th costal cartilage

External oblique muscle

**Internal oblique muscle**

Anterior superior iliac spine

External oblique muscle (cut)

**Inguinal ligament**

Cremaster muscle

**Fig. 200: Middle Layer of Abdominal Musculature: Internal Oblique Muscle**

NOTE: 1) on the right side, the external oblique muscle has been severed and reflected to expose the right internal oblique muscle. On the left side, the anterior layer of the rectus sheath has been incised longitudinally to expose the left rectus abdominis muscle with its tendinous intersections and the small pyramidalis muscle.

2) the muscle fibers of the internal oblique muscle arise from the inguinal ligament, the iliac crest and the lumbar aponeurosis. They insert into the lower ribs above, and into an aponeurosis which contributes to the formation of the rectus sheath medially. Inferiorly, the aponeurosis of the internal oblique along with the aponeurosis of the transversus abdominis muscle forms the conjoint tendon, which is also known as the inguinal falx (shown, but not labelled). The conjoint tendon inserts into the pubic crest along with the lower end of the rectus sheath, thereby helping to provide strength to the inherently weak inguinal-pubic region.

3) the cremaster muscle. This muscular covering over the outer surface of the spermatic cord in the male represents an extension of the internal oblique (also possibly the transversus abdominis). It originates on the inguinal ligament and, after its fibers loop around the spermatic cord, inserts onto the pubis. Upon contraction this muscle lifts the testis within the scrotum toward the subcutaneous inguinal ring.

Fig. 200

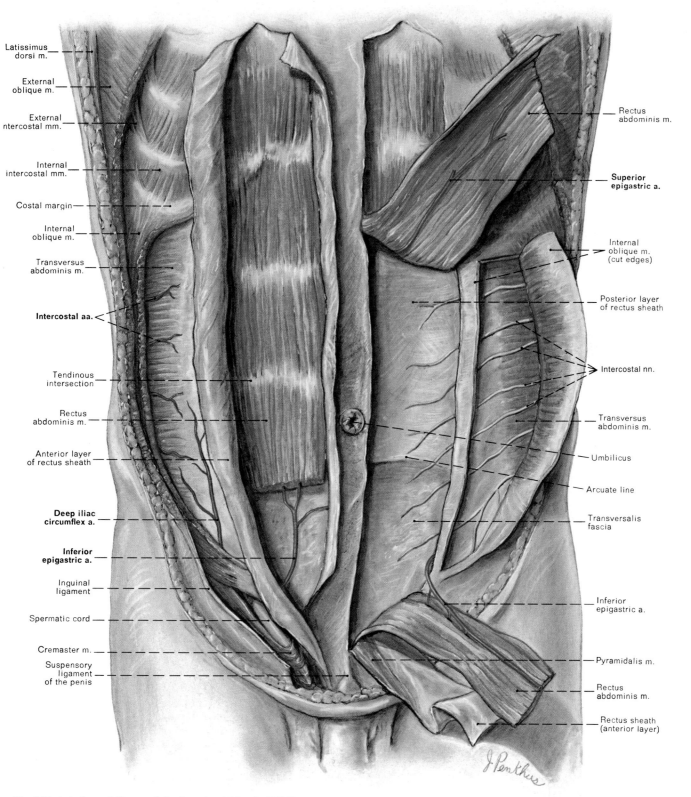

Latissimus dorsi m.

External oblique m.

External intercostal mm.

Internal intercostal mm.

Costal margin

Internal oblique m.

Transversus abdominis m.

**Intercostal aa.**

Tendinous intersection

Rectus abdominis m.

Anterior layer of rectus sheath

**Deep iliac circumflex a.**

**Inferior epigastric a.**

Inguinal ligament

Spermatic cord

Cremaster m.

Suspensory ligament of the penis

Rectus abdominis m.

**Superior epigastric a.**

Internal oblique m. (cut edges)

Posterior layer of rectus sheath

Intercostal nn.

Transversus abdominis m.

Umbilicus

Arcuate line

Transversalis fascia

Inferior epigastric a.

Pyramidalis m.

Rectus abdominis m.

Rectus sheath (anterior layer)

*J. Penkhus*

**Fig. 201: Arteries and Nerves of the Anterior Abdominal Wall**

NOTE: 1) on each side the first two layers of muscle (external oblique and internal oblique muscles) have been removed, since the vessels and nerves supplying the musculature of the anterior abdominal wall course between the internal oblique and transversus abdominis muscles.

2) thoracic nerves T7 to T12 and the 1st lumbar nerve (ilioinguinal and iliohypogastric nn.) supply the anterior abdominal musculature in their segmental course around the body.

3) in addition to segmental branches of the intercostal arteries, the deep circumflex iliac artery and the inferior epigastric artery also supply the abdominal muscles. This latter artery anastomoses with the superior epigastric artery within the rectus abdominis muscle.

Fig. 201   III

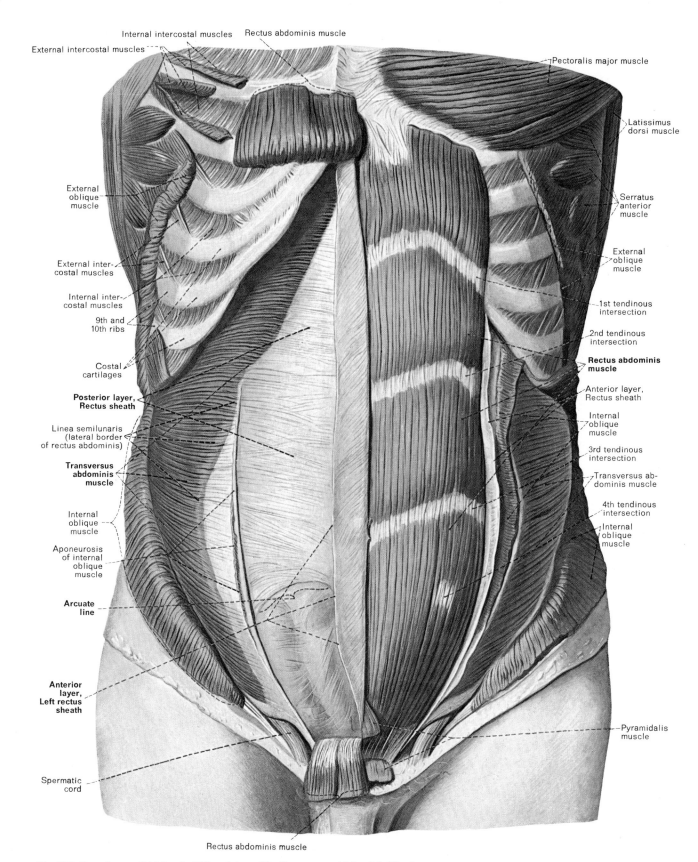

**Fig. 202: Deep Layer of Abdominal Musculature: The Transversus Abdominis Muscle**

NOTE: 1) on the right, the external and internal oblique and rectus abdominis muscles have been resected demonstrating the transversus abdominis muscle. On the left, the rectus abdominis muscle remains intact but the small pyramidalis muscle was severed to show the insertion of the left rectus.

2) on the right, the posterior layer of the rectus sheath is exposed, while on the left, the anterior layer of the sheath has been opened to demonstrate the muscle. Below the arcuate line, the posterior sheath of the rectus abdominis is wanting, and the overlying rectus muscle lies directly anterior to the transversalis fascia.

Fig. 202

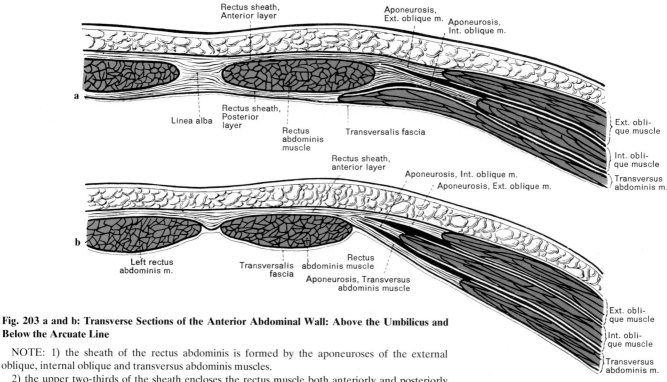

**Fig. 203 a and b: Transverse Sections of the Anterior Abdominal Wall: Above the Umbilicus and Below the Arcuate Line**

NOTE: 1) the sheath of the rectus abdominis is formed by the aponeuroses of the external oblique, internal oblique and transversus abdominis muscles.

2) the upper two-thirds of the sheath encloses the rectus muscle both anteriorly and posteriorly (a). To accomplish this, the internal oblique aponeurosis splits. Part of this aponeurosis joins the aponeurosis of the external oblique to form the anterior layer, while the other portion joins the aponeurosis of the transversus abdominis to form the posterior layer.

3) the lower one-third of the sheath (b), below the arcuate line, is deficient posteriorly, since the aponeuroses of all three muscles pass anterior to the rectus abdominis muscle.

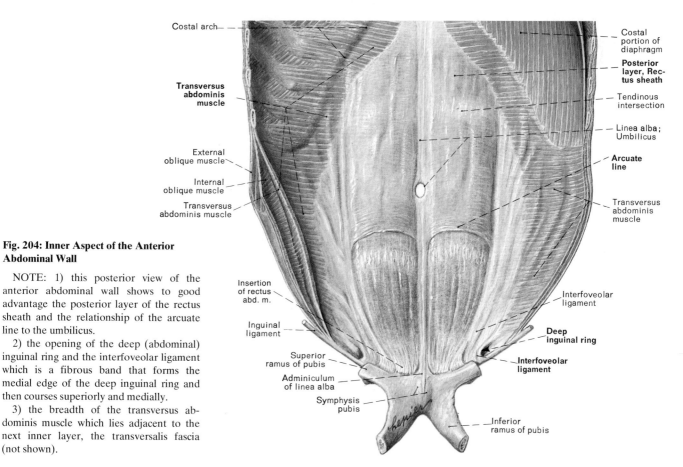

**Fig. 204: Inner Aspect of the Anterior Abdominal Wall**

NOTE: 1) this posterior view of the anterior abdominal wall shows to good advantage the posterior layer of the rectus sheath and the relationship of the arcuate line to the umbilicus.

2) the opening of the deep (abdominal) inguinal ring and the interfoveolar ligament which is a fibrous band that forms the medial edge of the deep inguinal ring and then courses superiorly and medially.

3) the breadth of the transversus abdominis muscle which lies adjacent to the next inner layer, the transversalis fascia (not shown).

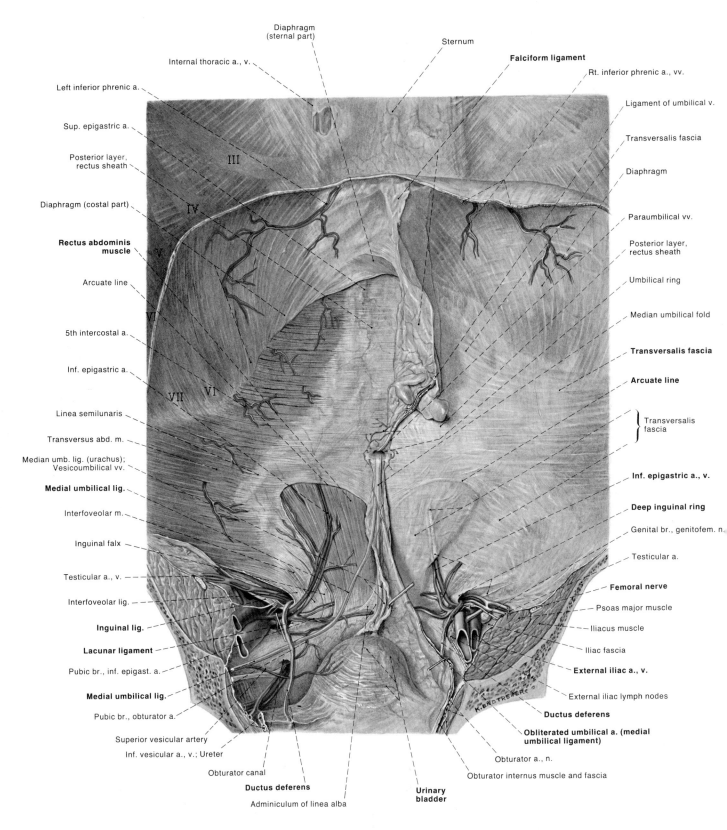

**Fig. 205: The Vessels and Umbilical Ligaments on the Inner Aspect of the Anterior Abdominal Wall**

NOTE: 1) the course of the *median umbilical ligament* (remnant of the urachus) and the two *medial umbilical ligaments* (remnants of the umbilical arteries) from their origins in the pelvis to the umbilicus. When covered with peritoneum, these structures are called umbilical folds;

2) that the two *lateral umbilical folds* represent peritoneal reflections over the inferior epigastric vessels;

3) the abdominal inguinal rings through each of which course the ductus deferens and the testicular artery and vein;

4) the passage of the external iliac artery and vein beneath the inguinal ligament on each side, thereby achieving the anterior aspect of the thigh, where the vessels become the femoral artery and vein.

Fig. 205

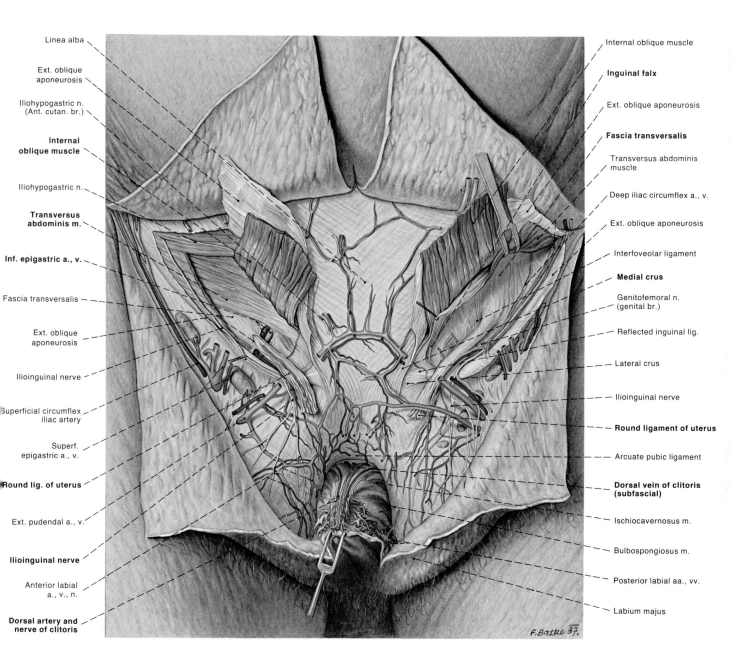

Linea alba

Ext. oblique aponeurosis

Iliohypogastric n. (Ant. cutan. br.)

**Internal oblique muscle**

Iliohypogastric n.

**Transversus abdominis m.**

**Inf. epigastric a., v.**

Fascia transversalis

Ext. oblique aponeurosis

Ilioinguinal nerve

Superficial circumflex iliac artery

Superf. epigastric a., v.

**Round lig. of uterus**

Ext. pudendal a., v.

**Ilioinguinal nerve**

Anterior labial a., v., n.

**Dorsal artery and nerve of clitoris**

Internal oblique muscle

**Inguinal falx**

Ext. oblique aponeurosis

**Fascia transversalis**

Transversus abdominis muscle

Deep iliac circumflex a., v.

Ext. oblique aponeurosis

Interfoveolar ligament

**Medial crus**

Genitofemoral n. (genital br.)

Reflected inguinal lig.

Lateral crus

Ilioinguinal nerve

**Round ligament of uterus**

Arcuate pubic ligament

**Dorsal vein of clitoris (subfascial)**

Ischiocavernosus m.

Bulbospongiosus m.

Posterior labial aa., vv.

Labium majus

F. Batke 37.

**Fig. 206: The Inguinal Region of the Anterior Abdominal Wall in the Female**

NOTE: 1) that in this anterior view, the left (reader's right) inguinal canal has been completely opened by severing the overlying transversus abdominis and internal oblique muscles, as well as the lower lateral portion of the aponeurosis of the external oblique muscle;

2) that the female inguinal canal contains the round ligament of the uterus and the artery and vein which supply that ligament. The ilioinguinal branch of the L-1 spinal nerve, along with the genital branch of the genitofemoral nerve (L-1 and L-2), both emerge from the superficial inguinal ring with the round ligament;

3) that although the genital branch of the genitofemoral nerve enters the inguinal canal with the round ligament at the deep inguinal ring, the ilioinguinal nerve does not. It joins with the contents of the inguinal canal just deep to the aponeurosis of the external oblique;

4) that the ilioinguinal nerve and the genital branch of the genitofemoral nerve, in the female, both supply sensory innervation to the inguinal region and to the labia majora;

5) that the round ligament, when leaving the superficial inguinal ring, splits into a number of fibrous strands which then become enmeshed in the subcutaneous folds of the labium majus on each side. The labia majora are the homologues of the scrotal sacs in the male;

6) the inferior epigastric artery and vein coursing just medial to the deep inguinal ring, as they do in the male;

7) that the principal superficial vessels of the inguinal region are the superficial iliac circumflex, superficial epigastric, and the external pudendal arteries and veins.

Fig. 206   III

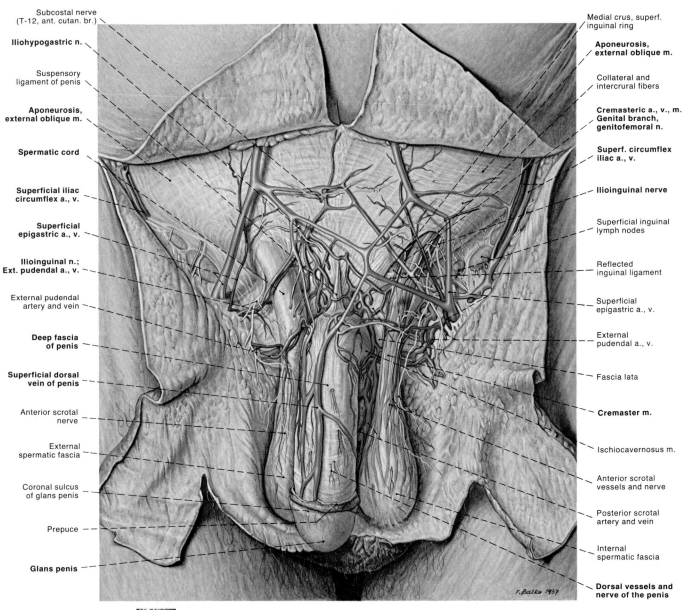

**Fig. 207:** The Superficial Inguinal Region and the Scrotum in the Male

Subcostal nerve (T-12, ant. cutan. br.)
Iliohypogastric n.
Suspensory ligament of penis
**Aponeurosis, external oblique m.**
**Spermatic cord**
**Superficial iliac circumflex a., v.**
**Superficial epigastric a., v.**
**Ilioinguinal n.; Ext. pudendal a., v.**
External pudendal artery and vein
**Deep fascia of penis**
**Superficial dorsal vein of penis**
Anterior scrotal nerve
External spermatic fascia
Coronal sulcus of glans penis
Prepuce
**Glans penis**

Medial crus, superf. inguinal ring
**Aponeurosis, external oblique m.**
Collateral and intercrural fibers
**Cremasteric a., v., m. Genital branch, genitofemoral n.**
**Superf. circumflex iliac a., v.**
**Ilioinguinal nerve**
Superficial inguinal lymph nodes
Reflected inguinal ligament
Superficial epigastric a., v.
External pudendal a., v.
Fascia lata
**Cremaster m.**
Ischiocavernosus m.
Anterior scrotal vessels and nerve
Posterior scrotal artery and vein
Internal spermatic fascia
**Dorsal vessels and nerve of the penis**

F. Batke 1937

**Fig. 207: The Superficial Inguinal Region and the Scrotum in the Male**

NOTE: 1) that the skin and fascial layers have been removed from the inguinal region, exposing the two superficial inguinal rings. The two scrotal sacs have been opened, exposing the testes and the course of the spermatic cord from the scrotum to the superficial inguinal ring;

2) the *iliohypogastric nerve* penetrating the aponeurosis of the external oblique just above the superficial inguinal ring, and the ilio-inguinal nerve emerging from the ring to supply the inguinal region and continuing into the scrotum as the anterior scrotal nerve;

3) that comparable superficial vessels supply the inguinal region in the male, as in the female (Fig. 206). These are the superficial iliac circumflex, superficial epigastric, and external pudendal.

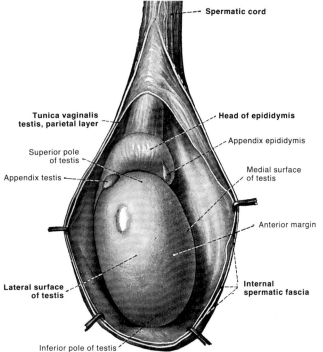

**Spermatic cord**
**Tunica vaginalis testis, parietal layer**
Superior pole of testis
Appendix testis
**Head of epididymis**
Appendix epididymis
Medial surface of testis
Anterior margin
**Lateral surface of testis**
**Internal spermatic fascia**
Inferior pole of testis

**Fig. 208: Right Testis and Epididymis (Anterior View)**

NOTE that the testis is suspended by its efferent duct system which consists of the head, body and tail of the epididymis, and that this eventually leads to the ductus deferens (see Fig. 211).

Figs. 207, 208

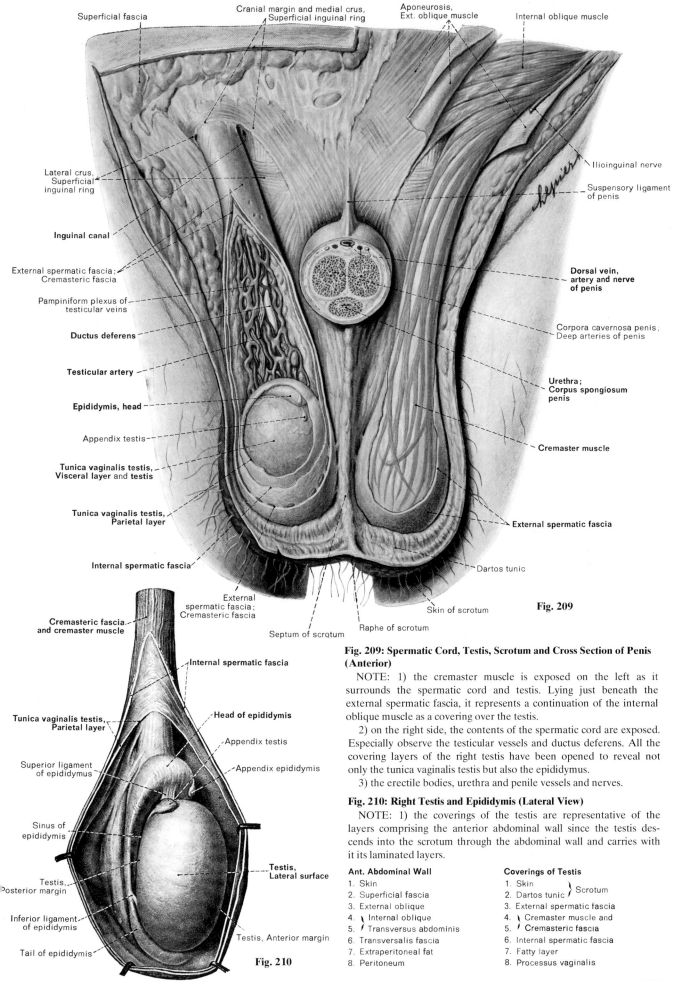

Superficial fascia

Cranial margin and medial crus,
Superficial inguinal ring

Aponeurosis,
Ext. oblique muscle

Internal oblique muscle

Lateral crus,
Superficial
inguinal ring

Ilioinguinal nerve

Suspensory ligament
of penis

Inguinal canal

External spermatic fascia;
Cremasteric fascia

Pampiniform plexus of
testicular veins

Ductus deferens

Dorsal vein,
artery and nerve
of penis

Testicular artery

Corpora cavernosa penis;
Deep arteries of penis

Epididymis, head

Urethra;
Corpus spongiosum
penis

Appendix testis

Tunica vaginalis testis,
Visceral layer and testis

Cremaster muscle

Tunica vaginalis testis,
Parietal layer

Internal spermatic fascia

External spermatic fascia

External
spermatic fascia;
Cremasteric fascia

Dartos tunic

Skin of scrotum

Fig. 209

Septum of scrotum

Raphe of scrotum

Cremasteric fascia
and cremaster muscle

Internal spermatic fascia

Head of epididymis

Tunica vaginalis testis,
Parietal layer

Appendix testis

Appendix epididymis

Superior ligament
of epididymus

Sinus of
epididymis

Testis,
Posterior margin

Testis,
Lateral surface

Inferior ligament
of epididymis

Testis, Anterior margin

Tail of epididymis

Fig. 210

**Fig. 209: Spermatic Cord, Testis, Scrotum and Cross Section of Penis
(Anterior)**

NOTE: 1) the cremaster muscle is exposed on the left as it
surrounds the spermatic cord and testis. Lying just beneath the
external spermatic fascia, it represents a continuation of the internal
oblique muscle as a covering over the testis.

2) on the right side, the contents of the spermatic cord are exposed.
Especially observe the testicular vessels and ductus deferens. All the
covering layers of the right testis have been opened to reveal not
only the tunica vaginalis testis but also the epididymus.

3) the erectile bodies, urethra and penile vessels and nerves.

**Fig. 210: Right Testis and Epididymis (Lateral View)**

NOTE: 1) the coverings of the testis are representative of the
layers comprising the anterior abdominal wall since the testis descends into the scrotum through the abdominal wall and carries with
it its laminated layers.

| **Ant. Abdominal Wall** | **Coverings of Testis** |
|---|---|
| 1. Skin | 1. Skin ⎫ Scrotum |
| 2. Superficial fascia | 2. Dartos tunic ⎭ |
| 3. External oblique | 3. External spermatic fascia |
| 4. ⎫ Internal oblique | 4. ⎫ Cremaster muscle and |
| 5. ⎭ Transversus abdominis | 5. ⎭ Cremasteric fascia |
| 6. Transversalis fascia | 6. Internal spermatic fascia |
| 7. Extraperitoneal fat | 7. Fatty layer |
| 8. Peritoneum | 8. Processus vaginalis |

Figs. 209, 210    III

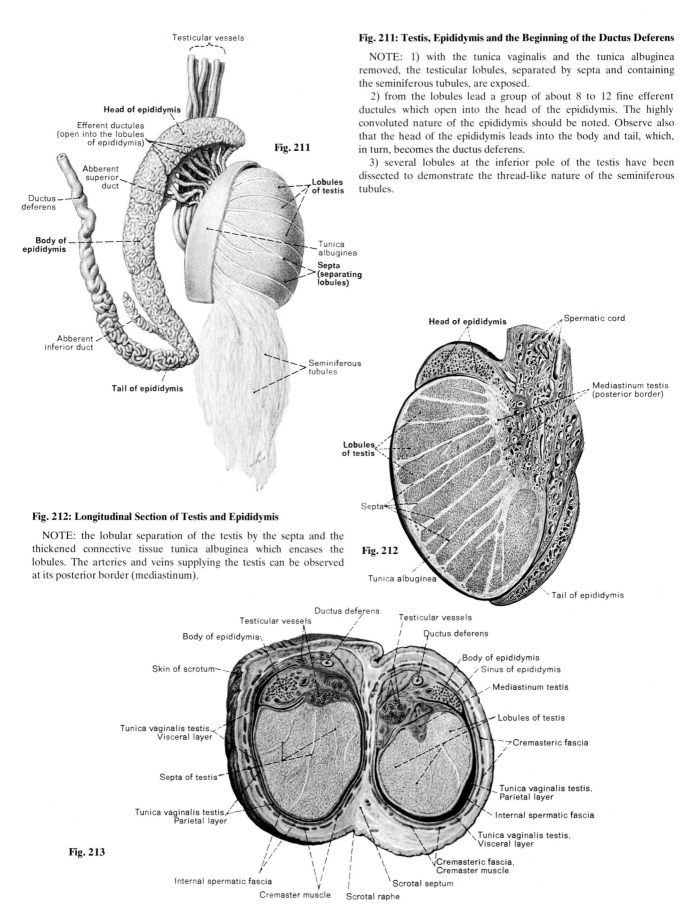

Testicular vessels

**Head of epididymis**

Efferent ductules
(open into the lobules
of epididymis)

Abberent
superior
duct

Ductus
deferens

**Body of
epididymis**

Abberent
inferior duct

**Tail of epididymis**

**Fig. 211**

**Lobules
of testis**

Tunica
albuginea

**Septa
(separating
lobules)**

Seminiferous
tubules

### Fig. 211: Testis, Epididymis and the Beginning of the Ductus Deferens

NOTE: 1) with the tunica vaginalis and the tunica albuginea removed, the testicular lobules, separated by septa and containing the seminiferous tubules, are exposed.

2) from the lobules lead a group of about 8 to 12 fine efferent ductules which open into the head of the epididymis. The highly convoluted nature of the epididymis should be noted. Observe also that the head of the epididymis leads into the body and tail, which, in turn, becomes the ductus deferens.

3) several lobules at the inferior pole of the testis have been dissected to demonstrate the thread-like nature of the seminiferous tubules.

### Fig. 212: Longitudinal Section of Testis and Epididymis

NOTE: the lobular separation of the testis by the septa and the thickened connective tissue tunica albuginea which encases the lobules. The arteries and veins supplying the testis can be observed at its posterior border (mediastinum).

Head of epididymis

Spermatic cord

Mediastinum testis
(posterior border)

**Lobules
of testis**

Septa

**Fig. 212**

Tunica albuginea

Tail of epididymis

Ductus deferens

Testicular vessels

Body of epididymis

Testicular vessels

Ductus deferens

Skin of scrotum

Body of epididymis

Sinus of epididymis

Mediastinum testis

Lobules of testis

Cremasteric fascia

Tunica vaginalis testis,
Visceral layer

Septa of testis

Tunica vaginalis testis,
Parietal layer

Tunica vaginalis testis,
Parietal layer

Internal spermatic fascia

Tunica vaginalis testis,
Visceral layer

Cremasteric fascia,
Cremaster muscle

Internal spermatic fascia

Cremaster muscle

Scrotal raphe

Scrotal septum

**Fig. 213**

### Fig. 213: Cross Section of Testis and Scrotum

NOTE: the scrotum is divided by the median raphe and septum into two lateral compartments, each surrounding an ovoid-shaped testis. The two scrotal compartments do not communicate.

Figs. 211, 212, 213

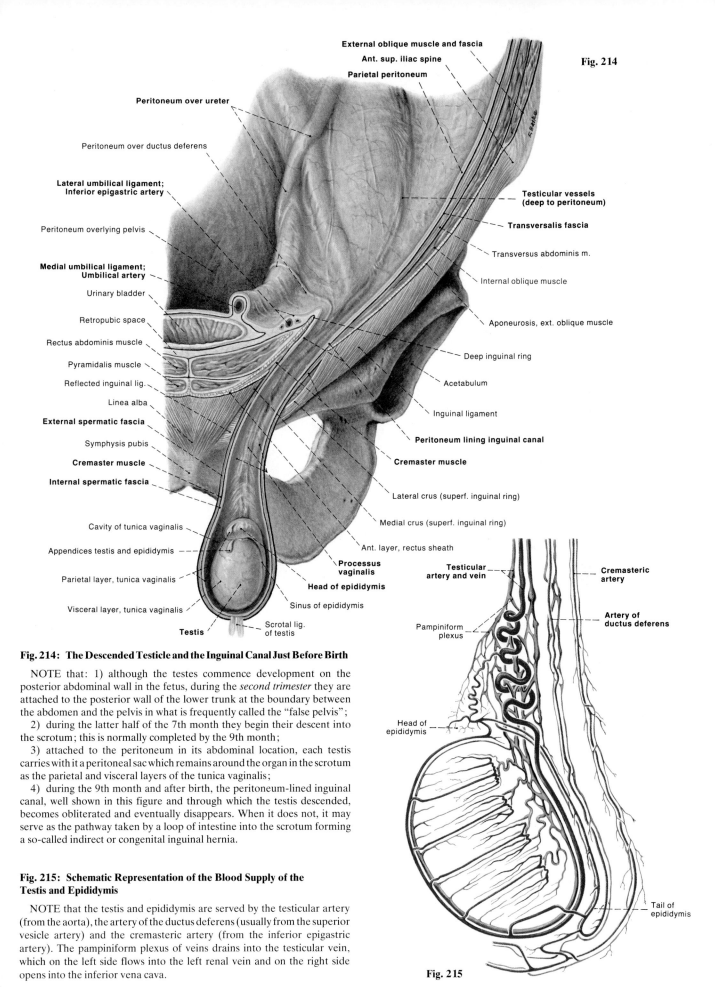

**External oblique muscle and fascia**
**Ant. sup. iliac spine**
**Parietal peritoneum**

Fig. 214

**Peritoneum over ureter**

Peritoneum over ductus deferens

**Lateral umbilical ligament;**
**Inferior epigastric artery**

Peritoneum overlying pelvis

**Medial umbilical ligament;**
**Umbilical artery**

Urinary bladder

Retropubic space

Rectus abdominis muscle

Pyramidalis muscle

Reflected inguinal lig.

Linea alba

**External spermatic fascia**

Symphysis pubis

**Cremaster muscle**

**Internal spermatic fascia**

Cavity of tunica vaginalis

Appendices testis and epididymis

Parietal layer, tunica vaginalis

Visceral layer, tunica vaginalis

**Testis**

**Testicular vessels**
**(deep to peritoneum)**

**Transversalis fascia**

Transversus abdominis m.

Internal oblique muscle

Aponeurosis, ext. oblique muscle

Deep inguinal ring

Acetabulum

Inguinal ligament

**Peritoneum lining inguinal canal**

**Cremaster muscle**

Lateral crus (superf. inguinal ring)

Medial crus (superf. inguinal ring)

Ant. layer, rectus sheath

**Processus**
**vaginalis**

**Head of epididymis**

Sinus of epididymis

Scrotal lig.
of testis

**Testicular**
**artery and vein**

**Cremasteric**
**artery**

**Artery of**
**ductus deferens**

Pampiniform
plexus

Head of
epididymis

Tail of
epididymis

**Fig. 215**

**Fig. 214: The Descended Testicle and the Inguinal Canal Just Before Birth**

NOTE that: 1) although the testes commence development on the posterior abdominal wall in the fetus, during the *second trimester* they are attached to the posterior wall of the lower trunk at the boundary between the abdomen and the pelvis in what is frequently called the "false pelvis";

2) during the latter half of the 7th month they begin their descent into the scrotum; this is normally completed by the 9th month;

3) attached to the peritoneum in its abdominal location, each testis carries with it a peritoneal sac which remains around the organ in the scrotum as the parietal and visceral layers of the tunica vaginalis;

4) during the 9th month and after birth, the peritoneum-lined inguinal canal, well shown in this figure and through which the testis descended, becomes obliterated and eventually disappears. When it does not, it may serve as the pathway taken by a loop of intestine into the scrotum forming a so-called indirect or congenital inguinal hernia.

**Fig. 215: Schematic Representation of the Blood Supply of the Testis and Epididymis**

NOTE that the testis and epididymis are served by the testicular artery (from the aorta), the artery of the ductus deferens (usually from the superior vesicle artery) and the cremasteric artery (from the inferior epigastric artery). The pampiniform plexus of veins drains into the testicular vein, which on the left side flows into the left renal vein and on the right side opens into the inferior vena cava.

Figs. 214, 215      **III**

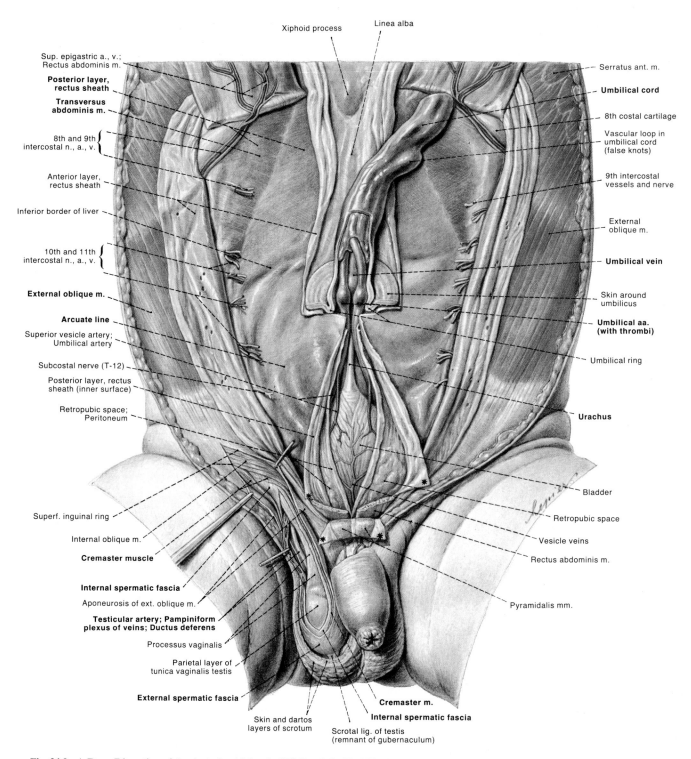

Xiphoid process    Linea alba

Sup. epigastric a., v.;
Rectus abdominis m.

**Posterior layer,
rectus sheath**

**Transversus
abdominis m.**

8th and 9th
intercostal n., a., v.

Anterior layer,
rectus sheath

Inferior border of liver

10th and 11th
intercostal n., a., v.

**External oblique m.**

**Arcuate line**

Superior vesicle artery;
Umbilical artery

Subcostal nerve (T-12)

Posterior layer, rectus
sheath (inner surface)

Retropubic space;
Peritoneum

Superf. inguinal ring

Internal oblique m.

**Cremaster muscle**

**Internal spermatic fascia**

Aponeurosis of ext. oblique m.

**Testicular artery; Pampiniform
plexus of veins; Ductus deferens**

Processus vaginalis

Parietal layer of
tunica vaginalis testis

**External spermatic fascia**

Skin and dartos
layers of scrotum

Scrotal lig. of testis
(remnant of gubernaculum)

Serratus ant. m.

**Umbilical cord**

8th costal cartilage

Vascular loop in
umbilical cord
(false knots)

9th intercostal
vessels and nerve

External
oblique m.

**Umbilical vein**

Skin around
umbilicus

**Umbilical aa.
(with thrombi)**

Umbilical ring

**Urachus**

Bladder

Retropubic space

Vesicle veins

Rectus abdominis m.

Pyramidalis mm.

**Cremaster m.**

**Internal spermatic fascia**

**Fig. 216: A Deep Dissection of the Anterior Abdominal Wall and the Umbilical Region in the Newborn**

NOTE: 1) that the anterior layer of the rectus sheath has been severed and reflected laterally on each side. The two rectus abdominis muscles have been severed near the symphysis pubis and reflected superiorly (almost out of view) in order to reveal the posterior layer of the rectus sheath. Observe the arcuate line.

2) that an incision has been made in the linea alba between the umbilical ring and the symphysis pubis exposing the apex of the bladder, the urachus, the five umbilical arteries and the single umbilical vein.

3) that the anterior aspect of the right spermatic cord and right scrotal sac have been opened to uncover the ductus deferens and the testis, the latter structure surrounded by the tunica vaginalis testis.

4) the severed umbilical cord which is usually between one and two centimeters in diameter and about 50 centimeters (20 inches) long. It contains the two umbilical arteries and the umbilical vein which are surrounded by a mucoid form of connective tissue called Wharton's jelly. Frequently the umbilical vessels form harmless loops in the cord called "false knots" (see as bulges in this figure). More rarely looping of the cord may be of some functional significance and such "true knots" may alter the circulation to and from the fetus, causing vascular obstruction.

5) the bulges in the umbilical arteries. These are *in situ* blood clots, called thrombi, which occlude the arteries, but which are probably postmortem phenomena in this instance.

Fig. 216

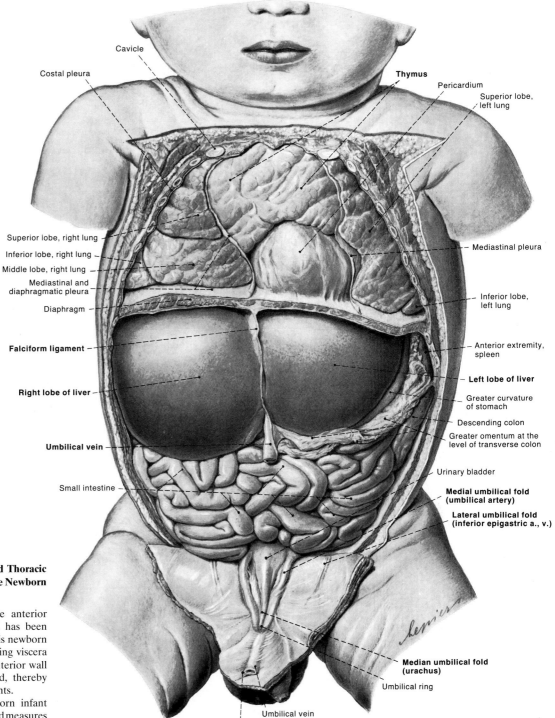

Cavicle

Costal pleura

**Thymus**

Pericardium

Superior lobe,
left lung

Superior lobe, right lung

Inferior lobe, right lung

Middle lobe, right lung

Mediastinal and
diaphragmatic pleura

Diaphragm

**Falciform ligament**

**Right lobe of liver**

**Umbilical vein**

Small intestine

Mediastinal pleura

Inferior lobe,
left lung

Anterior extremity,
spleen

**Left lobe of liver**

Greater curvature
of stomach

Descending colon

Greater omentum at the
level of transverse colon

Urinary bladder

**Medial umbilical fold
(umbilical artery)**

**Lateral umbilical fold
(inferior epigastric a., v.)**

**Median umbilical fold
(urachus)**

Umbilical ring

Umbilical vein

Falciform ligament

**Fig. 217: The Abdominal and Thoracic
Viscera Observed** *In Situ* **in the Newborn
Child**

NOTE: 1) that the entire anterior
thoracic and abdominal wall has been
removed from the trunk in this newborn
child, uncovering the underlying viscera
in both cavities. The lower anterior wall
has been reflected downward, thereby
exposing the umbilical ligaments.

2) that the average newborn infant
weighs about 3300 gr (7 lbs) and measures
about 50 cm (20 inches) from the top of
the head to the sole of the foot, and the
umbilicus is located about 1.5 cm below
the mid-point of this crown-heel length.

3) that the transverse diameter of the abdominal cavity in the newborn is greatest above the umbilicus, principally due to the inordinate proportion of the abdomen occupied by the liver. Observe that a greater area (than in the adult) of the anterior surface of both lobes lies immediately deep to the abdominal musculature and that the ribs (cut away in this figure) afford less protection to the upper abdomen.

4) that the average weight of the liver in the newborn is about 120 gr, and it constitutes 4 percent of the body weight at birth. In the adult, the liver weighs 12 to 13 times its weight at birth, but accounts for only 2.5 to 3.5 percent of the total body weight.

5) that most of the anterior surface of the stomach lies deep to the left lobe of the liver, allowing only a small portion of the greater curvature to be visible. The left lobe of the liver almost reaches the spleen.

6) that the loops of intestine form an oval-shaped mass, the greatest diameter of which is transverse in contrast to the adult in which it is vertical.

7) the broad-based truncated shape of the thoracic cavity and the large size of the thymus which weighs about 10 gr at birth (it accounts for 0.42 percent of body weight at birth, compared to 0.03 to 0.05 percent in the adult).

8) that the facts mentioned in 2, 3, 4, 6, and 7 are taken from: Crelin, Edmund S., *Functional Anatomy of the Newborn,* Yale University Press, New Haven, 1973. This is an excellent and short monograph (87 pages) which would be of benefit for any medical student to read.

Fig. 217    **III**

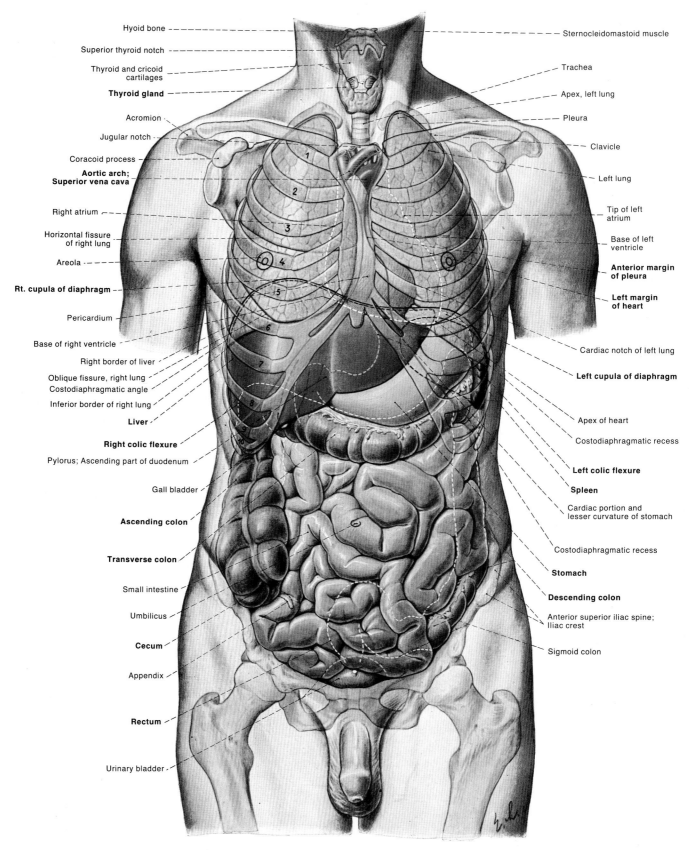

**Fig. 218: Frontal View of Thoracic and Abdominal Viscera**

NOTE that the surface projections of the heart, stomach, gall bladder, spleen, transverse colon, descending and sigmoid colon, rectum, and urinary bladder are indicated by white broken outlines. The limits of the pleura are shown as solid blue lines and the spleen as a purple broken line. The gall bladder is shown as a broken blue line.

Fig. 218

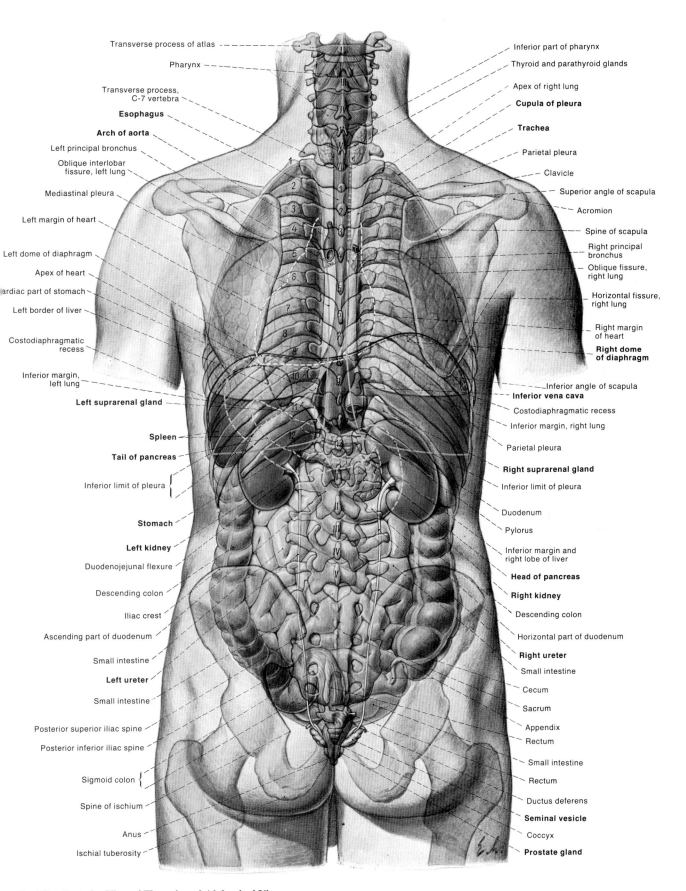

Transverse process of atlas
Pharynx
Transverse process, C-7 vertebra
**Esophagus**
**Arch of aorta**
Left principal bronchus
Oblique interlobar fissure, left lung
Mediastinal pleura
Left margin of heart
Left dome of diaphragm
Apex of heart
Cardiac part of stomach
Left border of liver
Costodiaphragmatic recess
Inferior margin, left lung
**Left suprarenal gland**
**Spleen**
**Tail of pancreas**
Inferior limit of pleura
**Stomach**
**Left kidney**
Duodenojejunal flexure
Descending colon
Iliac crest
Ascending part of duodenum
Small intestine
**Left ureter**
Small intestine
Posterior superior iliac spine
Posterior inferior iliac spine
Sigmoid colon
Spine of ischium
Anus
Ischial tuberosity

Inferior part of pharynx
Thyroid and parathyroid glands
Apex of right lung
**Cupula of pleura**
**Trachea**
Parietal pleura
Clavicle
Superior angle of scapula
Acromion
Spine of scapula
Right principal bronchus
Oblique fissure, right lung
Horizontal fissure, right lung
Right margin of heart
**Right dome of diaphragm**
Inferior angle of scapula
**Inferior vena cava**
Costodiaphragmatic recess
Inferior margin, right lung
Parietal pleura
**Right suprarenal gland**
Inferior limit of pleura
Duodenum
Pylorus
Inferior margin and right lobe of liver
**Head of pancreas**
**Right kidney**
Descending colon
Horizontal part of duodenum
**Right ureter**
Small intestine
Cecum
Sacrum
Appendix
Rectum
Small intestine
Rectum
Ductus deferens
**Seminal vesicle**
Coccyx
**Prostate gland**

**Fig. 219:  Posterior View of Thoracic and Abdominal Viscera**

   NOTE that the surface projections of the heart, stomach and duodenum are shown as white broken lines, the body and tail of the pancreas as yellow broken lines, the liver as brown broken lines, the superior pole of the spleen as a purple broken line, and the limits of the pleura as solid blue lines.

Fig. 219     III

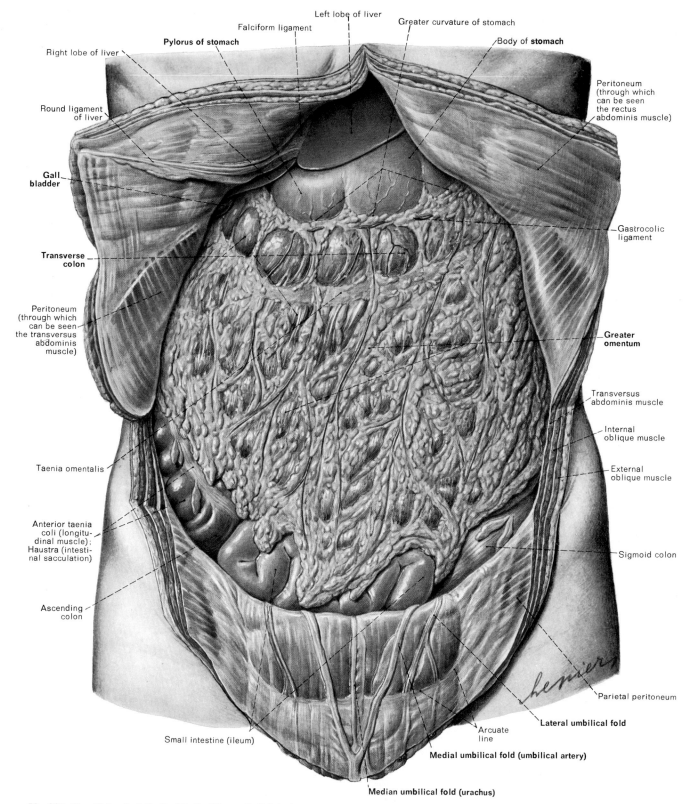

**Fig. 220: The Abdominal Cavity (1), the Viscera Left Intact**

Labels on figure:
Right lobe of liver
Round ligament of liver
Gall bladder
Transverse colon
Peritoneum (through which can be seen the transversus abdominis muscle)
Taenia omentalis
Anterior taenia coli (longitudinal muscle); Haustra (intestinal sacculation)
Ascending colon
Small intestine (ileum)
**Pylorus of stomach**
Falciform ligament
Left lobe of liver
Greater curvature of stomach
Body of **stomach**
Peritoneum (through which can be seen the rectus abdominis muscle)
Gastrocolic ligament
**Greater omentum**
Transversus abdominis muscle
Internal oblique muscle
External oblique muscle
Sigmoid colon
Parietal peritoneum
**Lateral umbilical fold**
Arcuate line
**Medial umbilical fold (umbilical artery)**
Median umbilical fold (urachus)

NOTE: 1) the greater omentum, which attaches along the greater curvature of the stomach, covers most of the intestines like an apron, and extends inferiorly almost as far as the pelvis.

2) the falciform ligament and round ligament of the liver (ligamentum teres). The falciform ligament is a remnant of the ventral mesogastrium. It extends between the liver and the anterior wall and separates the left and right lobes of the liver. The round ligament is the remains of the obliterated umbilical vein.

3) on the inner surface of the anterior wall identify

a) *the median umbilical fold* = the remains of the urachus, which in the fetus extends between the bladder and the umbilicus.

b) *the medial umbilical folds* = the obliterated umbilical arteries, which, before birth, coursed from the common iliac arteries to the umbilicus.

c) *the lateral umbilical folds* = which represent a reflection of peritoneum over the inferior epigastric vessels.

Fig. 220

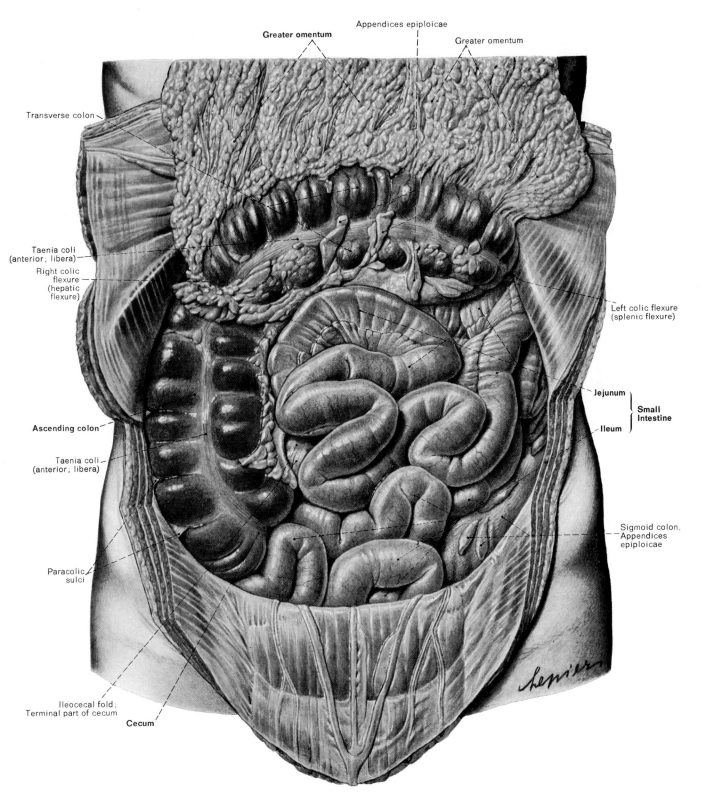

Greater omentum   Appendices epiploicae   Greater omentum

Transverse colon

Taenia coli
(anterior; libera)

Right colic
flexure
(hepatic
flexure)

Left colic flexure
(splenic flexure)

Jejunum
Small
Intestine
Ileum

Ascending colon

Taenia coli
(anterior, libera)

Sigmoid colon,
Appendices
epiploicae

Paracolic
sulci

Ileocecal fold;
Terminal part of cecum

Cecum

**Fig. 221: The Abdominal Cavity (2), the Ascending Colon and the Transverse Colon and its Mesocolon**

NOTE: 1) with the greater omentum reflected superiorly, the transverse colon comes into view as it crosses the abdominal cavity from right to left, in continuity with the ascending colon on the right and the descending colon (not shown in this figure; see Figs. 261 and 262) on the left. Observe the longitudinal muscles (taeniae) along the outer surface of the colon. Since these muscles are shorter than the other coats of the large intestine, they cause sacculations which are called haustrae.

2) that small, smooth irregular fatty masses called appendices epiploicae are suspended from the large intestine, thereby assisting in its identification.

3) below the mesocolon (inframesocolic) can be seen the small intestine which consists of three portions, the duodenum (see Figs. 246–248), jejunum and ileum. The outer walls of the small intestine are smooth and glistening and are not sacculated.

4) the small intestine measures about 22 feet in length, commencing at the pyloric end of the stomach and terminating at the ileocecal junction, which marks the commencement of the large intestine.

Fig. 221   **III**

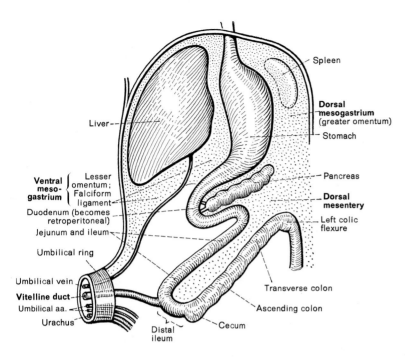

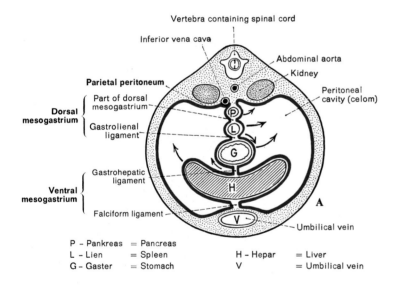

P – Pankreas = Pancreas
L – Lien = Spleen
G – Gaster = Stomach

H – Hepar = Liver
V = Umbilical vein

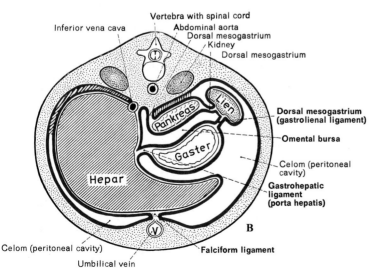

Figs. 222, 223 A, 223 B

## Fig. 222: The Developing Gastrointestinal Organs and their Mesenteries

NOTE: 1) as the primitive gastrointestinal tube develops within the abdominal celom, it is suspended to the body wall by primitive peritoneal reflections, both ventrally and dorsally. The early peritoneal attachments to the expanding stomach are called the ventral mesogastrium and dorsal mesogastrium, while the dorsal mesentery develops on the posterior aspect of the primitive small and large intestine.

2) the embryonic liver develops into the ventral mesogastrium, thereby dividing this ventral peritoneal attachment into:

a) a portion between the anterior body wall and the liver which eventually becomes the falciform ligament, and

b) a portion between the liver and the stomach which becomes the lesser omentum.

3) on the dorsal aspect:

a) the pancreas develops in relation to the primitive duodenum, both of which lose their mesenteries during gut rotation to become retroperitoneal;

b) the dorsal mesogastrium, attaching along the greater curvature of the stomach and rotating with the stomach, becomes the greater omentum. This eventually encases the transverse colon;

c) the dorsal mesentery remains attached to the small intestine, while the ascending and descending colon become displaced to the right and left side respectively, becoming adherent to the posterior body wall;

d) the sigmoid colon usually retains its mesentery while that of the rectum becomes obliterated.

4) near the cecal end of the small intestine the developing G.I. canal communicates with the vitelline duct. After birth, this duct usually becomes resorbed; when it persists (2% of cases), it results in a diverticulum of the ileum called Meckel's diverticulum.

## Cross Sectional Diagram of Development of Mesogastria
## Fig. 223 A: Early Stage (about six weeks)

NOTE: 1) the primitive peritoneal reflections are indicated in red. The arrows show the direction of growth and, therefore, of movement by the various organs to achieve the positions shown in Fig. 223 B.

2) at this early stage, the peritoneum completely surrounds the organs in the upper abdominal region (visceral peritoneum) and attaches peripherally to the body wall (parietal peritoneum). Attaching along the posterior border of the stomach, the dorsal mesogastrium then surrounds the spleen and pancreas. Anterior to the stomach, the liver becomes interposed between the stomach and the anterior body wall. This forms the gastrohepatic ligament (also called lesser omentum) between the lesser curvature of the stomach and the liver, and the falciform ligament between the liver and the anterior body wall.

## Cross Sectional Diagram of Development of Mesogastria
## Fig. 223 B: Late Fetal Stage

NOTE: 1) with the rotation of the organs (in the direction of the arrows in Fig. 223 A), the liver grows into the celomic cavity toward the right and contacts the inferior vena cava, while the stomach rotates such that its dorsal mesogastrium (greater curvature) is shifted to the left. The pancreas and spleen still retain their position posterior to the stomach.

2) the reflection of dorsal mesogastrium between the stomach and spleen becomes established as the gastrolienal ligament while one layer of mesogastrium surrounding the pancreas (and duodenum) fuses to the posterior body wall. This latter development fixates these two organs with a layer of peritoneum on their anterior surface, causing them to become retroperitoneal. The omental bursa also develops posterior to the stomach and anterior to the pancreas.

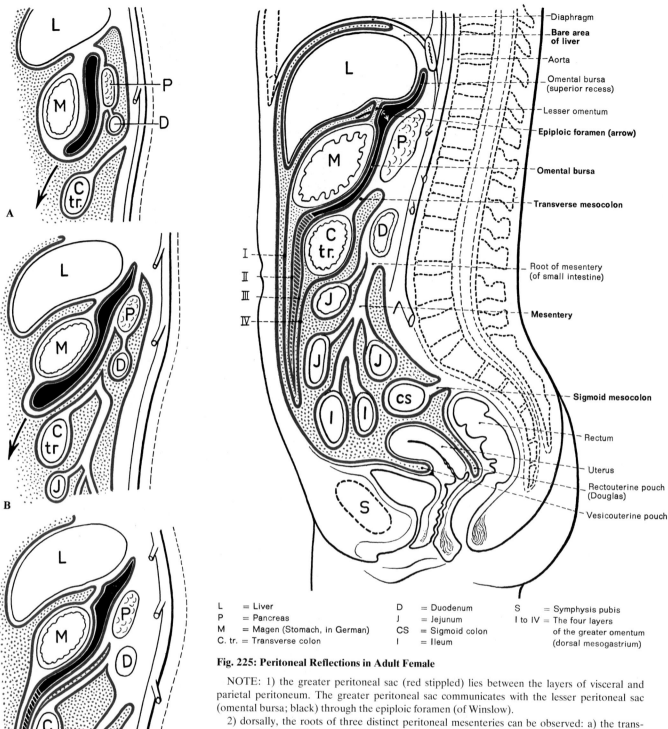

| | | | | | | |
|---|---|---|---|---|---|---|
| L | = Liver | D | = Duodenum | S | = Symphysis pubis |
| P | = Pancreas | J | = Jejunum | I to IV | = The four layers |
| M | = Magen (Stomach, in German) | CS | = Sigmoid colon | | of the greater omentum |
| C. tr. | = Transverse colon | I | = Ileum | | (dorsal mesogastrium) |

**Fig. 225: Peritoneal Reflections in Adult Female**

NOTE: 1) the greater peritoneal sac (red stippled) lies between the layers of visceral and parietal peritoneum. The greater peritoneal sac communicates with the lesser peritoneal sac (omental bursa; black) through the epiploic foramen (of Winslow).

2) dorsally, the roots of three distinct peritoneal mesenteries can be observed: a) the transverse mesocolon, b) the mesentery surrounding the small intestine, and c) the sigmoid mesocolon.

3) behind the stomach and transverse colon, observe the retroperitoneal pancreas and duodenum. Note also that a portion of the liver is not surrounded by peritoneum (bare area of the liver) and lies adjacent to the diaphragm.

**Fig. 224 A, B, & C: Stages in the Development of the Omental Bursa (Sagittal Diagrams)**

NOTE: 1) at four weeks the dorsal border of the stomach (Magen, M) grows faster than the ventral border assisting in rotation of the stomach on its long axis. The greater curvature and its dorsal mesogastrium becomes directed to the left, while the lesser curvature and the ventral mesogastrium is directed to the right.

2) by eight weeks (Fig. 224 A) the omental bursa (black) forms behind the stomach between the two leaves of dorsal mesogastrium. The pancreas and duodenum are still surrounded by dorsal mesentery. As gut rotation continues the dorsal mesogastrium extends inferiorly (Fig. 224 B, arrow) to form the greater omentum which becomes a double reflection (4 leaves) of the dorsal mesogastrium "trapping" the cavity of the omental bursa between the 2nd and 3rd leaves.

3) continued development (Fig. 224 C) results in a further descent of the greater omentum over the abdominal viscera and a fusion (cross-hatched) of the 2nd and 3rd leaves inferiorly.

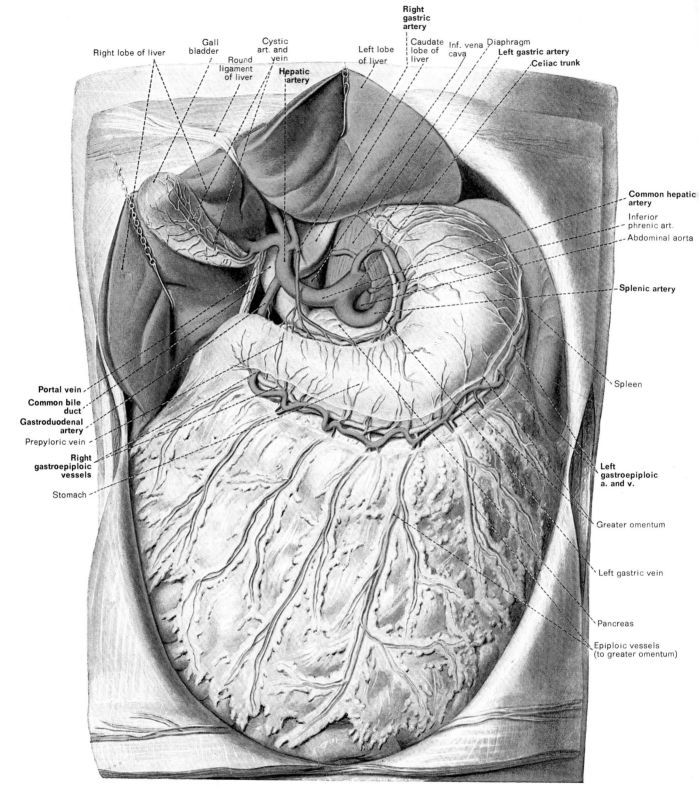

Right lobe of liver
Gall bladder
Round ligament of liver
Cystic art. and vein
Hepatic artery
Left lobe of liver
Right gastric artery
Caudate lobe of liver
Inf. vena cava
Diaphragm
Left gastric artery
Celiac trunk

Common hepatic artery
Inferior phrenic art.
Abdominal aorta
Splenic artery
Spleen
Left gastroepiploic a. and v.
Greater omentum
Left gastric vein
Pancreas
Epiploic vessels (to greater omentum)

Portal vein
Common bile duct
Gastroduodenal artery
Prepyloric vein
Right gastroepiploic vessels
Stomach

**Fig. 226: The Abdominal Cavity (3): The Celiac Trunk and its Branches**

NOTE: 1) the right and left lobes of the liver have been elevated and the lesser omentum has been removed between the lesser curvature of the stomach and the liver to reveal the celiac trunk and its branches and three major structures at the porta hepatis, the hepatic artery, portal vein and common bile duct.

2) the celiac trunk lies anterior to the 12th thoracic vertebra and almost immediately divides into the left gastric artery, and the hepatic and splenic arteries:

a) the left gastric artery courses along the lesser curvature of the stomach and anastomoses with the right gastric branch of the hepatic artery;

b) the hepatic artery courses to the right and gives off the gastroduodenal artery before dividing to enter the lobes of the liver;

c) the splenic artery courses to the left toward the hilum of the spleen;

d) the gastroduodenal artery gives rise to the right gastroepiploic artery which follows along the greater curvature of the stomach to anastomose with the left gastroepiploic branch of the splenic artery.

Fig. 226

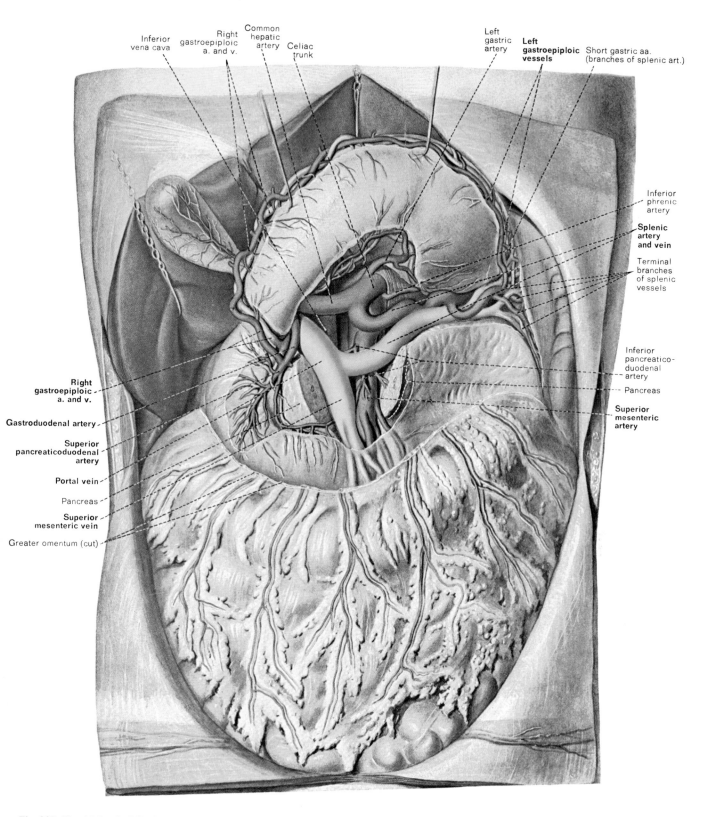

Inferior vena cava — Right gastroepiploic a. and v. — Common hepatic artery — Celiac trunk — Left gastric artery — **Left gastroepiploic vessels** — Short gastric aa. (branches of splenic art.)

Inferior phrenic artery

**Splenic artery and vein**

Terminal branches of splenic vessels

Inferior pancreatico-duodenal artery

Pancreas

**Superior mesenteric artery**

**Right gastroepiploic a. and v.**

**Gastroduodenal artery**

**Superior pancreaticoduodenal artery**

**Portal vein**

**Pancreas**

**Superior mesenteric vein**

**Greater omentum (cut)**

**Fig. 227: The Abdominal Cavity (4): The Splenic Vessels and Formation of the Portal Vein**

NOTE: 1) the attachment of the greater omentum has been cut along the greater curvature of the stomach. The stomach has been lifted to expose its posterior surface and the underlying pancreas, duodenum and blood vessels. A portion of the body of the pancreas has been removed to reveal the formation of the portal vein by the junction of the splenic and superior mesenteric veins.

2) the splenic artery in its tortuous course across the left upper abdomen to the hilum of the spleen. Observe also how the gastroduodenal artery lies posterior to the pyloric end of the stomach and divides into the right gastroepiploic artery and the superior pancreaticoduodenal artery. The origin of the left gastroepiploic artery from the splenic is also visible.

3) the root of the superior mesenteric artery as it branches from the abdominal aorta just below the celiac trunk.

Fig. 227    **III**

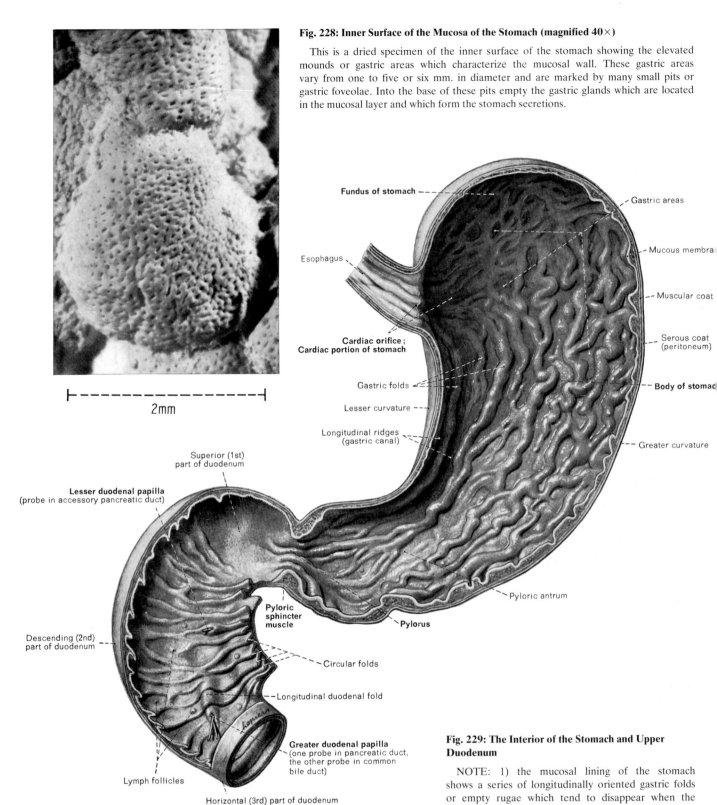

**Fig. 228: Inner Surface of the Mucosa of the Stomach (magnified 40×)**

This is a dried specimen of the inner surface of the stomach showing the elevated mounds or gastric areas which characterize the mucosal wall. These gastric areas vary from one to five or six mm. in diameter and are marked by many small pits or gastric foveolae. Into the base of these pits empty the gastric glands which are located in the mucosal layer and which form the stomach secretions.

2mm

Fundus of stomach

Gastric areas

Mucous membra

Esophagus

Muscular coat

Serous coat (peritoneum)

Cardiac orifice; Cardiac portion of stomach

Body of stomac

Gastric folds

Lesser curvature

Longitudinal ridges (gastric canal)

Greater curvature

Superior (1st) part of duodenum

Lesser duodenal papilla (probe in accessory pancreatic duct)

Pyloric antrum

Pyloric sphincter muscle

Pylorus

Descending (2nd) part of duodenum

Circular folds

Longitudinal duodenal fold

Greater duodenal papilla (one probe in pancreatic duct, the other probe in common bile duct)

Lymph follicles

Horizontal (3rd) part of duodenum

**Fig. 229: The Interior of the Stomach and Upper Duodenum**

NOTE: 1) the mucosal lining of the stomach shows a series of longitudinally oriented gastric folds or empty rugae which tend to disappear when the stomach is full and distended. These folds are more regular along the lesser curvature and form the grooved gastric canal. The concept that food travels along this canal (magenstrasse) is not correct.

2) the surface of the first portion of the duodenum (superior) is smooth, whereas the circular ridges characteristic of the small intestine can be seen to commence in the second or descending portion of the duodenum.

3) the pyloric junction of the stomach with the duodenum. A circular muscle, the pyloric sphincter, guards this junction. It diminishes significantly in size the lumen of the gastrointestinal tract at this point. The pylorus is to the right of midline at the level of the 1st lumbar vertebra.

4) the openings in the wall of the duodenum. The greater duodenal papilla serves as the site of the openings of both the common bile duct and the main pancreatic duct. The accessory pancreatic duct opens two centimeters more proximally through the lesser duodenal papilla.

Figs. 228, 229

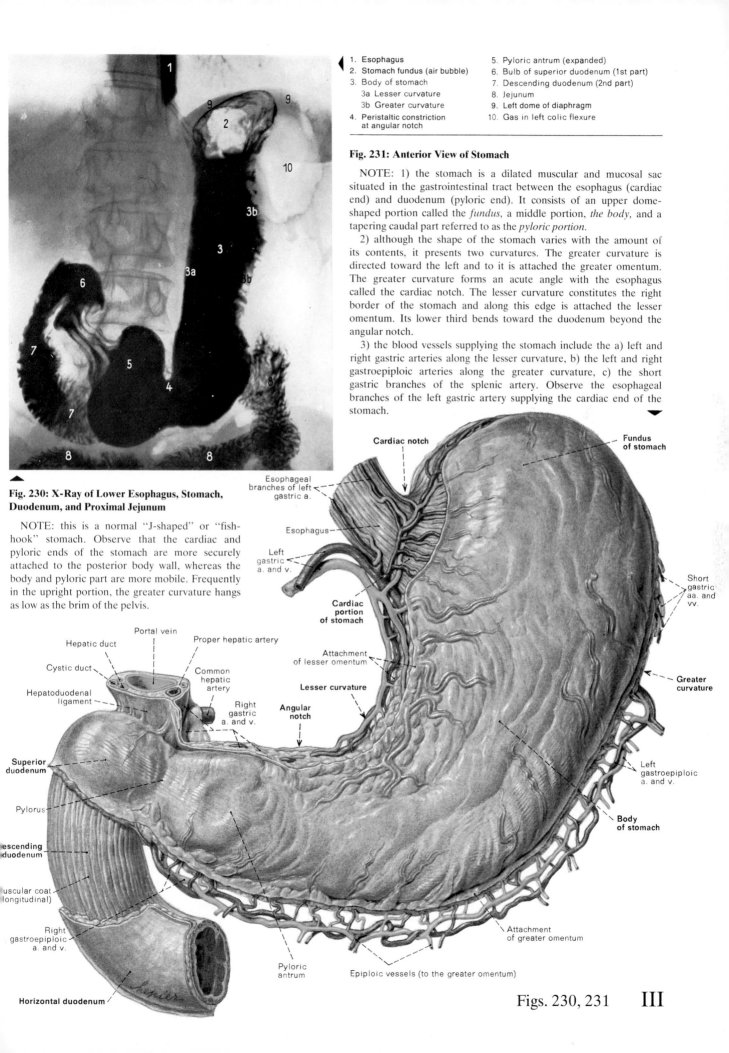

1. Esophagus
2. Stomach fundus (air bubble)
3. Body of stomach
    3a Lesser curvature
    3b Greater curvature
4. Peristaltic constriction
    at angular notch
5. Pyloric antrum (expanded)
6. Bulb of superior duodenum (1st part)
7. Descending duodenum (2nd part)
8. Jejunum
9. Left dome of diaphragm
10. Gas in left colic flexure

**Fig. 231: Anterior View of Stomach**

NOTE: 1) the stomach is a dilated muscular and mucosal sac situated in the gastrointestinal tract between the esophagus (cardiac end) and duodenum (pyloric end). It consists of an upper dome-shaped portion called the *fundus,* a middle portion, *the body,* and a tapering caudal part referred to as the *pyloric portion.*

2) although the shape of the stomach varies with the amount of its contents, it presents two curvatures. The greater curvature is directed toward the left and to it is attached the greater omentum. The greater curvature forms an acute angle with the esophagus called the cardiac notch. The lesser curvature constitutes the right border of the stomach and along this edge is attached the lesser omentum. Its lower third bends toward the duodenum beyond the angular notch.

3) the blood vessels supplying the stomach include the a) left and right gastric arteries along the lesser curvature, b) the left and right gastroepiploic arteries along the greater curvature, c) the short gastric branches of the splenic artery. Observe the esophageal branches of the left gastric artery supplying the cardiac end of the stomach.

**Fig. 230: X-Ray of Lower Esophagus, Stomach, Duodenum, and Proximal Jejunum**

NOTE: this is a normal "J-shaped" or "fish-hook" stomach. Observe that the cardiac and pyloric ends of the stomach are more securely attached to the posterior body wall, whereas the body and pyloric part are more mobile. Frequently in the upright portion, the greater curvature hangs as low as the brim of the pelvis.

Cardiac notch

Fundus of stomach

Esophageal branches of left gastric a.

Esophagus

Left gastric a. and v.

Cardiac portion of stomach

Short gastric aa. and vv.

Attachment of lesser omentum

Greater curvature

Lesser curvature

Angular notch

Portal vein

Hepatic duct

Proper hepatic artery

Cystic duct

Common hepatic artery

Hepatoduodenal ligament

Right gastric a. and v.

Superior duodenum

Left gastroepiploic a. and v.

Pylorus

Body of stomach

Descending duodenum

Muscular coat (longitudinal)

Right gastroepiploic a. and v.

Attachment of greater omentum

Horizontal duodenum

Pyloric antrum

Epiploic vessels (to the greater omentum)

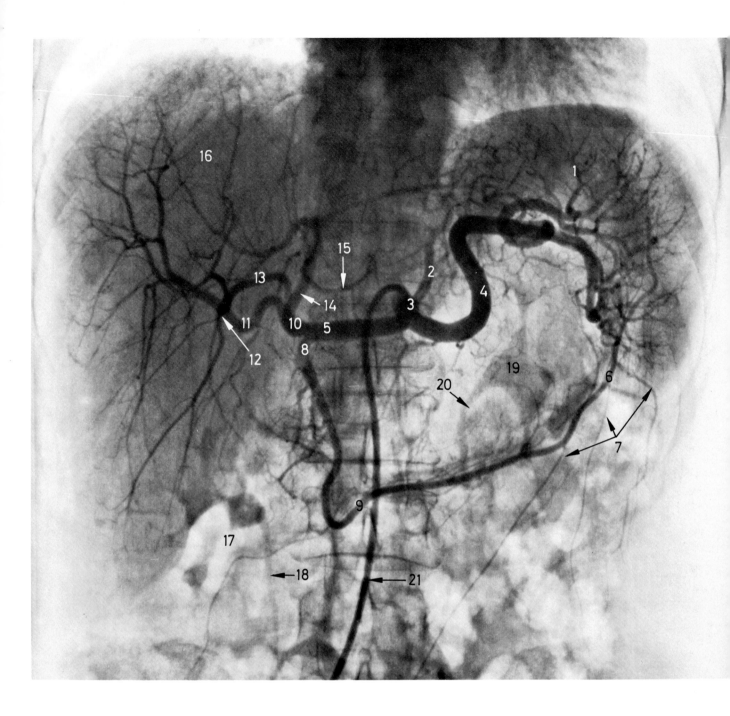

**Fig. 232: A Celiac Trunk Arteriogram**

NOTE: 1) that this figure is a positive print from an X-ray taken of the upper abdomen following the injection of a contrast medium through a catheter (*21*, arrow), which was introduced into the abdominal aorta and directed upward to the point where the celiac trunk (*3*) branches from the aorta. The principal subbranches of the celiac trunk, therefore, can be visualized.

2) the three primary vessels arising from the celiac trunk (*3*) are the *left gastric artery* (*2*), the *splenic artery* (*4*) which is directed in a tortuous pattern toward the spleen (*1*), and the *common hepatic artery* (*5*) which courses almost directly to the right.

3) that from one of the inferior hilar branches of the splenic artery arises the left gastroepiploic artery (*6*), which then gives origin to epiploic arteries (*7*, arrows) which descend to supply the greater omentum. The left gastroepiploic (*6*) courses along the greater curvature of the stomach to anastomose with the right gastroepiploic artery (*9*). This latter vessel arises from the gastroduodenal artery (*8*) which, in turn, courses inferiorly as a major vessel derived from the common hepatic artery (*5*).

4) that beyond the origin of the gastroduodenal artery (*8*) the common hepatic artery (*5*) is called the proper hepatic artery (*10*).

5) that the proper hepatic artery (*10*) soon divides into the *right hepatic artery* (*11*), from which branches the cystic artery (*12*) which supplies the gall bladder, the *middle hepatic artery* (*13*), and the *left hepatic artery* (*14*, arrow). The hepatic vessels, of course, supply the liver (*16*).

6) that from the right hepatic artery (*14*) in this individual branches the right gastric artery (*15*, arrow). Just as frequently the right gastric artery is found arising from the common hepatic artery (*5*). The right gastric artery courses around the lesser curvature of the stomach to anastomose with the left gastric (*2*). The latter vessel is one of the original branches of the celiac trunk.

7) that inferiorly can be seen the right renal pelvis (*17*) and the right ureter (*18*, arrow). Observe that because of the liver, these structures on the right side are significantly lower than the left renal pelvis (*19*) and the origin of the left ureter (*20*, arrow).

Fig. 232

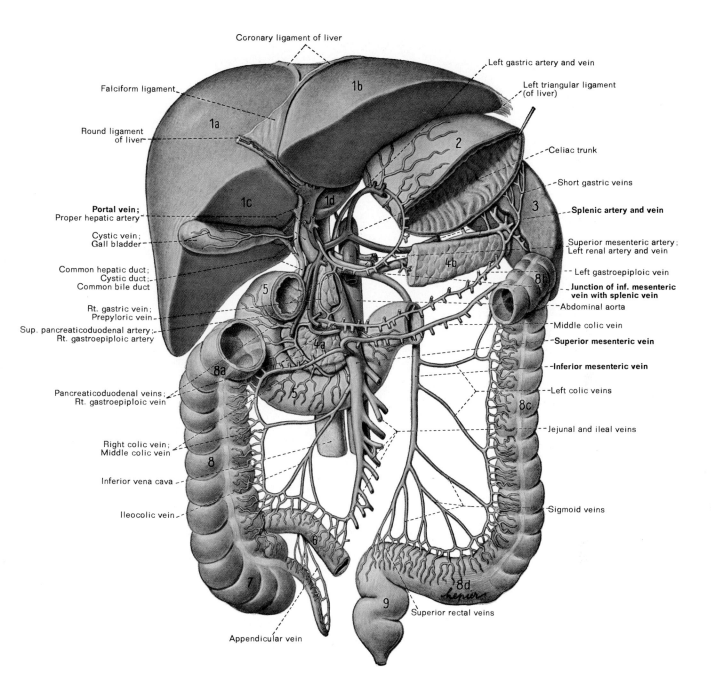

Coronary ligament of liver

Falciform ligament

Round ligament of liver

**Portal vein;** Proper hepatic artery

Cystic vein; Gall bladder

Common hepatic duct; Cystic duct; Common bile duct

Rt. gastric vein; Prepyloric vein

Sup. pancreaticoduodenal artery; Rt. gastroepiploic artery

Pancreaticoduodenal veins; Rt. gastroepiploic vein

Right colic vein; Middle colic vein

Inferior vena cava

Ileocolic vein

Appendicular vein

Left gastric artery and vein

Left triangular ligament (of liver)

Celiac trunk

Short gastric veins

**Splenic artery and vein**

Superior mesenteric artery; Left renal artery and vein

Left gastroepiploic vein

**Junction of inf. mesenteric vein with splenic vein**

Abdominal aorta

Middle colic vein

**Superior mesenteric vein**

**Inferior mesenteric vein**

Left colic veins

Jejunal and ileal veins

Sigmoid veins

Superior rectal veins

### Fig. 233: Abdominal Portal System of Veins

NOTE: 1) the abdominal portal system of veins drains venous blood from the gastro-intestinal tract, the gall bladder, pancreas and spleen through the liver via the large portal vein. This is done in order to subject this venous blood to the various functions of the liver before it is returned to the general systemic circulation by way of the hepatic veins into the inferior vena cava.

2) the portal vein is formed by the union of the superior mesenteric vein and the splenic vein. The inferior mesenteric vein drains into the splenic vein. At the esophageal end of the stomach (esophageal veins) and at the distal end of the rectum (inferior rectal veins), the portal system of veins anastomoses with the systemic veins. Certain disease states which may cause a reduction of blood flow through the liver result in greater use of these anastomotic channels in the return of blood in the portal system.

3) the functions of the liver are numerous, varied and vital to life. The liver secretes bile which is then stored in the gall bladder and released when food appears in the duodenum. Bile aids in the digestion and absorption of fats. The liver converts glucose to glycogen, stores the glycogen and then reconverts it to glucose again when needed. Further, the liver is involved in the synthesis of Vitamin A, heparin, prothrombin, fibrinogen and other substances. It functions also in detoxification of substances in the blood. It is involved in the breakdown of hemoglobin and stores both iron and copper.

1a Right lobe of liver
1b Left lobe of liver
1c Quadrate lobe of liver
1d Caudate lobe of liver
2 Stomach
3 Spleen
4a Head of pancreas
4b Tail of pancreas
5 Duodenum
6 Ileum
7 Cecum
8 Ascending colon
8a Right colic flexure
8b Left colic flexure
8c Descending colon
8d Sigmoid colon
9 Rectum
↑ = Junction of sup. mesenteric v. and splenic vein to form portal vein

Fig. 233   III

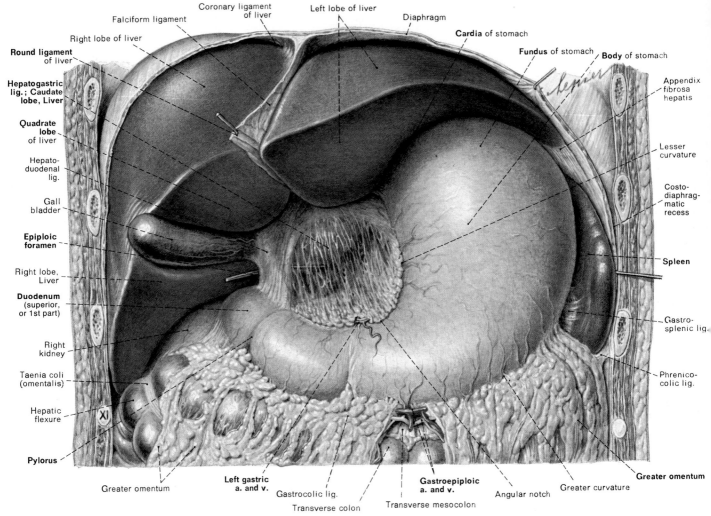

**Fig. 234: The Lesser Omentum, Stomach, Liver and Spleen**

NOTE: 1) with the liver elevated, a probe has been inserted through the epiploic foramen into the vestibule of the omental bursa. By way of this opening, the greater peritoneal sac communicates with the lesser peritoneal sac. Observe that the lesser omentum consists of the hepatogastric and hepatoduodenal ligaments.

2) the epiploic foramen is situated just caudal to the liver and readily admits two fingers. It is bound superiorly by the caudate lobe of the liver, inferiorly by the superior or 1st part of the duodenum, posteriorly by the inferior vena cava, and anteriorly by the lesser omentum which ensheathes the structures of the porta hepatis (hepatic artery, portal vein and bile ducts).

3) the greater omentum extends along the greater curvature from the spleen to the duodenum. The gall bladder is situated between the right and quadrate lobes of the liver and projects just beyond the inferior border of the liver, thereby coming into contact directly with the anterior abdominal wall at this site.

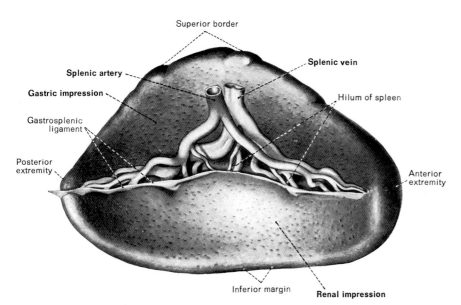

**Fig. 235: The Spleen, Visceral Surface**

NOTE that the spleen is situated in the left hypochondriac region between the fundus of the stomach and the diaphragm. Its visceral surface shows the contours of the organs related to it. A gastric impression and a renal impression conform to the shapes of the stomach and left kidney. Additionally, the left colic flexure, the tail of the pancreas and the left adrenal gland, which overlies the left kidney, are related to this visceral surface.

Figs. 234, 235

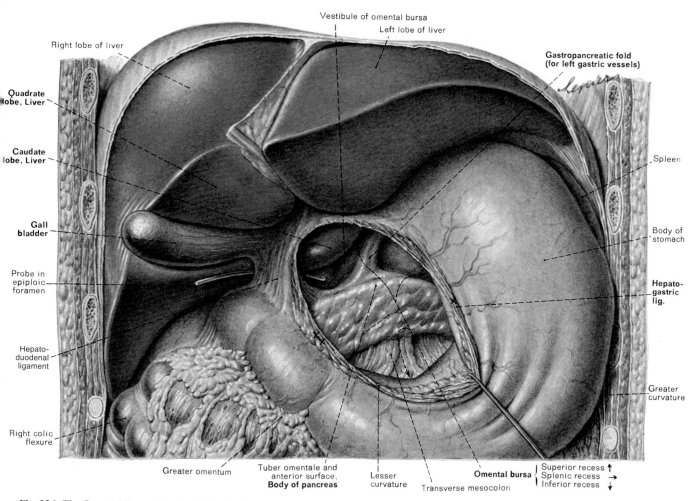

**Fig. 236: The Omental Bursa, Caudate Lobe of Liver and Body of Pancreas**

NOTE: 1) the liver has been elevated and the lesser curvature of the stomach has been pulled down and to the left in order to enlarge the exposure obtained by opening the omental bursa through the hepatogastric ligament (indicated by X and XX). The superior, splenic and inferior recesses of this bursa have been indicated by the arrows.

2) the portion of the omental bursa adjacent to the epiploic foramen is called the vestibule. Observe the gastropancreatic fold which crosses the dorsal wall of the bursa. This fold is formed by a reflection of peritoneum covering the left gastric artery which courses (from its origin on the celiac trunk) to the left of the superior recess of the omental bursa to achieve its destination, the lesser curvature of the stomach.

3) exposure of the omental bursa in this manner reveals the caudate lobe of the liver which can be seen situated on the dorsal surface of the liver's right lobe as well as the anterior surface of the body of the pancreas coursing transversely behind the stomach.

4) the left lobe of the liver overlies the lesser curvature, the fundus and part of the body of the stomach. While the caudate lobe is situated to the right of the esophagus (not visible in this figure), the quadrate lobe, which lies between the fossa of the gall bladder and the round ligament, comes into contact with the pylorus and the first part of the duodenum.

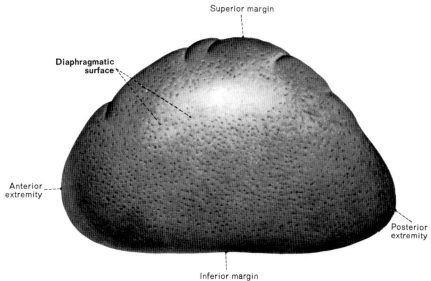

**Fig. 237: The Spleen, Diaphragmatic Surface**

NOTE: the diaphragmatic surface of the spleen is directed posterolaterally. It is smooth and convex and conforms to the concave abdominal surface of the adjacent diaphragm. Although the normal adult spleen may vary considerably in size from 100 grams to 400 grams, its proximity to the 9th, 10th and 11th ribs of the left side makes it vulnerable to costal fractures in this region.

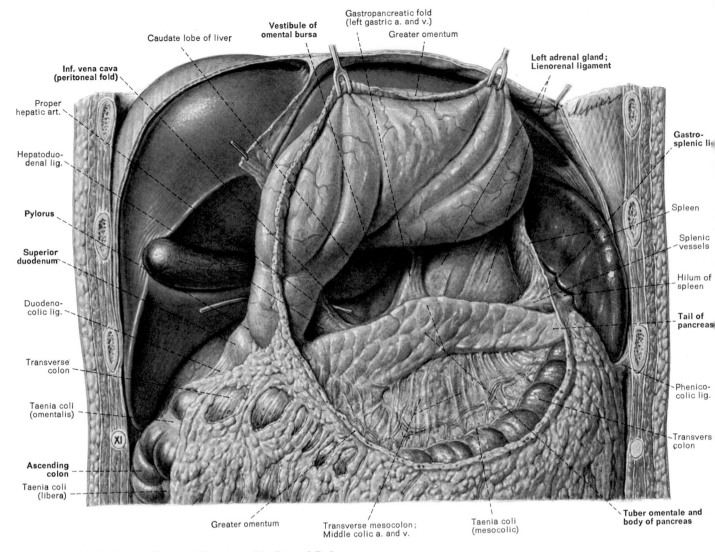

Inf. vena cava (peritoneal fold)

Caudate lobe of liver

**Vestibule of omental bursa**

Gastropancreatic fold (left gastric a. and v.)

Greater omentum

Left adrenal gland; Lienorenal ligament

Proper hepatic art.

Hepatoduo-denal lig.

**Gastro-splenic li**

**Pylorus**

**Superior duodenum**

Spleen

Splenic vessels

Hilum of spleen

Duodeno-colic lig.

**Tail of pancreas**

Transverse colon

Taenia coli (omentalis)

XI

Phenico-colic lig.

**Ascending colon**

Taenia coli (libera)

Transvers colon

Greater omentum

Transverse mesocolon; Middle colic a. and v.

Taenia coli (mesocolic)

**Tuber omentale and body of pancreas**

## Fig. 238: The Omental Bursa and Structures of the Stomach Bed

NOTE: 1) the attachment of the greater omentum has been cut along the entire greater curvature of the stomach and the stomach has been elevated to expose the dorsal wall of the omental bursa.

2) the transverse course of the pancreas across the posterior abdomen and the pointed direction of the tail of the pancreas toward the hilum of the spleen.

3) the severed peritoneal reflection between the stomach and the spleen, the gastrosplenic ligament and its conti-nuation from the spleen to the kidney, the lienorenal liga-ment. Covering the upper pole of the left kidney, observe the adrenal gland.

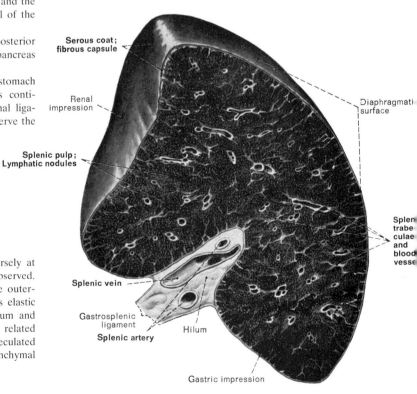

Serous coat; fibrous capsule

Renal impression

Splenic pulp; Lymphatic nodules

Diaphragmati surface

Splen trabe culae and blood vesse

Splenic vein

Gastrosplenic ligament

**Splenic artery**

Hilum

Gastric impression

## Fig. 239: Spleen, Cross Section

NOTE: 1) the spleen has been sectioned transversely at the hilum where the severed splenic vessels can be observed.

2) covering the spleen are two external coats. The outer-most is a serous coat and beneath this is the fibrous elastic capsule. The serous coat derives from the peritoneum and is continuous at the hilum with the peritoneal folds related to the spleen. The fibrous, elastic coat invests the trabeculated soft masses of splenic pulp which compose the parenchymal tissue of the organ.

Figs. 238, 239

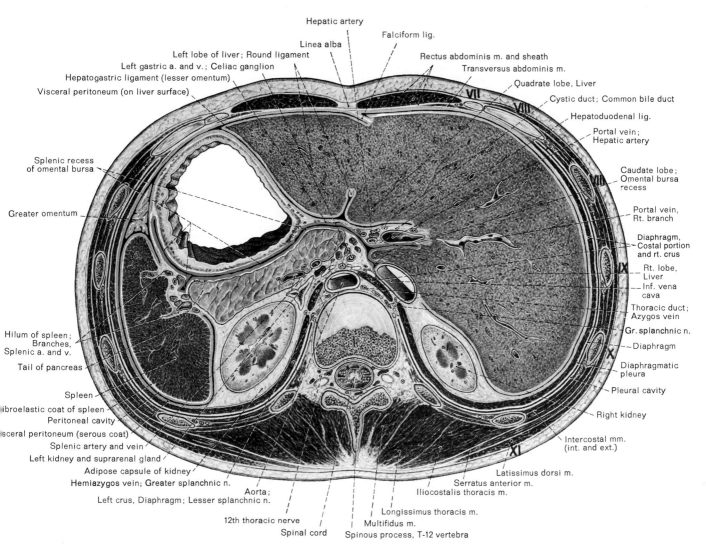

Fig. 240: Transverse Section Through the Upper Abdomen (between T-12 and L-1)

NOTE: in light red is outlined the peritoneum of the greater peritoneal cavity while in dark red is the peritoneum of the omental bursa or lesser peritoneal cavity.

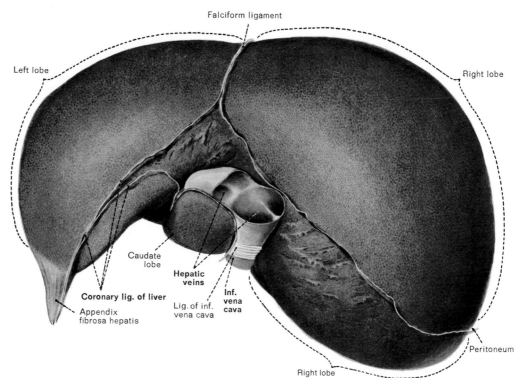

Fig. 241: Dorsocranial View of Liver

NOTE: 1) the visceral peritoneum closely adheres to the surface of the liver and is called the coronary ligament. Between the two leaves of the coronary ligament a portion of the liver is devoid of peritoneum. This is called the bare area of the liver and it is in direct contact with the diaphragm.

2) the hepatic veins as they converge superiorly from the liver lobes to empty into the inferior vena cava; this latter vessel lies in its sulcus on the posterior surface of the liver.

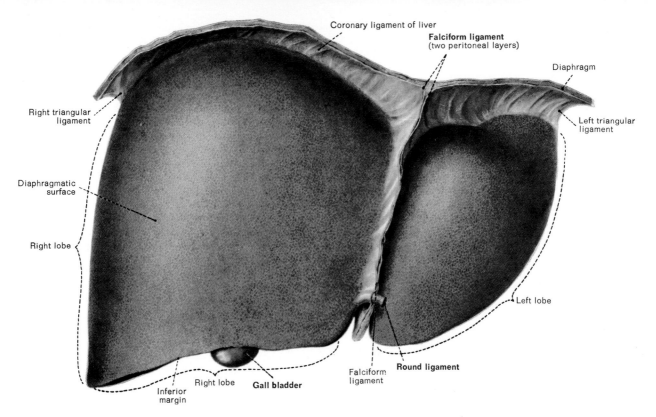

Fig. 242: Anterior Surface of the Liver (with Diaphragmatic Attachment)

NOTE: 1) the falciform ligament (derived from the ventral mesogastrium) separates the large right from the smaller left lobe of the liver. It contains the fibrous cord called the round ligament of the liver which is the resultant structure from the obliteration of the umbilical vein.

2) the fundus of the gall bladder extending below the sharply angled hepatic inferior margin.

Fig. 243: Posterior (Visceral) Surface of Liver and the Gall Bladder

NOTE: 1) the impressions made by the esophagus and stomach on the left lobe of the liver and the right kidney, right suprarenal gland, duodenum and transverse colon on the right lobe.

2) the sulcus formed by the inferior vena cava, which subdivides the caudate lobe from the right lobe. The gall bladder along with the portal vein, hepatic artery and common bile duct bound the quadrate lobe.

3) the continuity of the round ligament (umbilical vein) with the ligamentum venosum (ductus venosus).

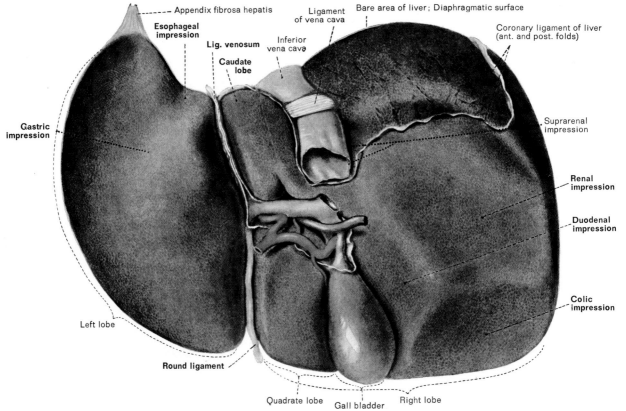

Figs. 242, 243

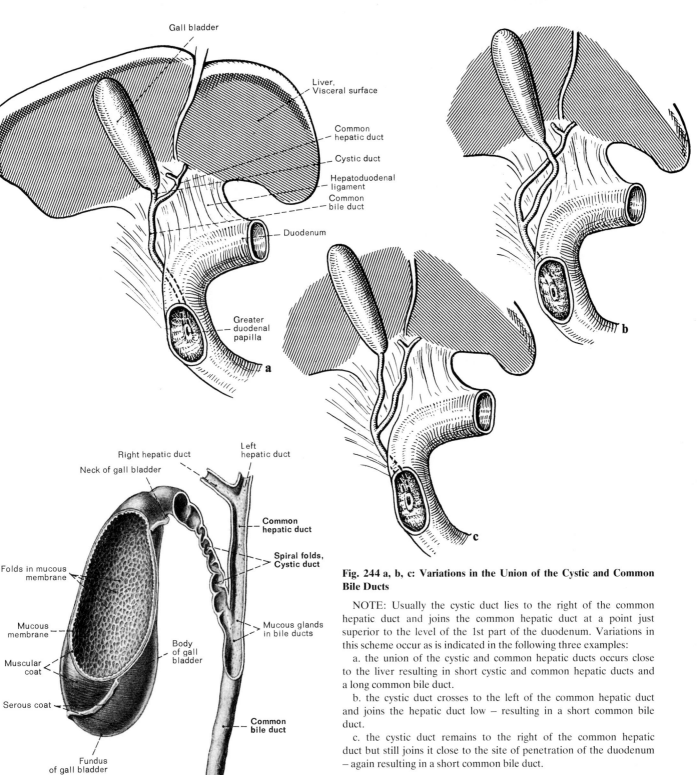

Gall bladder

Liver,
Visceral surface

Common
hepatic duct

Cystic duct

Hepatoduodenal
ligament

Common
bile duct

Duodenum

Greater
duodenal
papilla

**a**

**b**

**c**

Right hepatic duct

Left
hepatic duct

Neck of gall bladder

**Common
hepatic duct**

**Spiral folds,
Cystic duct**

Folds in mucous
membrane

Mucous
membrane

Muscular
coat

Serous coat

Body
of gall
bladder

Mucous glands
in bile ducts

**Common
bile duct**

Fundus
of gall bladder

Circular
duodenal folds

Lymph nodes

**Pancreatic
duct**

Longitudinal
duodenal folds

Greater
duodenal papilla

Orifice of
pancreatic duct

**Fig. 244 a, b, c: Variations in the Union of the Cystic and Common Bile Ducts**

NOTE: Usually the cystic duct lies to the right of the common hepatic duct and joins the common hepatic duct at a point just superior to the level of the 1st part of the duodenum. Variations in this scheme occur as is indicated in the following three examples:

a. the union of the cystic and common hepatic ducts occurs close to the liver resulting in short cystic and common hepatic ducts and a long common bile duct.

b. the cystic duct crosses to the left of the common hepatic duct and joins the hepatic duct low – resulting in a short common bile duct.

c. the cystic duct remains to the right of the common hepatic duct but still joins it close to the site of penetration of the duodenum – again resulting in a short common bile duct.

**Fig. 245: The Gall Bladder and Biliary Duct System**

NOTE: 1) the wall of the gall bladder has been opened to reveal the meshwork characteristic of the surface of the mucosal layer. The pear-shaped gall bladder stores bile which reaches it from the liver. Its capacity is about 35 cc.

2) the spiral nature of the cystic duct which leads from the neck of the gall bladder. Normally the cystic duct measures about $1^{1}/_{2}$ inches long and joins the common hepatic duct (which also is about $1^{1}/_{2}$ inches long) to form the common bile duct. The common bile duct descends about 3 inches to open into the 2nd or descending portion of the duodenum.

3) at its point of entrance into the duodenum (the greater duodenal papilla), the common bile duct is joined by the main pancreatic duct (duct of Wirsung).

Figs. 244 a – c, 245    **III**

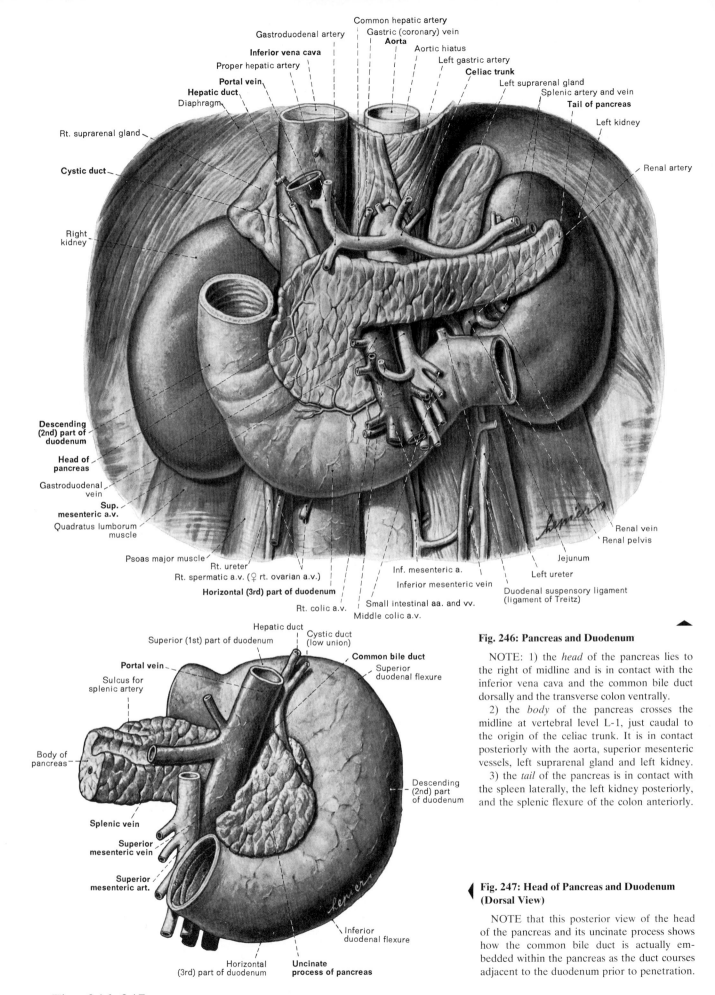

Common hepatic artery
Gastroduodenal artery
Gastric (coronary) vein
**Aorta**
Inferior vena cava
Aortic hiatus
Proper hepatic artery
Left gastric artery
**Portal vein**
**Celiac trunk**
**Hepatic duct**
Left suprarenal gland
Diaphragm
Splenic artery and vein
**Tail of pancreas**
Rt. suprarenal gland
Left kidney
**Cystic duct**
Renal artery
Right kidney
**Descending (2nd) part of duodenum**
**Head of pancreas**
Gastroduodenal vein
**Sup. mesenteric a.v.**
Quadratus lumborum muscle
Renal vein
Renal pelvis
Psoas major muscle
Jejunum
Rt. ureter
Left ureter
Rt. spermatic a.v. (♀ rt. ovarian a.v.)
Inf. mesenteric a.
Inferior mesenteric vein
Duodenal suspensory ligament (ligament of Treitz)
**Horizontal (3rd) part of duodenum**
Rt. colic a.v.
Small intestinal aa. and vv.
Middle colic a.v.

Hepatic duct
Superior (1st) part of duodenum
Cystic duct (low union)
**Common bile duct**
**Portal vein**
Superior duodenal flexure
Sulcus for splenic artery
Body of pancreas
Descending (2nd) part of duodenum
**Splenic vein**
**Superior mesenteric vein**
**Superior mesenteric art.**
Inferior duodenal flexure
Horizontal (3rd) part of duodenum
**Uncinate process of pancreas**

Figs. 246, 247

### Fig. 246: Pancreas and Duodenum

NOTE: 1) the *head* of the pancreas lies to the right of midline and is in contact with the inferior vena cava and the common bile duct dorsally and the transverse colon ventrally.

2) the *body* of the pancreas crosses the midline at vertebral level L-1, just caudal to the origin of the celiac trunk. It is in contact posteriorly with the aorta, superior mesenteric vessels, left suprarenal gland and left kidney.

3) the *tail* of the pancreas is in contact with the spleen laterally, the left kidney posteriorly, and the splenic flexure of the colon anteriorly.

### Fig. 247: Head of Pancreas and Duodenum (Dorsal View)

NOTE that this posterior view of the head of the pancreas and its uncinate process shows how the common bile duct is actually embedded within the pancreas as the duct courses adjacent to the duodenum prior to penetration.

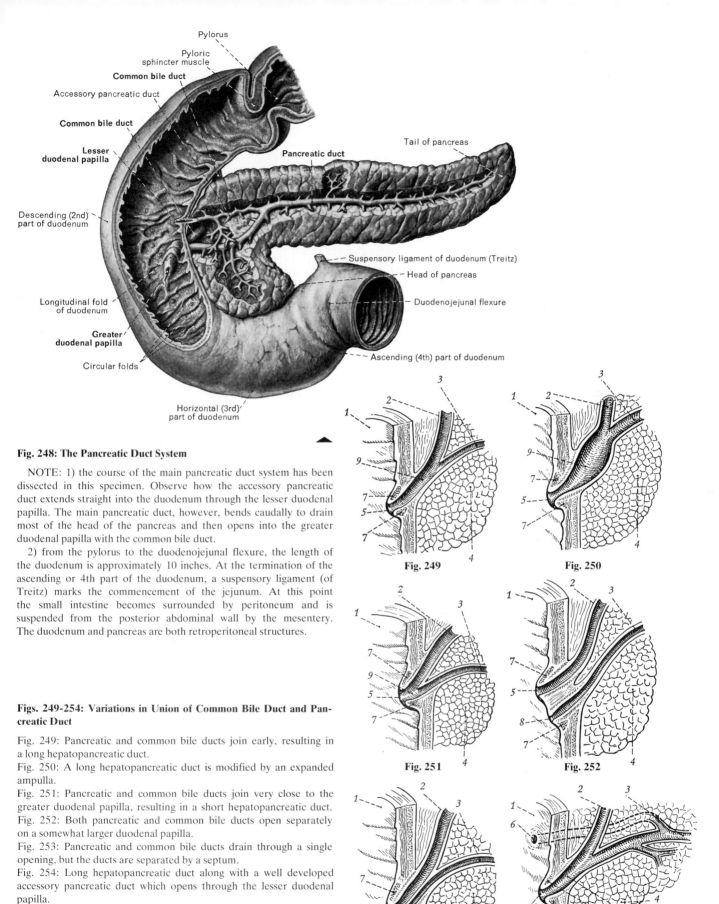

Fig. 248: The Pancreatic Duct System

NOTE: 1) the course of the main pancreatic duct system has been dissected in this specimen. Observe how the accessory pancreatic duct extends straight into the duodenum through the lesser duodenal papilla. The main pancreatic duct, however, bends caudally to drain most of the head of the pancreas and then opens into the greater duodenal papilla with the common bile duct.

2) from the pylorus to the duodenojejunal flexure, the length of the duodenum is approximately 10 inches. At the termination of the ascending or 4th part of the duodenum, a suspensory ligament (of Treitz) marks the commencement of the jejunum. At this point the small intestine becomes surrounded by peritoneum and is suspended from the posterior abdominal wall by the mesentery. The duodenum and pancreas are both retroperitoneal structures.

Figs. 249-254: Variations in Union of Common Bile Duct and Pancreatic Duct

Fig. 249: Pancreatic and common bile ducts join early, resulting in a long hepatopancreatic duct.
Fig. 250: A long hepatopancreatic duct is modified by an expanded ampulla.
Fig. 251: Pancreatic and common bile ducts join very close to the greater duodenal papilla, resulting in a short hepatopancreatic duct.
Fig. 252: Both pancreatic and common bile ducts open separately on a somewhat larger duodenal papilla.
Fig. 253: Pancreatic and common bile ducts drain through a single opening, but the ducts are separated by a septum.
Fig. 254: Long hepatopancreatic duct along with a well developed accessory pancreatic duct which opens through the lesser duodenal papilla.

| | |
|---|---|
| 1 Duodenum | 6 Accessory pancreatic duct (Santorini) |
| 2 Common bile duct | 7 Sphincter (Oddi) at duodenal papilla |
| 3 Pancreatic duct (Wirsung) | 8 Pancreatic duct separate opening |
| 4 Pancreas | 9 Hepatopancreatic duct |
| 5 Greater duodenal papilla | |

Figs. 248–254    III

## Fig. 255: X-Ray of the Upper Gastrointestinal Tract.

NOTE: 1) that this figure is a positive print made from an X-ray film and, thus, the contrast medium appears black instead of the conventional white.

2) the sites of junction of the tubular organs comprising the upper gastrointestinal tract. The esophageal orifice at the cardiac end of the stomach (*1 a*) is closed. Observe that this is at the T-11 vertebral level.

3) that the pylorus of the stomach (not numbered) is the narrowed region leading into the superior part of the duodenum (*4*). The superior (*4*), descending (*5 a*), horizontal (*5 b*) and ascending (*5 c*) parts of the duodenum are easily recognizable, as is the duodenojejunal junction (*5 d*).

4) that the contrast medium outlines the internal circular folds or plicae of the jejunum (*6*) and also identifies a peristaltic contraction wave (*7 a, 7 b*).

1  Esophagus. 1a. Cardia closed, contrast medium in creases of mucous membrane
2  Fundus of stomach (filled)
3a Lesser curvature of stomach with longitudinal mucosal folds
3b Greater curvature with gastric folds and areas
4  Duodenal bulb, superior part of duodenum
5a Descending part of duodenum
5b Horizontal part of duodenum
5c Ascending part of duodenum
5d Duodenojejunal flexure
6  Jejunum with circular plicae
7  Peristaltic contraction wave from 7a to 7b

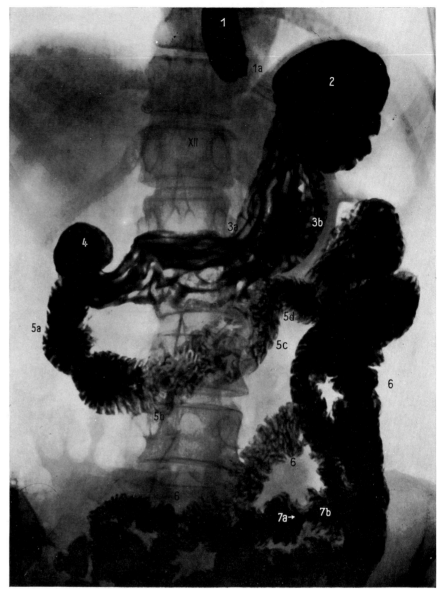

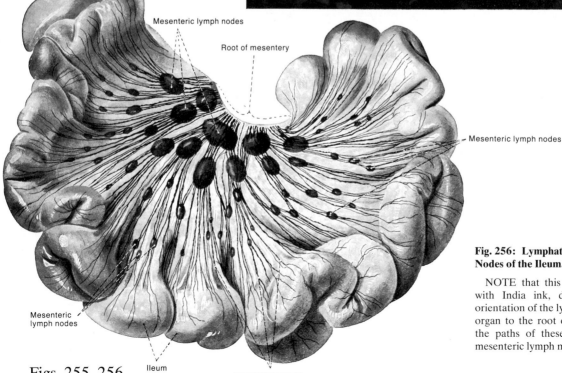

## Fig. 256: Lymphatic Vessels and Nodes of the Ileum.

NOTE that this loop of ileum, injected with India ink, demonstrates the radial orientation of the lymphatic vessels from the organ to the root of the mesentery. Along the paths of these vessels are found the mesenteric lymph nodes.

Figs. 255, 256

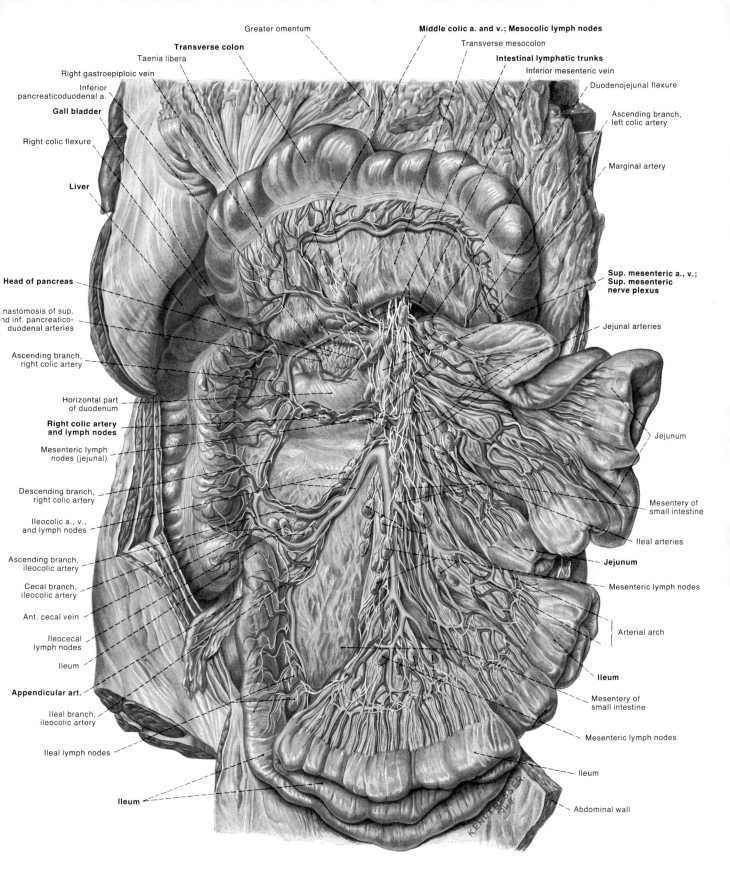

Greater omentum

Middle colic a. and v.; Mesocolic lymph nodes

Transverse colon

Transverse mesocolon

Taenia libera

Intestinal lymphatic trunks

Right gastroepiploic vein

Inferior mesenteric vein

Inferior pancreaticoduodenal a.

Duodenojejunal flexure

Gall bladder

Ascending branch, left colic artery

Right colic flexure

Marginal artery

Liver

Head of pancreas

Sup. mesenteric a., v.; Sup. mesenteric nerve plexus

Anastomosis of sup. and inf. pancreatico-duodenal arteries

Jejunal arteries

Ascending branch, right colic artery

Horizontal part of duodenum

Right colic artery and lymph nodes

Jejunum

Mesenteric lymph nodes (jejunal)

Descending branch, right colic artery

Mesentery of small intestine

Ileocolic a., v., and lymph nodes

Ileal arteries

Ascending branch, ileocolic artery

Jejunum

Cecal branch, ileocolic artery

Mesenteric lymph nodes

Ant. cecal vein

Arterial arch

Ileocecal lymph nodes

Ileum

Appendicular art.

Ileum

Ileal branch, ileocolic artery

Mesentery of small intestine

Ileal lymph nodes

Mesenteric lymph nodes

Ileum

Ileum

Abdominal wall

**Fig. 257: Abdominal Cavity (5); Lymph Nodes, Vessels and Nerves Serving the Jejunum, Ileum, Ascending and Transverse Colon**

NOTE that: 1) the transverse colon has been lifted to reveal its mesocolon along with the retroperitoneal head of the pancreas and duodenum. The loops of jejunum and ileum have been reflected to the left to show the root of the mesentery with its complex network of lymphatics, blood vessels and autonomic nerves.

2) chains of mesenteric lymph nodes follow the ileal and jejunal branches of the superior mesenteric artery and vein, as well as the ileocolic, right colic and middle colic branches of the same vessel.

3) the lymphatics from both the small and large intestine drain centrally and superiorly, eventually to interconnect with pre-aortic chains of nodes.

Fig. 257    III

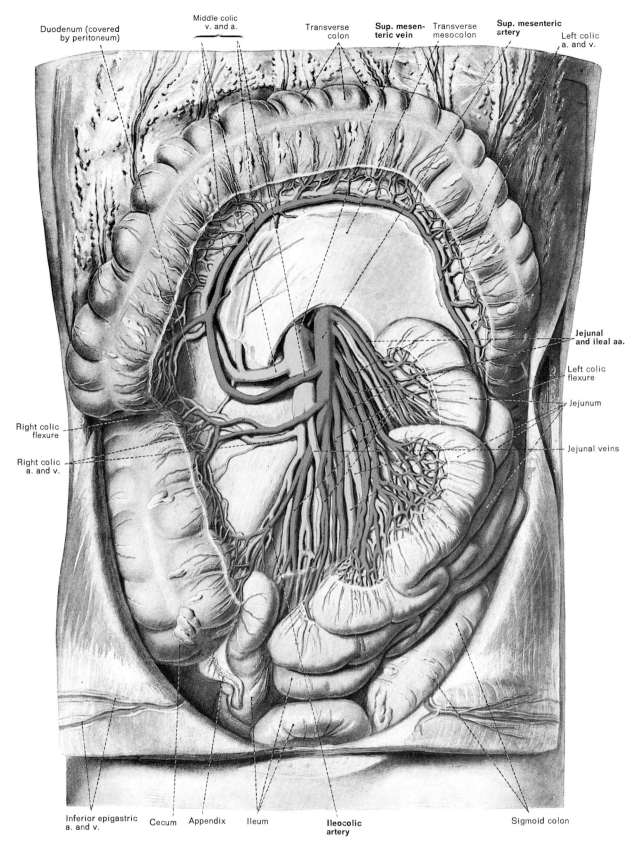

Duodenum (covered by peritoneum) · Middle colic v. and a. · Transverse colon · **Sup. mesenteric vein** · Transverse mesocolon · **Sup. mesenteric artery** · Left colic a. and v.

Jejunal and ileal aa.

Left colic flexure

Jejunum

Jejunal veins

Right colic flexure

Right colic a. and v.

Inferior epigastric a. and v. · Cecum · Appendix · Ileum · **Ileocolic artery** · Sigmoid colon

**Fig. 258: Abdominal Cavity (6): Superior Mesenteric Vessels and Branches**

NOTE: 1) the transverse colon has been turned upward and the small intestine was pushed to the left. The peritoneal attachment along the coils of small intestine and colon has been dissected to reveal the branches of the superior mesenteric vessels which supply the small intestine, ascending colon and transverse colon.

2) the intestinal arteries (jejunal and ileal) branch from the left side of the superior mesenteric artery. There are about 12 of these vessels and they are distributed to the jejunum and ileum.

3) branching from the right side of the superior mesenteric artery are the ileocolic (to the ileocecal region), right colic (to the ascending colon) and middle colic (transverse colon) arteries. Observe the elaborate branching of these vessels and the rich anastomoses which exist among them.

Fig. 258

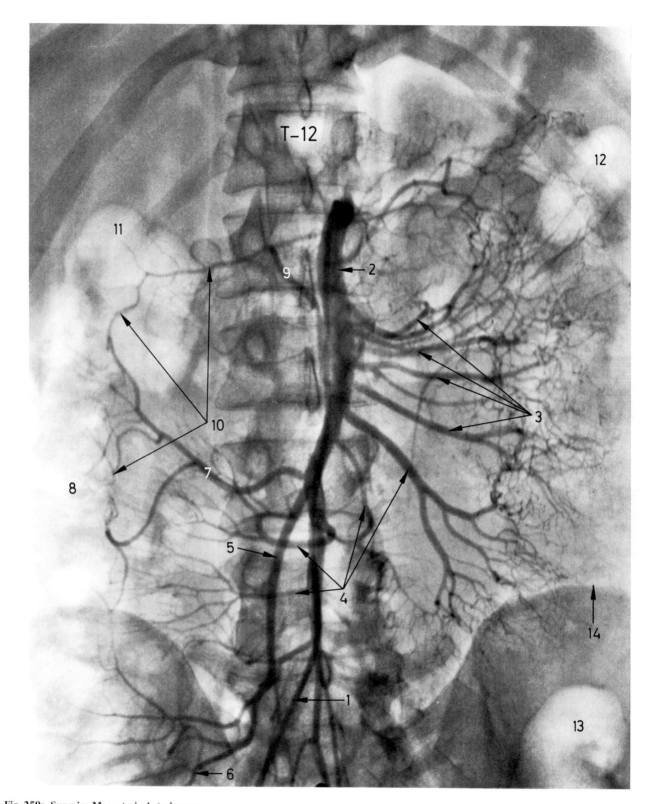

**Fig. 259: Superior Mesenteric Arteriogram**

NOTE: 1) that a catheter (*1*) has been inserted into the common iliac artery and through the abdominal aorta to the point of branching of the superior mesenteric artery (*2*). Contrast medium was injected in order to allow visualization of the principal branches of that vessel. The original radiograph was converted into a positive print.

2) the jejunal (*3*) and ileal (*4*) arteries branching as a sequence of vessels (about fifteen in number) which supply all of the small intestine beyond the duodenum.

3) the ileocolic artery (*5*) and its appendicular branch (*6*), the right colic (*7*), and middle colic (*9*) arteries which supply the cecum, ascending colon (*8*) and transverse colon. Observe that anastomoses among these vessels close to the colon contribute to the formation of the marginal artery (*10*).

4) that other structures can be identified for orientation. These are the right colic flexure (*11*), the left colic flexure (*12*), the sigmoid colon (*13*), the body of the T-12 vertebra and the iliac crest (*14*).

Fig. 259    **III**

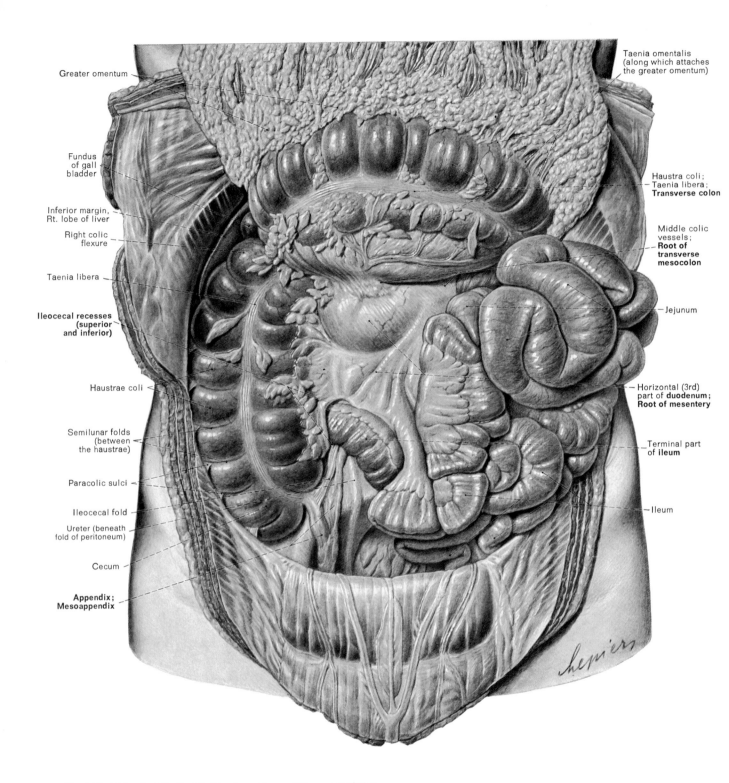

Greater omentum

Taenia omentalis
(along which attaches
the greater omentum)

Fundus
of gall
bladder

Haustra coli;
Taenia libera;
**Transverse colon**

Inferior margin,
Rt. lobe of liver

Middle colic
vessels;
**Root of
transverse
mesocolon**

Right colic
flexure

Taenia libera

Jejunum

Ileocecal recesses
(superior
and inferior)

Horizontal (3rd)
part of **duodenum;
Root of mesentery**

Haustrae coli

Semilunar folds
(between
the haustrae)

Terminal part
of **ileum**

Paracolic sulci

Ileum

Ileocecal fold

Ureter (beneath
fold of peritoneum)

Cecum

**Appendix;
Mesoappendix**

**Fig. 260: Abdominal Cavity (7): The Ascending and Transverse Colon**

NOTE: 1) the greater omentum has been reflected superiorly and the jejunum and ileum have been pulled to the left in order to expose the root of the mesentery of the small intestine on the right side.

2) the horizontal (3rd) part of the duodenum which is retroperitoneal and which is covered by the smooth and glistening peritoneum. Observe also the distal portion of the ileum at its junction with the cecum. At this ileocecal junction, identify the ileocecal fold, the appendix and the mesoappendix. The appendix may extend cranially behind the cecum, toward the left and behind the ileum, or as demonstrated here, inferiorly over the pelvic brim.

3) the transverse colon and the small intestine beyond the duodenal junction are more mobile than most other organs because they are attached to the transverse mesocolon and the mesentery.

4) the retroperitoneal position of the right ureter as it descends over the pelvic brim on its course toward the bladder in the pelvis.

Fig. 260

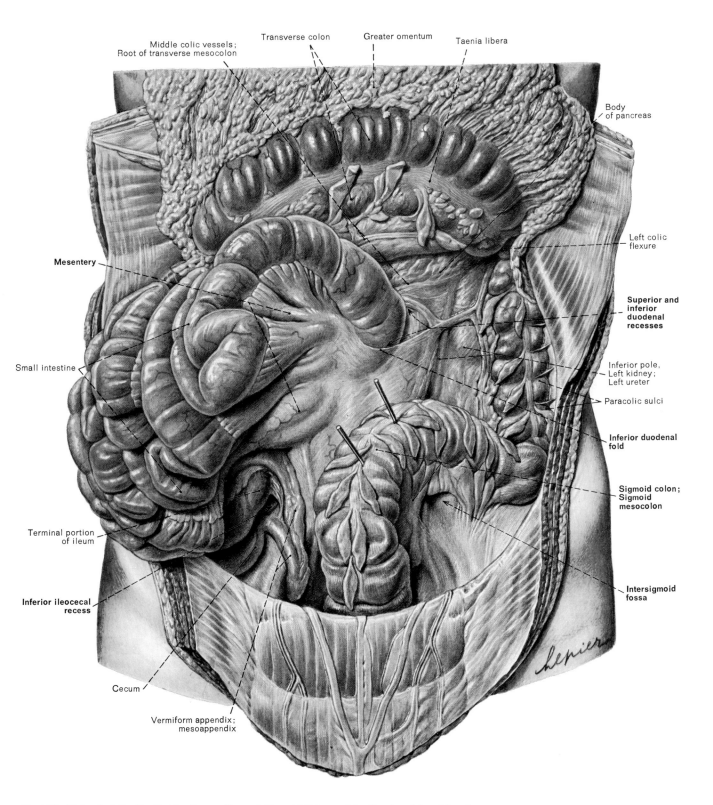

Middle colic vessels;
Root of transverse mesocolon

Transverse colon

Greater omentum

Taenia libera

Body
of pancreas

Left colic
flexure

Mesentery

Superior and
inferior
duodenal
recesses

Inferior pole,
Left kidney;
Left ureter

Small intestine

Paracolic sulci

Inferior duodenal
fold

Sigmoid colon;
Sigmoid
mesocolon

Terminal portion
of ileum

Inferior ileocecal
recess

Intersigmoid
fossa

Cecum

Vermiform appendix;
mesoappendix

**Fig. 261: Abdominal Cavity (8): The Descending and Sigmoid Colon and the Duodenojejunal Junction**

NOTE: 1) the transverse colon and greater omentum have been reflected superiorly and the jejunum and ileum have been pulled to the right to reveal the duodenojejunal junction and the descending and sigmoid colon.

2) as the ascending (4th) part of the duodenum becomes jejunum, and the small intestine acquires a mesentery at that site, there frequently are found duodenal fossae or recesses situated in relation to the junction. Look for the inferior and superior duodenal recesses (present in over 50% of the cases). These are of importance because they represent possible sites of intestinal herniae within the abdomen.

3) the mobility of the sigmoid colon because of its mesocolic attachment, in contrast to the descending colon which is more fixed to the posterior wall of the abdomen. Observe the intersigmoid fossa located behind the sigmoid mesocolon and between it and the peritoneum reflected over the external iliac vessels.

Fig. 261    III

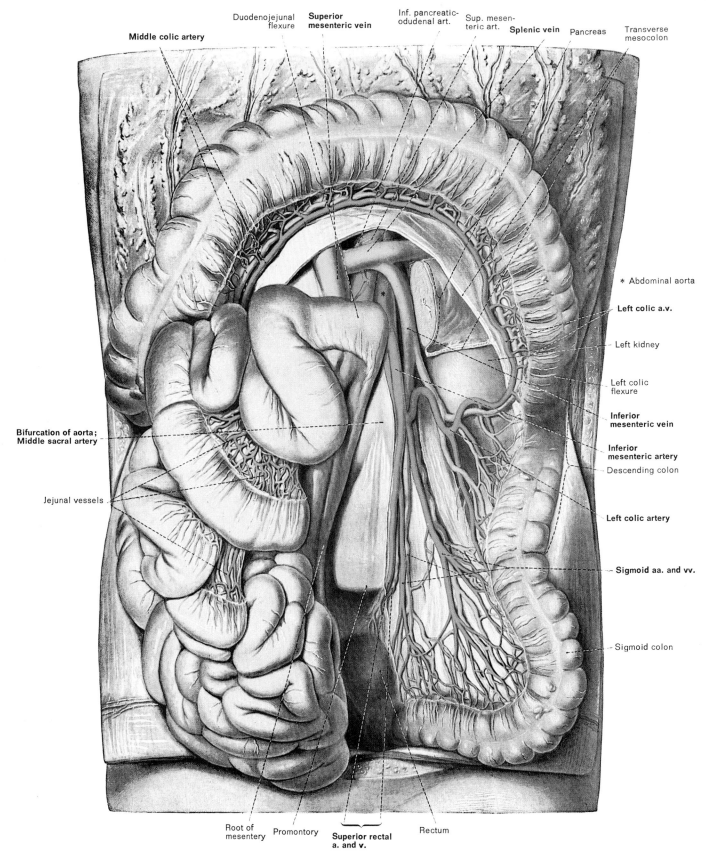

Middle colic artery

Duodenojejunal flexure

**Superior mesenteric vein**

Inf. pancreatic-odudenal art.

Sup. mesen-teric art.

**Splenic vein**

Pancreas

Transverse mesocolon

\* Abdominal aorta

**Left colic a.v.**

Left kidney

Left colic flexure

**Inferior mesenteric vein**

**Inferior mesenteric artery**

Descending colon

**Left colic artery**

**Sigmoid aa. and vv.**

Sigmoid colon

Bifurcation of aorta; Middle sacral artery

Jejunal vessels

Root of mesentery

Promontory

**Superior rectal a. and v.**

Rectum

**Fig. 262: Abdominal Cavity (9): The Inferior Mesenteric Vessels and Branches**

NOTE: 1) the small intestine has been pushed to the right side of the abdomen to reveal the origin of the inferior mesenteric artery from the aorta, and the drainage of the inferior mesenteric vein into the splenic vein. Also a portion of the body of the pancreas and transverse mesocolon was removed to show these relationships more clearly.

2) the inferior mesenteric artery supplies the descending colon via the left colic artery. Observe the anastomosis around the margin of the large bowel between the left colic artery and the middle colic artery. Somewhat lower, the inferior mesenteric gives rise to the sigmoid arteries and the superior rectal vessels.

3) the bifurcation of the abdominal aorta retroperitoneally and the middle sacral artery descending in the midline.

Fig. 262

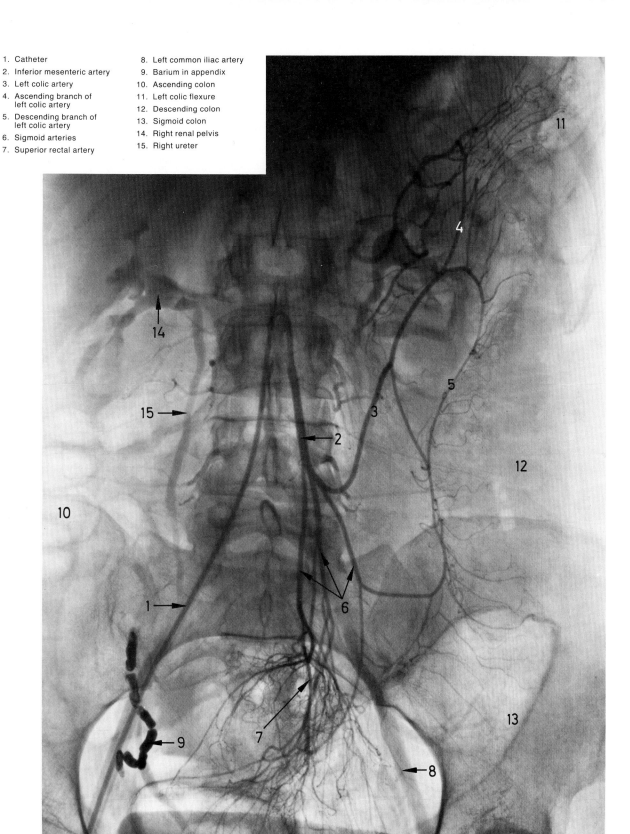

1. Catheter
2. Inferior mesenteric artery
3. Left colic artery
4. Ascending branch of left colic artery
5. Descending branch of left colic artery
6. Sigmoid arteries
7. Superior rectal artery
8. Left common iliac artery
9. Barium in appendix
10. Ascending colon
11. Left colic flexure
12. Descending colon
13. Sigmoid colon
14. Right renal pelvis
15. Right ureter

**Fig. 263: An Inferior Mesenteric Arteriogram**

NOTE that: 1) a catheter *(1)* has been inserted through the right internal iliac artery and directed superiorly into the abdominal aorta to the point of origin of the inferior mesenteric artery *(2)*. A contrast medium was then injected into that artery in order to demonstrate its field of distribution;

2) the branches of the inferior mesenteric artery *(2)* shown in this arteriogram are quite normal. The left colic artery *(3)* shows both an ascending *(4)* and a descending branch *(5)*;

3) several sigmoid arteries *(6)* supply the sigmoid colon *(13)*, and these anastomose above with branches of the left colic artery *(3)* and below with the superior rectal artery *(7)*.

Fig. 263    III

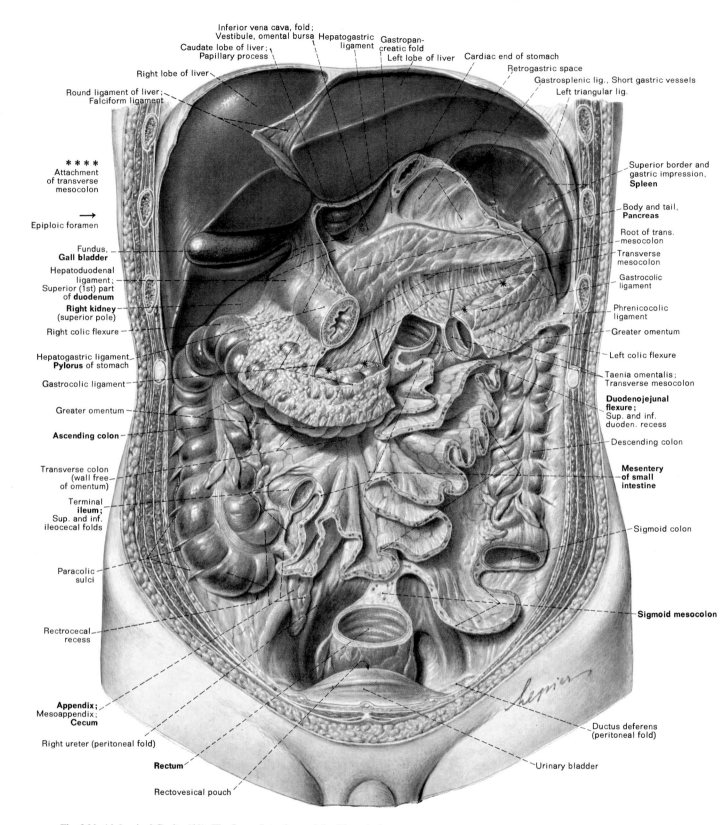

Inferior vena cava, fold;
Vestibule, omental bursa
Caudate lobe of liver;
Papillary process
Right lobe of liver
Round ligament of liver;
Falciform ligament
Hepatogastric ligament
Gastropan-creatic fold
Left lobe of liver
Cardiac end of stomach
Retrogastric space
Gastrosplenic lig., Short gastric vessels
Left triangular lig.

* * * *
Attachment of transverse mesocolon

→
Epiploic foramen

Fundus, **Gall bladder**

Hepatoduodenal ligament;
Superior (1st) part of **duodenum**

**Right kidney** (superior pole)

Right colic flexure

Hepatogastric ligament
**Pylorus** of stomach

Gastrocolic ligament

Greater omentum

**Ascending colon**

Transverse colon (wall free of omentum)

Terminal **ileum;**
Sup. and inf. ileocecal folds

Paracolic sulci

Rectrocecal recess

**Appendix;**
Mesoappendix;
**Cecum**

Right ureter (peritoneal fold)

**Rectum**

Rectovesical pouch

Superior border and gastric impression, **Spleen**

Body and tail, **Pancreas**

Root of trans. mesocolon

Transverse mesocolon

Gastrocolic ligament

Phrenicocolic ligament

Greater omentum

Left colic flexure

Taenia omentalis;
Transverse mesocolon

**Duodenojejunal flexure;**
Sup. and inf. duoden. recess

Descending colon

**Mesentery of small intestine**

Sigmoid colon

**Sigmoid mesocolon**

Ductus deferens (peritoneal fold)

Urinary bladder

**Fig. 264: Abdominal Cavity (10): The Large Intestine and the Mesenteries**

NOTE: 1) the stomach was cut just proximal to the pylorus and the small intestine was severed at the duodenojejunal junction and at the distal ileum and then removed by cutting the mesentery. A portion of the transverse colon was removed along with the greater omentum, and the sigmoid colon was resected to reveal its mesocolon.

2) the mesentery of the small intestine extends obliquely across the posterior abdominal wall from the duodenojejunal flexure to the ilocecal junction. In this distance of about 6 to 7 inches, the mesentery is thrown into many folds to accommodate all the loops of jejunum and ileum.

3) the ascending and descending colon is fused to the posterior abdominal wall, while the transverse and sigmoid colon are suspended by their respective mesocolons.

4) that the vessels and nerves supplying the small intestine course *between* the layers of the mesentery to achieve the organ.

Fig. 264

**Fig. 265: The Ileocecal Junction**

NOTE: 1) the terminal ileum, cecum and lower ascending colon have been opened anteriorly to reveal the ileocecal junction and the opening of the vermiform appendix.

2) the leaves of the ileocecal valve have been separated. Observe that this valve is formed by two reflected folds of the wall of the large intestine. These folds unite and then project further around the large intestine as the frenulum.

3) the orifice of the appendix opens into the cecum, although the position and the direction of the appendix are quite variable. Observe the semilunar folds, the sacculations (haustrae) and longitudinal muscle bands (taeniae) which characterize the large intestine.

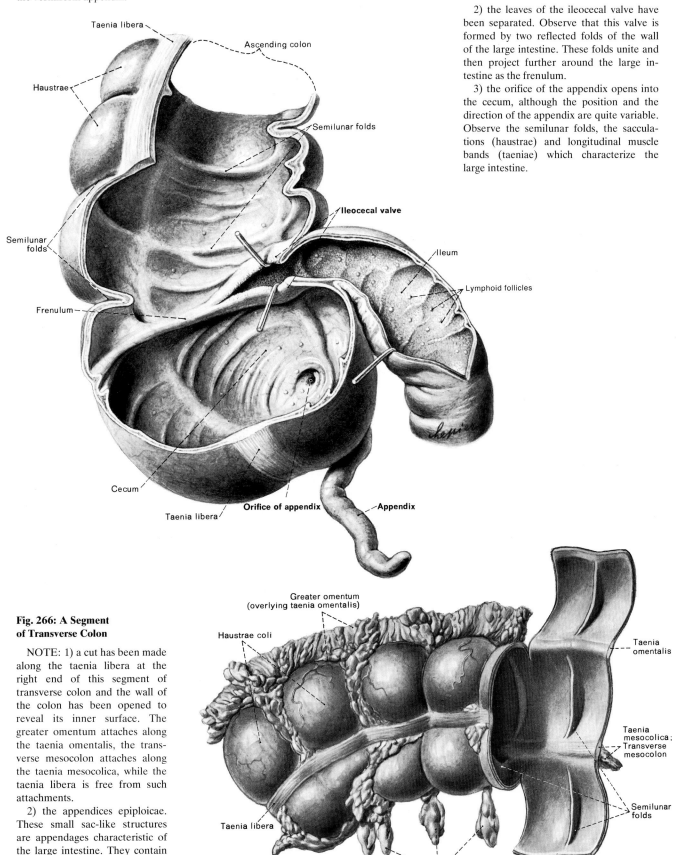

**Fig. 266: A Segment of Transverse Colon**

NOTE: 1) a cut has been made along the taenia libera at the right end of this segment of transverse colon and the wall of the colon has been opened to reveal its inner surface. The greater omentum attaches along the taenia omentalis, the transverse mesocolon attaches along the taenia mesocolica, while the taenia libera is free from such attachments.

2) the appendices epiploicae. These small sac-like structures are appendages characteristic of the large intestine. They contain fat and their function is unknown.

Figs. 265, 266     III

**Fig. 267: The Inner Surface of the Rectum and Anal Canal**

NOTE: 1) at about the level of the 3rd sacral vertebra, the sigmoid colon becomes the rectum. Measuring about 5 inches in length, the rectum then becomes the anal canal which is the terminal $1^1/_2$ inches of the intestinal tract. The rectum is dilated near its junction with the anal canal, giving rise to the rectal ampulla.

2) the internal mucosa of the rectum is thrown into transverse folds of which there are usually three in number. They are also known as the valves of Houston.

3) below the rectal ampulla, the mucosa of the anal canal shows a series of longitudinal folds called the anal colums (columns of Morgagni). Each of these folds usually possesses an artery and vein, and between the anal columns are small fossae called the anal sinuses. The veins in this region are dilated and tortuous and can become varicosed, giving rise to a condition called hemorrhoids or piles.

4) distal to the anal column is an abrupt zone of epithelial transition. The stratified squamous of the distalmost part of the anal canal becomes the simple columnar of the rectum. This transition line can be identified in a living person and is referred to as Hilton's line.

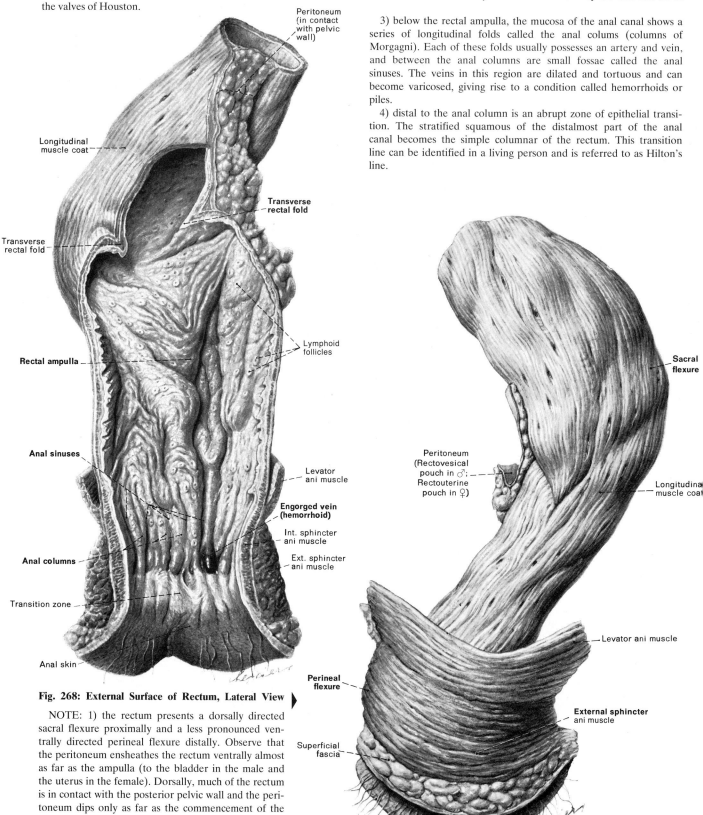

**Fig. 268: External Surface of Rectum, Lateral View**

NOTE: 1) the rectum presents a dorsally directed sacral flexure proximally and a less pronounced ventrally directed perineal flexure distally. Observe that the peritoneum ensheathes the rectum ventrally almost as far as the ampulla (to the bladder in the male and the uterus in the female). Dorsally, much of the rectum is in contact with the posterior pelvic wall and the peritoneum dips only as far as the commencement of the sacral flexure.

2) the fibers of the levator ani muscle (which forms the floor of the pelvis) surround the rectum and are

(con't next page)

Figs. 267, 268

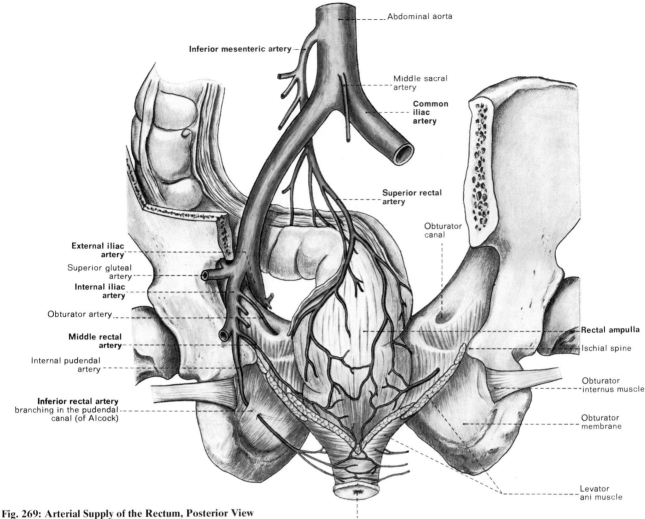

Abdominal aorta

Inferior mesenteric artery

Middle sacral artery

Common iliac artery

Superior rectal artery

Obturator canal

External iliac artery

Superior gluteal artery

Internal iliac artery

Obturator artery

Middle rectal artery

Internal pudendal artery

Inferior rectal artery branching in the pudendal canal (of Alcock)

Rectal ampulla

Ischial spine

Obturator internus muscle

Obturator membrane

Levator ani muscle

Anus

**Fig. 269: Arterial Supply of the Rectum, Posterior View**

NOTE: 1) this posterior view of the arterial supply of the rectum shows the superior rectal artery which branches from the inferior mesenteric artery, and distributes to the rectum as far as the ampulla. The middle rectal artery coming off the internal iliac artery and the inferior rectal artery branching from the internal pudendal artery supply the more caudal parts of the rectum.

2) from the bifurcation of the aorta, the middle sacral artery descends down the midline of the sacrum. The common iliac arteries branch into external and internal iliac vessels. From the internal iliac (hypogastric), many of the pelvic organs derive their blood supply.

3) the internal pudendal artery coursing within the pudendal canal (of Alcock). The inferior rectal artery branches from the internal pudendal within this canal.

**Fig. 270: Distribution Pattern of the Rectal Arteries**

This figure shows the distribution of the superior, middle and inferior rectal arteries as they supply the rectum and the anal canal. Observe that the region of distribution of the superior rectal artery is much greater than either the middle or inferior rectal arteries. Note the rich anastomoses among these three vessels.

Superior rectal artery

Middle rectal artery

Inferior rectal artery

continued distally as the external sphincter ani muscle. The internal sphincter ani muscle (seen in Figure 267) is composed of smooth muscle and really represents a thickening of the inner circular muscle layer in the wall of the rectum. Observe also the outer longitudinal (smooth) muscle layer.

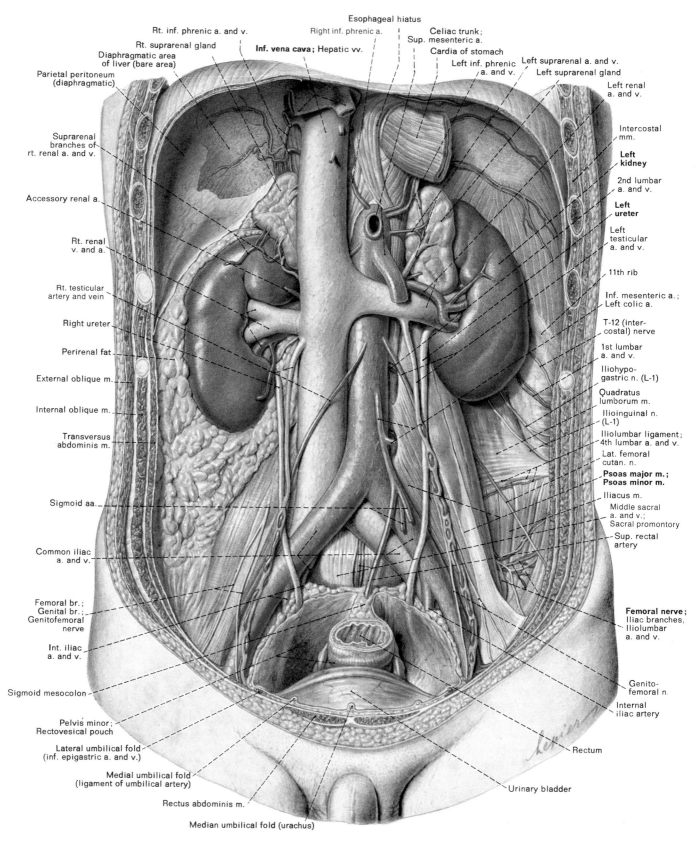

Rt. inf. phrenic a. and v.
Rt. suprarenal gland
Diaphragmatic area
of liver (bare area)
Parietal peritoneum
(diaphragmatic)

Esophageal hiatus
Right inf. phrenic a.
Inf. vena cava; Hepatic vv.

Celiac trunk;
Sup. mesenteric a.
Cardia of stomach
Left inf. phrenic
a. and v.
Left suprarenal a. and v.
Left suprarenal gland

Left renal
a. and v.

Suprarenal
branches of
rt. renal a. and v.

Intercostal
mm.
Left
kidney
2nd lumbar
a. and v.
Left
ureter
Left
testicular
a. and v.

Accessory renal a.

Rt. renal
v. and a.

Rt. testicular
artery and vein

11th rib

Inf. mesenteric a.;
Left colic a.

Right ureter

Perirenal fat

External oblique m.

Internal oblique m.

Transversus
abdominis m.

Sigmoid aa.

Common iliac
a. and v.

Femoral br.;
Genital br.;
Genitofemoral
nerve

Int. iliac
a. and v.

Sigmoid mesocolon

Pelvis minor;
Rectovesical pouch

Lateral umbilical fold
(inf. epigastric a. and v.)

Medial umbilical fold
(ligament of umbilical artery)

Rectus abdominis m.

Median umbilical fold (urachus)

T-12 (inter-
costal) nerve
1st lumbar
a. and v.
Iliohypo-
gastric n. (L-1)
Quadratus
lumborum m.
Ilioinguinal n.
(L-1)
Iliolumbar ligament;
4th lumbar a. and v.
Lat. femoral
cutan. n.
Psoas major m.;
Psoas minor m.
Iliacus m.
Middle sacral
a. and v.;
Sacral promontory
Sup. rectal
artery

Femoral nerve;
Iliac branches,
Iliolumbar
a. and v.

Genito-
femoral n.
Internal
iliac artery

Rectum

Urinary bladder

**Fig. 273: The Abdominal Cavity (13): The Posterior Abdominal Wall**

NOTE: 1) the kidneys, ureters, suprarenal glands, and the great vessels and their branches. The kidneys extend between vertebral levels T-12 and L-3. The ureters commence on the posterior aspect of the hilum of the kidneys, course inferiorly over the pelvic brim near the bifurcation of the common iliac arteries, eventually to terminate in the bladder.

2) the suprarenal glands as they cap the upper pole of each kidney. These are highly vascular and vital glands of internal secretion (endocrine).

3) the aorta which enters the abdomen through the aortic hiatus (T-12). The inferior vena cava lies to the right of the vertebral column. It is formed by the confluence of the two common iliac veins (at about L-5) and passes through the caval opening of the diaphragm.

Fig. 273

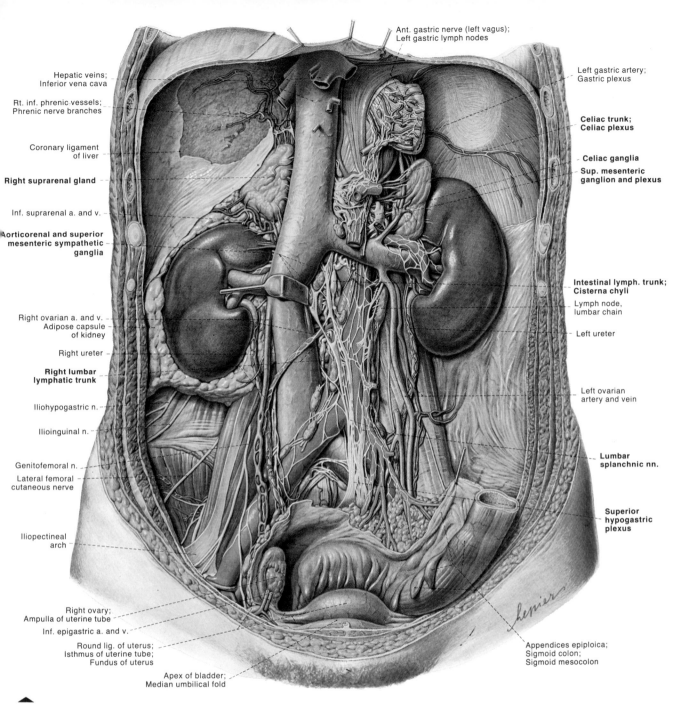

Hepatic veins;
Inferior vena cava

Rt. inf. phrenic vessels;
Phrenic nerve branches

Coronary ligament
of liver

**Right suprarenal gland**

Inf. suprarenal a. and v.

Aorticorenal and superior
mesenteric sympathetic
ganglia

Right ovarian a. and v.
Adipose capsule
of kidney

Right ureter

**Right lumbar
lymphatic trunk**

Iliohypogastric n.

Ilioinguinal n.

Genitofemoral n.
Lateral femoral
cutaneous nerve

Iliopectineal
arch

Right ovary;
Ampulla of uterine tube

Inf. epigastric a. and v.

Round lig. of uterus;
Isthmus of uterine tube;
Fundus of uterus

Apex of bladder;
Median umbilical fold

Ant. gastric nerve (left vagus);
Left gastric lymph nodes

Left gastric artery;
Gastric plexus

**Celiac trunk;
Celiac plexus**

**Celiac ganglia**
**Sup. mesenteric
ganglion and plexus**

**Intestinal lymph. trunk;
Cisterna chyli**

Lymph node,
lumbar chain

Left ureter

Left ovarian
artery and vein

**Lumbar
splanchnic nn.**

**Superior
hypogastric
plexus**

Appendices epiploica;
Sigmoid colon;
Sigmoid mesocolon

---

▲

### Fig. 274: Abdominal Cavity (14): Lymphatics and Nerves of the Posterior Abdominal Wall

NOTE: 1) that lymphatic channels draining pelvic and posterior abdominal wall structures course along iliac nodes to right and left chains of lumbar nodes which parallel the aorta. These lumbar trunks are joined by intestinal trunks draining the G. I. tract in helping to form the cysterna chyli;

2) the sympathetic ganglia and plexuses which are found in relation to the abdominal aorta and its branches.

### Fig. 275: Posterior Abdominal Wall in 5 Month Fetus

NOTE the lobulated appearance of the fetal kidneys. Even at birth this lobulation is obvious, but as maturation proceeds the surface slowly becomes smooth. Observe the large suprarenal glands and ureters, and the location of the testes.

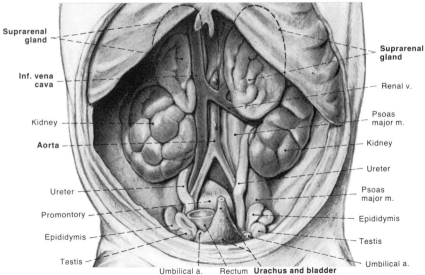

Suprarenal
gland

Inf. vena
cava

Kidney

**Aorta**

Ureter

Promontory

Epididymis

Testis

**Suprarenal
gland**

Renal v.

Psoas
major m.

Kidney

Ureter

Psoas
major m.

Epididymis

Testis

Umbilical a.

Umbilical a.    Rectum    **Urachus and bladder**

Figs. 274, 275    III

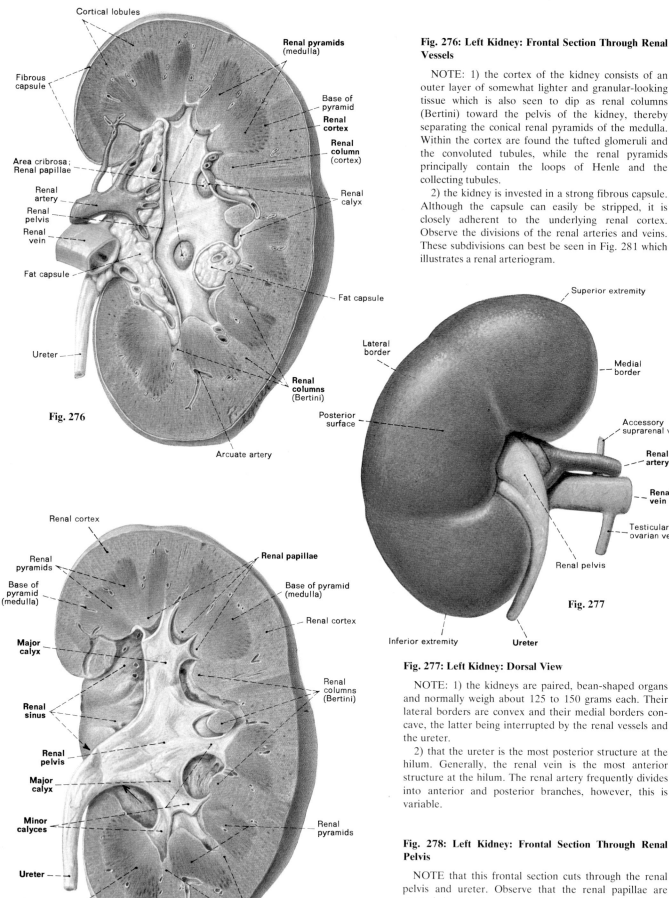

**Fig. 276 (Left Kidney: Frontal Section Through Renal Vessels)**

Labels: Cortical lobules · Fibrous capsule · Area cribrosa; Renal papillae · Renal artery · Renal pelvis · Renal vein · Fat capsule · Ureter · Fig. 276 · Arcuate artery · **Renal pyramids** (medulla) · Base of pyramid · **Renal cortex** · **Renal column** (cortex) · Renal calyx · Fat capsule · **Renal columns** (Bertini)

**Fig. 278 (Left Kidney: Frontal Section Through Renal Pelvis)**

Labels: Renal cortex · Renal pyramids · Base of pyramid (medulla) · **Major calyx** · **Renal sinus** · **Renal pelvis** · **Major calyx** · **Minor calyces** · **Ureter** · Renal pyramid (medulla) · Renal cortex · **Renal papillae** · Base of pyramid (medulla) · Renal cortex · Renal columns (Bertini) · Renal pyramids · Renal columns · Fig. 278

**Fig. 277 (Left Kidney: Dorsal View)**

Labels: Superior extremity · Medial border · Lateral border · Posterior surface · Accessory suprarenal vein · **Renal artery** · **Renal vein** · Testicular or ovarian vein · Renal pelvis · Inferior extremity · Ureter · Fig. 277

### Fig. 276: Left Kidney: Frontal Section Through Renal Vessels

NOTE: 1) the cortex of the kidney consists of an outer layer of somewhat lighter and granular-looking tissue which is also seen to dip as renal columns (Bertini) toward the pelvis of the kidney, thereby separating the conical renal pyramids of the medulla. Within the cortex are found the tufted glomeruli and the convoluted tubules, while the renal pyramids principally contain the loops of Henle and the collecting tubules.

2) the kidney is invested in a strong fibrous capsule. Although the capsule can easily be stripped, it is closely adherent to the underlying renal cortex. Observe the divisions of the renal arteries and veins. These subdivisions can best be seen in Fig. 281 which illustrates a renal arteriogram.

### Fig. 277: Left Kidney: Dorsal View

NOTE: 1) the kidneys are paired, bean-shaped organs and normally weigh about 125 to 150 grams each. Their lateral borders are convex and their medial borders concave, the latter being interrupted by the renal vessels and the ureter.

2) that the ureter is the most posterior structure at the hilum. Generally, the renal vein is the most anterior structure at the hilum. The renal artery frequently divides into anterior and posterior branches, however, this is variable.

### Fig. 278: Left Kidney: Frontal Section Through Renal Pelvis

NOTE that this frontal section cuts through the renal pelvis and ureter. Observe that the renal papillae are cupped by small collecting tubes, the minor calyces. Several minor calyces unite to form a mayor calyx, while the renal pelvis is formed by the union of two or three major calyces. Leading from the renal pelvis is the somewhat more narrowed ureter.

Figs. 276, 277, 278

## Fig. 279: Retrograde Pyelogram

NOTE: 1) a radioopaque substance has been introduced into each ureter and forced in a retrograde manner into the renal pelvis, major calyces and minor calyces of each side. Observe that into the minor calyces project the renal papillae (5), resulting in radiolucent invaginations into the radioopaque minor calyces.

2) the shadow of the superior extremity of the left kidney extending to the top of the body of the T-12 vertebra, while the right kidney is somewhat more inferior.

3) the lateral margins of the psoas major muscles. The ureters course toward the pelvis along the anterior surfaces of these muscles.

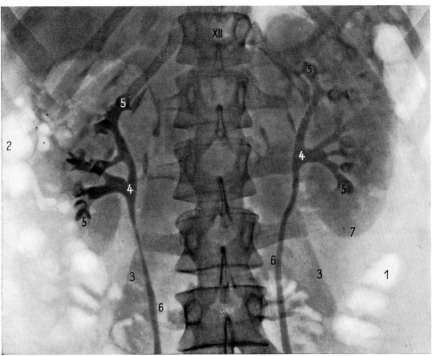

| | | | |
|---|---|---|---|
| 1 Descending colon | 3 Psoas major muscle | 5 Renal papilla | 7 Inferior pole of |
| 2 Ascending colon | (lateral border) | 6 Ureter | left kidney |
| | 4 Renal pelvis | | XII 12th thoracic vertebra |

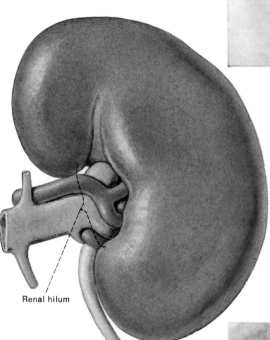

Renal hilum

## Fig. 280: Left Kidney: Ventral View

NOTE: 1) although the stem of the renal artery initially lies dorsal to the stem of the renal vein at the hilum, the renal artery divides into anterior and posterior branches. The anterior branch generally enters the kidney ventral to the renal vein, as is shown in this figure.

2) the anterior surfaces of the kidneys are covered by peritoneum and are in relationship to more ventrally located abdominal organs. In contrast, their posterior surfaces lie adjacent to the musculature of the posterior abdominal wall and the diaphragm.

| | | | |
|---|---|---|---|
| 1 Stomach | 3 Right renal artery | 5 Interlobular arteries | XII 12th thoracic |
| 2 Superior (1st) part | 4 Interlobar arteries | K Catheter | vertebra |
| of duodenum | | | |

## Fig. 281: Arteriogram of Right Renal Artery and its Branches

NOTE: 1) an arterial catheter (K) has been inserted into the femoral artery, passed through the abdominal aorta and into the right renal artery. Observe the division of the renal artery successively into interlobar arteries (4).

2) as the interlobar arteries reach the junction of the renal cortex and medulla, they arch over the bases of the pyramids forming the arcuate arteries (not numbered in this figure). From the arcuate arteries branch a series of interlobular arteries which extend through the afferent arterioles which enter the renal glomeruli.

3) the stomach (1) and superior (1st) part of the duodenum (2) which are filled with air.

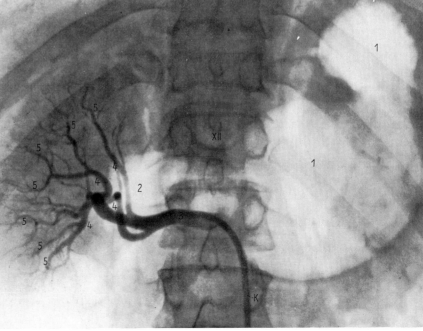

Figs. 279, 280, 281    III

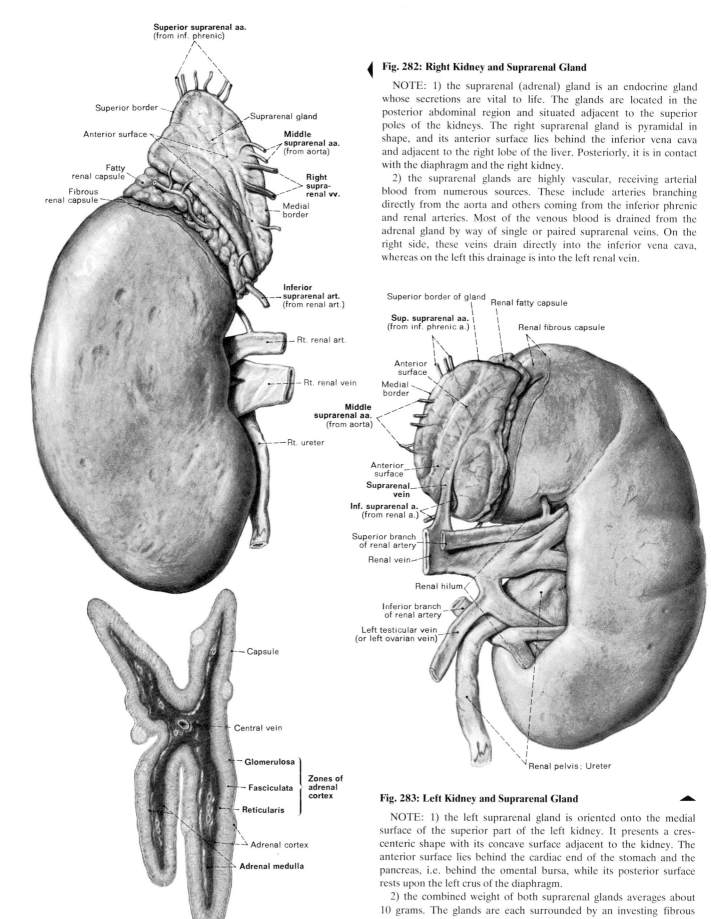

**Superior suprarenal aa.**
(from inf. phrenic)

Superior border

Anterior surface

Fatty renal capsule

Fibrous renal capsule

Suprarenal gland

**Middle suprarenal aa.**
(from aorta)

**Right supra-renal vv.**

Medial border

**Inferior suprarenal art.**
(from renal art.)

Rt. renal art.

Rt. renal vein

Rt. ureter

Capsule

Central vein

**Glomerulosa**

**Fasciculata**

**Reticularis**

Zones of adrenal cortex

Adrenal cortex

**Adrenal medulla**

### Fig. 282: Right Kidney and Suprarenal Gland

NOTE: 1) the suprarenal (adrenal) gland is an endocrine gland whose secretions are vital to life. The glands are located in the posterior abdominal region and situated adjacent to the superior poles of the kidneys. The right suprarenal gland is pyramidal in shape, and its anterior surface lies behind the inferior vena cava and adjacent to the right lobe of the liver. Posteriorly, it is in contact with the diaphragm and the right kidney.

2) the suprarenal glands are highly vascular, receiving arterial blood from numerous sources. These include arteries branching directly from the aorta and others coming from the inferior phrenic and renal arteries. Most of the venous blood is drained from the adrenal gland by way of single or paired suprarenal veins. On the right side, these veins drain directly into the inferior vena cava, whereas on the left this drainage is into the left renal vein.

Superior border of gland

Renal fatty capsule

**Sup. suprarenal aa.**
(from inf. phrenic a.)

Renal fibrous capsule

Anterior surface

Medial border

**Middle suprarenal aa.**
(from aorta)

Anterior surface

**Suprarenal vein**

**Inf. suprarenal a.**
(from renal a.)

Superior branch of renal artery

Renal vein

Renal hilum

Inferior branch of renal artery

Left testicular vein
(or left ovarian vein)

Renal pelvis ; Ureter

### Fig. 283: Left Kidney and Suprarenal Gland

NOTE: 1) the left suprarenal gland is oriented onto the medial surface of the superior part of the left kidney. It presents a crescenteric shape with its concave surface adjacent to the kidney. The anterior surface lies behind the cardiac end of the stomach and the pancreas, i.e. behind the omental bursa, while its posterior surface rests upon the left crus of the diaphragm.

2) the combined weight of both suprarenal glands averages about 10 grams. The glands are each surrounded by an investing fibrous capsule, around which is a variable amount of areolar tissue.

### Fig. 284: Section Through Suprarenal Gland

NOTE that the suprarenal gland is composed of an inner medulla and outer cortex. The cells of the medulla secrete epinephrine while the adrenal cortex secretes adrenal corticosteroids.

Figs. 282, 283, 284

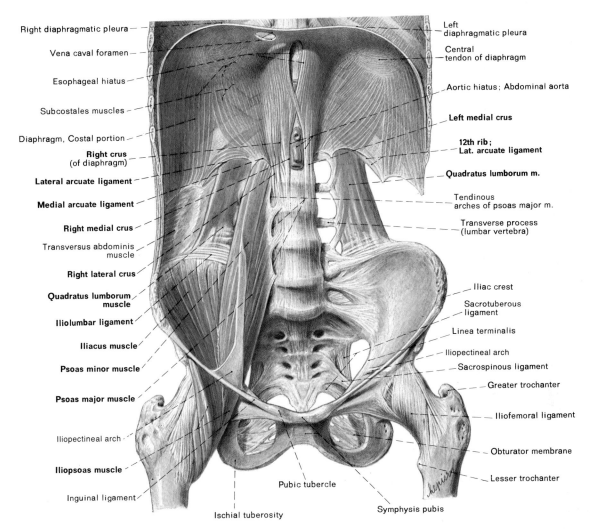

Right diaphragmatic pleura —
Vena caval foramen —
Esophageal hiatus —
Subcostales muscles —
Diaphragm, Costal portion —
**Right crus** (of diaphragm)
**Lateral arcuate ligament** —
**Medial arcuate ligament** —
**Right medial crus** —
Transversus abdominis muscle —
**Right lateral crus** —
**Quadratus lumborum muscle**
**Iliolumbar ligament** —
**Iliacus muscle** —
**Psoas minor muscle** —
**Psoas major muscle** —
Iliopectineal arch —
**Iliopsoas muscle** —
Inguinal ligament —

Left diaphragmatic pleura
Central tendon of diaphragm
Aortic hiatus; Abdominal aorta
**Left medial crus**
**12th rib; Lat. arcuate ligament**
**Quadratus lumborum m.**
Tendinous arches of psoas major m.
Transverse process (lumbar vertebra)
Iliac crest
Sacrotuberous ligament
Linea terminalis
Iliopectineal arch
Sacrospinous ligament
Greater trochanter
Iliofemoral ligament
Obturator membrane
Lesser trochanter

Ischial tuberosity
Pubic tubercle
Symphysis pubis

## Fig. 285: The Diaphragm and Posterior Abdominal Wall Muscles

NOTE: 1) the posterior attachments of the diaphragm include a) the right and left crura which arise from the anterior and lateral aspects of the bodies of the upper 3 or 4 lumbar vertebrae, b) the right and left medial arcuate ligaments which are thickenings in the psoas fascia, and c) the lateral arcuate ligaments along the 12th rib overlying the quadratus lumborum muscle.

2) the psoas major and minor muscles descending from the lumbar vertebrae to join the iliacus in the lateral wall of the pelvis to insert onto the lesser trochanter of the femur. The iliopsoas is the most powerful flexor of the thigh at the hip joint.

3) the rectangular quadratus lumborum intervening between the 12th rib, the transverse processes of the lumbar vertebrae and the posteromedial iliac crest.

## Fig. 286: Posterior View of Diaphragm

NOTE: 1) the posterior half of the bony thorax (ribs and vertebral column) has been removed to reveal the diaphragm from behind. Observe that the caval opening is to the right of midline and more superior to those transmitting the esophagus and aorta.

2) that from their origin around the thoracic outlet, the muscular fibers of the diaphragm converge to insert into a central tendon. Observe the dome-shape of the diaphragm on each side and that the right dome extends more superiorly into the thoracic cavity because of the large right lobe of the liver.

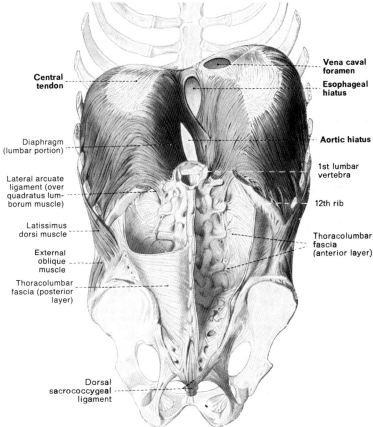

**Central tendon**
Diaphragm (lumbar portion)
Lateral arcuate ligament (over quadratus lumborum muscle)
Latissimus dorsi muscle
External oblique muscle
Thoracolumbar fascia (posterior layer)
Dorsal sacrococcygeal ligament

**Vena caval foramen**
**Esophageal hiatus**
**Aortic hiatus**
1st lumbar vertebra
12th rib
Thoracolumbar fascia (anterior layer)

Figs. 285, 286    **III**

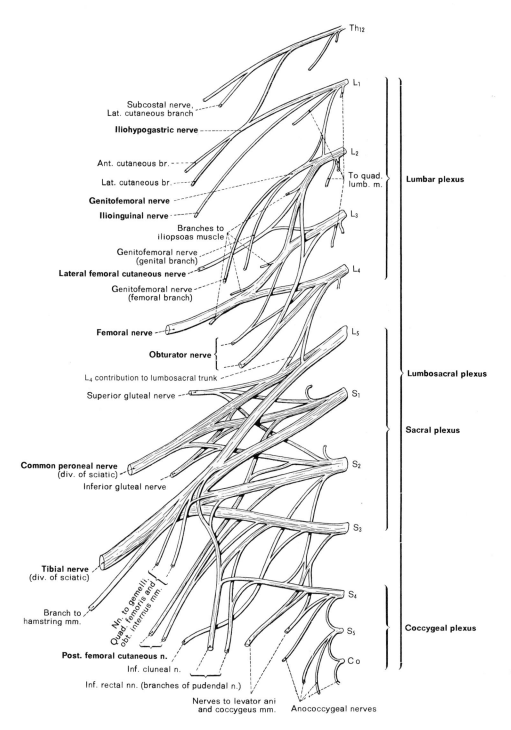

**Fig. 287: Diagram of the Lumbar, Sacral, Pudendal and Coccygeal Nerve Plexuses**

NOTE: 1) the 12th thoracic (subcostal) and 1st lumbar nerves are distributed principally to the lower abdominal wall. The anterior rami of the remaining segmental nerves of the lumbosacral plexus innervate the muscles and skin of the pelvis, perineum and lower extremity. $L_1$ divides into the iliohypogastric and ilioinguinal nerves.

2) $L_2$, $L_3$ and $L_4$ are the principal segments forming the lumbar plexus. $L_1$ contributes some fibers to the genitofemoral nerve. The main peripheral nerves derived from these segments include:

    a) the genitofemoral nerve               ($L_1$, $L_2$)        c) the obturator nerve     ($L_2$, $L_3$, $L_4$)
    b) the lateral femoral cutaneous nerve     ($L_2$, $L_3$)        d) femoral nerve        ($L_2$, $L_3$, $L_4$)

3) $L_5$, $S_1$, $S_2$ and $S_3$ with some contribution from $L_4$ form the sacral plexus. The principal peripheral nerves derived from these segments include:

    a) the superior gluteal nerve         ($L_4$, $L_5$, $S_1$)                        common peroneal nerve ($L_4$, $L_5$, $S_1$, $S_2$)
    b) the inferior gluteal nerve          ($L_5$, $S_1$, $S_2$)     c) the sciatic nerve $\Big\{$ tibial nerve             ($L_4$, $L_5$, $S_1$, $S_2$, $S_3$)
                                              d) the posterior femoral cutaneous nerve     ($S_1$, $S_2$, $S_3$)

4) $S_2$, $S_3$ and $S_4$ also contribute to the pudendal plexus while $S_4$, $S_5$ and the coccygeal nerve form fine nerve filaments which innervate the skin of the anococcygeal region. The pudendal nerve is the main sensory and motor nerve of the perineum. Other sensory (inferior cluneal) and motor (nerve to levator ani and coccygeus muscles) branches of the pudendal plexus also come from sacral segments.

Fig. 287

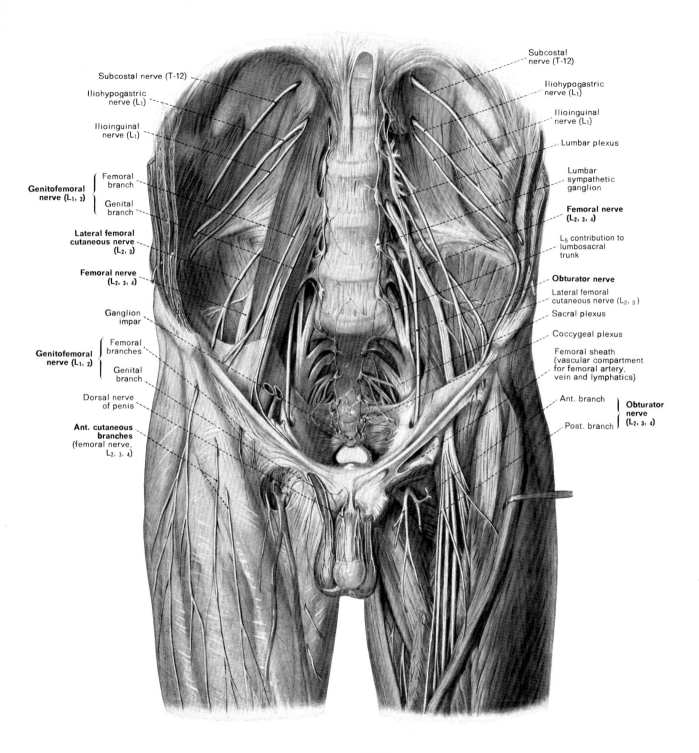

Subcostal nerve (T-12)
Iliohypogastric nerve (L₁)
Ilioinguinal nerve (L₁)

Genitofemoral nerve (L₁, ₂) { Femoral branch / Genital branch }

Lateral femoral cutaneous nerve (L₂, ₃)

Femoral nerve (L₂, ₃, ₄)

Ganglion impar

Genitofemoral nerve (L₁, ₂) { Femoral branches / Genital branch }

Dorsal nerve of penis

Ant. cutaneous branches (femoral nerve, L₂, ₃, ₄)

Subcostal nerve (T-12)
Iliohypogastric nerve (L₁)
Ilioinguinal nerve (L₁)
Lumbar plexus
Lumbar sympathetic ganglion
Femoral nerve (L₂, ₃, ₄)
L₅ contribution to lumbosacral trunk
Obturator nerve
Lateral femoral cutaneous nerve (L₂, ₃)
Sacral plexus
Coccygeal plexus
Femoral sheath (vascular compartment for femoral artery, vein and lymphatics)
Ant. branch } Obturator nerve (L₂, ₃, ₄)
Post. branch

**Fig. 288: The Lumbosacral Plexus: Posterior Abdominal Wall and Anterior Thigh**

NOTE: 1) on the left side, the psoas major and minor muscles have been removed in order to reveal the plexus of lumbar nerves more completely. As can be seen on the right side, these nerves emerge from the spinal cord and descend along the posterior abdominal wall within the substance of the psoas muscles. Observe that the 12th thoracic nerve (subcostal nerve) courses around the abdominal wall below the 12th rib.

2) the 1st lumbar nerve divides into an iliohypogastric and an ilioinguinal branch. The ilioinguinal nerve descends obliquely toward the iliac crest, penetrates through the transversus and internal oblique muscles to join the spermatic cord, becoming cutaneous at the superficial inguinal ring.

3) the genitofemoral nerve can be found coursing superficially on the surface of the psoas major muscle. It divides into a genital branch (which innervates the cremaster muscle and the skin of the scrotum) and a femoral branch (which is sensory to the upper anterior thigh.)

4) the femoral and obturator nerves. These nerves are derived from L₂, L₃ and L₄ and descend to innervate the anterior and medial groups of femoral muscles, respectively. The femoral nerve enters the thigh beneath the inguinal ligament, dividing into both motor and sensory branches, whereas the obturator nerve courses more medially through the obturator foramen to become the principal nerve of the adductor muscle group.

5) L₄ and L₅ nerve roots (lumbosacral trunk) join with the upper three sacral nerves to form the sacral plexus. From most of this plexus is derived the large sciatic nerve which leaves the pelvis through the greater sciatic foramen to achieve the gluteal region and the posterior aspect of the lower limb.

Fig. 288    III

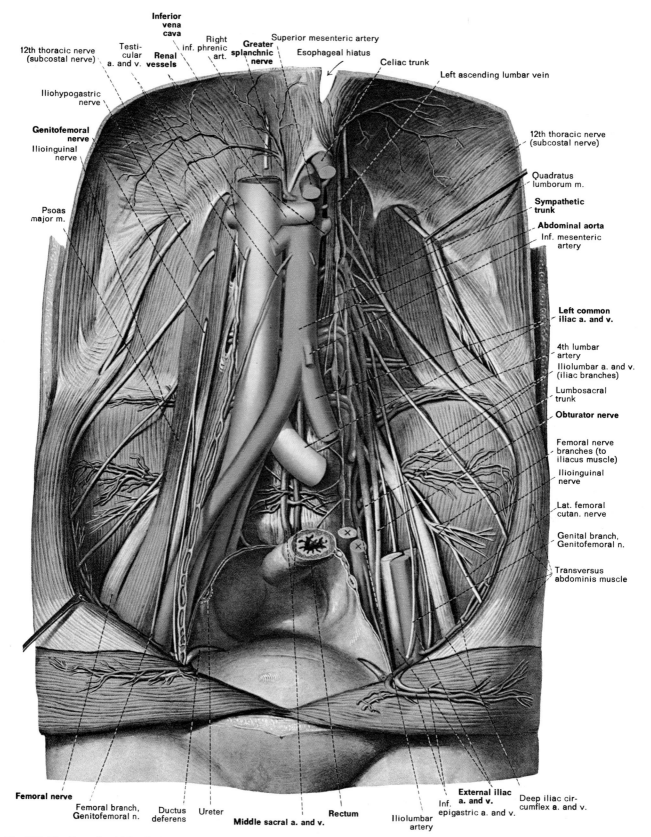

**Fig. 289: The Posterior Abdominal Vessels and Nerves**

NOTE: 1) the abdominal viscera have been removed as well as the psoas muscles on the left side. Observe the greater splanchnic nerves as they pierce the diaphragmatic crura to enter the abdomen. Also note the inferior phrenic arteries nearby. Identify the abdominal sympathetic chain of ganglia situated anterolaterally on the vertebral column.

2) the testicular arteries arising from the aorta just below the renal arteries. Inferiorly, the testicular artery and vein join the ductus deferens to enter the abdominal inguinal ring just lateral to the inferior epigastric vessels. Observe the middle sacral vessels descending into the pelvis in the midline. The middle sacral artery originates from the aorta at its bifurcation, whereas the vein usually drains into the left common iliac vein.

Fig. 289

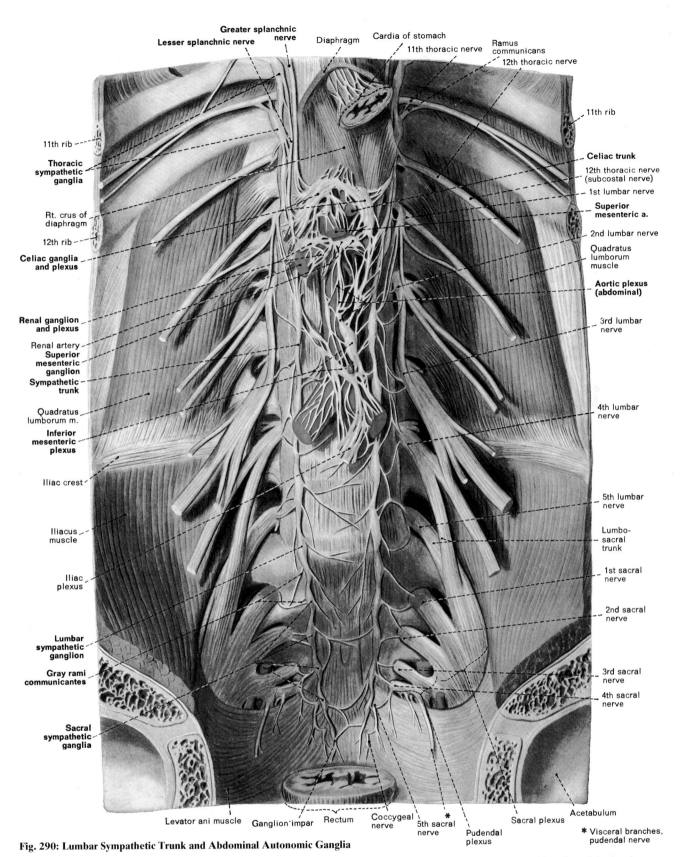

Greater splanchnic nerve
Lesser splanchnic nerve
Diaphragm
Cardia of stomach
11th thoracic nerve
Ramus communicans
12th thoracic nerve

11th rib
11th rib
Thoracic sympathetic ganglia
Celiac trunk
12th thoracic nerve (subcostal nerve)
1st lumbar nerve

Rt. crus of diaphragm
Superior mesenteric a.
12th rib
2nd lumbar nerve
Quadratus lumborum muscle
Celiac ganglia and plexus
Aortic plexus (abdominal)

Renal ganglion and plexus
3rd lumbar nerve
Renal artery
Superior mesenteric ganglion
Sympathetic trunk

Quadratus lumborum m.
4th lumbar nerve
Inferior mesenteric plexus

Iliac crest
5th lumbar nerve

Iliacus muscle
Lumbo-sacral trunk

Iliac plexus
1st sacral nerve

2nd sacral nerve

Lumbar sympathetic ganglion
Gray rami communicantes
3rd sacral nerve
4th sacral nerve

Sacral sympathetic ganglia

Levator ani muscle
Ganglion impar
Rectum
Coccygeal nerve
5th sacral nerve
*
Pudendal plexus
Sacral plexus
Acetabulum
* Visceral branches, pudendal nerve

**Fig. 290: Lumbar Sympathetic Trunk and Abdominal Autonomic Ganglia**

NOTE: 1) in addition to the two sympathetic chains of ganglia descending from the thorax through the abdomen and into the pelvis, the plexuses and their associated ganglia which overlie the major arteries branching from the aorta. Thus, the celiac plexuses along with the superior mesenteric, inferior mesenteric, renal, aortic and iliac plexuses form a dense network of autonomic fibers from which many of the abdominal and pelvic viscera receive sympathetic innervation.

2) the splanchnic nerves (containing preganglionic sympathetic fibers) as they join the upper abdominal ganglia where many of their fibers synapse with postganglionic sympathetic neurons.

3) that below L-2 only gray rami communicantes connect the ganglia of the sympathetic chain to the segmental nerves, since at these lower levels the rami consist only of postganglionic sympathetic fibers.

Fig. 290    III

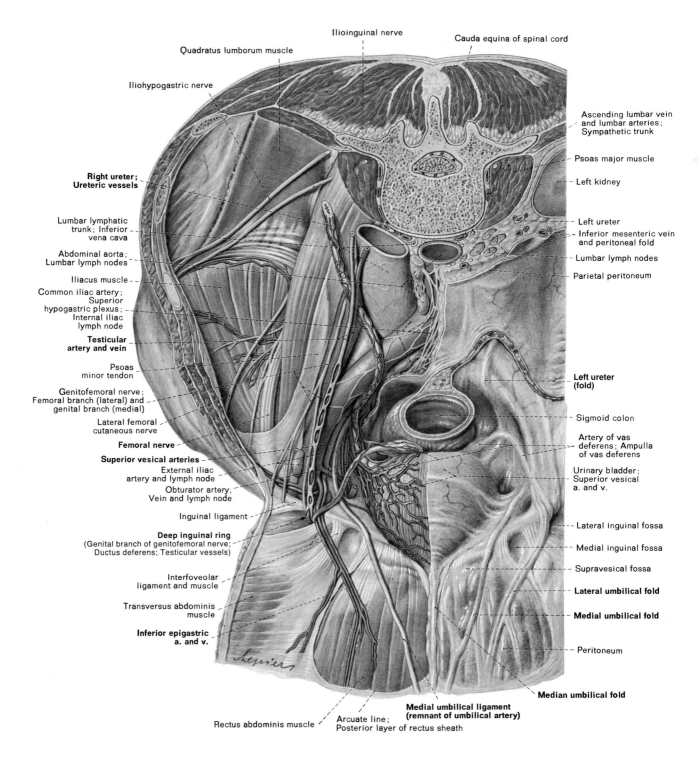

Quadratus lumborum muscle

Ilioinguinal nerve

Cauda equina of spinal cord

Iliohypogastric nerve

Ascending lumbar vein and lumbar arteries; Sympathetic trunk

Psoas major muscle

**Right ureter; Ureteric vessels**

Left kidney

Lumbar lymphatic trunk; Inferior vena cava

Left ureter

Inferior mesenteric vein and peritoneal fold

Abdominal aorta; Lumbar lymph nodes

Lumbar lymph nodes

Iliacus muscle

Parietal peritoneum

Common iliac artery; Superior hypogastric plexus; Internal iliac lymph node

**Testicular artery and vein**

Psoas minor tendon

**Left ureter (fold)**

Genitofemoral nerve; Femoral branch (lateral) and genital branch (medial)

Sigmoid colon

Lateral femoral cutaneous nerve

Artery of vas deferens; Ampulla of vas deferens

**Femoral nerve**

Urinary bladder; Superior vesical a. and v.

**Superior vesical arteries**

External iliac artery and lymph node

Obturator artery, Vein and lymph node

Lateral inguinal fossa

Medial inguinal fossa

Inguinal ligament

Supravesical fossa

**Deep inguinal ring** (Genital branch of genitofemoral nerve; Ductus deferens; Testicular vessels)

**Lateral umbilical fold**

Interfoveolar ligament and muscle

**Medial umbilical fold**

Transversus abdominis muscle

**Inferior epigastric a. and v.**

Peritoneum

Median umbilical fold

Rectus abdominis muscle

Arcuate line; Posterior layer of rectus sheath

**Medial umbilical ligament (remnant of umbilical artery)**

## Fig. 291: Vessels and Nerves of the Inferior Abdomen and Pelvis

NOTE: 1) the anterior abdominal wall has been incised vertically on both sides and reflected inferiorly, thereby exposing its inner (posterior) surface. The body has been transected through the lumbar region at the caudal end of the 3rd lumbar vertebra. On the right side, the peritoneum investing the abdominal cavity has been stripped away, whereas on the left it has been left intact.

2) this dissection reveals the intact male pelvic viscera viewed from above. Observe the course of the ureters as they cross the pelvic brim anterior to the common iliac arteries. Within the pelvis, the ureter curves medially toward the bladder. At the lateral angle of the bladder, the ductus deferens on its path to the seminal vesicle courses ventral to the ureter.

3) the convergence of the testicular vessels, ductus deferens and genital branch of the genitofemoral nerve (innervation of cremaster muscle) at the abdominal inguinal ring to form the spermatic cord of the inguinal canal.

4) the origins within the pelvis of the umbilical ligaments of the anterior abdominal wall: a) the median umbilical fold extending from the bladder to the umbilicus (urachus), b) the medial umbilical fold formed by a peritoneal reflection over the obliterated umbilical artery, and c) the lateral umbilical fold formed by peritoneum covering the inferior epigastric vessels.

5) the superior hypogastric plexus or presacral nerve lying anterior to the bifurcation of the aorta and descending behind the peritoneum into the pelvis.

Fig. 291

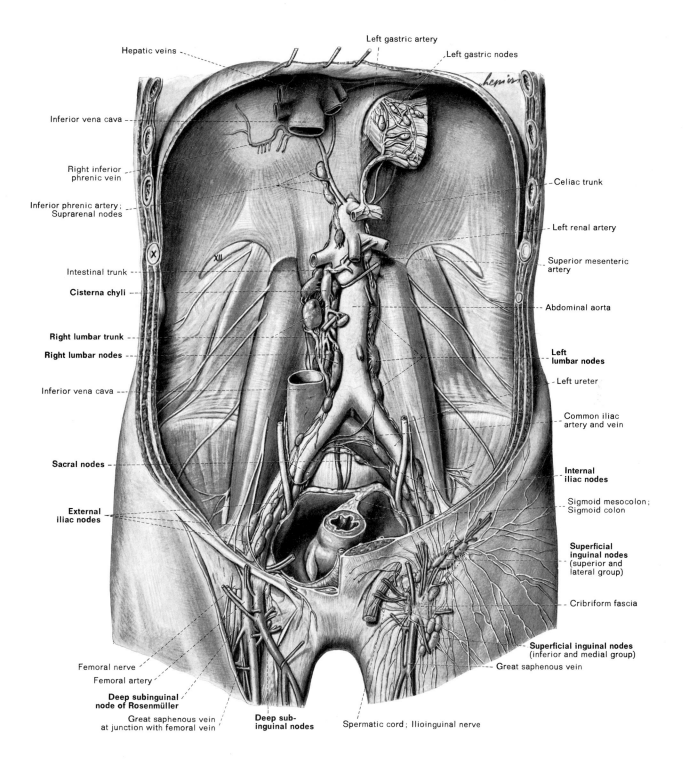

Hepatic veins

Left gastric artery

Left gastric nodes

Inferior vena cava

Right inferior phrenic vein

Inferior phrenic artery; Suprarenal nodes

Intestinal trunk

**Cisterna chyli**

**Right lumbar trunk**

**Right lumbar nodes**

Inferior vena cava

**Sacral nodes**

**External iliac nodes**

Femoral nerve

Femoral artery

**Deep subinguinal node of Rosenmüller**

Great saphenous vein at junction with femoral vein

**Deep sub-inguinal nodes**

Spermatic cord; Ilioinguinal nerve

Celiac trunk

Left renal artery

Superior mesenteric artery

Abdominal aorta

**Left lumbar nodes**

Left ureter

Common iliac artery and vein

**Internal iliac nodes**

Sigmoid mesocolon; Sigmoid colon

**Superficial inguinal nodes** (superior and lateral group)

Cribriform fascia

**Superficial inguinal nodes** (inferior and medial group)

Great saphenous vein

**Fig. 292: The Inguinal, Pelvic and Lumbar (Aortic) Lymph Nodes**

NOTE: 1) chains of lymph nodes from the inguinal region to the diaphragm lie along the paths of the major blood vessels. In the inguinal region, the superficial inguinal lymph nodes lie just distal to the inguinal ligament and in the subcutaneous superficial fascia. They range from 10 to 20 in number and receive drainage from the genitalia, perineum, gluteal region and the anterior abdominal wall. More deeply, the subinguinal nodes receive drainage from the lower extremity. One of the deep subinguinal nodes (node of Rosenmüller or Cloquet) lies in the femoral ring.

2) within the pelvis and abdomen, visceral lymph nodes lie close to the organs which they drain. These visceral nodes then channel lymph through chains of parietal nodes which generally are located along the paths of the major arteries and veins. Thus, external iliac, internal iliac (hypogastric) and common iliac nodes are located in proximity to these vessels in the pelvis.

3) along the posterior abdominal wall are found right and left lumbar chains which course along the sides of the abdominal aorta. Other groups of nodes, the preaortic, are arranged along the roots of the major unpaired branches of the aorta, forming the celiac and superior and inferior mesenteric node chains.

4) at about the level of the 2nd lumbar vertebra there is a confluence of lymph channels which forms a dilated sac, the cisterna chyli. This is located somewhat posterior and to the right of the aorta and marks the commencement of the thoracic duct.

Fig. 292    III

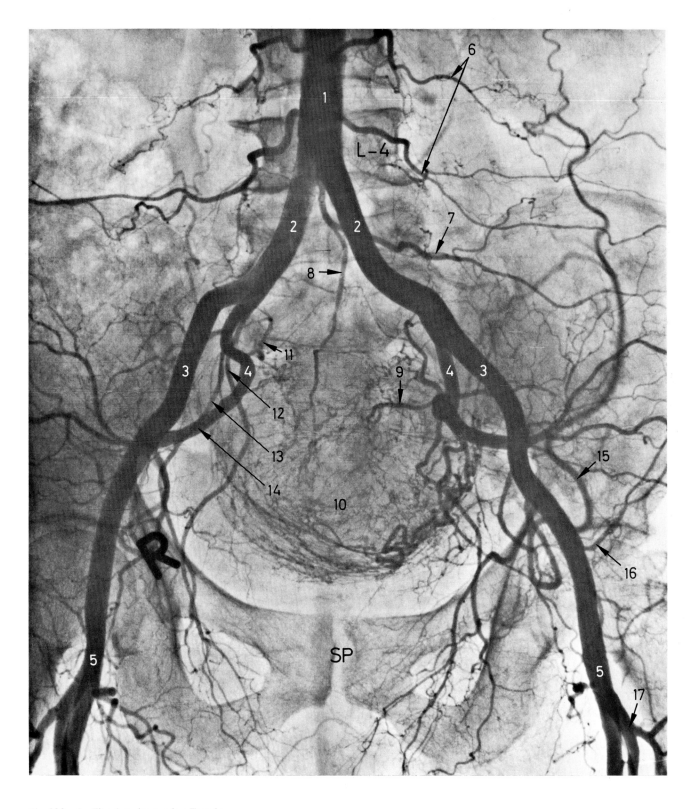

**Fig. 293: An Iliac Arteriogram in a Female**

NOTE that the bifurcation of the aorta (*1*) into the two common iliac arteries (*2*) occurs at the lower border of the body of the L 4 vertebra. The common iliac vessels branch into external (*3*) and internal (*4*) iliac arteries. The internal iliac artery (*4*) on each side serves a number of branches to the pelvis, perineum, and gluteal region, while the external iliac artery (*3*), after giving off the inferior epigastric (*15*) and deep circumflex iliac (*16*) arteries, becomes the femoral artery below the inguinal ligament.

| | | | | |
|---|---|---|---|---|
| 1. Abdominal aorta | 5. Femoral artery | 9. Uterine artery | 13. Internal pudendal artery | 17. Deep femoral artery |
| 2. Common iliac artery | 6. Lumbar arteries | 10. Uterus | 14. Superior gluteal artery | L 4 - 4 th lumbar vertebra |
| 3. External iliac artery | 7. Iliolumbar artery | 11. Lateral sacral artery | 15. Inferior epigastric artery | SP - Symphysis pubis |
| 4. Internal iliac artery | 8. Median sacral artery | 12. Obturator artery | 16. Deep circumflex iliac artery | |

Fig. 293

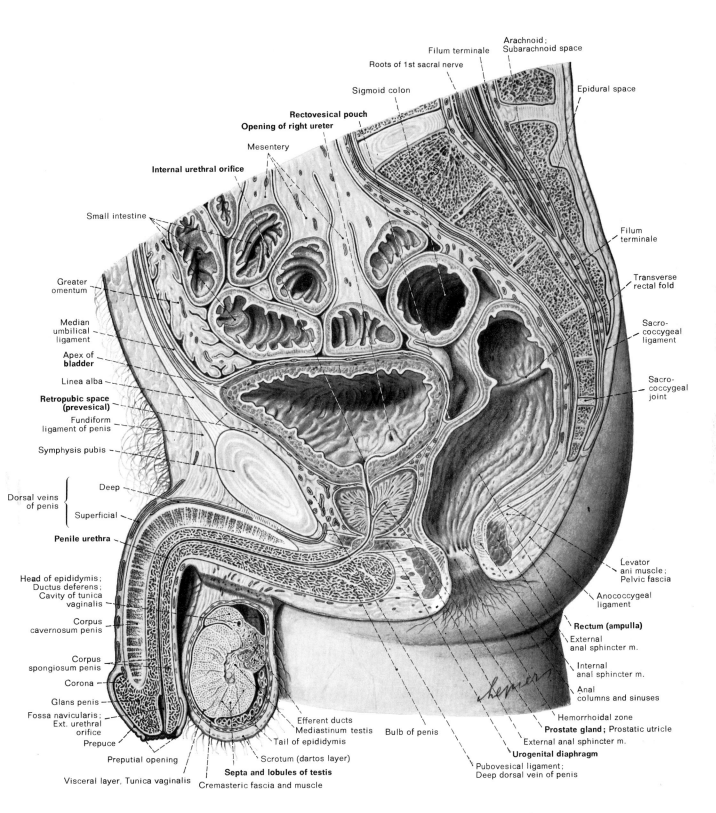

Arachnoid;
Subarachnoid space

Filum terminale

Roots of 1st sacral nerve

Sigmoid colon

Epidural space

**Rectovesical pouch**
**Opening of right ureter**

Mesentery

**Internal urethral orifice**

Filum
terminale

Small intestine

Transverse
rectal fold

Greater
omentum

Sacro-
coccygeal
ligament

Median
umbilical
ligament

Apex of
**bladder**

Sacro-
coccygeal
joint

Linea alba

**Retropubic space
(prevesical)**

Fundiform
ligament of penis

Symphysis pubis

Deep

Dorsal veins
of penis

Superficial

Levator
ani muscle;
Pelvic fascia

**Penile urethra**

Anococcygeal
ligament

Head of epididymis;
Ductus deferens;
Cavity of tunica
vaginalis

**Rectum (ampulla)**

External
anal sphincter m.

Corpus
cavernosum penis

Internal
anal sphincter m.

Corpus
spongiosum penis

Anal
columns and sinuses

Corona

Glans penis

Hemorrhoidal zone

Fossa navicularis;
Ext. urethral
orifice

**Prostate gland;** Prostatic utricle

External anal sphincter m.

Prepuce

**Urogenital diaphragm**

Efferent ducts
Mediastinum testis      Bulb of penis

Preputial opening

Pubovesical ligament;
Deep dorsal vein of penis

Tail of epididymis

Visceral layer, Tunica vaginalis

Scrotum (dartos layer)

**Septa and lobules of testis**

Cremasteric fascia and muscle

**Fig. 294: Median Sagittal Section of the Male Pelvis and Perineum Showing the Pelvic Viscera and the External Genitalia**

Fig. 294      **IV**

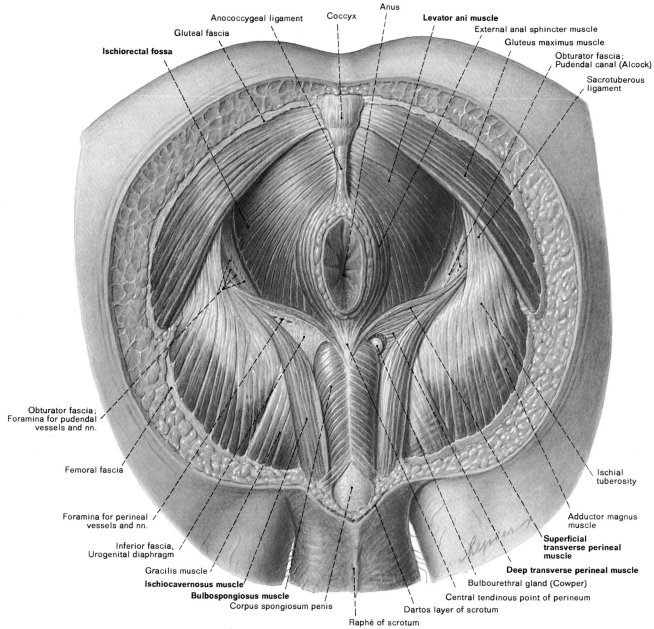

Anococcygeal ligament
Coccyx
Anus
Levator ani muscle
Gluteal fascia
External anal sphincter muscle
Gluteus maximus muscle
Ischiorectal fossa
Obturator fascia; Pudendal canal (Alcock)
Sacrotuberous ligament

Obturator fascia; Foramina for pudendal vessels and nn.

Femoral fascia

Ischial tuberosity

Foramina for perineal vessels and nn.

Adductor magnus muscle

Inferior fascia, Urogenital diaphragm

Superficial transverse perineal muscle

Gracilis muscle

Deep transverse perineal muscle

Ischiocavernosus muscle

Bulbourethral gland (Cowper)

Bulbospongiosus muscle

Central tendinous point of perineum

Corpus spongiosum penis

Dartos layer of scrotum

Raphé of scrotum

**Fig. 295: The Superficial Muscles of the Male Perineum**

**Fig. 296: Diagram of Frontal Section Through Male Pelvis and Perineum**

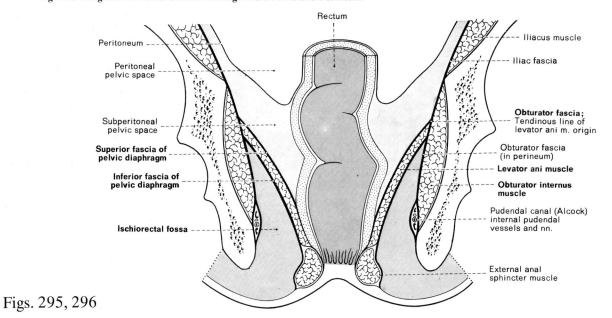

Rectum

Peritoneum

Iliacus muscle

Peritoneal pelvic space

Iliac fascia

Subperitoneal pelvic space

Obturator fascia; Tendinous line of levator ani m. origin

Superior fascia of pelvic diaphragm

Obturator fascia (in perineum)

Inferior fascia of pelvic diaphragm

Levator ani muscle

Obturator internus muscle

Pudendal canal (Alcock) internal pudendal vessels and nn.

Ischiorectal fossa

External anal sphincter muscle

Figs. 295, 296

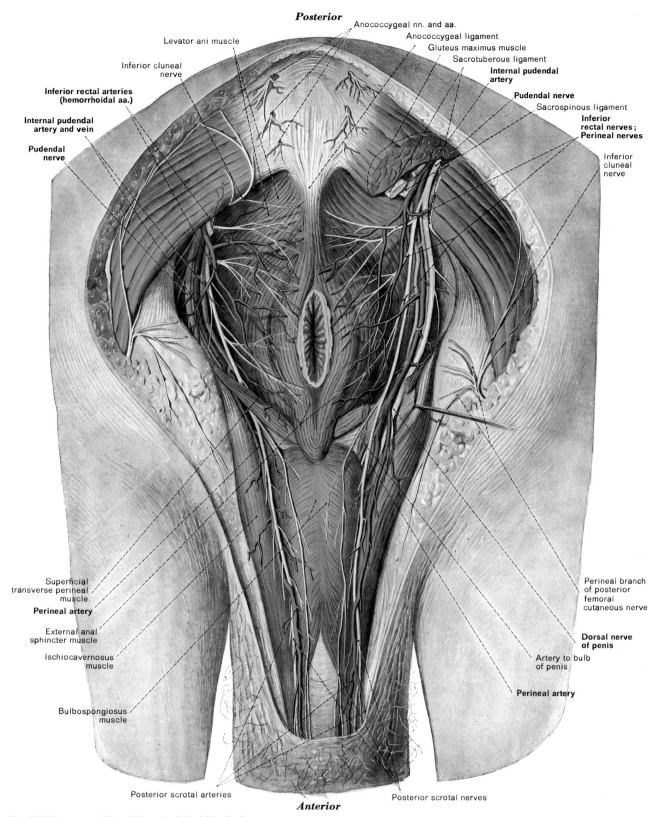

Posterior

Anococcygeal nn. and aa.
Anococcygeal ligament
Levator ani muscle
Gluteus maximus muscle
Inferior cluneal nerve
Sacrotuberous ligament
**Internal pudendal artery**
**Inferior rectal arteries (hemorrhoidal aa.)**
**Pudendal nerve**
Sacrospinous ligament
**Internal pudendal artery and vein**
**Inferior rectal nerves; Perineal nerves**
**Pudendal nerve**
Inferior cluneal nerve

Superficial transverse perineal muscle
Perineal branch of posterior femoral cutaneous nerve
**Perineal artery**
External anal sphincter muscle
**Dorsal nerve of penis**
Ischiocavernosus muscle
Artery to bulb of penis
**Perineal artery**
Bulbospongiosus muscle

Posterior scrotal arteries
Posterior scrotal nerves

Anterior

**Fig. 297: Nerves and Blood Vessels of the Male Perineum**

NOTE: 1) the skin of the male perineum as well as the fat of the ischiorectal fossae have been removed in order to expose the muscles, vessels and nerves of both the anal and urogenital regions of the perineum.

2) emerging from the pelvis through the lesser sciatic foramen by way of the pudendal canal (Alcock) are the internal pudendal vessels and the pudendal nerve. These structures enter the perineum at the lateral border of the ischiorectal fossa. There is an immediate branching of the inferior rectal (hemorrhoidal) vessels and nerves which course transversely across the ischiorectal fossa to supply the levator ani and external anal sphincter muscles.

3) the internal pudendal structures then continue anteriorly, pierce the urogenital diaphragm, and become the perineal vessels and nerve and the dorsal vessels and nerve of the penis. The muscles of the urogenital triangle are innervated by the perineal nerve, while the dorsal nerve of the penis is the principal sensory nerve of that organ.

Fig. 297    IV

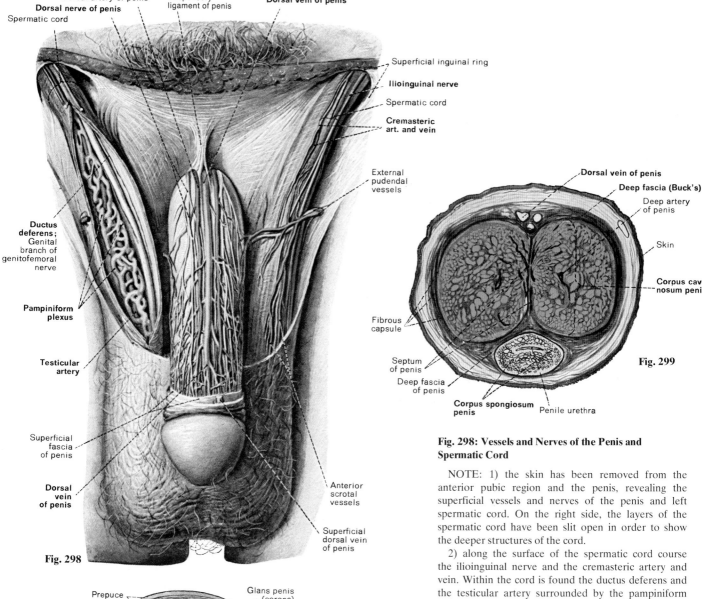

Dorsal artery of penis
**Dorsal nerve of penis**
Spermatic cord
Suspensory ligament of penis
**Dorsal vein of penis**

Superficial inguinal ring
**Ilioinguinal nerve**
Spermatic cord
**Cremasteric art. and vein**

External pudendal vessels

**Ductus deferens; Genital branch of genitofemoral nerve**

**Pampiniform plexus**

**Testicular artery**

Superficial fascia of penis

**Dorsal vein of penis**

Anterior scrotal vessels

Superficial dorsal vein of penis

**Fig. 298**

Dorsal vein of penis
**Deep fascia (Buck's)**
Deep artery of penis
Skin
**Corpus cavernosum penis**

Fibrous capsule

Septum of penis
Deep fascia of penis
**Corpus spongiosum penis**
Penile urethra

**Fig. 299**

### Fig. 298: Vessels and Nerves of the Penis and Spermatic Cord

NOTE: 1) the skin has been removed from the anterior pubic region and the penis, revealing the superficial vessels and nerves of the penis and left spermatic cord. On the right side, the layers of the spermatic cord have been slit open in order to show the deeper structures of the cord.

2) along the surface of the spermatic cord course the ilioinguinal nerve and the cremasteric artery and vein. Within the cord is found the ductus deferens and the testicular artery surrounded by the pampiniform plexus of veins.

3) beneath the superficial fascia of the penis and in the midline courses the unpaired dorsal vein of the penis. Along the sides of the vein, note the paired dorsal arteries and nerves of the penis.

### Cross Section of Penis

### Fig. 299: Section Through Middle of Penis

NOTE that the penis is composed principally of two laterally situated corpora cavernosa penis containing erectile tissue and one corpus spongiosum penis placed ventrally and in the midline containing the penile portion of the urethra. These are surrounded by a closely investing layer of deep fascia. During erection, blood fills the erectile tissue (as is seen in this cross section), causing them to become rigid. This engorgement exerts pressure on the veins and maintains the erection by preventing the blood from draining back into the general circulation.

### Fig. 300: Section at Neck of Glans Penis

This section is taken from the proximal part of the glans penis. Note that the corpora cavernosa penis becomes smaller distally, while the corona of the glans penis is formed by the spongy tissue of the corpus spongiosum penis.

### Fig. 301: Section Through Glans Penis

The expanded distal extremity of the corpus spongiosum penis is called the glans penis. At its distal end is the opening of the urethra. In the uncircumcised male, the glans penis is covered by a duplication of thin skin, the prepuce, which is attached to the glans penis ventrally by the frenulum.

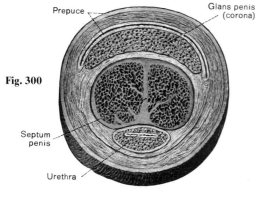

Prepuce
Glans penis (corona)

**Fig. 300**

Septum penis

Urethra

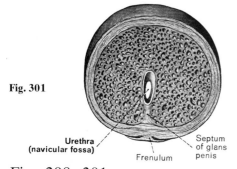

**Fig. 301**

**Urethra (navicular fossa)**
Septum of glans penis
Frenulum

Figs. 298–301

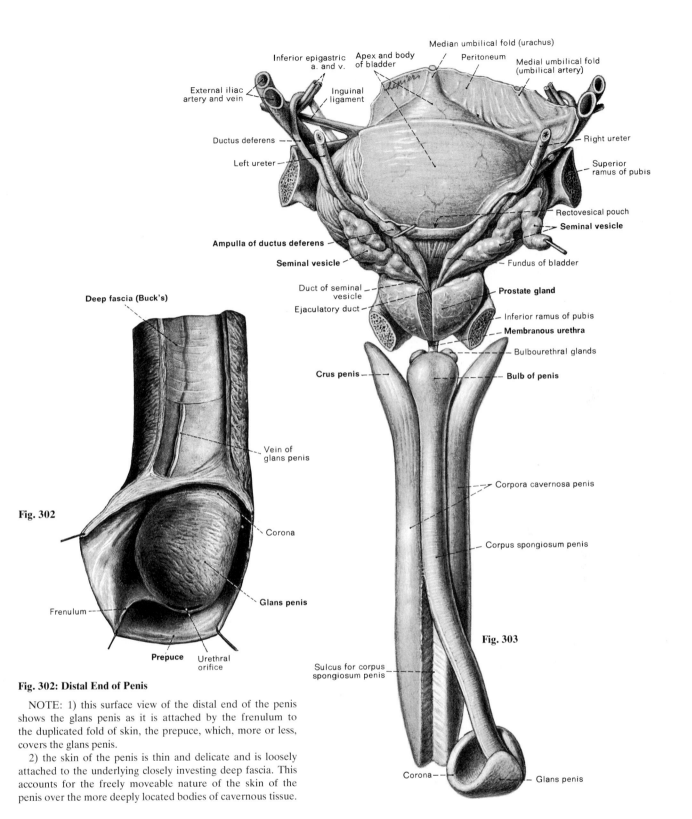

Median umbilical fold (urachus)
Peritoneum
Medial umbilical fold (umbilical artery)
Inferior epigastric a. and v.
Apex and body of bladder
External iliac artery and vein
Inguinal ligament
Ductus deferens
Left ureter
Right ureter
Superior ramus of pubis
Rectovesical pouch
**Seminal vesicle**
**Ampulla of ductus deferens**
**Seminal vesicle**
Fundus of bladder
Duct of seminal vesicle
**Prostate gland**
Ejaculatory duct
Inferior ramus of pubis
**Membranous urethra**
Bulbourethral glands
**Crus penis**
**Bulb of penis**

**Deep fascia (Buck's)**
Vein of glans penis
Corona
**Fig. 302**
Corona
**Glans penis**
Frenulum
**Prepuce**  Urethral orifice

Corpora cavernosa penis
Corpus spongiosum penis

**Fig. 303**

Sulcus for corpus spongiosum penis
Corona
Glans penis

**Fig. 302: Distal End of Penis**

NOTE: 1) this surface view of the distal end of the penis shows the glans penis as it is attached by the frenulum to the duplicated fold of skin, the prepuce, which, more or less, covers the glans penis.

2) the skin of the penis is thin and delicate and is loosely attached to the underlying closely investing deep fascia. This accounts for the freely moveable nature of the skin of the penis over the more deeply located bodies of cavernous tissue.

**Fig. 303: The Erectile Bodies of the Penis Attached to the Bladder and Other Organs by the Membranous Urethra**

NOTE: 1) the firmly investing deep fascia which surrounds the erectile bodies of the penis has been removed, and the distal portion of the corpus spongiosum penis (which contains the penile urethra) has been displaced from its position between the two corpora cavernosa penis.

2) the posterior surface of the bladder and prostate and the associated seminal vesicles, vasa deferens, and bulbourethral glands are also demonstrated. These structures all communicate with the urethra, the membranous portion of which is in continuity with the penile urethra.

3) the tapered crura of the corpora cavernosa penis diverge laterally at their base to become adherent to the ischial and pubic rami. They are surrounded by the fibers of the ischiocavernosus muscles. The base of the corpus spongiosum penis is also expanded and is called the bulb. It is enclosed by the bulbocavernosus muscle.

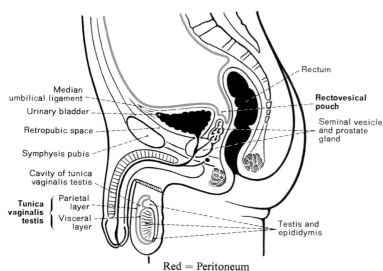

Fig. 304: The Inferior Reflection of Peritoneum over the Pelvic Organs

- Rectum

Median umbilical ligament

Urinary bladder

Retropubic space

Symphysis pubis

Cavity of tunica vaginalis testis

**Tunica vaginalis testis** { Parietal layer / Visceral layer

**Rectovesical pouch**

Seminal vesicle and prostate gland

Testis and epididymis

Red = Peritoneum

## Fig. 304: The Inferior Reflection of Peritoneum over the Pelvic Organs

NOTE: 1) the inferior extent of the peritoneum anteriorly when the bladder is empty is to the level of the symphysis pubis, whereas when the bladder is full the peritoneum is elevated as much as 3 or 4 inches superior to the symphysis pubis. Between the rectum and the bladder the peritoneum forms the rectovesical pouch.

2) in the scrotum, the visceral and parietal layers of the tunica vaginalis testis also enclose a cavity lined by peritoneum.

3) that the prostate and bladder may be reached anteriorly by means of a suprapubic approach, and inferiorly by ascending through the perineum, in front of the rectum. By either route, these organs may be achieved without entering the peritoneal cavity.

## Fig. 305: The Male Pelvic Organs Viewed from the Left Side

NOTE that the peritoneum has been removed from the left side of the bladder and rectum.

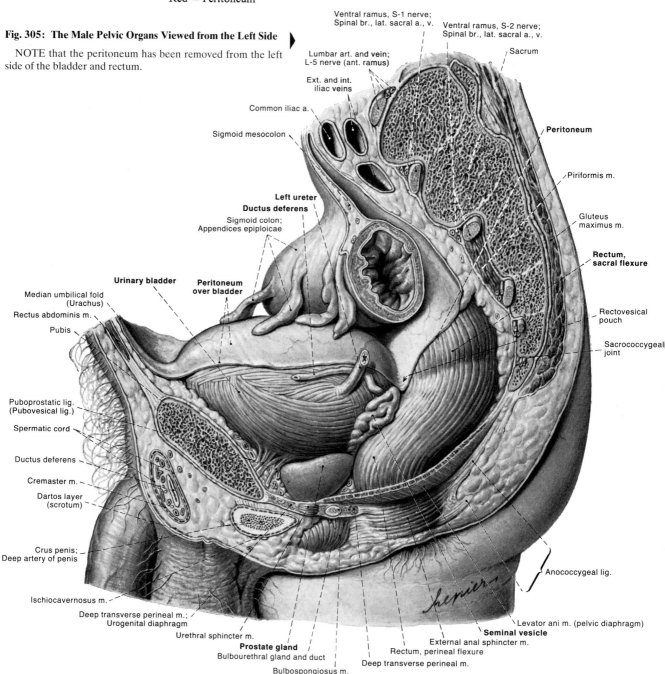

Ventral ramus, S-1 nerve; Spinal br., lat. sacral a., v.

Ventral ramus, S-2 nerve; Spinal br., lat. sacral a., v.

Lumbar art. and vein; L-5 nerve (ant. ramus)

Sacrum

Ext. and int. iliac veins

Common iliac a.

Sigmoid mesocolon

**Peritoneum**

Piriformis m.

Gluteus maximus m.

**Left ureter**
**Ductus deferens**

Sigmoid colon; Appendices epiploicae

**Rectum, sacral flexure**

**Urinary bladder**

Median umbilical fold (Urachus)

Rectus abdominis m.

Pubis

**Peritoneum over bladder**

Rectovesical pouch

Sacrococcygeal joint

Puboprostatic lig. (Pubovesical lig.)

Spermatic cord

Ductus deferens

Cremaster m.

Dartos layer (scrotum)

Crus penis; Deep artery of penis

Ischiocavernosus m.

Anococcygeal lig.

Deep transverse perineal m.; Urogenital diaphragm

Urethral sphincter m.

**Prostate gland**
Bulbourethral gland and duct

Bulbospongiosus m.

Levator ani m. (pelvic diaphragm)
**Seminal vesicle**

External anal sphincter m.

Rectum, perineal flexure

Deep transverse perineal m.

Figs. 304, 305

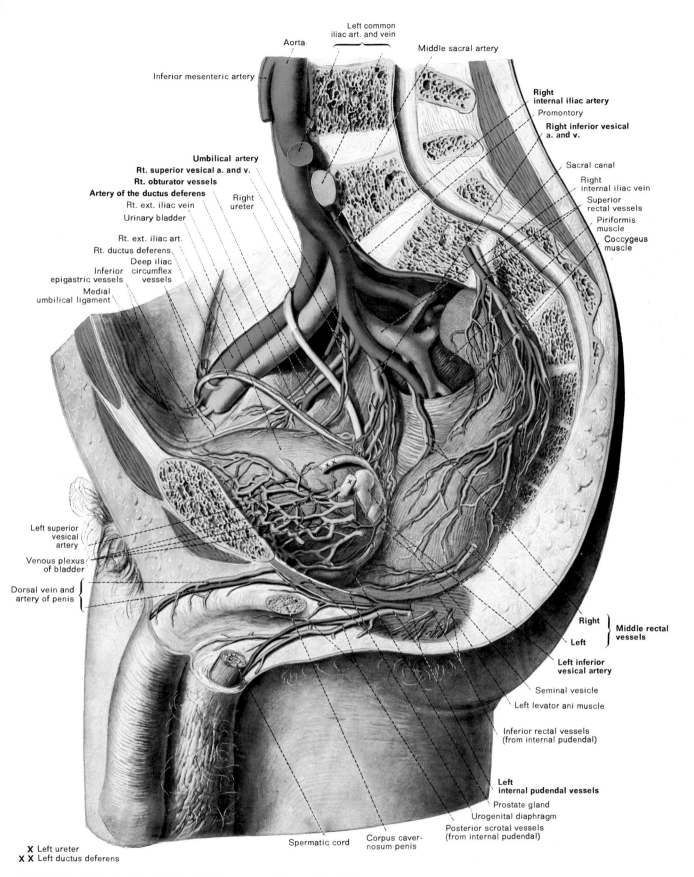

Aorta

Left common iliac art. and vein

Middle sacral artery

Inferior mesenteric artery

**Right internal iliac artery**

Promontory

**Right inferior vesical a. and v.**

Sacral canal

Right internal iliac vein

Superior rectal vessels

Piriformis muscle

**Coccygeus muscle**

**Umbilical artery**
**Rt. superior vesical a. and v.**
**Rt. obturator vessels**
**Artery of the ductus deferens**
Rt. ext. iliac vein
Urinary bladder

Right ureter

Rt. ext. iliac art.
Rt. ductus deferens
Deep iliac circumflex vessels
Inferior epigastric vessels
Medial umbilical ligament

Left superior vesical artery

Venous plexus of bladder

Dorsal vein and artery of penis

**Right**
**Middle rectal vessels**
**Left**

**Left inferior vesical artery**

Seminal vesicle

Left levator ani muscle

Inferior rectal vessels (from internal pudendal)

**Left internal pudendal vessels**

Prostate gland

Urogenital diaphragm

Posterior scrotal vessels (from internal pudendal)

Spermatic cord

Corpus cavernosum penis

**X** Left ureter
**X X** Left ductus deferens

**Fig. 306: Blood Vessels of the Male Pelvis, Perineum and External Genitalia**

NOTE: 1) the aorta bifurcates into the common iliac arteries which then divide into the external and internal iliac arteries. The external iliac becomes the chief arterial trunk of the lower extremity, while the internal iliac artery supplies the organs of the pelvis and perineum.

2) the branches of the internal iliac artery include visceral and parietal vessels. The *visceral* branches are (a) the umbilical (from which is derived the superior vesical artery), (b) the inferior vesical, (c) the artery of the vas deferens (uterine in the female) and, (d) the middle rectal. The *parietal* branches include (a) the iliolumbar, (b) lateral sacral, (c) superior gluteal, (d) inferior gluteal, (e) obturator, and (f) internal pudendal.

Fig. 306    IV

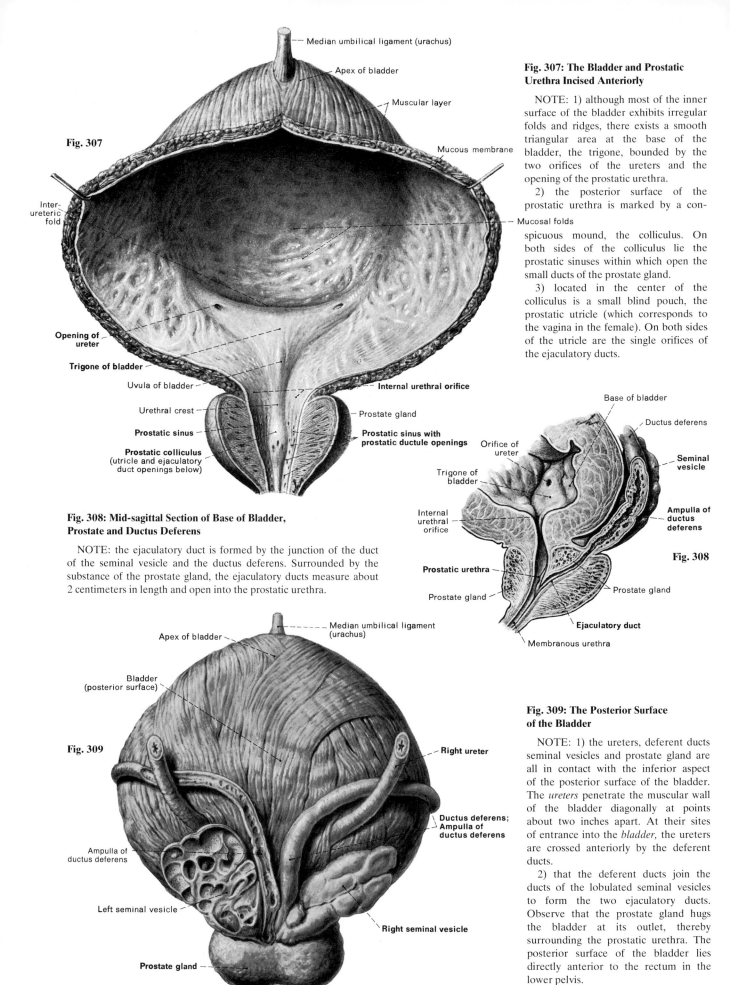

Fig. 307

Median umbilical ligament (urachus)

Apex of bladder

Muscular layer

Mucous membrane

Inter-
ureteric
fold

Mucosal folds

Opening of
ureter

Trigone of bladder

Uvula of bladder

Internal urethral orifice

Urethral crest

Prostate gland

Prostatic sinus

Prostatic sinus with
prostatic ductule openings

Prostatic colliculus
(utricle and ejaculatory
duct openings below)

## Fig. 307: The Bladder and Prostatic Urethra Incised Anteriorly

NOTE: 1) although most of the inner surface of the bladder exhibits irregular folds and ridges, there exists a smooth triangular area at the base of the bladder, the trigone, bounded by the two orifices of the ureters and the opening of the prostatic urethra.

2) the posterior surface of the prostatic urethra is marked by a conspicuous mound, the colliculus. On both sides of the colliculus lie the prostatic sinuses within which open the small ducts of the prostate gland.

3) located in the center of the colliculus is a small blind pouch, the prostatic utricle (which corresponds to the vagina in the female). On both sides of the utricle are the single orifices of the ejaculatory ducts.

## Fig. 308: Mid-sagittal Section of Base of Bladder, Prostate and Ductus Deferens

NOTE: the ejaculatory duct is formed by the junction of the duct of the seminal vesicle and the ductus deferens. Surrounded by the substance of the prostate gland, the ejaculatory ducts measure about 2 centimeters in length and open into the prostatic urethra.

Base of bladder

Ductus deferens

Orifice of
ureter

Seminal
vesicle

Trigone of
bladder

Internal
urethral
orifice

Ampulla of
ductus
deferens

Fig. 308

Prostatic urethra

Prostate gland

Prostate gland

Ejaculatory duct

Membranous urethra

Median umbilical ligament
(urachus)

Apex of bladder

Bladder
(posterior surface)

Fig. 309

Right ureter

Ductus deferens;
Ampulla of
ductus deferens

Ampulla of
ductus deferens

Left seminal vesicle

Right seminal vesicle

Prostate gland

## Fig. 309: The Posterior Surface of the Bladder

NOTE: 1) the ureters, deferent ducts seminal vesicles and prostate gland are all in contact with the inferior aspect of the posterior surface of the bladder. The *ureters* penetrate the muscular wall of the bladder diagonally at points about two inches apart. At their sites of entrance into the *bladder*, the ureters are crossed anteriorly by the deferent ducts.

2) that the deferent ducts join the ducts of the lobulated seminal vesicles to form the two ejaculatory ducts. Observe that the prostate gland hugs the bladder at its outlet, thereby surrounding the prostatic urethra. The posterior surface of the bladder lies directly anterior to the rectum in the lower pelvis.

Figs. 307, 308, 309

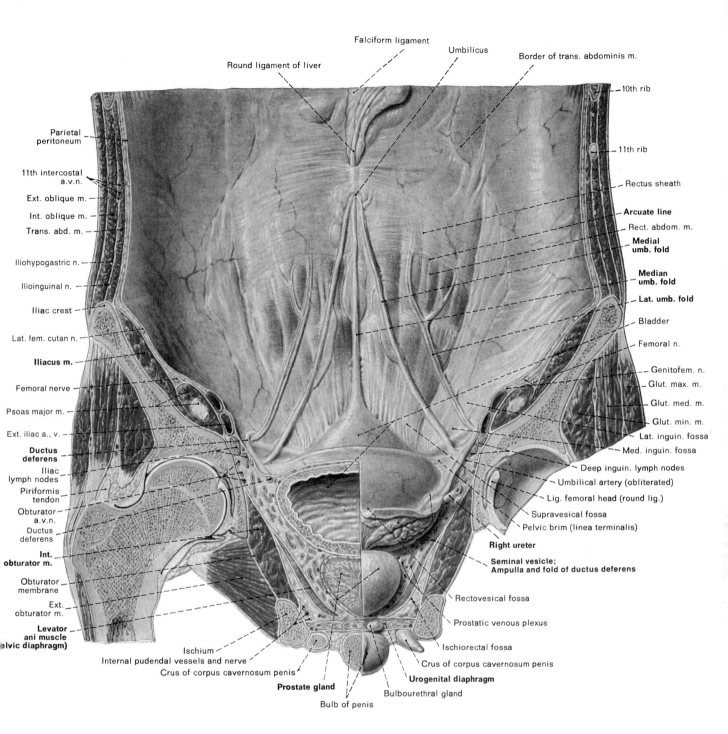

Falciform ligament
Round ligament of liver
Umbilicus
Border of trans. abdominis m.

Parietal peritoneum

11th intercostal a.v.n.
Ext. oblique m.
Int. oblique m.
Trans. abd. m.

Iliohypogastric n.
Ilioinguinal n.
Iliac crest
Lat. fem. cutan n.
**Iliacus m.**
Femoral nerve
Psoas major m.
Ext. iliac a., v.
**Ductus deferens**
Iliac lymph nodes
Piriformis tendon
Obturator a.v.n.
Ductus deferens
**Int. obturator m.**
Obturator membrane
Ext. obturator m.
**Levator ani muscle (pelvic diaphragm)**

— 10th rib
— 11th rib
— Rectus sheath
**Arcuate line**
Rect. abdom. m.
**Medial umb. fold**
**Median umb. fold**
**Lat. umb. fold**
Bladder
Femoral n.
Genitofem. n.
Glut. max. m.
Glut. med. m.
Glut. min. m.
Lat. inguin. fossa
Med. inguin. fossa
Deep inguin. lymph nodes
Umbilical artery (obliterated)
Lig. femoral head (round lig.)
Supravesical fossa
Pelvic brim (linea terminalis)
**Right ureter**
**Seminal vesicle; Ampulla and fold of ductus deferens**
Rectovesical fossa
Prostatic venous plexus
Ischiorectal fossa
Crus of corpus cavernosum penis
**Urogenital diaphragm**
Bulbourethral gland

Ischium
Internal pudendal vessels and nerve
Crus of corpus cavernosum penis
**Prostate gland**
Bulb of penis

**Fig. 310: The Posterior Aspect of the Ventral Abdominal Wall and the Male Pelvic Organs**

NOTE: 1) the inner aspect of the anterior abdominal wall shows the courses of the umbilical ligaments and the round ligament of the liver, as well as the smooth contours of the rectus abdominis muscle and the arcuate line, which marks the inferior limit of the posterior layer of the rectus sheath.

2) the frontal section through the bones of the pelvis and the femur. Observe the expanded wings (alae) of each ilium which extend laterally to reach the skin as the iliac crest. The wings of the ilia bound the greater (or false) pelvis. On their internal or pelvic surface lie the iliacus and psoas muscles along with the iliac vessels and the various nerves of the lumbar plexus. Their external surface is directed toward the gluteal region.

3) that the lesser (or true) pelvis lies below the pelvic brim. It is restricted by bone and bounds more snugly the pelvic organs (bladder, prostate, seminal vesicle, etc.). Inferiorly the pelvic organs are separated from the perineum by the pelvic diaphragm (levator ani muscles) and, to a lesser extent, the urogenital diaphragm (deep transverse perineal muscles).

4) the reflection of peritoneum as it invests the inner surface of the anterior abdominal wall, curves over the superior surface of the bladder and dips somewhat posterior to the bladder (rectovesical pouch) to come into contact with the seminal vesicles and deferent ducts.

5) the obturator internus muscle which covers much of the inner surface of the lateral wall of the true pelvis. Extending into the perineum, this muscle also forms the lateral boundary of the ischiorectal fossa.

Fig. 310    IV

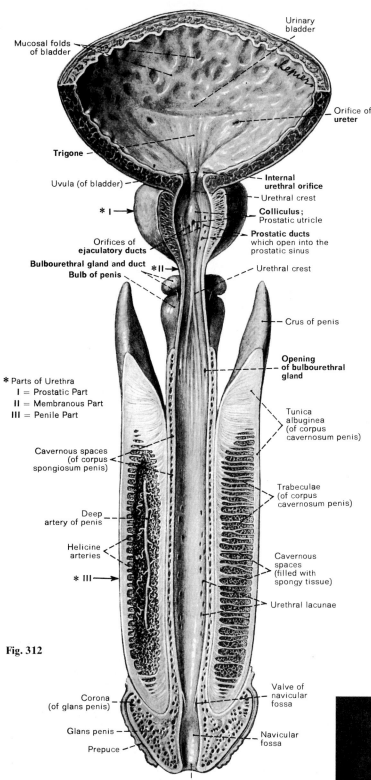

Mucosal folds of bladder

Urinary bladder

Orifice of **ureter**

**Trigone**

Uvula (of bladder)

**Internal urethral orifice**

Urethral crest

**Colliculus; Prostatic utricle**

*I →

Orifices of **ejaculatory ducts**

**Prostatic ducts** which open into the prostatic sinus

**Bulbourethral gland and duct**
**Bulb of penis**

*II →

Urethral crest

Crus of penis

**Opening of bulbourethral gland**

*Parts of Urethra
I = Prostatic Part
II = Membranous Part
III = Penile Part

Tunica albuginea (of corpus cavernosum penis)

Cavernous spaces (of corpus spongiosum penis)

Trabeculae (of corpus cavernosum penis)

Deep artery of penis

Helicine arteries

*III →

Cavernous spaces (filled with spongy tissue)

Urethral lacunae

**Fig. 312**

Corona (of glans penis)

Glans penis

Prepuce

Valve of navicular fossa

Navicular fossa

**External urethral orifice**

### Fig. 311: Radiograph of Bladder, Seminal Vesicles, Deferent Ducts and Ejaculatory Ducts

NOTE: 1) this figure is a positive print of an X-ray. The bladder has been filled with air and appears light, whereas the images of the seminal vesicles, deferent ducts and ejaculatory ducts stand out as dark.

2) that the convoluted seminal vesicles, which secrete the seminal fluid, consist of coiled tubes 4−5 mm in diameter and 2 to 3 inches in length.

3) the shadows of the deferent ducts. These cross the bladder surface toward the midline to join the seminal vesicles forming the ejaculatory ducts.

Figs. 311, 312

### Fig. 312: The Male Urethra and its Associated Orifices

NOTE: 1) the male urethra is a canal that extends from its internal urethral orifice at the bladder to its external urethral orifice at the end of the glans penis. Since the male urethra transverses the prostate gland, the urogenital diaphragm (membrane) and the penis, it is divided into three parts: prostatic, membranous and penile.

2) urine passes through the urethra from the bladder. The urethra also transports the seminal fluid which is composed of a mixture of sperm from the testis and the secretions of the seminal vesicles and prostate. Just prior to ejaculation, the urethra is lubricated by a viscous fluid secreted by the bulbourethral glands (of Cowper). These glands are located in the urogenital diaphragm, but their ducts open about one inch or more distally into the penile urethra.

3) the total urethra measures between 7 and 8 inches in length. The prostatic urethra is about 1½ inches long, the membranous urethra about ½ inch and the penile urethra 5 to 6 inches. On its posterior wall, the *prostatic urethra* is marked by a ridge, the urethral crest and a mound, the colliculus. It receives the secretions of the ejaculatory ducts along with those of the prostate. Enlargement of the prostate, often occurring in older men, tends to constrict the urethra at this site and frequently results in difficulty in urination.

4) the *membranous urethra* is short and narrow. In its course through the urogenital diaphragm, it is completely surrounded by the circular fibers of the urethral sphincter muscle (see Figure 317). Since this important sphincter is under voluntary control, its relaxation initiates urination while its tonic contraction constricts the urethra and maintains urinary continence.

5) the penile (or spongy) portion of the urethra at once is surrounded by the bulb of the penis and, thus, the bulbospongiosus muscle. It traverses the penile shaft embedded within the corpus spongiosum penis. In its course, it receives the ducts of the bulbourethral glands. The internal surface of its distal half is marked by a number of small recesses, the urethral lacunae. The distal portion of the penile urethra is somewhat narrowed and its external urethral orifice simply a vertical slit.

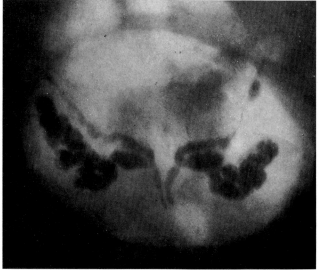

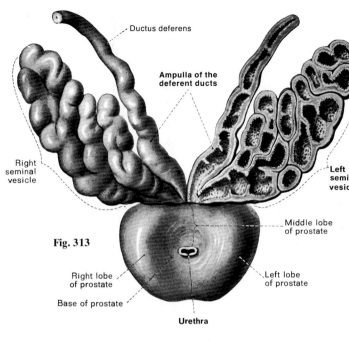

Fig. 313

- Ductus deferens
- Ampulla of the deferent ducts
- Right seminal vesicle
- **Left seminal vesicle**
- Middle lobe of prostate
- Right lobe of prostate
- Left lobe of prostate
- Base of prostate
- **Urethra**

## Fig. 313: The Prostate Gland, Seminal Vesicles and Ampullae of the Deferent Ducts (Superior View)

NOTE: the left seminal vesicle and ductus deferens were cut longitudinally, while the urethra was cut transversely just distal to the bladder. The prostate gland is conical in shape and normally measures just over 1½ inches across, 1 inch in thickness and slightly longer than 1 inch vertically. In the young adult male it weighs about 25 grams and is formed by two lateral lobes surrounding a middle lobe.

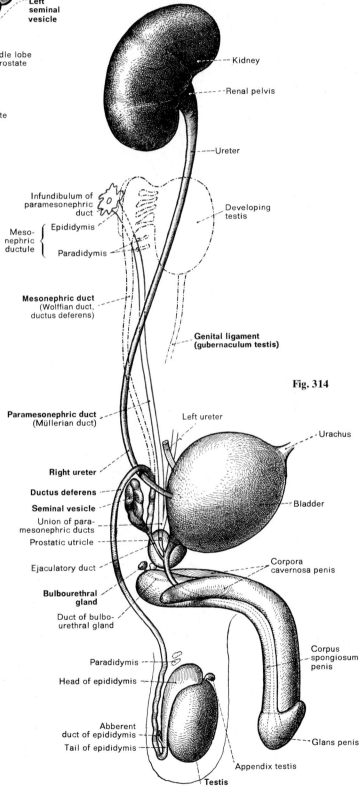

- Kidney
- Renal pelvis
- Ureter
- Developing testis
- Infundibulum of paramesonephric duct
- Meso-nephric ductule
  - Epididymis
  - Paradidymis
- **Mesonephric duct** (Wolffian duct, ductus deferens)
- **Genital ligament** (gubernaculum testis)
- Fig. 314
- **Paramesonephric duct** (Müllerian duct)
- Left ureter
- Urachus
- **Right ureter**
- **Ductus deferens**
- **Seminal vesicle**
- Union of para-mesonephric ducts
- Prostatic utricle
- Ejaculatory duct
- Bladder
- Corpora cavernosa penis
- **Bulbourethral gland**
- Duct of bulbo-urethral gland
- Corpus spongiosum penis
- Paradidymis
- Head of epididymis
- Abberent duct of epididymis
- Tail of epididymis
- Glans penis
- Appendix testis
- **Testis**

## Fig. 314: Diagram of the Male Genitourinary System

NOTE: 1) this figure shows:

a) the organs of the adult male genitourinary system;

b) the structures of the genital system prior to the descent of the testis (interrupted black lines);

c) those structures which partially or entirely became atrophic and disappeared during development (red lines).

2) the urinary system includes the *kidneys* which produce urine by filtration of the blood, the *ureters* which convey the urine to the *bladder,* where it is stored, and the *urethra* through which urine is discharged.

3) the adult male genital system includes the *testis* where sperm are generated, the *epididymis* and *ductus deferens* which transport the sperm to the *ejaculatory duct* where the *seminal vesicle* joins the genital system. The *prostate* and *bulbourethral glands* along with the ejaculatory ducts join the *urethra,* which then courses through the male copulatory organ, the *penis.*

4) embryologically, structures capable of developing into both male and female genital systems exist in all individuals. In the male, the Wolffian or mesonephric duct (which becomes the epididymis, vas deferens ejaculatory duct and seminal vesicle) and the penis, develop, while the paramesonephric or Müllerian duct becomes vestigial.

5) the testes are developed on the posterior abdominal wall and are attached by a fibrous genital ligament called the gubernaculum testis to the abdominal wall. As development continues, each testis gradually "migrates" from its site of formation, so that by the 5th month it comes to lie adjacent to the abdominal inguinal ring. The gubernaculum testis is still attached to anterior abdominal wall tissue, which by this time has evaginated as the developing scrotum. The testes then commence their descent through the inguinal canal, so that by the 8th month they usually lie in the scrotum. During this "migration", the testes pass behind the peritoneum but are attached to it by its peritoneal reflection, the processus vaginalis testis. This becomes the *tunica vaginalis testis.*

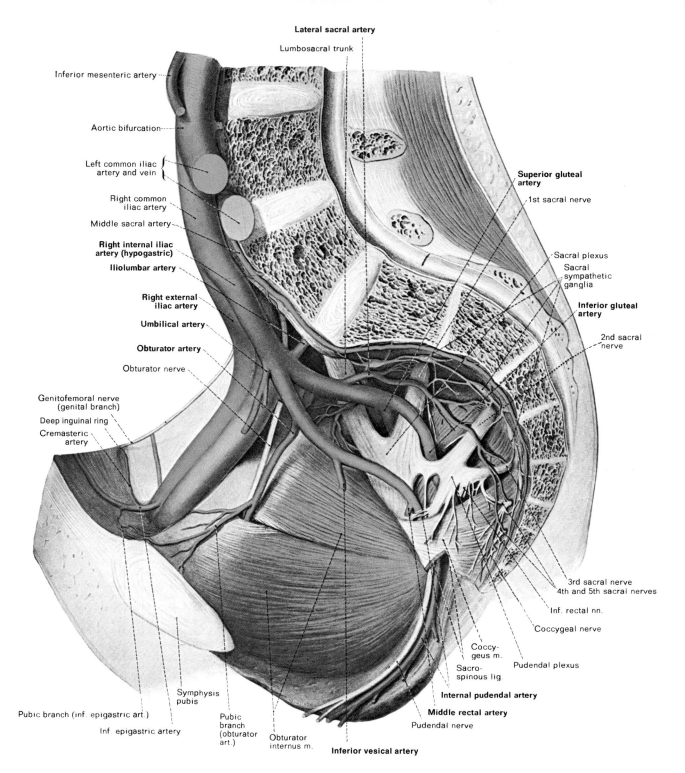

**Lateral sacral artery**

Lumbosacral trunk

Inferior mesenteric artery

Aortic bifurcation

Left common iliac
artery and vein

Right common
iliac artery

Middle sacral artery

**Right internal iliac
artery (hypogastric)**

**Iliolumbar artery**

**Right external
iliac artery**

**Umbilical artery**

**Obturator artery**

Obturator nerve

Genitofemoral nerve
(genital branch)

Deep inguinal ring

Cremasteric
artery

**Superior gluteal
artery**

1st sacral nerve

Sacral plexus

Sacral
sympathetic
ganglia

**Inferior gluteal
artery**

2nd sacral
nerve

3rd sacral nerve
4th and 5th sacral nerves

Inf. rectal nn.

Coccygeal nerve

Coccy-
geus m.

Sacro-
spinous lig.

Pudendal plexus

**Internal pudendal artery**

**Middle rectal artery**

Pudendal nerve

Pubic branch (inf. epigastric art.)

Inf. epigastric artery

Symphysis
pubis

Pubic
branch
(obturator
art.)

Obturator
internus m.

**Inferior vesical artery**

**Fig. 315: Blood Vessels and Nerves of the Pelvic Wall**

NOTE: 1) this is a mid-sagittal view of the right pelvic wall viewed from the left side. The pelvic viscera have been removed and the parietal blood vessels and nerves demonstrated.

2) the principal arteries of the pelvic wall are derived from the internal iliac artery. Although the branches of this vessel are quite variable, in at least 50% of cadavers it courses about 1½ inches toward the greater sciatic foramen before branching into a posterior division of 4 vessels and an anterior division of 6 vessels.

3) the four posterior division vessels include a) the *iliolumbar* which courses superiorly toward the iliac fossa, b) the *lateral sacral* which courses inferiorly, anastomoses with the middle sacral artery and supplies branches to the upper sacral foramina, c) the *superior gluteal* which is the largest of the branches of the internal iliac and which leaves the pelvis above the border of the piriformis muscle, and d) the *inferior gluteal* which leaves the pelvis below the piriformis muscle.

4) the anterior division of the internal iliac artery gives rise to four visceral arteries (umbilical, inferior vesical, middle rectal and uterine or deferential; see in Fig. 306). These are simply indicated by cut stumps in this figure. The two parietal vessels of this anterior division are the *obturator* artery which courses through the obturator canal to the medial thigh, and the long *internal pudendal* artery which leaves the pelvis through the greater sciatic foramen, crosses the ischial spine to reenter the pelvis by way of the lesser sciatic foramen. It then courses toward the perineum by way of the pudendal canal to supply the anal and urogenital triangles.

Fig. 315

## Fig. 316: The Muscular Floor of the Pelvis: Pelvic Diaphragm

NOTE: 1) with the pelvic organs removed, this superior view of the floor of the pelvis emphasizes the muscular nature of the pelvic outlet. The *pelvic diaphragm* consists of the levator ani and coccygeus muscles along with two fascial layers which cover the pelvic (supra-anal fascia) and perineal (infraanal fascia) surfaces of these muscles.

2) the muscles and fascial layers composing the pelvic diaphragm stretch across the pelvic floor in a concave sling-like manner, thereby forming a separation between the structures of the pelvis and those of the perineum below.

3) the more caudal part of this "sling" is formed by the two coccygeus muscles. Since these muscles stretch from the ischial spines to the sacrum and coccyx, they are sometimes referred to as the ischiococcygeus muscles. The mid and anterior portions of the "sling" are formed by the iliococcygeus and pubococcygeus muscles. These latter combine to form the levator ani muscle. The levator ani arises from the tendinous arc along the pelvic surface of the obturator internus and inserts into the anococcygeal raphé, the central point of the perineum, the external spincter and the lower segments of the coccyx.

4) in the male, the pelvic diaphragm is perforated by the anal canal and urethra.

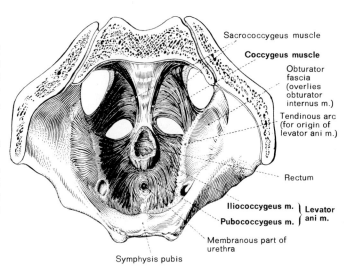

Sacrococcygeus muscle
**Coccygeus muscle**
Obturator fascia (overlies obturator internus m.)
Tendinous arc (for origin of levator ani m.)
Rectum
**Iliococcygeus m.** } Levator ani m.
**Pubococcygeus m.** }
Membranous part of urethra
Symphysis pubis

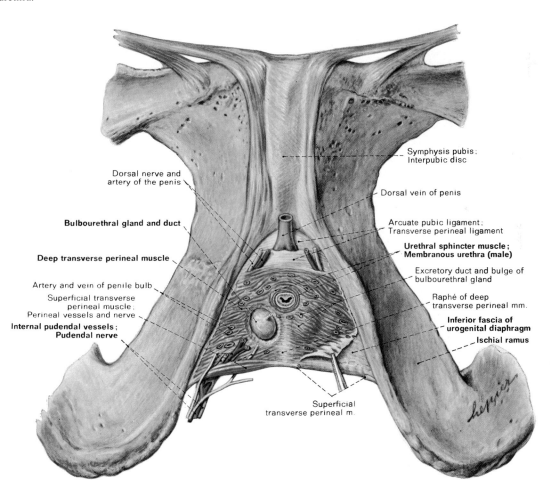

Dorsal nerve and artery of the penis
**Bulbourethral gland and duct**
**Deep transverse perineal muscle**
Artery and vein of penile bulb
Superficial transverse perineal muscle; Perineal vessels and nerve
**Internal pudendal vessels; Pudendal nerve**
Symphysis pubis; Interpubic disc
Dorsal vein of penis
Arcuate pubic ligament; Transverse perineal ligament
**Urethral sphincter muscle; Membranous urethra (male)**
Excretory duct and bulge of bulbourethral gland
Raphé of deep transverse perineal mm.
**Inferior fascia of urogenital diaphragm**
**Ischial ramus**
Superficial transverse perineal m.

## Fig. 317: The Urogenital Diaphragm; Deep Transverse Perineal Muscle (Male)

NOTE: 1) the deep transverse perineal muscle, which stretches between the rami of the ischium, is covered by fascia on both its internal (pelvic or superior) surface and its external (perineal or inferior) surface. As such, this muscle and these two fascial sheaths constitute the urogenital diaphragm.

2) the region between the superior and inferior fascial planes is frequently referred to as the deep perineal compartment (pouch, cleft or space). In the male it contains a) the deep transverse perineal muscle, b) the membranous sphincter of the urethra, c) the bulbourethral glands and ducts, d) the membranous urethra and e) the various branches of the internal pudendal vessels and nerves.

3) the urogenital diaphragm assists somewhat in strengthening the anterior portion of the levator ani muscle where, in the midline at the so-called genital hiatus, it is penetrated by the urethra in the male and the urethra and vagina in the female.

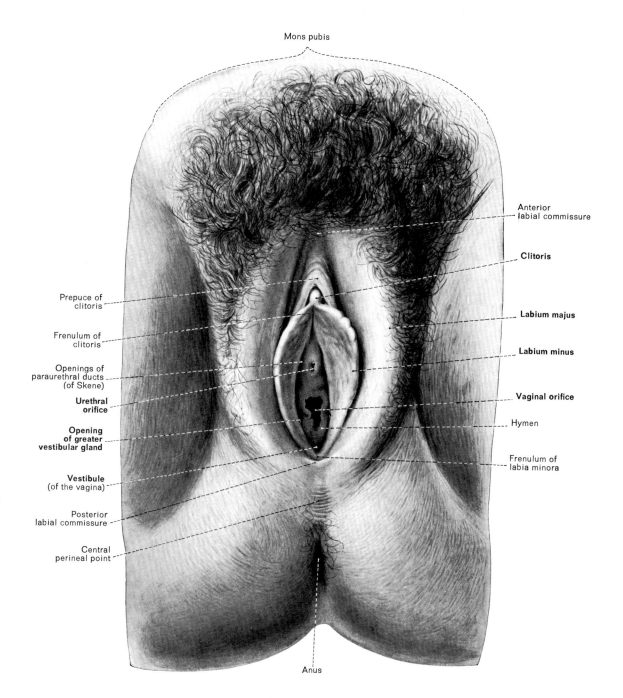

Mons pubis

Anterior labial commissure

Clitoris

Prepuce of clitoris

Labium majus

Frenulum of clitoris

Labium minus

Openings of paraurethral ducts (of Skene)

Urethral orifice

Vaginal orifice

Opening of greater vestibular gland

Hymen

Vestibule (of the vagina)

Frenulum of labia minora

Posterior labial commissure

Central perineal point

Anus

**Fig. 318: The External Genitalia of an 18 Year Old Virgin**

NOTE: 1) the female external genitalia include a) the labia majora, b) the labia minora, c) the clitoris and d) the vestibule of the vagina. The mons pubis, a rounded mound of adipose tissue anterior to the symphysis pubis and covered with hair in the adult, might also be considered an external genital structure. The orifices of the female perineum include the urethral orifice, the vaginal orifice, the two openings of the ducts of the greater vestibular glands, the orifices of the small paraurethral ducts (of Skene) and the anus.

2) the labia majora are two elongated folds of skin which form natural extensions from the mons pubis toward the anus. Although there is some variation in size and thickness dependent on age and obesity, the labia majora are in contact laterally with the thighs, unite both anteriorly and posteriorly to form integumentary commissures and represent the female homologous structures to the male scrotum. The anterior end of each labium majus receives the fibrous round ligament of the uterus as it leaves the superficial inguinal ring.

3) the labia minora are two thin folds of skin situated between the labia majora. Anteriorly, the labia minora commence at the glans clitoris, although small extensions of the labia pass over the dorsum of the clitoris to unite and form the prepuce. Posteriorly, the labia minora meet at the midline to form the frenulum of the labia.

4) the clitoris, homologous to the male penis, is an erectile organ and measures one inch or less in length. It is composed of two corpora cavernosa which are bound by dense connective tissue and which are attached by crura to the pubic rami; the crura are covered by small ischiocavernosus muscles. The clitoris is maintained by a suspensory ligament and capped by the glans.

5) the vestibule (of the vagina) is the region between the two labia minora. Into it open the urethra ventrally, the ducts of the greater vestibular glands bilaterally and the vagina. The vaginal orifice is partially closed in the virgin by a thin mucous membrane, the hymen, which separates the vestibule from the vagina proper. Generally, the hymen is ruptured at first copulation, however since its form and extent are quite variable, the establishment of virginity in this manner cannot be absolutely ascertained.

Fig. 318

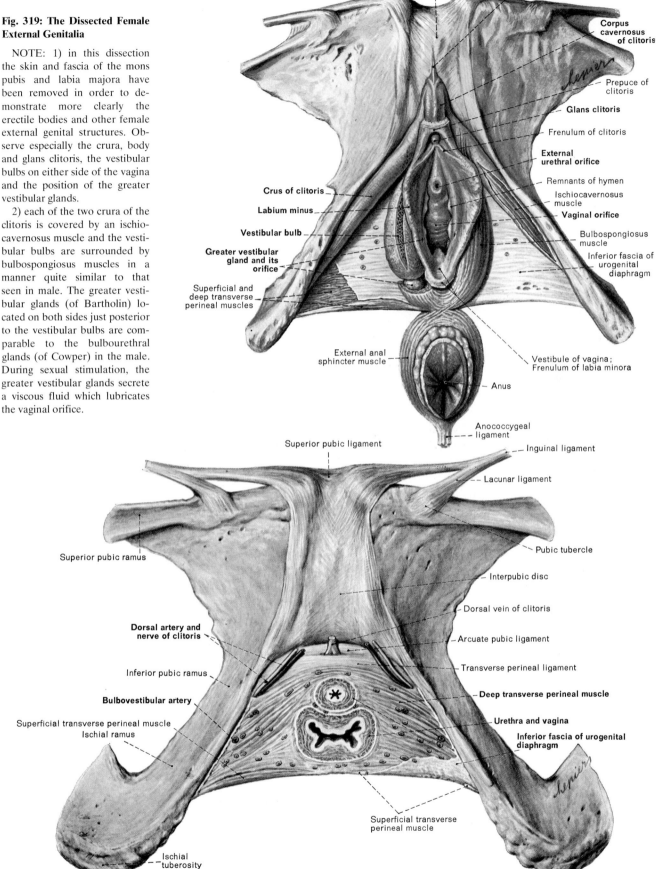

## Fig. 319: The Dissected Female External Genitalia

NOTE: 1) in this dissection the skin and fascia of the mons pubis and labia majora have been removed in order to demonstrate more clearly the erectile bodies and other female external genital structures. Observe especially the crura, body and glans clitoris, the vestibular bulbs on either side of the vagina and the position of the greater vestibular glands.

2) each of the two crura of the clitoris is covered by an ischiocavernosus muscle and the vestibular bulbs are surrounded by bulbospongiosus muscles in a manner quite similar to that seen in male. The greater vestibular glands (of Bartholin) located on both sides just posterior to the vestibular bulbs are comparable to the bulbourethral glands (of Cowper) in the male. During sexual stimulation, the greater vestibular glands secrete a viscous fluid which lubricates the vaginal orifice.

Symphysis pubis

Suspensory ligament of clitoris

**Corpus cavernosus of clitoris**

Prepuce of clitoris

**Glans clitoris**

Frenulum of clitoris

**External urethral orifice**

Remnants of hymen

Ischiocavernosus muscle

**Vaginal orifice**

Bulbospongiosus muscle

Inferior fascia of urogenital diaphragm

Crus of clitoris

Labium minus

Vestibular bulb

Greater vestibular gland and its orifice

Superficial and deep transverse perineal muscles

External anal sphincter muscle

Vestibule of vagina; Frenulum of labia minora

Anus

Anococcygeal ligament

Superior pubic ligament

Inguinal ligament

Lacunar ligament

Pubic tubercle

Interpubic disc

Dorsal vein of clitoris

Superior pubic ramus

**Dorsal artery and nerve of clitoris**

Inferior pubic ramus

Arcuate pubic ligament

Transverse perineal ligament

**Bulbovestibular artery**

**Deep transverse perineal muscle**

**Urethra and vagina**

**Inferior fascia of urogenital diaphragm**

Superficial transverse perineal muscle
Ischial ramus

Superficial transverse perineal muscle

Ischial tuberosity

## Fig. 320: The Urogenital Diaphragm in the Female

NOTE that in the female both the urethra and the vagina pass through the urogenital diaphragm. As in the male, the female urogenital diaphragm consists of the deep transverse perineal muscles and a layer of deep fascia on each of their superior and inferior surfaces. Observe the circular sphincter surrounding the membranous urethra.

Figs. 319, 320    IV

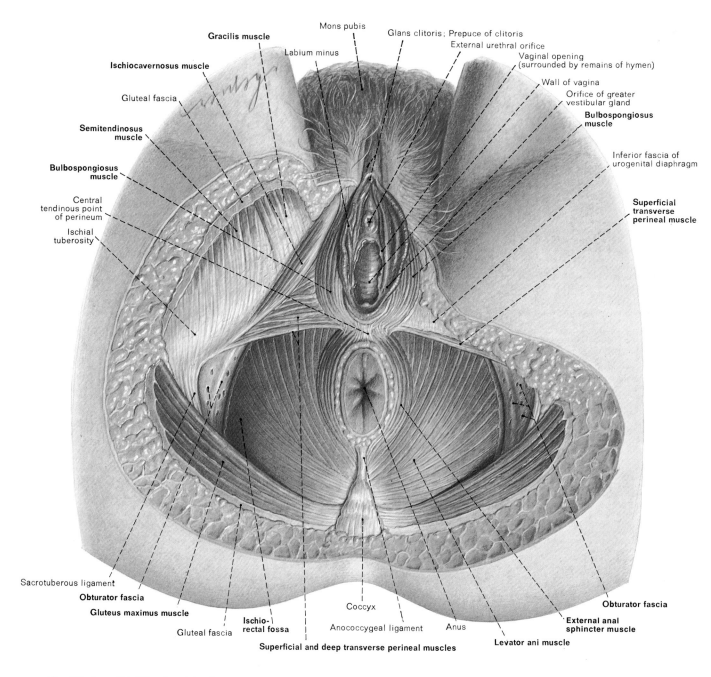

**Fig. 321: Superficial Muscles of the Female Perineum**

NOTE: 1) the perineum is a diamond-shaped region which is located inferior to the pelvis and separated from it by the muscular pelvic diaphragm. Four points limit the perineum: the symphysis pubis anteriorly; the tip of the coccyx posteriorly; and the two ischial tuberosities laterally. A line drawn transversely across the perineum between the two ischial tuberosities, passing anterior to the anus through the central point of the perineum, divides the diamond-shaped region into an anterior urogenital region and a posterior anal region.

2) the urogenital region contains the external genital organs and the associated muscles and glands. A description of this region frequently refers to a superficial and deep perineal compartment (space, pouch). Simply stated the superficial perineal compartment lies superficial to the inferior layer of fascia of the urogenital diaphragm and contains the ischiocavernosus, bulbocavernosus and superficial transverse perineal muscle, plus a number of other structures related to the external genitalia. It is traversed by the perineal vessels and nerves and is limited superficially by a layer of deep fascia, the external perineal fascia which stretches just deep to Colles' fascia. The deep perineal compartment is that space enclosed between the superior and inferior layers of fascia of the urogenital diaphragm. Thus, it contains the deep transverse perineal und urethral sphincter muscles (plus the bulbourethral glands in the male) and is traversed by the urethra and vagina in the female and the urethra in the male.

3) the anal region is situated posterior to the urogenital region. The anus, surrounded by the external anal sphincter muscle is located about 1½ inches anterior to the tip of the coccyx. A large portion of the anal region of the perineum is occupied on each side by the fat-filled ischiorectal fossae. Each fossa is wedge-shaped with the base of the wedge directed inferiorly toward the skin. The medial wall of the ischiorectal fossa is formed by the levator ani muscle, the lateral wall being the fascia over the obturator internus muscle. Recesses of each ischiorectal fossa extend anteriorly, adjacent (superior) to the urogenital diaphragm.

Fig. 321

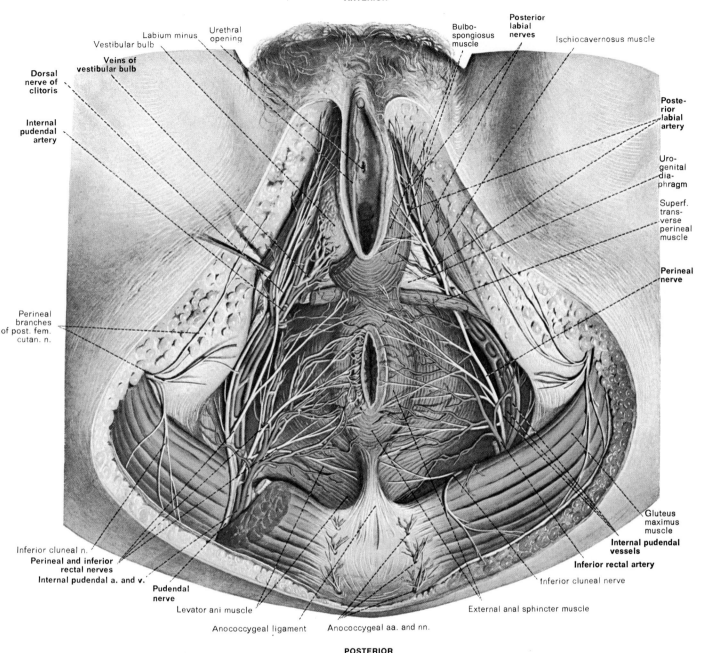

Dorsal nerve of clitoris

Internal pudendal artery

**Veins of vestibular bulb**

Labium minus

Urethral opening

Vestibular bulb

Bulbo-spongiosus muscle

**Posterior labial nerves**

Ischiocavernosus muscle

**Poste-rior labial artery**

Uro-genital dia-phragm

Superf. trans-verse perineal muscle

**Perineal nerve**

Perineal branches of post. fem. cutan. n.

Gluteus maximus muscle

**Internal pudendal vessels**

**Inferior rectal artery**

Inferior cluneal nerve

External anal sphincter muscle

Inferior cluneal n.

**Perineal and inferior rectal nerves**

**Internal pudendal a. and v.**

**Pudendal nerve**

Levator ani muscle

Anococcygeal ligament

Anococcygeal aa. and nn.

## Fig. 322: Nerves and Blood Vessels of the Female Perineum

NOTE: 1) in this dissection the skin and superficial fascia have been removed from both the urogenital and anal regions of the female perineum. The ischiorectal fossae have been cleared of fat as well.

2) the principal nerve from which most of the branches which innervate the perineum are derived is the *pudendal nerve*. It originates in the sacral cord and contains fibers of the $S_2$, $S_3$ and $S_4$ segments. In its course within the pelvis, it is joined by the *internal pudendal artery* and *vein* at the lower border of the piriformis muscle at the greater sciatic foramen. Together the vessels and nerve leave the pelvis through the greater sciatic foramen, cross the ischial spine (sacrospinous ligament) to enter the pelvis once again through the lesser sciatic foramen.

3) the pudendal structures achieve the perineum from the pelvis by way of the pudendal canal (of Alcock) which courses beneath the fascia of the obturator internus muscle. Within the perineum, the pudendal structures are first seen at the lateral wall of the ischiorectal fossa. At this point the *inferior rectal vessels* and nerves branch and cross the ischiorectal fossa toward the midline, thereby supplying the levator ani and external anal sphincter muscles along with the other structures in the anal region.

4) continuing anteriorly the pudendal nerve and internal pudendal vessels approach the urogenital diaphragm to become the perineal vessels and nerve. Upon entering the urogenital region, superficial and deep branches supply the structures of the superficial and deep perineal compartments.

5) the superficial perineal branches in the female supply the labia majora and the external genital structures, while the deep branches supply the muscles of the urogenital region, the vestibular bulb and the clitoris.

Fig. 322    IV

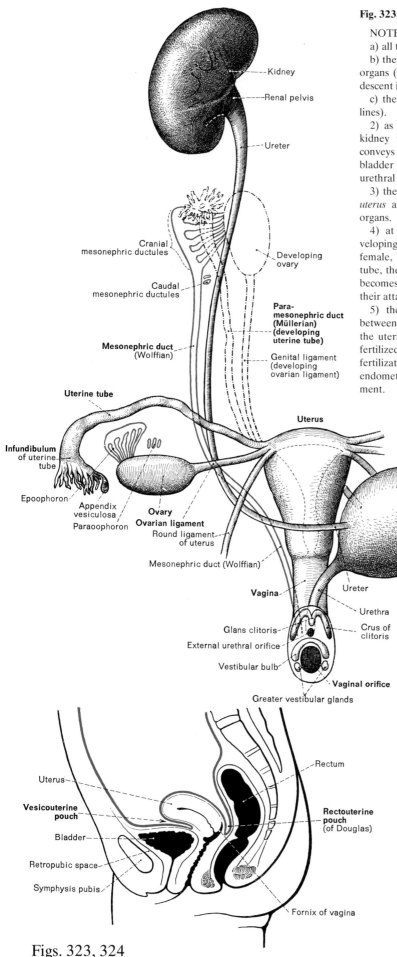

## Fig. 323: Diagram of the Female Genitourinary System

NOTE: 1) this figure shows:

a) all the organs of the adult female genitourinary system;

b) the structures and relevant positions of the female genital organs (gonad and ovarian ligament and uterine tube) prior to their descent into the pelvis (interrupted black lines); and

c) the structures which became atrophic during development (red lines).

2) as in the male, the urinary system of the female includes the kidney which produces urine from the blood, the ureter which conveys the urine to the bladder where it is stored. Leading from the bladder is the urethra through which urine passes to the external urethral orifice during micturition.

3) the adult female genital system includes the *ovary, uterine tube, uterus* and *vagina,* plus the associated glands and external genital organs.

4) at one time during development, structures capable of developing into both male and female genital systems existed. In the female, the Müllerian or paramesonephric duct forms the uterine tube, the uterus and vagina, while the Wolffian or mesonephric duct becomes vestigial. Also the developing gonads become ovaries, while their attachments become the ovarian ligaments.

5) the ovaries produce ova which are discharged periodically between adolescence and the menopause. The ova are captured by the uterine tube where fertilization may occur. If this happens, the fertilized ovum is transported to the uterus and about a week after fertilization, implantation occurs in the wall of the uterus. The endometrium nourishes the embryo in this early period of development.

## Fig. 324: Diagram of Peritoneal Reflections Over Female Pelvic Organs (Mid-Sagittal Section)

Peritoneum in red

NOTE: 1) that the parietal peritoneum is reflected over the free abdominal surfaces of the pelvic organs. Observe that as the uterus and vagina are interposed between the bladder and rectum, that peritoneal pouches are formed between the bladder and the uterus (vesicouterine) and between the rectum and the uterus (rectouterine pouch of Douglas).

2) the vesicouterine pouch is relatively shallow. The forward tilt or inclination of the uterus (anteversion) toward the superior surface of the bladder reduces the potential size of the vesicouterine pouch. This fossa does not extend as far inferiorly as the vagina, whereas the deeper rectouterine pouch dips to the posterior surface of the fornix of the vagina. This important anatomical relationship stresses the fact that the fornix of the vagina is separated from the peritoneal cavity only by the thin vaginal wall and the peritoneum.

Figs. 323, 324

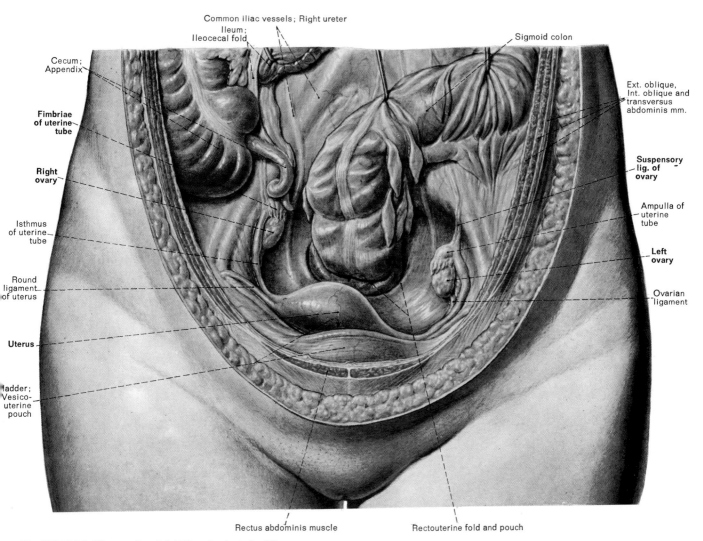

Common iliac vessels; Right ureter
Ileum;
Ileocecal fold
Sigmoid colon
Cecum;
Appendix
Ext. oblique,
Int. oblique and
transversus
abdominis mm.
**Fimbriae
of uterine
tube**
Suspensory
lig. of
ovary
**Right
ovary**
Ampulla of
uterine
tube
Isthmus
of uterine
tube
**Left
ovary**
Round
ligament
of uterus
Ovarian
ligament
**Uterus**
Bladder;
Vesico-
uterine
pouch
Rectus abdominis muscle
Rectouterine fold and pouch

**Fig. 325: Pelvic Viscera of an Adult Female: Anterior View**

NOTE: 1) that the ovaries are situated on the posterolateral aspect of the true pelvis on each side. Having descended from the posterior abdominal wall to their location just below the pelvic brim, the ovaries are held in position by ligamentous attachments. The suspensory ligament transmits the ovarian vessels and nerves.

2) the position of the uterus interposed between the bladder and rectum. Observe that the uterus is frequently located somewhat to one or the other side of the midline.

3) the fimbriae of the uterine tubes as they extend from the ampullae of the tubes to encircle the upper medial surfaces of the ovaries. These tubes vary from 3 to 6 inches in length and, as extensions of the uterus, they convey the ova to the uterus. It is within the uterine tube that fertilization of the ovum usually occurs.

**Fig. 326: Utero-Salpingogram**

By means of a cannula (K) placed in the vagina, radiopaque material has been injected into the uterus and uterine tubes (salpinx). Observe the narrow lumen of the isthmus of the uterine tubes and note how the tubes enlarge at the ampullae. On the specimen's left side (reader's right side), even the fimbriated end of the tube is discernible, while on the specimen's right side (reader's left side) a small portion of the radiopaque material has been forced into the pelvis through the opening of the uterine tube.

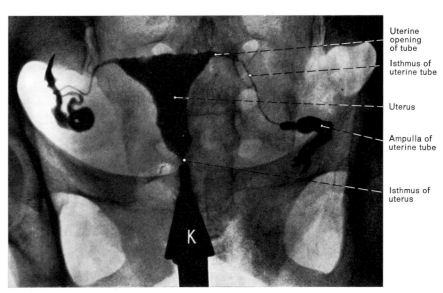

Uterine
opening
of tube

Isthmus of
uterine tube

Uterus

Ampulla of
uterine tube

Isthmus of
uterus

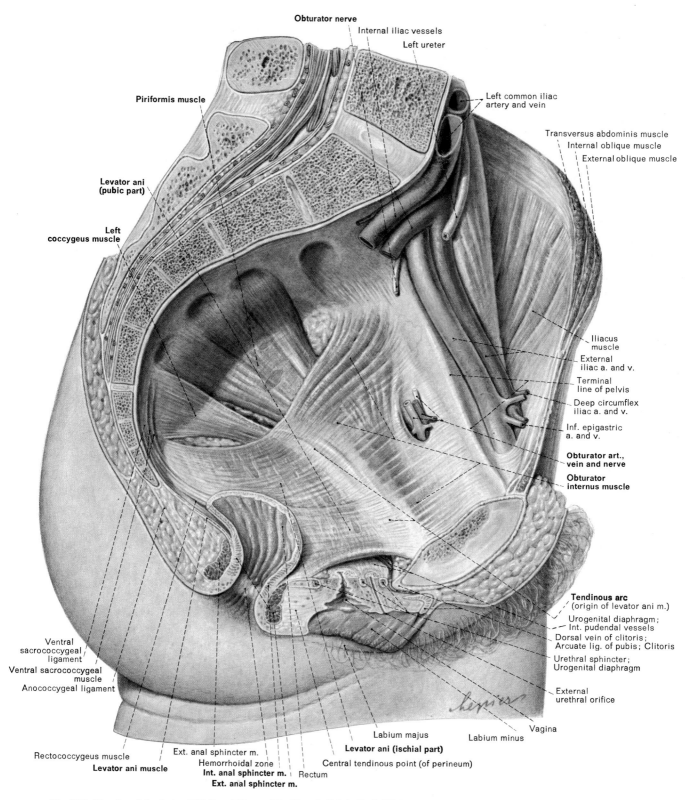

**Fig. 327: Muscles of the Lateral Wall and Floor of the Female Pelvis (Left Side)**

NOTE: 1) the lateral wall of the true pelvis is covered principally by the piriformis and obturator internus muscles while the floor of the pelvis is formed by both the pubic and ischial portions of the levator ani muscle and, more posteriorly, by the coccygeus muscle.

2) although the *piriformis muscle* arises from the ventral surface of the 2nd, 3rd and 4th sacral vertebrae, it is frequently studied with the gluteal muscles because its fibers converge and leave the pelvis through the greater sciatic foramen. The *obturator internus muscle*, covered by its fascia, has an extensive origin on the inner surface of the lateral and anterior wall of the true bony pelvis. It surrounds the obturator foramen (note the obturator vessels and nerve) and its fibers converge to form a tendon which passes out of the pelvis to enter the gluteal region through the lesser sciatic foramen.

3) both the pubic and ischial portions of the *levator ani* muscle arise principally from the tendinous arc of the obturator internus fascia. Observe the *internal* and *external* anal sphincters surrounding the anal orifice.

Fig. 327

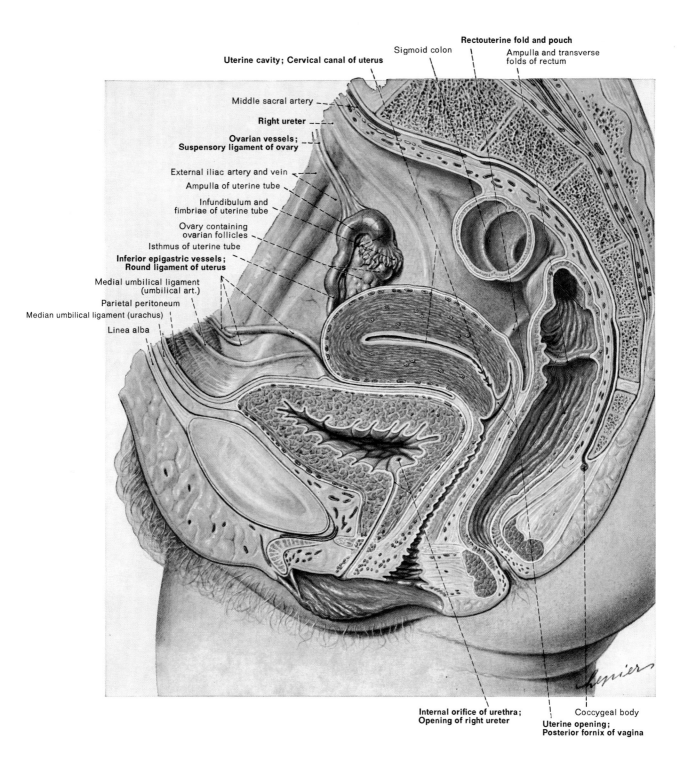

Uterine cavity; Cervical canal of uterus

Sigmoid colon

**Rectouterine fold and pouch**

Ampulla and transverse folds of rectum

Middle sacral artery

**Right ureter**

**Ovarian vessels; Suspensory ligament of ovary**

External iliac artery and vein

Ampulla of uterine tube

Infundibulum and fimbriae of uterine tube

Ovary containing ovarian follicles

Isthmus of uterine tube

**Inferior epigastric vessels; Round ligament of uterus**

Medial umbilical ligament (umbilical art.)

Parietal peritoneum

Median umbilical ligament (urachus)

Linea alba

Internal orifice of urethra; Opening of right ureter

Coccygeal body

Uterine opening; Posterior fornix of vagina

**Fig. 328: The Adult Female Pelvis. Median Sagittal Section**

NOTE: 1) this medial view of the right half of the female pelvis illustrates the relationships among the bladder, uterus and vagina, rectum, ovary and uterine tube. Observe the immediate retropubic position of the empty *bladder* and the relatively short course of the female *urethra*, which leads from the bladder through the urogenital diaphragm to open in the midline, anterior to the vagina and between the labia minora.

2) the opening between the vagina and the uterus. An extension of the vagina, the posterior fornix, reaches enough superiorly to lie just in front of the rectouterine pouch (of Douglas) and separated from it only by the vaginal wall. Note the interposition of the vagina and uterus between the bladder and rectum. The pear-shaped uterus is so positioned over the superior surface of the empty bladder that when the woman is standing erect, the uterus is horizontal.

3) that the round ligament is directed laterally and anteriorly to enter the abdominal inguinal ring and the course of the inferior epigastric vessels in relation to this ligament. Likewise observe the course of the ovarian vessels within the suspensory ligament of the ovary and their important relationship to the descending ureter on the posterolateral wall of the pelvis.

4) the sigmoid flexure of the large bowel and the relatively direct course of the rectum toward the anal canal. The peritoneum is reflected over the anterior surface of the rectum, thereby lining the rectouterine pouch.

Fig. 328    **IV**

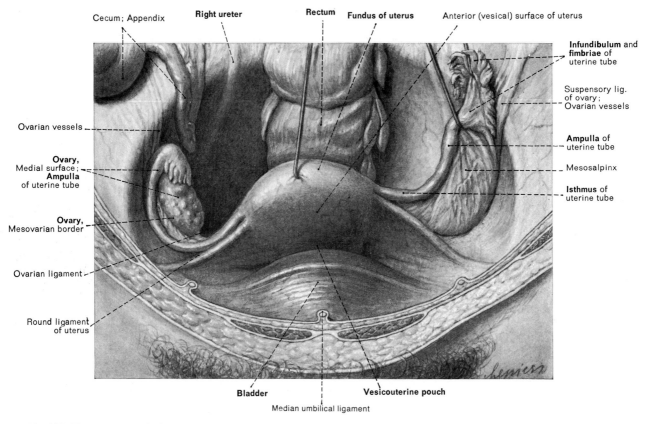

Cecum; Appendix    **Right ureter**    **Rectum**    **Fundus of uterus**    Anterior (vesical) surface of uterus

**Infundibulum** and **fimbriae** of uterine tube

Suspensory lig. of ovary; Ovarian vessels

Ovarian vessels

**Ampulla** of uterine tube

**Ovary,** Medial surface; **Ampulla** of uterine tube

Mesosalpinx

**Ovary,** Mesovarian border

**Isthmus** of uterine tube

Ovarian ligament

Round ligament of uterus

**Bladder**    **Vesicouterine pouch**

Median umbilical ligament

**Fig. 329: The Female Pelvic Organs: Anterosuperior View**

Observe that the body of the uterus has been elevated, thereby exposing the vesicouterine pouch and demonstrating the broad ligaments.

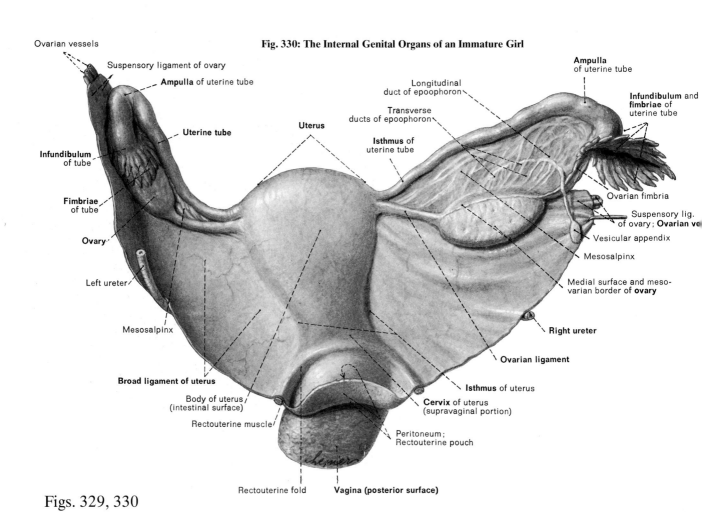

**Fig. 330: The Internal Genital Organs of an Immature Girl**

Ovarian vessels

Suspensory ligament of ovary

**Ampulla** of uterine tube

Longitudinal duct of epoophoron

**Ampulla** of uterine tube

**Uterine tube**

**Infundibulum** and **fimbriae** of uterine tube

Transverse ducts of epoophoron

Uterus

**Infundibulum** of tube

**Isthmus** of uterine tube

**Fimbriae** of tube

Ovarian fimbria

Suspensory lig. of ovary; **Ovarian ve**

**Ovary**

Vesicular appendix

Left ureter

Mesosalpinx

Medial surface and mesovarian border of **ovary**

Mesosalpinx

**Right ureter**

**Broad ligament of uterus**

**Ovarian ligament**

Body of uterus (intestinal surface)

**Isthmus** of uterus

Rectouterine muscle

**Cervix** of uterus (supravaginal portion)

Peritoneum; Rectouterine pouch

Rectouterine fold    **Vagina (posterior surface)**

Figs. 329, 330

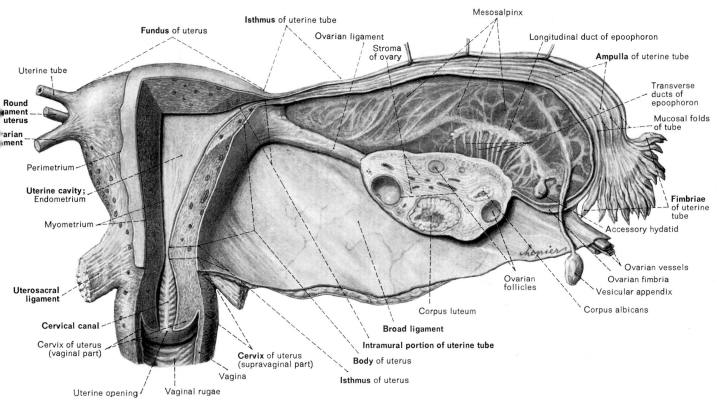

Fig. 331: **Frontal Section of Uterus, Uterine Tube and Ovary**

NOTE: 1) the vagina communicates with the pelvic cavity through the uterus and the uterine tube. The lumen of this pathway varies in diameter, and its most narrow sites are the isthmus of the uterus and the intrauterine (intramural) portion of the uterine tube.

2) the uterus consists of the cervix (vaginal and supravaginal portions) and the body of the uterus. These are interconnected by the isthmus. The attachments of the uterus include a) the broad ligaments which are mesentery-like attachments to the lateral margins of the uterus, b) the fibrous round ligament of the uterus and the ligament of the ovary attached just below the uterine tube, c) the uterosacral ligaments and d) the lateral cervical or cardinal ligaments (not shown in this figure). The cardinal ligaments are generally regarded as the principal ligamentous support of the uterus and upper vagina.

Fig. 332: **Arterial Supply to Female Pelvic Genital Organs**

NOTE: 1) the principal vessels supplying the female pelvic genital organs are the uterine arteries from the internal iliac vessels and the ovarian arteries which stem directly from the aorta. The uterine and ovarian arteries anastomose freely along both lateral borders of the uterus.

2) inferiorly, the uterine artery also anastomoses with the arterial supply to the vagina. Frequently, the vaginal arteries branch directly from the uterine, however, they may branch from the inferior vesical artery or even directly from the internal iliac artery.

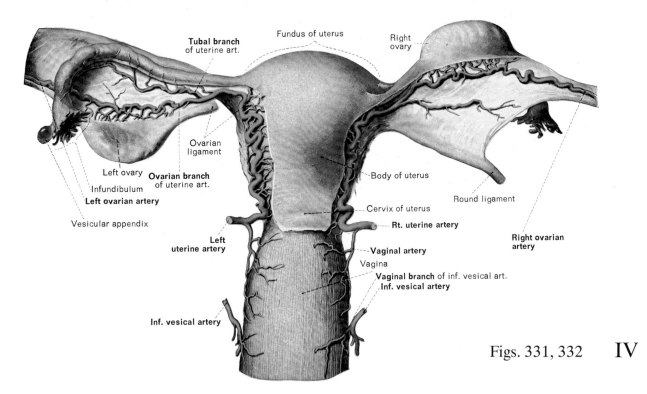

Figs. 331, 332    **IV**

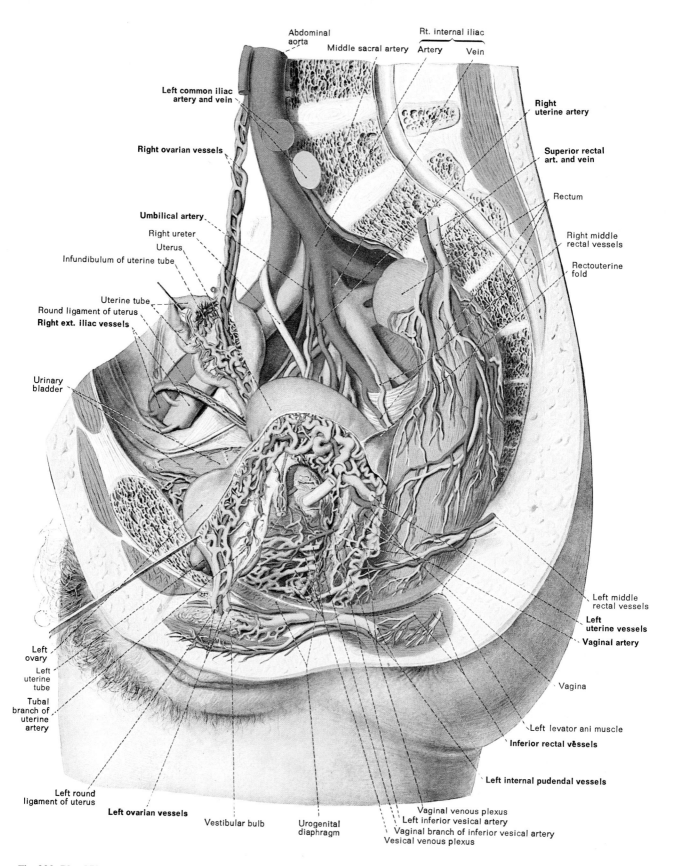

**Fig. 333: Blood Vessels of the Female Pelvis and Genital System**

NOTE: 1) the left half of the pelvis has been removed while most of the female pelvic organs are still in place. Observe the dense plexuses of veins. These include the ovarian, uterine, vaginal and vesical plexuses which accompany their respective arteries and which drain the pelvic organs.

2) with the exception of the *ovarian artery* which is derived from the aorta and the *superior rectal artery* (hemorrhoidal) which branches from the inferior mesenteric, all the other arteries supplying blood to the pelvic organs, perineum and genital tract are derived from the *internal iliac artery* or its branches. Observe the anastomosis among the superior, middle and inferior rectal vessels.

3) the descending course of the ureter over the pelvic brim from the posterior abdominal wall. In its path it crosses the external iliac artery and vein, as does the round ligament of the uterus more inferiorly.

Fig. 333

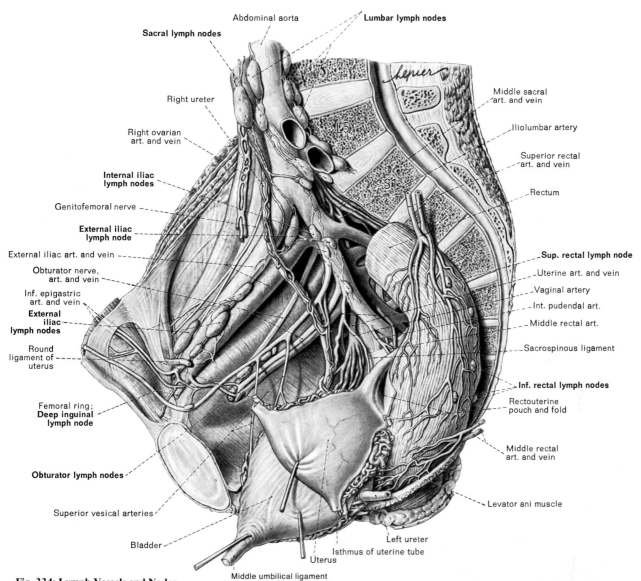

Abdominal aorta
Lumbar lymph nodes
Sacral lymph nodes
Right ureter
Right ovarian art. and vein
Internal iliac lymph nodes
Genitofemoral nerve
External iliac lymph node
External iliac art. and vein
Obturator nerve, art. and vein
Inf. epigastric art. and vein
External iliac lymph nodes
Round ligament of uterus
Femoral ring; Deep inguinal lymph node
Obturator lymph nodes
Superior vesical arteries
Bladder
Middle umbilical ligament
Uterus
Isthmus of uterine tube
Left ureter
Levator ani muscle
Middle rectal art. and vein
Rectouterine pouch and fold
Inf. rectal lymph nodes
Sacrospinous ligament
Middle rectal art.
Int. pudendal art.
Vaginal artery
Uterine art. and vein
Sup. rectal lymph node
Rectum
Superior rectal art. and vein
Iliolumbar artery
Middle sacral art. and vein

## Fig. 334: Lymph Vessels and Nodes of the Female Pelvis

NOTE: 1) as a rule, the lymph nodes of the pelvis lie along the course of the major vessels. Generally, the lymphatics drain superiorly and posteriorly to achieve the right and left lumbar lymphatic chain of nodes which lie upon the psoas major muscles on both sides of the aorta.

2) the lymphatics of the bladder drain laterally to the external iliac nodes and posteriorly to the internal iliac nodes. These latter lymphatic channels and nodes also receive lymph from the fundus and body of the uterus in the female and the prostate and seminal vesicles in the male. Lymphatics of the cervix and vagina drain into both the external and internal iliac nodes.

## Fig. 335: Lymphograph of Pelvis and Lumbar Region

This lymphograph displays the lymphatic channels from the deeper femoral vessels and nodes, which course superiorly through to the lumbar and aortic nodes. Observe the profuse network along the iliac vessels and the concentration of nodes in the deep inguinal region.

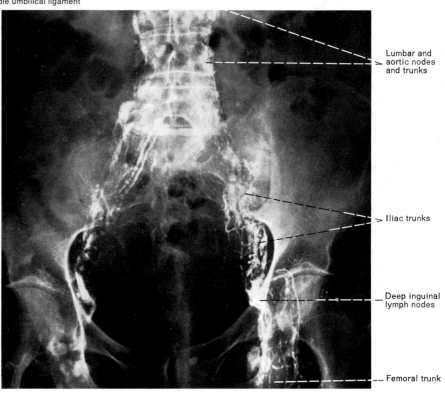

Lumbar and aortic nodes and trunks

Iliac trunks

Deep inguinal lymph nodes

Femoral trunk

Figs. 334, 335    **IV**

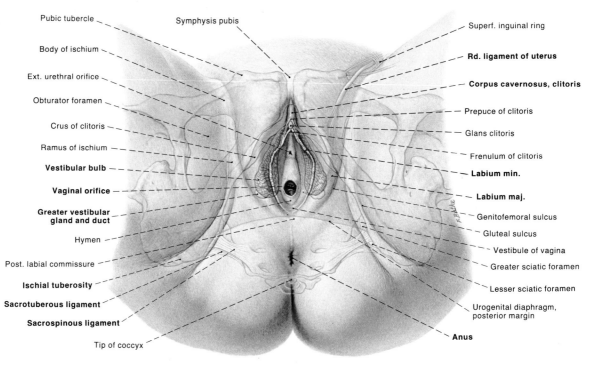

Pubic tubercle

Symphysis pubis

Superf. inguinal ring

Body of ischium

**Rd. ligament of uterus**

Ext. urethral orifice

**Corpus cavernosus, clitoris**

Obturator foramen

Prepuce of clitoris

Crus of clitoris

Glans clitoris

Ramus of ischium

Frenulum of clitoris

**Vestibular bulb**

**Labium min.**

**Vaginal orifice**

**Labium maj.**

**Greater vestibular gland and duct**

Genitofemoral sulcus

Gluteal sulcus

Hymen

Vestibule of vagina

Post. labial commissure

Greater sciatic foramen

**Ischial tuberosity**

Lesser sciatic foramen

**Sacrotuberous ligament**

Urogenital diaphragm, posterior margin

**Sacrospinous ligament**

**Anus**

Tip of coccyx

**Fig. 336: Projection of External Female Genitalia on Bony Structures of the Pelvis**

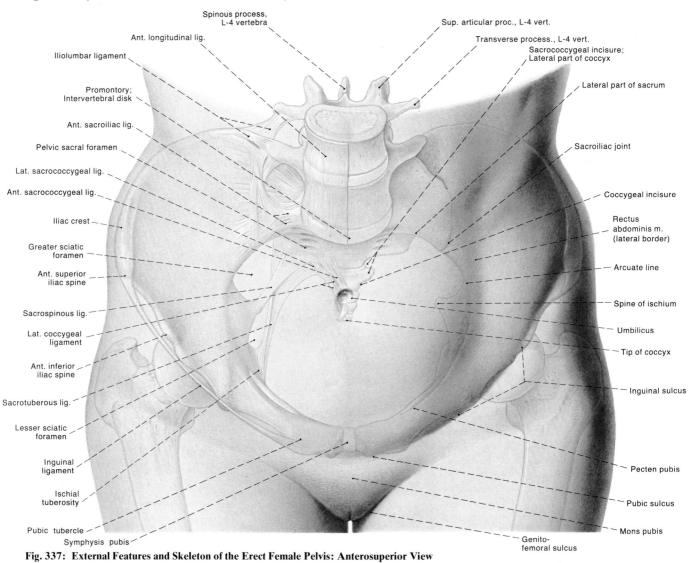

Spinous process, L-4 vertebra

Sup. articular proc., L-4 vert.

Ant. longitudinal lig.

Transverse process., L-4 vert.

Iliolumbar ligament

Sacrococcygeal incisure; Lateral part of coccyx

Promontory; Intervertebral disk

Lateral part of sacrum

Ant. sacroiliac lig.

Pelvic sacral foramen

Sacroiliac joint

Lat. sacrococcygeal lig.

Coccygeal incisure

Ant. sacrococcygeal lig.

Rectus abdominis m. (lateral border)

Iliac crest

Greater sciatic foramen

Arcuate line

Ant. superior iliac spine

Spine of ischium

Sacrospinous lig.

Umbilicus

Lat. coccygeal ligament

Tip of coccyx

Ant. inferior iliac spine

Inguinal sulcus

Sacrotuberous lig.

Lesser sciatic foramen

Inguinal ligament

Pecten pubis

Ischial tuberosity

Pubic sulcus

Pubic tubercle

Mons pubis

Symphysis pubis

Genito-femoral sulcus

**Fig. 337: External Features and Skeleton of the Erect Female Pelvis: Anterosuperior View**

Figs. 336, 337

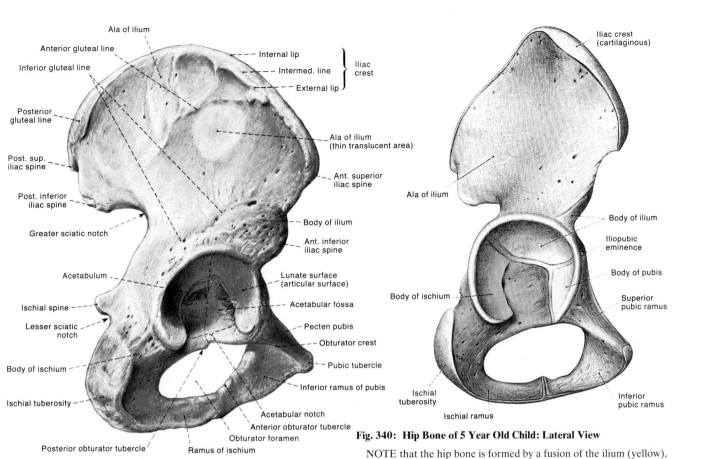

Fig. 338: Lateral View of the Adult Right Hip Bone

**Fig. 340: Hip Bone of 5 Year Old Child: Lateral View**

NOTE that the hip bone is formed by a fusion of the ilium (yellow), ischium (green) and pubis (blue). Although ossification of the inferior pubic ramus occurs during the 7th or 8th year, complete fusion of the three bones at the acetabulum occurs sometime between the 15th and 20th year.

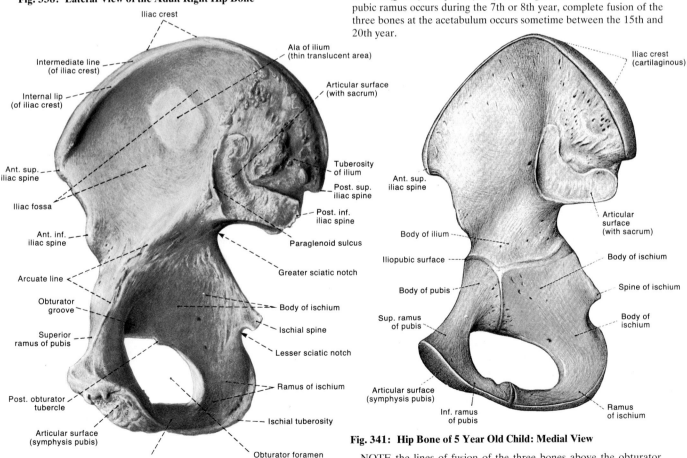

**Fig. 339: Medial View of the Adult Right Hip Bone**

**Fig. 341: Hip Bone of 5 Year Old Child: Medial View**

NOTE the lines of fusion of the three bones above the obturator foramen and of the inferior pubic ramus and the ischial ramus below that foramen.

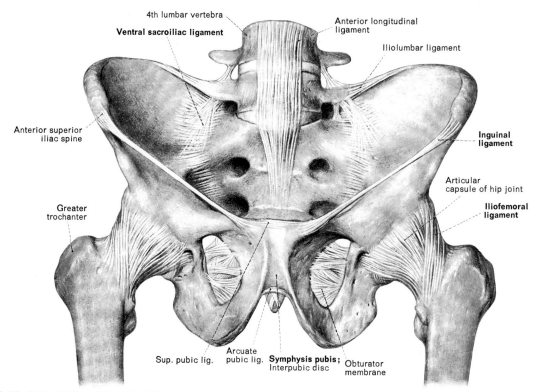

Fig. 342: The Male Pelvis and Associated Ligaments: Anterior Aspect

NOTE that the pelvis is formed by the articulation of the left and right hip bones anteriorly at the symphysis pubis and posteriorly with the sacrum and coccyx of the vertebral column. The articulations inferiorly of the pelvis with the two femora allow the weight of the head, trunk and upper extremities to be transmitted to the lower limbs, thereby maintaining the upright posture characteristic of the human being.

Fig. 343: The Female Pelvis with Joints and Ligaments: Posterior Aspect

NOTE that broad ligamentous bands articulate the two hip bones posteriorly with the sacrum and coccyx. This sacroiliac joint is bound by the extremely strong dorsal sacroiliac ligament. Attaching the sacrum to the ischial tuberosity is the broad sacrotuberous ligament. Additionally, the sacrospinous ligament stretches between the sacrum and the ischium (ischial spine).

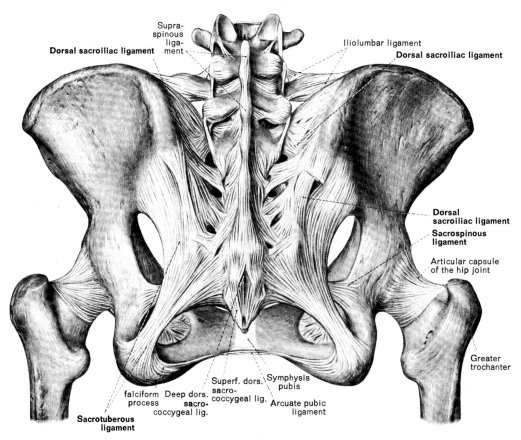

Figs. 342, 343

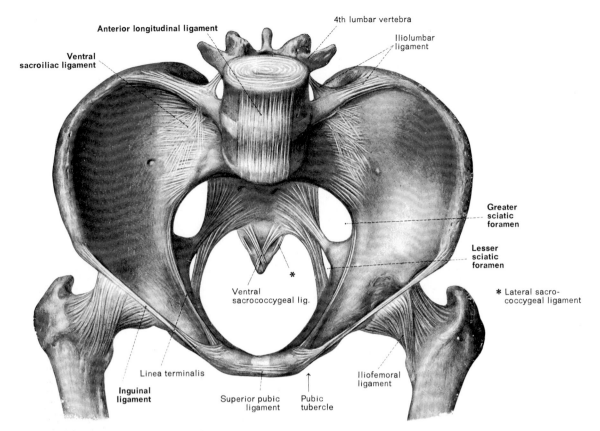

Fig. 344: The Male Pelvis and Ligaments Viewed from Above

NOTE that the size of both the pelvic inlet (superior aperture of the minor pelvis) and inferior outlet of the male pelvis is smaller than that in the female (see Figure 345 below). Thus, the minor pelvis is deeper and narrower in the male and its cavity has a smaller capacity than a female. In the male, however, the pelvic bones are thicker and heavier and generally the major pelvis (above the pelvic brim) is larger than in the female.

Fig. 345: The Female Pelvis and Ligaments Viewed from Above

NOTE that in addition to having wider diameters, both the pelvic inlet and outlet of the female pelvis minor are more circular in shape than in the male. The female pelvic bones are more delicate and the sacrum less curved. The larger capacity of the true pelvis in the female, and the fact that the female hormones of pregnancy tend to relax the pelvic ligaments serve to facilitate the function of child bearing.

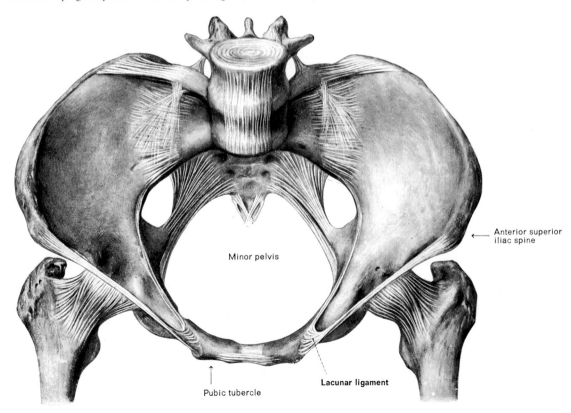

Figs. 344, 345    IV

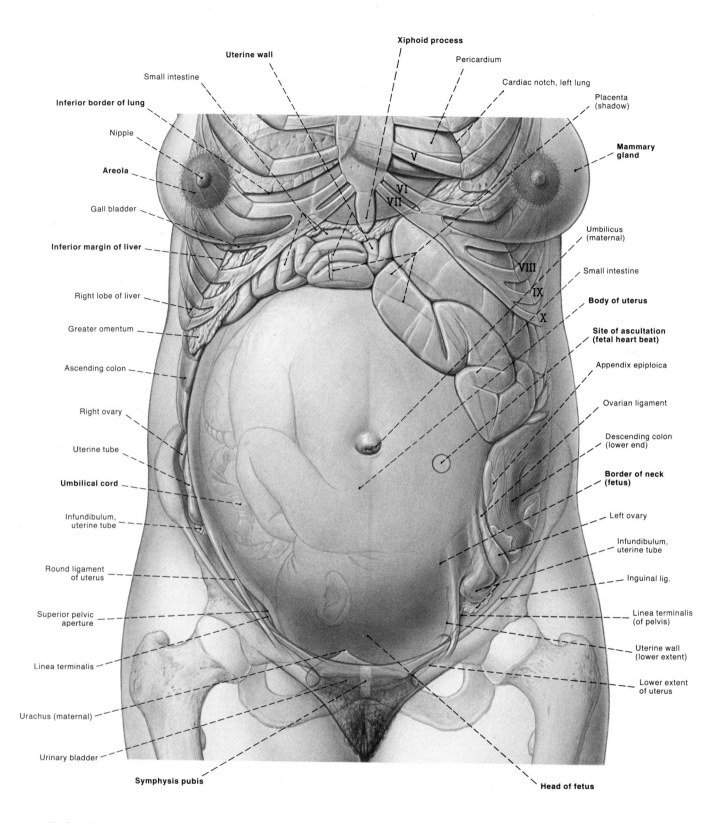

Xiphoid process

Uterine wall

Pericardium

Small intestine

Cardiac notch, left lung

Inferior border of lung

Placenta (shadow)

Nipple

V

**Mammary gland**

**Areola**

VI

VII

Gall bladder

**Inferior margin of liver**

VIII

Umbilicus (maternal)

Small intestine

Right lobe of liver

IX

**Body of uterus**

Greater omentum

X

**Site of ascultation (fetal heart beat)**

Ascending colon

Appendix epiploica

Right ovary

Ovarian ligament

Uterine tube

Descending colon (lower end)

**Umbilical cord**

**Border of neck (fetus)**

Infundibulum, uterine tube

Left ovary

Infundibulum, uterine tube

Round ligament of uterus

Inguinal lig.

Superior pelvic aperture

Linea terminalis (of pelvis)

Linea terminalis

Uterine wall (lower extent)

Urachus (maternal)

Lower extent of uterus

Urinary bladder

**Symphysis pubis**

**Head of fetus**

**Fig. 346: Diagrammatic Projection of Abdominal and Pelvic Organs in a Pregnant Woman Shortly Before Giving Birth: Anterior View**

NOTE that: 1) in the maternal abdomen, the full-term fetus is in a characteristically longitudinal posture, with the dorsum of the fetal head and back oriented toward the mother's anterior abdominal wall. This type of cephalic longitudinal presentation occurs in 95% of births, while longitudinal pelvic presentation (breech) occurs in about 3% of births. In about 1% of births, a transverse presentation of the fetus occurs, with one of the shoulders as the presenting part *(Reid, 1962, A Textbook of Obstetrics, W. B. Saunders Co. Publ.)*;

2) as the fetus grows, the maternal uterus enlarges. By the end of the 3rd month, the uterus occupies most of the pelvis, extending as gestation continues, higher and higher within the abdomen. Near the end of pregnancy, it occupies most of the abdomen, reaching above the costal margin, nearly to the xiphoid process;

3) the maternal liver, stomach and intestines are displaced upward, while the diaphragm is elevated and the dimensions of the thoracic cavity broadened. The breasts enlarge considerably through a proliferation of its glandular tissue in advance of lactation, and the areolar region around the nipple becomes more darkly pigmented.

Fig. 346

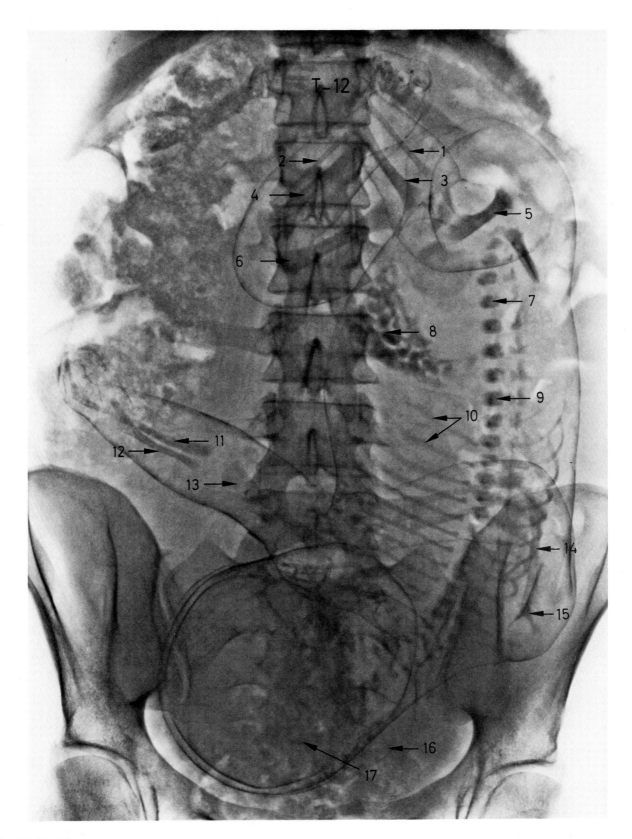

**Fig. 347: Fetal Roentgenogram**

NOTE the body contours of this near-term fetus *in utero* and a number of the ossifying fetal bones. Observe that the uterus extends to the maternal T-12 vertebral body level.

| | | | |
|---|---|---|---|
| 1. Right fibula | 6. Left femur | 10. Ribs | 14. Right humerus |
| 2. Left fibula | 7. L-5 vertebra | 11. Left ulna | 15. Right scapula |
| 3. Right tibia | 8. Small intestine (fetal) | 12. Left radius | 16. External ear |
| 4. Left tibia | 9. L-1 vertebra | 13. Left humerus | 17. Fetal head |
| 5. Right femur | | | |

Fig. 347    IV

Fig. 348

1. Iliac crest
2. Gas bubble in colon
3. Ala of ilium
4. Lateral part of sacrum
5. Sacroiliac joint
6. Post. inf. iliac spine
7. Ant. sup. iliac spine
8. Ant. inf. iliac spine
9. Lunate surface of acetabulum
10. Spine of ischium
11. Greater trochanter
12. Intertrochanteric crest
13. Lesser trochanter
14. Ischial tuberosity
15. Superior ramus of pubis
16. Symphysis pubis
17. Inferior ramus of pubis
18. Obturator foramen
19. Neck of femur
20. Head of femur
21. Fovea on head of femur
22. Acetabular fossa
23. Greater sciatic notch
24. Iliopubic eminence
25. Transverse process L-5 vertebra
26. Gas bubble in colon

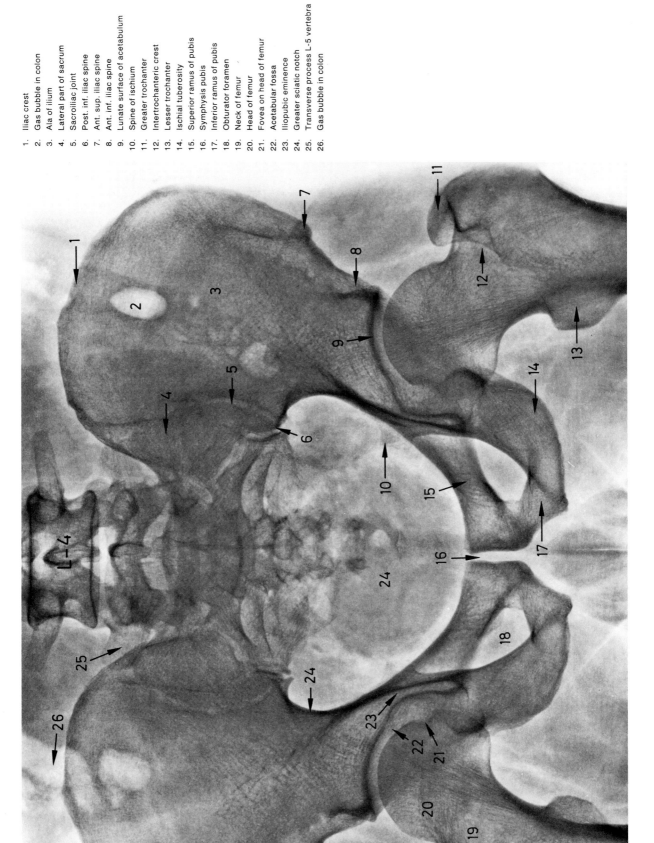

**Fig. 348: Radiograph of the Pelvis and the Sacroiliac and Hip Joints**

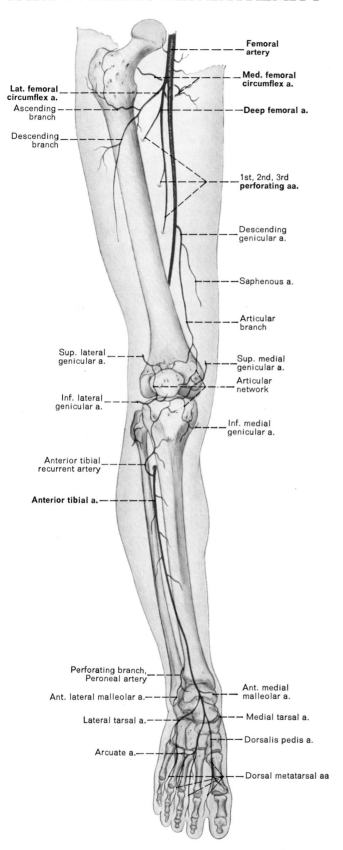

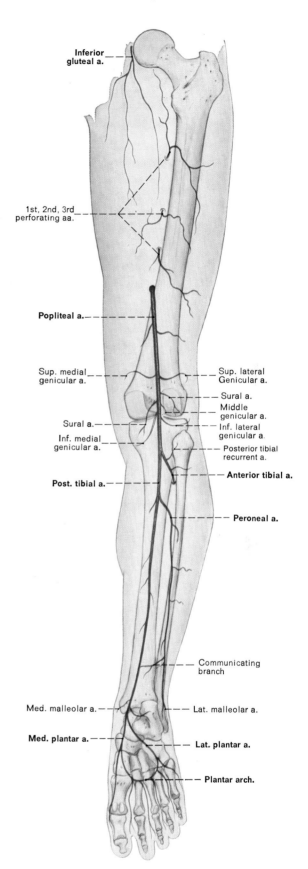

**Fig. 349: Arteries and Bones of the Lower Limb (Anterior View)**

NOTE the anastomoses in the hip and knee regions, and the perforating branches of the deep femoral artery. In the anterior leg, the anterior tibial artery descends between the tibia and fibula to achieve the malleolar region and dorsum of the foot.

**Fig. 350: Arteries and Bones of the Lower Limb (Posterior View)**

NOTE the branches of the popliteal artery at the knee, and the artery's continuation as the posterior tibial. In the foot this vessel becomes the medial and lateral plantar arteries, which join the plantar arch.

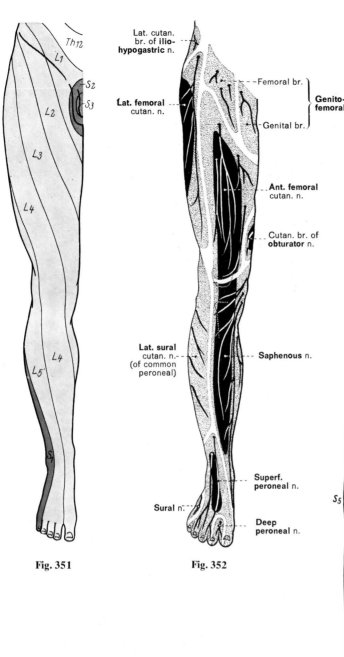

**Fig. 351**

**Fig. 352**

Lat. cutan.
br. of ilio-
hypogastric n.

Lat. femoral
cutan. n.

Femoral br.
Genito-
femoral n.
Genital br.

Ant. femoral
cutan. n.

Cutan. br. of
obturator n.

Lat. sural
cutan. n.
(of common
peroneal)

Saphenous n.

Superf.
peroneal n.

Sural n.

Deep
peroneal n.

### Fig. 351: Dermatomes of the Anterior Aspect of the Lower Extremity

NOTE that as a rule the lumbar segments of the spinal cord supply the cutaneous innervation to the anterior aspect of the lower extremity, and that the dermatomes are segmentally arranged in order from L-1 to S-1. Observe that the genital region is supplied by the sacral segments.

### Fig. 352: The Distribution of Cutaneous Nerves: Anterior Aspect of the Lower Extremity

The segmental distribution of the cutaneous nerves supplying the anterior aspect of the lower extremity is as follows:

| | |
|---|---|
| iliohypogastric nerve: | $(T_{12})$, $L_1$ |
| genitofemoral nerve: | $L_1$, $L_2$ |
| lateral femoral cutaneous nerve: | $L_2$, $L_3$ |
| femoral nerve: | $L_2$, $L_3$, $L_4$ |
| obturator nerve: | $L_2$, $L_3$, $L_4$ |
| saphenous nerve (femoral): | $L_2$, $L_3$, $L_4$ |
| deep peroneal (cutaneous br.): | $L_4$, $L_5$ |
| superficial peroneal: | $L_4$, $L_5$, $S_1$ |
| lateral sural cutaneous n.: | $L_5$, $S_1$, $S_2$ |
| (common peroneal n.) | |
| sural nerve (tibial): | $S_1$, $S_2$ |

### Fig. 353: Dermatomes of the Posterior Aspect of the Lower Extremity

NOTE that the skin on the posterior aspect of the lower extremity receives its sensory innervation principally from L5, S1 and S2. Observe, however, how the posterior medial border of the limb consecutively has the L1, L2, L3 and L4 segments represented. Segments S3, S4 and S5 are more limited to the perineal and anal regions.

### Fig. 354: The Distribution of Cutaneous Nerves: Posterior Aspect of the Lower Extremity

NOTE: 1) the principal nerve supplying cutaneous innervation to the posterior aspect of the thigh is the posterior femoral cutaneous nerve (S1, S2, S3). The skin of the medial calf is supplied by the saphenous (femoral) nerve (L2, L3, L4), while the lateral calf receives the sural nerve (S1, S2).

2) the heel of the foot is innervated by the tibial nerve through S1 and S2 segments, and the plantar surface of the foot receives L4 and L5 fibers medially (medial plantar nerve) and S1 and S2 laterally (lateral plantar nerve).

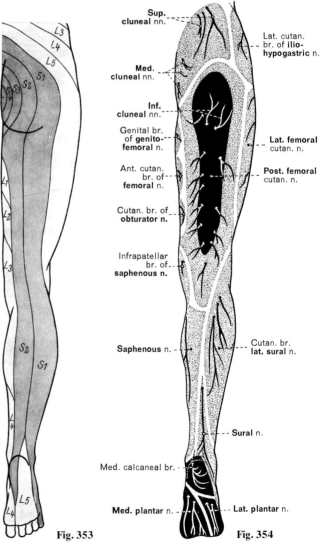

Sup.
cluneal nn.

Lat. cutan.
br. of ilio-
hypogastric n.

Med.
cluneal nn.

Inf.
cluneal nn.

Genital br.
of genito-
femoral n.

Lat. femoral
cutan. n.

Ant. cutan.
br. of
femoral n.

Post. femoral
cutan. n.

Cutan. br. of
obturator n.

Infrapatellar
br. of
saphenous n.

Saphenous n.

Cutan. br.
lat. sural n.

Sural n.

Med. calcaneal br.

Med. plantar n.

Lat. plantar n.

**Fig. 353**

**Fig. 354**

Figs. 351–354

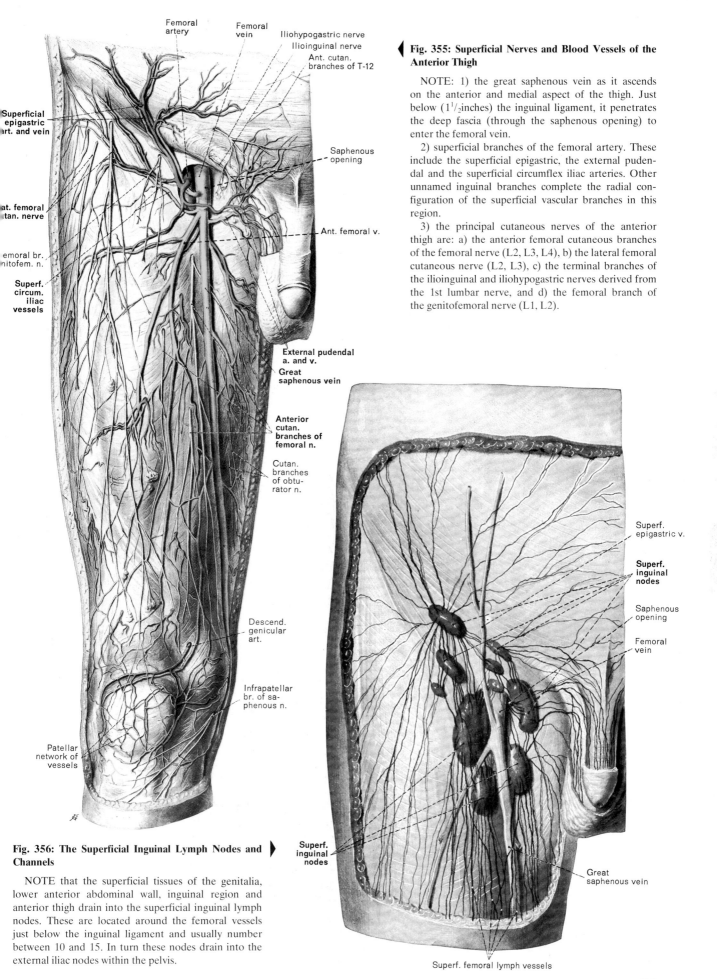

**Fig. 355: Superficial Nerves and Blood Vessels of the Anterior Thigh**

NOTE: 1) the great saphenous vein as it ascends on the anterior and medial aspect of the thigh. Just below (1½inches) the inguinal ligament, it penetrates the deep fascia (through the saphenous opening) to enter the femoral vein.

2) superficial branches of the femoral artery. These include the superficial epigastric, the external pudendal and the superficial circumflex iliac arteries. Other unnamed inguinal branches complete the radial configuration of the superficial vascular branches in this region.

3) the principal cutaneous nerves of the anterior thigh are: a) the anterior femoral cutaneous branches of the femoral nerve (L2, L3, L4), b) the lateral femoral cutaneous nerve (L2, L3), c) the terminal branches of the ilioinguinal and iliohypogastric nerves derived from the 1st lumbar nerve, and d) the femoral branch of the genitofemoral nerve (L1, L2).

Labels for Fig. 355:
- Femoral artery
- Femoral vein
- Iliohypogastric nerve
- Ilioinguinal nerve
- Ant. cutan. branches of T-12
- Superficial epigastric art. and vein
- Saphenous opening
- at. femoral tan. nerve
- Ant. femoral v.
- emoral br. nitofem. n.
- Superf. circum. iliac vessels
- External pudendal a. and v.
- Great saphenous vein
- Anterior cutan. branches of femoral n.
- Cutan. branches of obturator n.
- Descend. genicular art.
- Infrapatellar br. of saphenous n.
- Patellar network of vessels

**Fig. 356: The Superficial Inguinal Lymph Nodes and Channels**

NOTE that the superficial tissues of the genitalia, lower anterior abdominal wall, inguinal region and anterior thigh drain into the superficial inguinal lymph nodes. These are located around the femoral vessels just below the inguinal ligament and usually number between 10 and 15. In turn these nodes drain into the external iliac nodes within the pelvis.

Labels for Fig. 356:
- Superf. epigastric v.
- Superf. inguinal nodes
- Saphenous opening
- Femoral vein
- Superf. inguinal nodes
- Great saphenous vein
- Superf. femoral lymph vessels

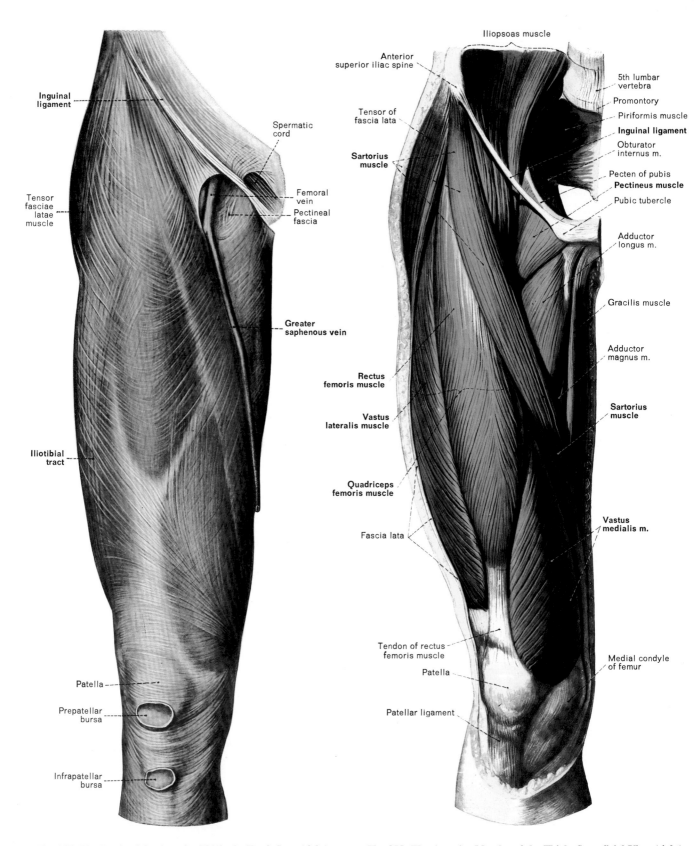

**Fig. 357: The Fascia of the Anterior Thigh, the Fascia Lata (right)**

NOTE: 1) the dense fascia which invests the muscles of the hip and thigh is called the fascia lata. It is attached above to the ischial and pubic rami and inguinal ligament anteriorly, the crest of the ilium laterally and the ischial tuberosity, sacrotuberous ligament, sacrum and coccyx posteriorly.

2) in the inguinal region the fascia lata is pierced by the greater saphenous vein, and inferiorly it extends to the investing fascia below the knee.

**Fig. 358: The Anterior Muscles of the Thigh: Superficial View (right)**

NOTE: 1) the long narrow sartorius muscle which arises on the anterior superior iliac spine and passes obliquely across the anterior femoral muscles to insert on the medial aspect of the body of the tibia. The sartorius flexes the thigh and rotates it laterally. It also flexes the knee and rotates it medially.

2) the quadriceps muscle forms the bulk of the anterior femoral muscles, and both the sartorius and quadriceps are innervated by the femoral nerve.

Figs. 357, 358

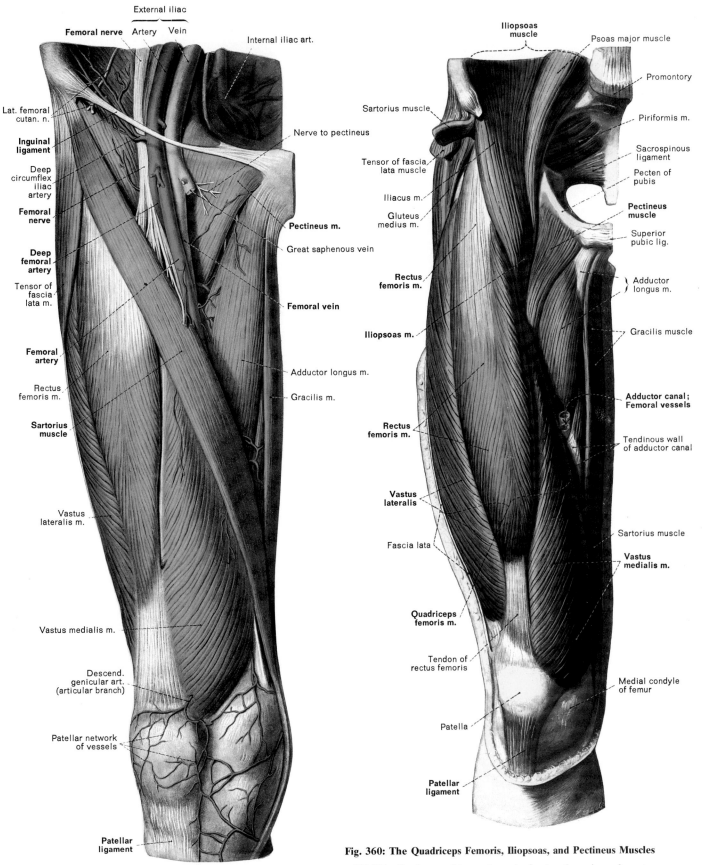

**Fig. 359: The Femoral Triangle**

NOTE: the boundaries of the femoral triangle are the inguinal ligament, the sartorius muscle and the medial border of the adductor longus. The floor is formed by the iliopsoas and pectineus muscles. The femoral nerve, artery and vein descend beneath the inguinal ligament and traverse the femoral triangle.

**Fig. 360: The Quadriceps Femoris, Iliopsoas, and Pectineus Muscles**

NOTE: 1) the quadriceps femoris (rectus femoris and vastus lateralis, intermedius and medialis) as it converges inferiorly to form a powerful tendon which encases the patella and which is inserted onto the tuberosity of the tibia. The entire quadriceps extends the leg, while the rectus femoris also flexes the thigh.

2) the iliopsoas muscle is a powerful flexor of the thigh and inserts on the lesser trochanter.

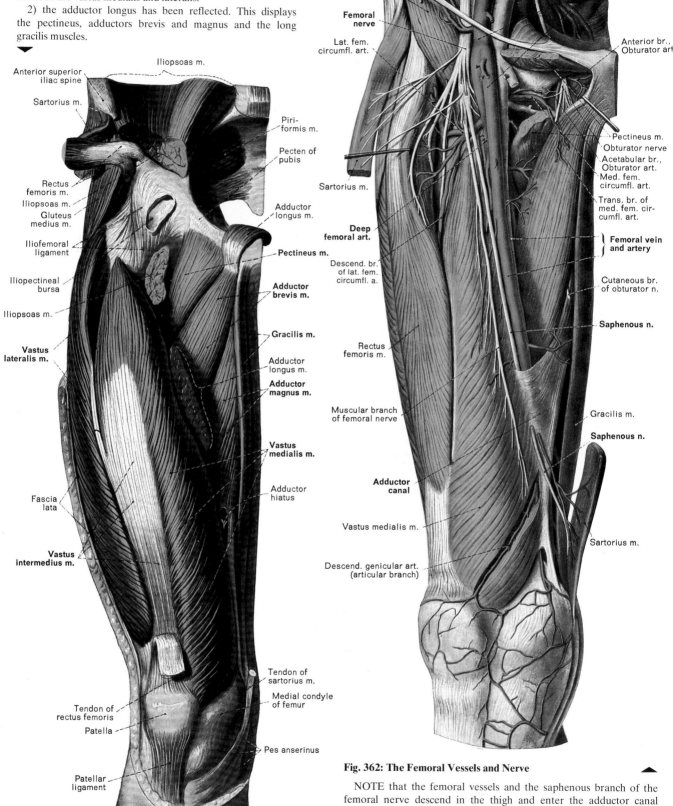

**Fig. 361: The Intermediate Layer of Anterior and Medial Thigh Muscles**

NOTE: 1) that the rectus femoris and iliopsoas muscles are cut to reveal the underlying vastus intermedius situated between the vastus medialis and lateralis.

2) the adductor longus has been reflected. This displays the pectineus, adductors brevis and magnus and the long gracilis muscles.

▼

Iliopsoas m.

Anterior superior iliac spine

Sartorius m.

Piri-formis m.

Pecten of pubis

Rectus femoris m.
Iliopsoas m.
Gluteus medius m.

Adductor longus m.

Iliofemoral ligament

Pectineus m.

Iliopectineal bursa

Adductor brevis m.

Iliopsoas m.

Gracilis m.

**Vastus lateralis m.**

Adductor longus m.

**Adductor magnus m.**

**Vastus medialis m.**

Adductor hiatus

Fascia lata

**Vastus intermedius m.**

Tendon of sartorius m.

Medial condyle of femur

Tendon of rectus femoris

Patella

Pes anserinus

Patellar ligament

Obturator nerve

Iliopsoas m.

**Femoral artery**

**Femoral nerve**

Lat. fem. circumfl. art.

Anterior br., Obturator art.

Sartorius m.

Pectineus m.
Obturator nerve
Acetabular br., Obturator art.
Med. fem. circumfl. art.
Trans. br. of med. fem. circumfl. art.

**Deep femoral art.**

Descend. br. of lat. fem. circumfl. a.

**Femoral vein and artery**

Cutaneous br. of obturator n.

Rectus femoris m.

**Saphenous n.**

Muscular branch of femoral nerve

Gracilis m.

**Saphenous n.**

**Adductor canal**

Vastus medialis m.

Sartorius m.

Descend. genicular art. (articular branch)

**Fig. 362: The Femoral Vessels and Nerve**

NOTE that the femoral vessels and the saphenous branch of the femoral nerve descend in the thigh and enter the adductor canal (of Hunter). Whereas the saphenous nerve then penetrates the overlying fascia to reach the superficial leg region, the vessels continue through the adductor magnus to reach the popliteal fossa on the posterior aspect.

Figs. 361, 362

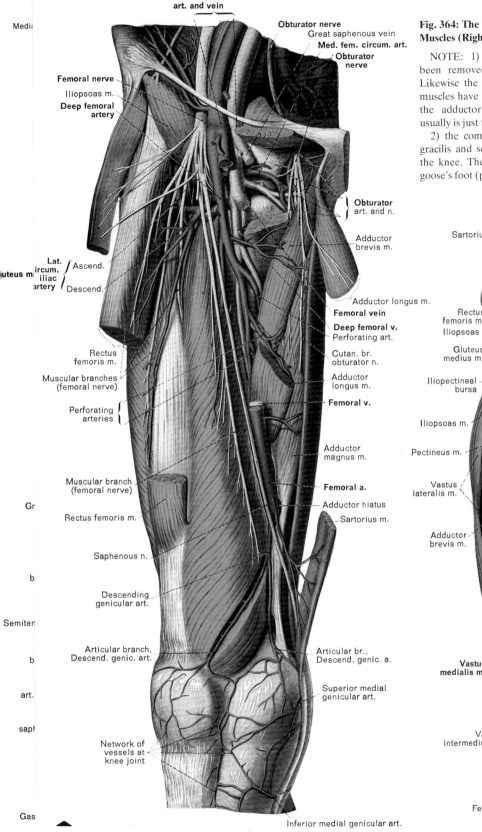

Left figure (Fig. 363) labels:

Medial (partial, left edge)

Femoral art. and vein

Obturator nerve
Great saphenous vein
Med. fem. circum. art.
Obturator nerve

Femoral nerve
Iliopsoas m.
Deep femoral artery

Obturator art. and n.

Adductor brevis m.

Lat. circum. iliac artery { Ascend. / Descend.

Gluteus m. (partial, left edge)

Adductor longus m.
Femoral vein
Deep femoral v.
Perforating art.
Cutan. br. obturator n.
Adductor longus m.
Femoral v.

Rectus femoris m.
Muscular branches (femoral nerve)
Perforating arteries

Gr (partial, left edge)

Muscular branch (femoral nerve)
Rectus femoris m.

Adductor magnus m.

Femoral a.

Adductor hiatus
Sartorius m.

Saphenous n.

Descending genicular art.

Semiten (partial, left edge)

b (partial, left edge)

art. (partial, left edge)

saph (partial, left edge)

Articular branch, Descend. genic. art.

Articular br., Descend. genic. a.

Superior medial genicular art.

Network of vessels at knee joint

Gas (partial, left edge)

Inferior medial genicular art.

**Fig. 363: The Femoral and Obturator Nerves and the Deep Femoral Artery**

NOTE that the obturator nerve supplies the adductor muscles, the gracilis and the obturator externus (not shown), while the femoral nerve innervates all the other anterior thigh muscles. The largest branch of the femoral artery is the deep femoral artery from which generally both the medial and lateral femoral circumflex arteries arise. Observe the femoral vessels disappearing in the femoral canal.

**Fig. 364: The Deep Layer of Anterior and Medial Thigh Muscles (Right)**

NOTE: 1) the rectus femoris and vastus medialis have been removed, thereby revealing the shaft of the femur. Likewise the adductors longus and brevis and the pectineus muscles have been reflected, exposing the obturator externus, the adductor magnus and the adductor minimus (which usually is just the upper portion of the adductor magnus).

2) the common insertion of the tendons of the sartorius, gracilis and semitendinosus muscles on the medial aspect of the knee. The diverging nature of this insertion resembles a goose's foot (pes anserinus). ▼

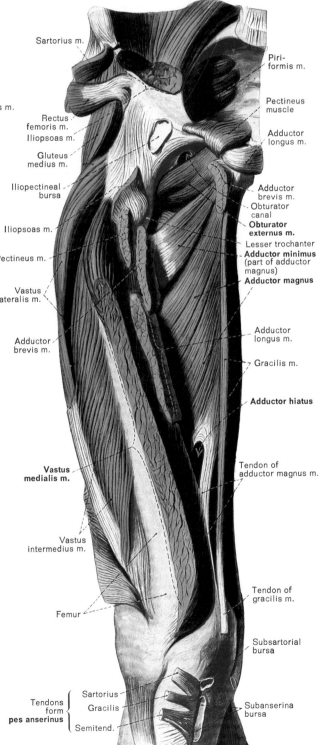

Right figure (Fig. 364) labels:

Sartorius m.
Piriformis m.
Pectineus muscle
Adductor longus m.

Rectus femoris m.
Iliopsoas m.
Gluteus medius m.

Iliopectineal bursa

Iliopsoas m.

Pectineus m.

Vastus lateralis m.

Adductor brevis m.

Adductor brevis m.
Obturator canal
Obturator externus m.
Lesser trochanter
Adductor minimus (part of adductor magnus)
Adductor magnus

Adductor longus m.
Gracilis m.

Adductor hiatus

Tendon of adductor magnus m.

**Vastus medialis m.**

Vastus intermedius m.

Tendon of gracilis m.

Femur

Subsartorial bursa

Tendons form pes anserinus { Sartorius / Gracilis / Semitend.

Subanserina bursa

Figs. 363, 364    V

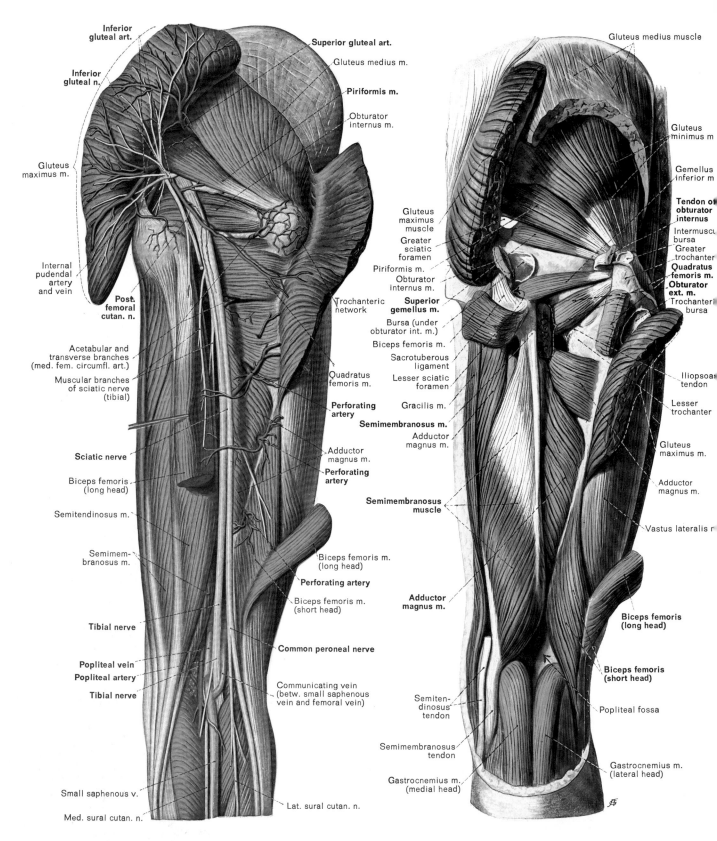

**Fig. 369: Deep Nerves and Vessels of the Gluteal Region and Posterior Thigh**

NOTE: 1) the course of the sciatic nerve as it passes through the greater sciatic foramen in the gluteal region, inferior to the piriformis muscle, lateral to the ischial tuberosity and under cover of the gluteus maximus muscle.

2) the superior and inferior gluteal arteries and the posterior femoral cutaneous nerve. In the thigh, observe the perforating arteries and the fact that the sciatic nerve splits to become the tibial and common peroneal nerves.

**Fig. 370: Deep Muscles of the Gluteal Region and Posterior Thigh**

NOTE: 1) in the gluteal region, the quadratus femoris has been reflected, revealing the obturator externus muscle. Also the tendon of the obturator internus muscle (between the gemelli) has been severed.

2) in the thigh, the common tendon of the long head of the biceps femoris and semitendinosus has been cut, thereby exposing the origin of the semimembranosus, the breadth of the adductor magnus, and the short head of the biceps femoris.

Figs. 369, 370

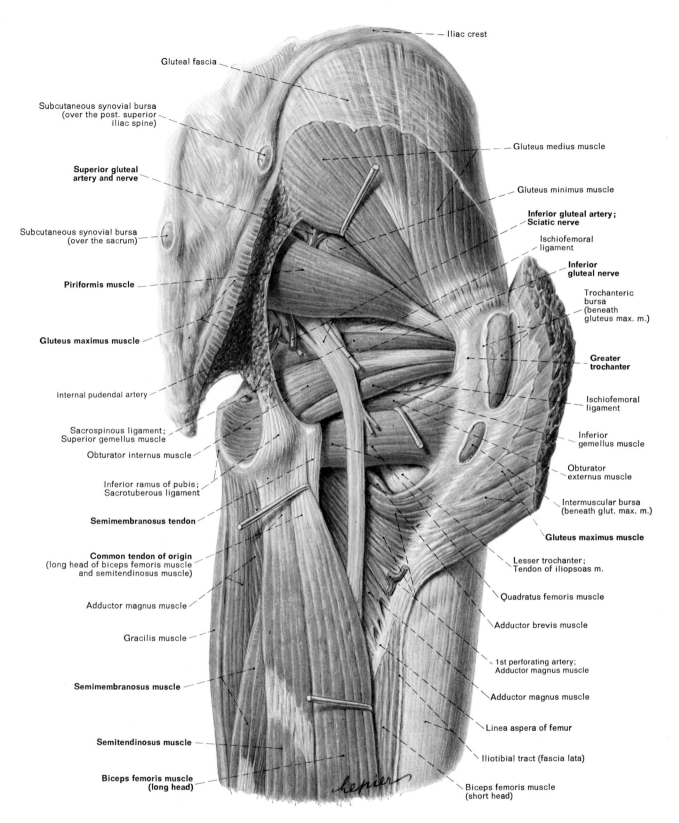

Iliac crest

Gluteal fascia

Subcutaneous synovial bursa
(over the post. superior
iliac spine)

**Superior gluteal
artery and nerve**

Subcutaneous synovial bursa
(over the sacrum)

**Piriformis muscle**

**Gluteus maximus muscle**

Internal pudendal artery

Sacrospinous ligament;
Superior gemellus muscle

Obturator internus muscle

Inferior ramus of pubis;
Sacrotuberous ligament

**Semimembranosus tendon**

**Common tendon of origin**
(long head of biceps femoris muscle
and semitendinosus muscle)

Adductor magnus muscle

Gracilis muscle

**Semimembranosus muscle**

**Semitendinosus muscle**

**Biceps femoris muscle
(long head)**

Gluteus medius muscle

Gluteus minimus muscle

**Inferior gluteal artery;
Sciatic nerve**

Ischiofemoral
ligament

**Inferior
gluteal nerve**

Trochanteric
bursa
(beneath
gluteus max. m.)

**Greater
trochanter**

Ischiofemoral
ligament

Inferior
gemellus muscle

Obturator
externus muscle

Intermuscular bursa
(beneath glut. max. m.)

**Gluteus maximus muscle**

Lesser trochanter;
Tendon of iliopsoas m.

Quadratus femoris muscle

Adductor brevis muscle

1st perforating artery;
Adductor magnus muscle

Adductor magnus muscle

Linea aspera of femur

Iliotibial tract (fascia lata)

Biceps femoris muscle
(short head)

Lepier

**Fig. 371: The Middle and Deep Gluteal Muscles and the Sciatic Nerve**

NOTE: 1) with the gluteal muscles exposed by the reflection of the gluteus maximus muscle, one can appreciate that the centrally located piriformis muscle is the key structure in understanding the anatomy of this region. This muscle, as do most of the other structures which leave the pelvis to enter the gluteal region, passes through the greater sciatic foramen. The nerves and vessels which enter the gluteal region from the pelvis are situated either above the piriformis or below it. The important sciatic nerve enters the gluteal region below the piriformis muscle.

2) through their insertions on or around the greater trochanter, many of the gluteal muscles laterally rotate the femur. The most powerful lateral rotator is the gluteus maximus which is also the most powerful extensor of the thigh at the hip joint.

3) the origin of the hamstring muscles from the ischial tuberosity. The semitendinosus and long head of the biceps femoris have a common tendon of origin deep to which arises the semimembranosus muscle.

Fig. 371    V

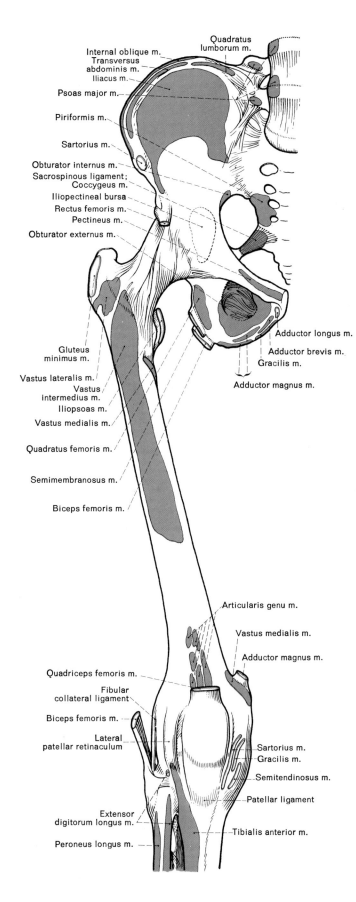

Fig. 372 labels (left figure, from top):
Internal oblique m.
Transversus abdominis m.
Iliacus m.
Quadratus lumborum m.
Psoas major m.
Piriformis m.
Sartorius m.
Obturator internus m.
Sacrospinous ligament; Coccygeus m.
Iliopectineal bursa
Rectus femoris m.
Pectineus m.
Obturator externus m.
Gluteus minimus m.
Vastus lateralis m.
Vastus intermedius m.
Iliopsoas m.
Vastus medialis m.
Quadratus femoris m.
Semimembranosus m.
Biceps femoris m.
Adductor longus m.
Adductor brevis m.
Gracilis m.
Adductor magnus m.
Articularis genu m.
Vastus medialis m.
Adductor magnus m.
Quadriceps femoris m.
Fibular collateral ligament
Biceps femoris m.
Lateral patellar retinaculum
Sartorius m.
Gracilis m.
Semitendinosus m.
Patellar ligament
Extensor digitorum longus m.
Tibialis anterior m.
Peroneus longus m.

**Fig. 372: Anterior View of Right Pelvis and Femur Showing Muscle Attachments**

Figs. 372, 373

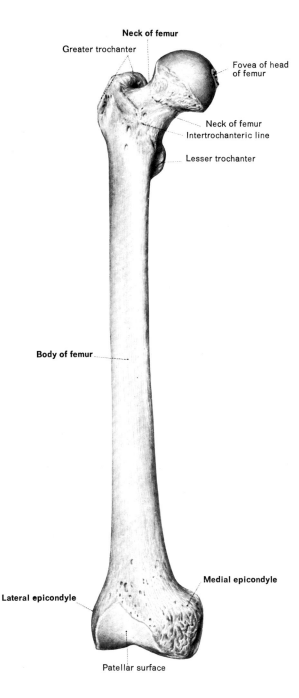

Fig. 373 labels (right figure):
Neck of femur
Greater trochanter
Fovea of head of femur
Neck of femur
Intertrochanteric line
Lesser trochanter
Body of femur
Medial epicondyle
Lateral epicondyle
Patellar surface

**Fig. 373: Right Femur: Anterior View**

NOTE: 1) the femur is the longest and largest bone in the body and serves to transmit to the tibia and feet the weight of the trunk, upper extremity and head. It consists of a proximal extremity or head, the body or shaft and a distal extremity which is enlarged by two condyles.

2) the spherical head of the femur fits into the acetabulum of the pelvis. This articulation is protected by the capsule of the hip joint which is further strengthened by several ligaments. Below the head of the femur is the somewhat narrowed femoral neck. The superior aspect of the shaft is marked by two prominent tubercles, the greater and lesser trochanters.

3) the anterior surface of the body of the femur is smooth and its proximal 2/3rds gives origin to the vastus intermedius muscle.

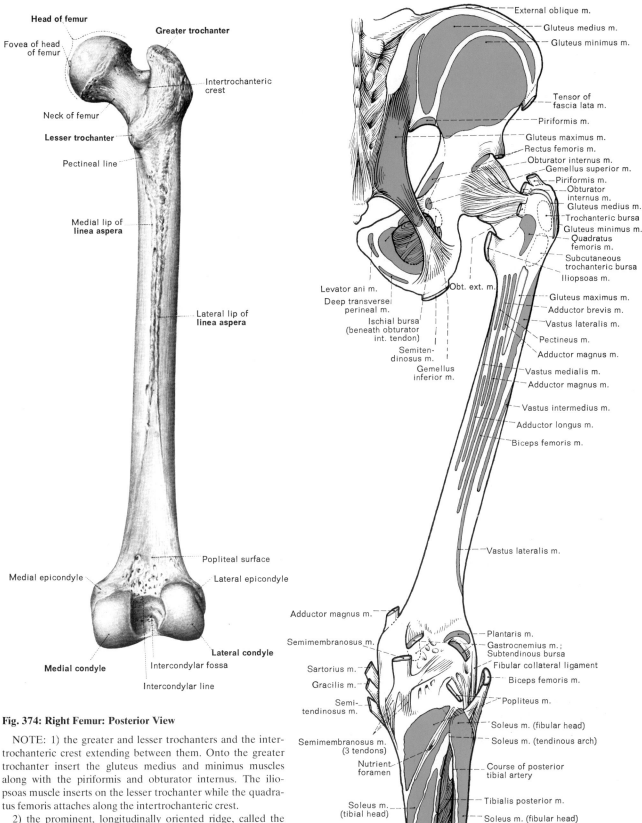

**Fig. 374: Right Femur: Posterior View**

NOTE: 1) the greater and lesser trochanters and the intertrochanteric crest extending between them. Onto the greater trochanter insert the gluteus medius and minimus muscles along with the piriformis and obturator internus. The iliopsoas muscle inserts on the lesser trochanter while the quadratus femoris attaches along the intertrochanteric crest.

2) the prominent, longitudinally oriented ridge, called the linea aspera along the posterior surface of the body of the femur. This likewise serves for muscle attachments.

3) the medial and lateral condyles and epicondyles inferiorly. The condyles articulate with the tibia and the intercondyloid fossa affords attachment to the cruciate ligaments.

**Fig. 375: Posterior View of Right Pelvis and Femur Showing Muscle Attachments**

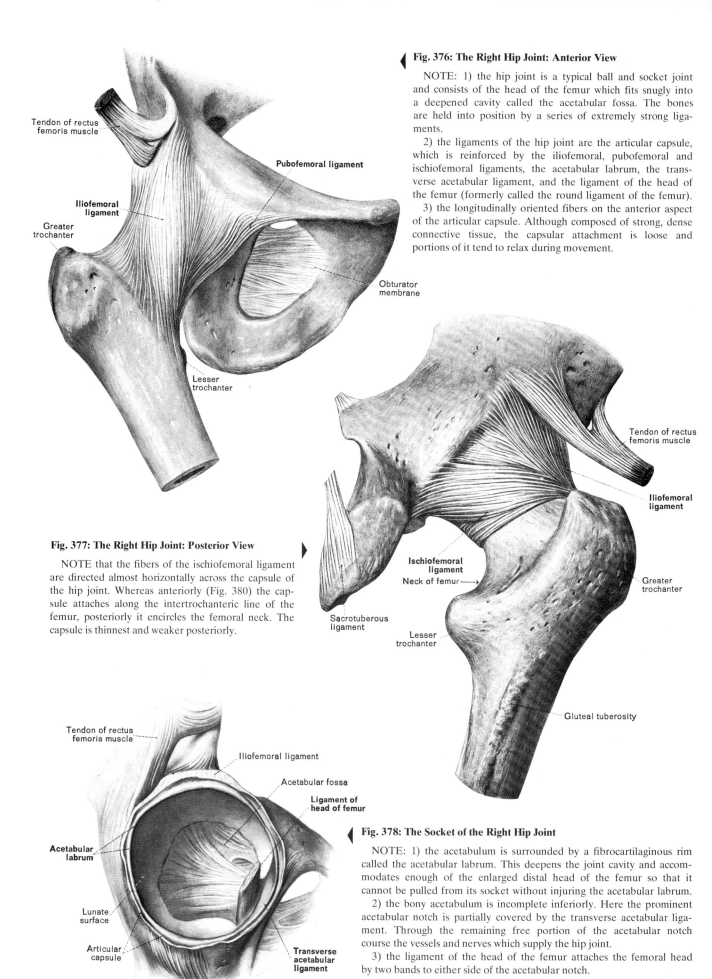

Tendon of rectus
femoris muscle

Pubofemoral ligament

Iliofemoral
ligament

Greater
trochanter

Obturator
membrane

Lesser
trochanter

### Fig. 376: The Right Hip Joint: Anterior View

NOTE: 1) the hip joint is a typical ball and socket joint and consists of the head of the femur which fits snugly into a deepened cavity called the acetabular fossa. The bones are held into position by a series of extremely strong ligaments.

2) the ligaments of the hip joint are the articular capsule, which is reinforced by the iliofemoral, pubofemoral and ischiofemoral ligaments, the acetabular labrum, the transverse acetabular ligament, and the ligament of the head of the femur (formerly called the round ligament of the femur).

3) the longitudinally oriented fibers on the anterior aspect of the articular capsule. Although composed of strong, dense connective tissue, the capsular attachment is loose and portions of it tend to relax during movement.

Tendon of rectus
femoris muscle

Iliofemoral
ligament

Ischiofemoral
ligament

Neck of femur →

Greater
trochanter

Sacrotuberous
ligament

Lesser
trochanter

Gluteal tuberosity

### Fig. 377: The Right Hip Joint: Posterior View

NOTE that the fibers of the ischiofemoral ligament are directed almost horizontally across the capsule of the hip joint. Whereas anteriorly (Fig. 380) the capsule attaches along the intertrochanteric line of the femur, posteriorly it encircles the femoral neck. The capsule is thinnest and weaker posteriorly.

Tendon of rectus
femoris muscle

Iliofemoral ligament

Acetabular fossa

Ligament of
head of femur

Acetabular
labrum

Lunate
surface

Articular
capsule

Transverse
acetabular
ligament

### Fig. 378: The Socket of the Right Hip Joint

NOTE: 1) the acetabulum is surrounded by a fibrocartilaginous rim called the acetabular labrum. This deepens the joint cavity and accommodates enough of the enlarged distal head of the femur so that it cannot be pulled from its socket without injuring the acetabular labrum.

2) the bony acetabulum is incomplete inferiorly. Here the prominent acetabular notch is partially covered by the transverse acetabular ligament. Through the remaining free portion of the acetabular notch course the vessels and nerves which supply the hip joint.

3) the ligament of the head of the femur attaches the femoral head by two bands to either side of the acetabular notch.

Figs. 376, 377, 378

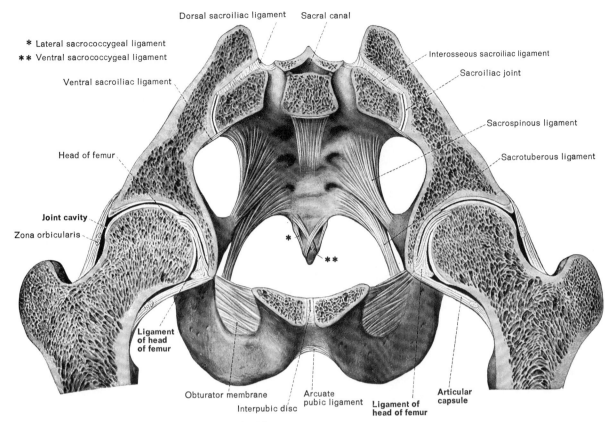

* Lateral sacrococcygeal ligament
** Ventral sacrococcygeal ligament

Dorsal sacroiliac ligament

Sacral canal

Interosseous sacroiliac ligament

Sacroiliac joint

Ventral sacroiliac ligament

Sacrospinous ligament

Sacrotuberous ligament

Head of femur

**Joint cavity**

Zona orbicularis

**Ligament of head of femur**

Obturator membrane

Interpubic disc

Arcuate pubic ligament

**Ligament of head of femur**

**Articular capsule**

**Fig. 379: Frontal Section of the Pelvis Showing Both Hip Joints**

**Fig. 380: Anterior Exposure of the Right Hip Joint**

NOTE that the anterior aspect of the articular capsule of the hip joint has been opened close to the rounded acetabular labrum. This exposes the cartilage covered head of the femur within the joint cavity. Observe the ligament of the femoral head which is attached to the femur at a site where the cartilage is lacking. This depression is called the fovea of the femoral head.

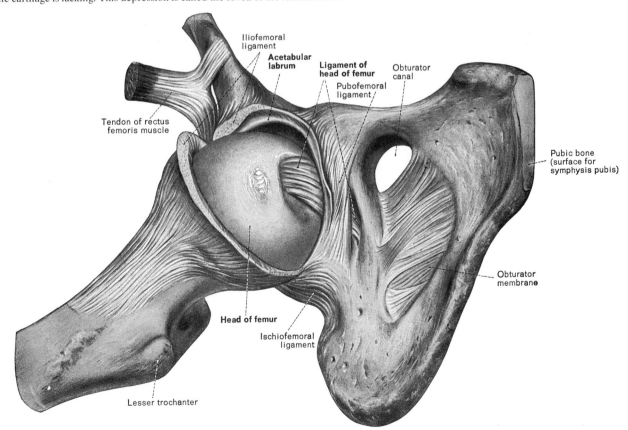

Iliofemoral ligament

**Acetabular labrum**

**Ligament of head of femur**

Obturator canal

Pubofemoral ligament

Tendon of rectus femoris muscle

Pubic bone (surface for symphysis pubis)

Obturator membrane

**Head of femur**

Ischiofemoral ligament

Lesser trochanter

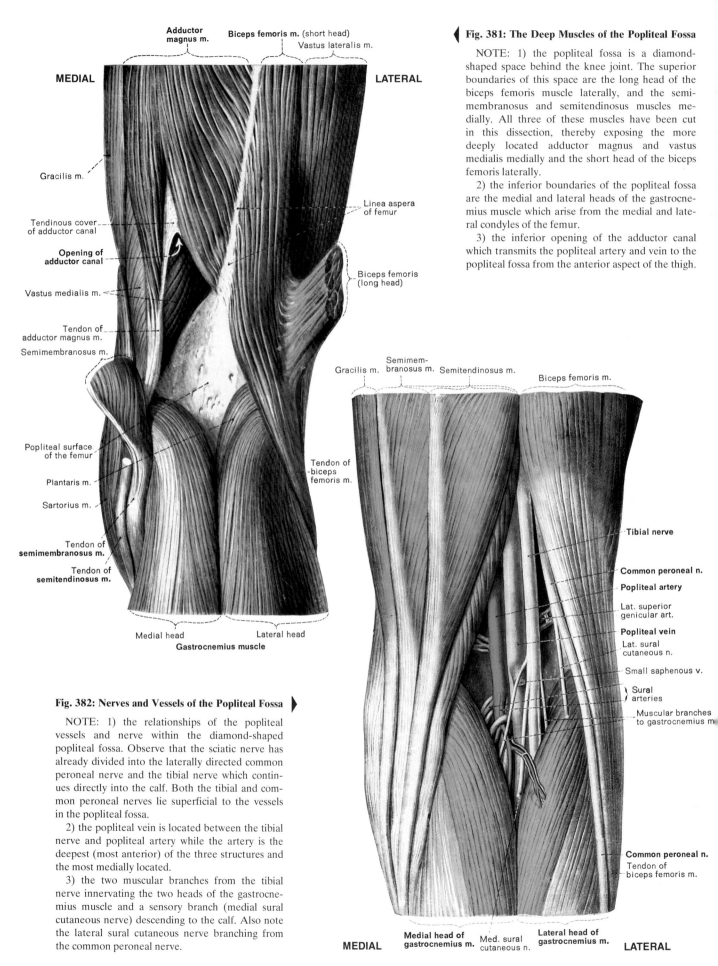

**Adductor magnus m.**

**Biceps femoris m.** (short head)

Vastus lateralis m.

MEDIAL

LATERAL

Gracilis m.

Tendinous cover of adductor canal

Linea aspera of femur

**Opening of adductor canal**

Vastus medialis m.

Biceps femoris (long head)

Tendon of adductor magnus m.

Semimembranosus m.

Popliteal surface of the femur

Plantaris m.

Sartorius m.

Tendon of **semimembranosus m.**

Tendon of **semitendinosus m.**

Medial head

Lateral head

**Gastrocnemius muscle**

Gracilis m.

Semimembranosus m.

Semitendinosus m.

Biceps femoris m.

Tendon of biceps femoris m.

**Tibial nerve**

**Common peroneal n.**

**Popliteal artery**

Lat. superior genicular art.

**Popliteal vein**

Lat. sural cutaneous n.

Small saphenous v.

Sural arteries

Muscular branches to gastrocnemius m.

**Common peroneal n.**

Tendon of biceps femoris m.

Medial head of **gastrocnemius m.**

Med. sural cutaneous n.

Lateral head of **gastrocnemius m.**

MEDIAL

LATERAL

### Fig. 381: The Deep Muscles of the Popliteal Fossa

NOTE: 1) the popliteal fossa is a diamond-shaped space behind the knee joint. The superior boundaries of this space are the long head of the biceps femoris muscle laterally, and the semimembranosus and semitendinosus muscles medially. All three of these muscles have been cut in this dissection, thereby exposing the more deeply located adductor magnus and vastus medialis medially and the short head of the biceps femoris laterally.

2) the inferior boundaries of the popliteal fossa are the medial and lateral heads of the gastrocnemius muscle which arise from the medial and lateral condyles of the femur.

3) the inferior opening of the adductor canal which transmits the popliteal artery and vein to the popliteal fossa from the anterior aspect of the thigh.

### Fig. 382: Nerves and Vessels of the Popliteal Fossa

NOTE: 1) the relationships of the popliteal vessels and nerve within the diamond-shaped popliteal fossa. Observe that the sciatic nerve has already divided into the laterally directed common peroneal nerve and the tibial nerve which continues directly into the calf. Both the tibial and common peroneal nerves lie superficial to the vessels in the popliteal fossa.

2) the popliteal vein is located between the tibial nerve and popliteal artery while the artery is the deepest (most anterior) of the three structures and the most medially located.

3) the two muscular branches from the tibial nerve innervating the two heads of the gastrocnemius muscle and a sensory branch (medial sural cutaneous nerve) descending to the calf. Also note the lateral sural cutaneous nerve branching from the common peroneal nerve.

Figs. 381, 382

## Fig. 383: Arteriogram of Lower Femoral and Popliteal Arteries

NOTE: 1) this arteriogram shows the arterial tree of the lower third of the thigh and the upper third of the calf. Note the course of the femoral artery as it becomes the popliteal artery just above the intercondylar fossa in the popliteal space. The genicular arteries supplying the knee joint, and the sural arteries descending to supply both superficial and muscular tissues in the calf can be seen arising from the popliteal artery.

2) below the popliteal fossa the popliteal artery becomes the posterior tibial artery. Soon, the anterior tibial artery branches from the posterior tibial to course toward the anterior compartment in the leg, while the posterior tibial continues to descend in the posterior compartment. About 3 inches below the knee the peroneal artery arises from the posterior tibial artery and descends in the lateral portion of the deep calf.

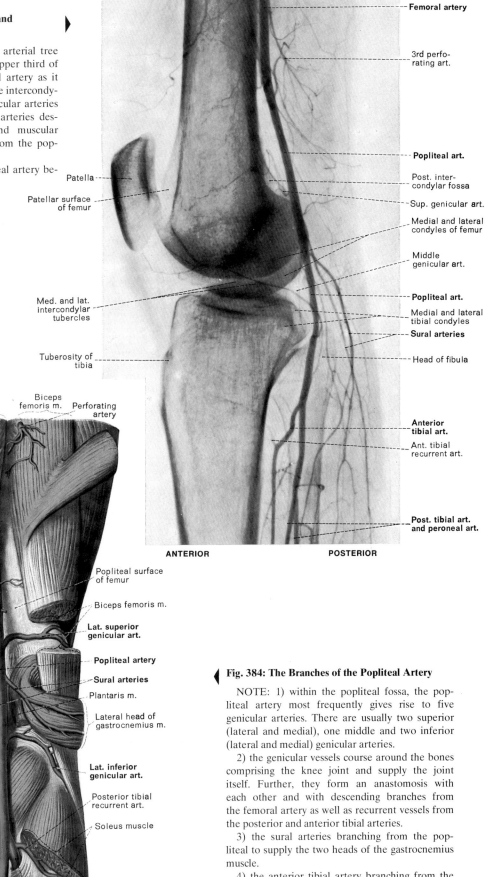

Femoral artery

3rd perforating art.

Patella

Patellar surface of femur

Popliteal art.

Post. intercondylar fossa

Sup. genicular art.

Medial and lateral condyles of femur

Middle genicular art.

Popliteal art.

Medial and lateral tibial condyles

Sural arteries

Head of fibula

Med. and lat. intercondylar tubercles

Tuberosity of tibia

Anterior tibial art.

Ant. tibial recurrent art.

Post. tibial art. and peroneal art.

**ANTERIOR**          **POSTERIOR**

Semimembranosus m.

Semitendinosus m.

Biceps femoris m.

Perforating artery

Popliteal surface of femur

Biceps femoris m.

Lat. superior genicular art.

Popliteal artery

Sural arteries

Plantaris m.

Lateral head of gastrocnemius m.

Descending genicular art.

Semimembranosus m.

Med. superior genicular art.

Middle genicular art.

Lat. inferior genicular art.

Posterior tibial recurrent art.

Soleus muscle

Medial head of gastrocnemius m.

Med. inferior genicular art.

Popliteus muscle

Soleus muscle

Posterior tibial artery

Anterior tibial artery

Peroneal artery

## Fig. 384: The Branches of the Popliteal Artery

NOTE: 1) within the popliteal fossa, the popliteal artery most frequently gives rise to five genicular arteries. There are usually two superior (lateral and medial), one middle and two inferior (lateral and medial) genicular arteries.

2) the genicular vessels course around the bones comprising the knee joint and supply the joint itself. Further, they form an anastomosis with each other and with descending branches from the femoral artery as well as recurrent vessels from the posterior and anterior tibial arteries.

3) the sural arteries branching from the popliteal to supply the two heads of the gastrocnemius muscle.

4) the anterior tibial artery branching from the posterior tibial and, penetrating an aperture above the interosseous membrane, achieves the anterior compartment. Somewhat lower, the peroneal artery also branches from the posterior tibial.

Figs. 383, 384    V

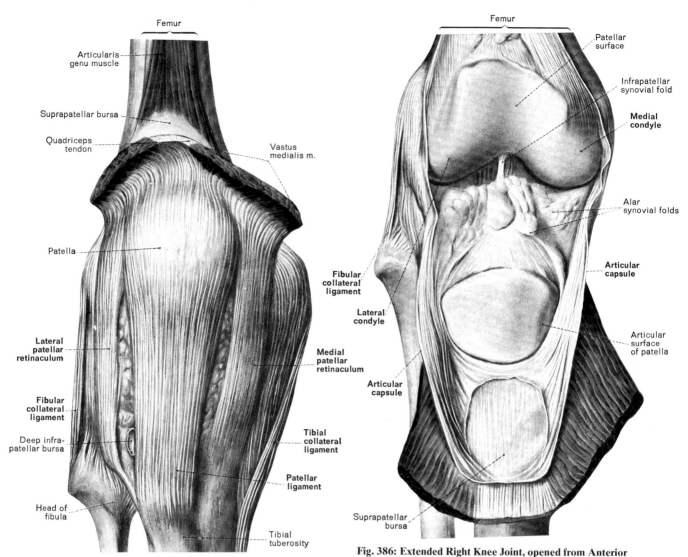

**Fig. 385: Right Knee Joint (Anterior View)**

Femur

Articularis genu muscle

Suprapatellar bursa

Quadriceps tendon

Vastus medialis m.

Patella

Lateral patellar retinaculum

Fibular collateral ligament

Deep infra-patellar bursa

Head of fibula

Tibial tuberosity

Medial patellar retinaculum

Tibial collateral ligament

Patellar ligament

Femur

Patellar surface

Infrapatellar synovial fold

**Medial condyle**

Alar synovial folds

**Articular capsule**

Articular surface of patella

Articular surface of patella

**Fibular collateral ligament**

**Lateral condyle**

**Articular capsule**

Suprapatellar bursa

**Fig. 386: Extended Right Knee Joint, opened from Anterior Side**

▶ **Fig. 387: Flexed Right Knee Joint (Anterior View) Showing Cruciate Ligaments**

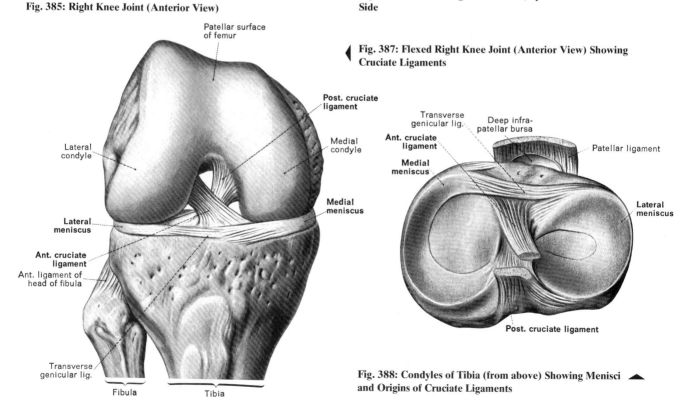

Patellar surface of femur

**Post. cruciate ligament**

Lateral condyle

Medial condyle

**Medial meniscus**

Lateral meniscus

**Ant. cruciate ligament**

Ant. ligament of head of fibula

Transverse genicular lig.

Fibula          Tibia

Transverse genicular lig.

Deep infra-patellar bursa

**Ant. cruciate ligament**

**Medial meniscus**

Patellar ligament

**Lateral meniscus**

**Post. cruciate ligament**

**Fig. 388: Condyles of Tibia (from above) Showing Menisci and Origins of Cruciate Ligaments** ◀

Figs. 385–388

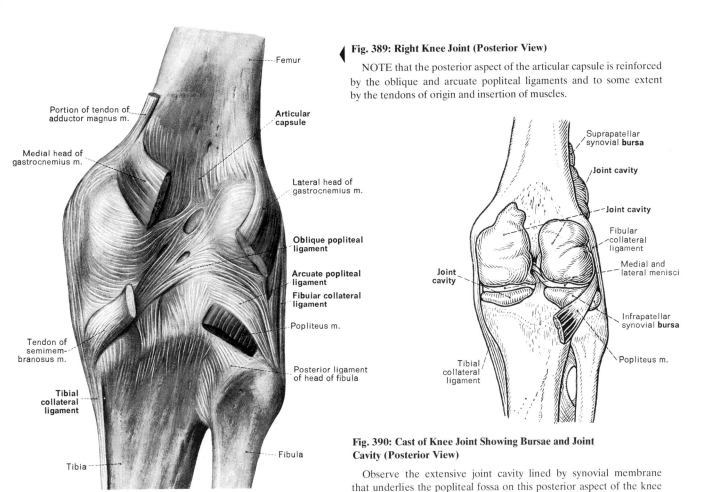

**Fig. 389: Right Knee Joint (Posterior View)**

NOTE that the posterior aspect of the articular capsule is reinforced by the oblique and arcuate popliteal ligaments and to some extent by the tendons of origin and insertion of muscles.

Labels for Fig. 389:
- Femur
- Portion of tendon of adductor magnus m.
- Medial head of gastrocnemius m.
- Articular capsule
- Lateral head of gastrocnemius m.
- Oblique popliteal ligament
- Arcuate popliteal ligament
- Fibular collateral ligament
- Popliteus m.
- Tendon of semimembranosus m.
- Posterior ligament of head of fibula
- Tibial collateral ligament
- Fibula
- Tibia

Labels for Fig. 390:
- Suprapatellar synovial bursa
- Joint cavity
- Joint cavity
- Fibular collateral ligament
- Medial and lateral menisci
- Joint cavity
- Infrapatellar synovial bursa
- Popliteus m.
- Tibial collateral ligament

**Fig. 390: Cast of Knee Joint Showing Bursae and Joint Cavity (Posterior View)**

Observe the extensive joint cavity lined by synovial membrane that underlies the popliteal fossa on this posterior aspect of the knee joint.

**Fig. 391: Sagittal Section of Right Knee Joint**

Labels for Fig. 391:
- Femur
- Quadriceps tendon
- Biceps femoris m.
- Suprapatellar bursa
- Articular surface of patella
- Patella
- Lateral head of gastrocnemius m.
- Lateral condyle of femur
- Prepatellar bursa (subcutan.)
- Infrapatellar fat pad
- Lateral meniscus (cut in 2 places)
- Patellar ligament
- Infrapatellar bursa
- Tibia

Labels for Fig. 392:
- Quadriceps tendon
- Suprapatellar bursa
- Prepatellar bursa
- Joint cavity
- Fibular collateral ligament
- Popliteus m.
- Joint cavity
- Lateral meniscus
- Patellar ligament
- Infrapatellar bursa

**Fig. 392: Cast of Knee Joint (Distended) Showing Bursae and Joint Cavity**

This lateral view of the distended synovial cavity of the knee joint demonstrates well that the synovial membrane of the knee joint is the most extensive of any joint in the body.

Figs. 389–392    V

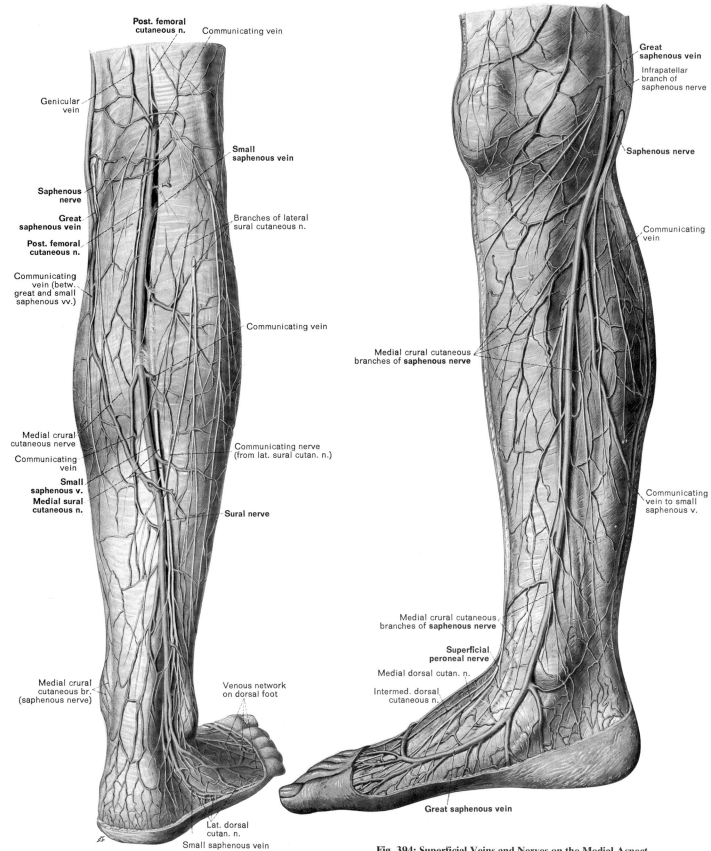

**Post. femoral cutaneous n.**

Communicating vein

Genicular vein

**Saphenous nerve**

**Great saphenous vein**

**Post. femoral cutaneous n.**

Communicating vein (betw. great and small saphenous vv.)

Medial crural cutaneous nerve

Communicating vein

**Small saphenous v.**

**Medial sural cutaneous n.**

Medial crural cutaneous br. (saphenous nerve)

**Small saphenous vein**

Lat. dorsal cutan. n.

Venous network on dorsal foot

**Small saphenous vein**

Branches of lateral sural cutaneous n.

Communicating vein

Communicating nerve (from lat. sural cutan. n.)

**Sural nerve**

**Great saphenous vein**

Infrapatellar branch of saphenous nerve

Saphenous nerve

Communicating vein

Medial crural cutaneous branches of **saphenous nerve**

Communicating vein to small saphenous v.

Medial crural cutaneous branches of **saphenous nerve**

**Superficial peroneal nerve**

Medial dorsal cutan. n.

Intermed. dorsal cutaneous n.

**Great saphenous vein**

**Fig. 393: Superficial Veins and Nerves of the Posterior Leg and Foot**

NOTE the small saphenous vein which forms on the dorsolateral aspect of the foot and ascends to the popliteal fossa, and the sural nerve which is formed by the junction of the medial sural cutaneous nerve and a communicating branch from the lateral sural cutaneous nerve.

**Fig. 394: Superficial Veins and Nerves on the Medial Aspect of the Leg and Foot**

NOTE the formation of the great saphenous vein on the medial aspect of the foot and its course anterior to the medial malleolus and up the medial aspect of the leg. Branches of the saphenous nerve accompany the great saphenous vein below the knee. The saphenous nerve is the largest branch of the femoral nerve.

Figs. 393, 394

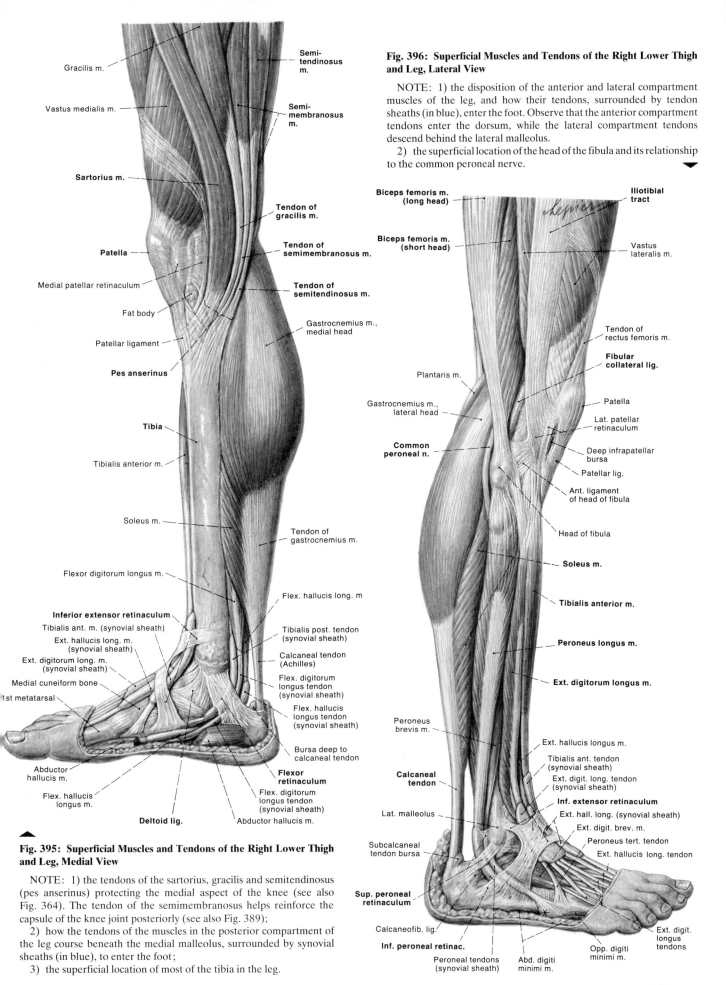

Gracilis m.

Vastus medialis m.

Sartorius m.

Patella

Medial patellar retinaculum

Fat body

Patellar ligament

Pes anserinus

Tibia

Tibialis anterior m.

Soleus m.

Flexor digitorum longus m.

Inferior extensor retinaculum
Tibialis ant. m. (synovial sheath)
Ext. hallucis long. m. (synovial sheath)
Ext. digitorum long. m. (synovial sheath)
Medial cuneiform bone
1st metatarsal

Abductor hallucis m.

Flex. hallucis longus m.

Deltoid lig.

Semi-tendinosus m.

Semi-membranosus m.

Tendon of gracilis m.

Tendon of semimembranosus m.

Tendon of semitendinosus m.

Gastrocnemius m., medial head

Flex. hallucis long. m

Tibialis post. tendon (synovial sheath)

Calcaneal tendon (Achilles)

Flex. digitorum longus tendon (synovial sheath)

Flex. hallucis longus tendon (synovial sheath)

Bursa deep to calcaneal tendon

Flexor retinaculum

Flex. digitorum longus tendon (synovial sheath)

Abductor hallucis m.

Tendon of gastrocnemius m.

**Fig. 395: Superficial Muscles and Tendons of the Right Lower Thigh and Leg, Medial View**

NOTE: 1) the tendons of the sartorius, gracilis and semitendinosus (pes anserinus) protecting the medial aspect of the knee (see also Fig. 364). The tendon of the semimembranosus helps reinforce the capsule of the knee joint posteriorly (see also Fig. 389);

2) how the tendons of the muscles in the posterior compartment of the leg course beneath the medial malleolus, surrounded by synovial sheaths (in blue), to enter the foot;

3) the superficial location of most of the tibia in the leg.

**Fig. 396: Superficial Muscles and Tendons of the Right Lower Thigh and Leg, Lateral View**

NOTE: 1) the disposition of the anterior and lateral compartment muscles of the leg, and how their tendons, surrounded by tendon sheaths (in blue), enter the foot. Observe that the anterior compartment tendons enter the dorsum, while the lateral compartment tendons descend behind the lateral malleolus.

2) the superficial location of the head of the fibula and its relationship to the common peroneal nerve.

Biceps femoris m. (long head)

Biceps femoris m. (short head)

Plantaris m.

Gastrocnemius m., lateral head

Common peroneal n.

Peroneus brevis m.

Calcaneal tendon

Lat. malleolus

Subcalcaneal tendon bursa

Sup. peroneal retinaculum

Calcaneofib. lig.

Inf. peroneal retinac.

Peroneal tendons (synovial sheath)

Abd. digiti minimi m.

Opp. digiti minimi m.

Ext. digit. longus tendons

Iliotibial tract

Vastus lateralis m.

Tendon of rectus femoris m.

Fibular collateral lig.

Patella

Lat. patellar retinaculum

Deep infrapatellar bursa

Patellar lig.

Ant. ligament of head of fibula

Head of fibula

Soleus m.

Tibialis anterior m.

Peroneus longus m.

Ext. digitorum longus m.

Ext. hallucis longus m.

Tibialis ant. tendon (synovial sheath)

Ext. digit. long. tendon (synovial sheath)

Inf. extensor retinaculum

Ext. hall. long. (synovial sheath)

Ext. digit. brev. m.

Peroneus tert. tendon

Ext. hallucis long. tendon

Figs. 395, 396  V

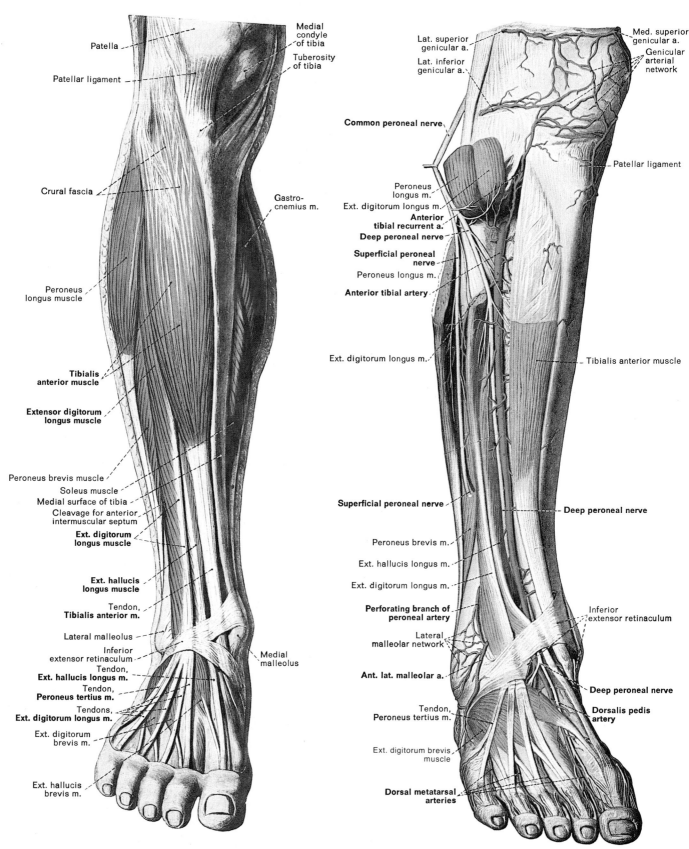

**Fig. 397: Muscles of the Anterior Compartment of the Leg**

NOTE: 1) the four anterior compartment muscles are the tibialis anterior, extensor hallucis longus, extensor digitorum longus and peroneus tertius.

2) the tibialis anterior dorsally flexes and supinates the foot. The other muscles extend the toes as well as dorsiflex the foot. Additionally, the extensor hallucis longus assists in supination, while the extensor digitorum longus and peroneus tertius are pronators.

**Fig. 398: Nerves and Arteries of the Anterior and Lateral Compartments of the Leg**

NOTE: 1) as the common peroneal nerve courses laterally around the head of the fibula, it divides into the superficial and deep peroneal nerves which innervate the muscles of the lateral and anterior compartments.

2) the deep peroneal nerve is joined by the anterior tibial artery which descends toward the foot.

Figs. 397, 398

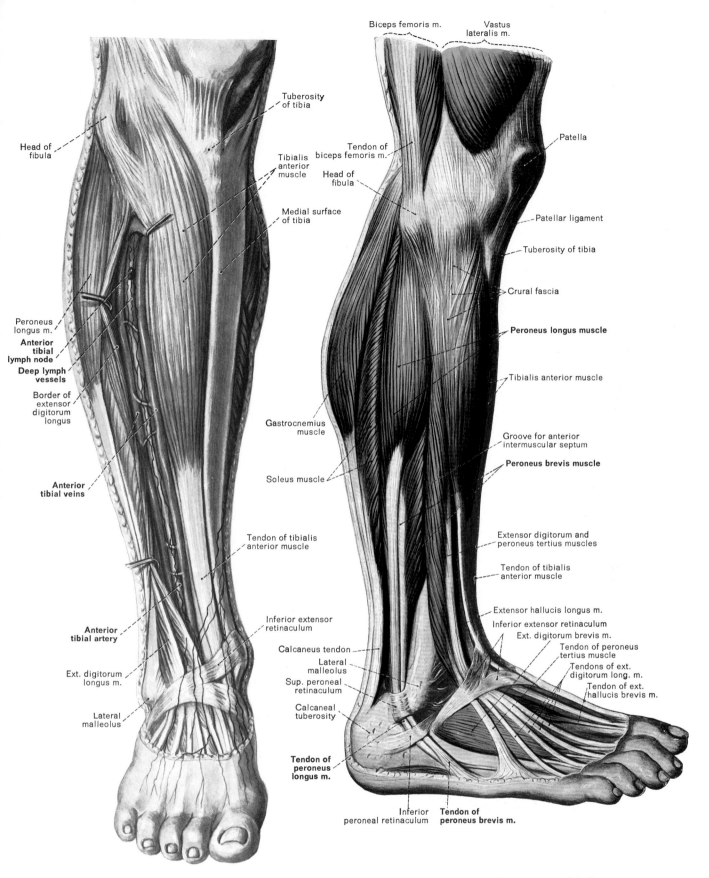

Biceps femoris m.
Vastus lateralis m.
Head of fibula
Tuberosity of tibia
Tibialis anterior muscle
Tendon of biceps femoris m.
Head of fibula
Medial surface of tibia
Patella
Patellar ligament
Tuberosity of tibia
Crural fascia
Peroneus longus m.
**Anterior tibial lymph node**
**Deep lymph vessels**
Border of extensor digitorum longus
**Peroneus longus muscle**
Tibialis anterior muscle
Gastrocnemius muscle
Groove for anterior intermuscular septum
**Peroneus brevis muscle**
**Anterior tibial veins**
Soleus muscle
**Anterior tibial artery**
Extensor digitorum and peroneus tertius muscles
Tendon of tibialis anterior muscle
Tendon of tibialis anterior muscle
Ext. digitorum longus m.
Extensor hallucis longus m.
Inferior extensor retinaculum
Ext. digitorum brevis m.
Inferior extensor retinaculum
Tendon of peroneus tertius muscle
Tendons of ext. digitorum long. m.
Tendon of ext. hallucis brevis m.
Lateral malleolus
Calcaneus tendon
Lateral malleolus
Sup. peroneal retinaculum
Calcaneal tuberosity
**Tendon of peroneus longus m.**
Inferior peroneal retinaculum
**Tendon of peroneus brevis m.**

**Fig. 399: Deep Lymphatic Channels and Nodes of the Anterior Leg**

NOTE that lymphatic channels from the dorsum of the foot course superiorly and collect along the path of the more deeply situated anterior tibial vessels and nerve. At times a lymph node can be found just ventral to the anterior tibial artery below the knee.

**Fig. 400: Muscles of the Lateral Compartment of the Leg**

NOTE that the peroneus longus and brevis occupy the lateral compartment of the leg. Their tendons descend into the foot behind the lateral malleolus. The peroneus longus tendon crosses the sole of the foot to insert on the base of the 1st metatarsal bone, while the peroneus brevis inserts directly onto the 5th metatarsal bone.

Figs. 399, 400     V

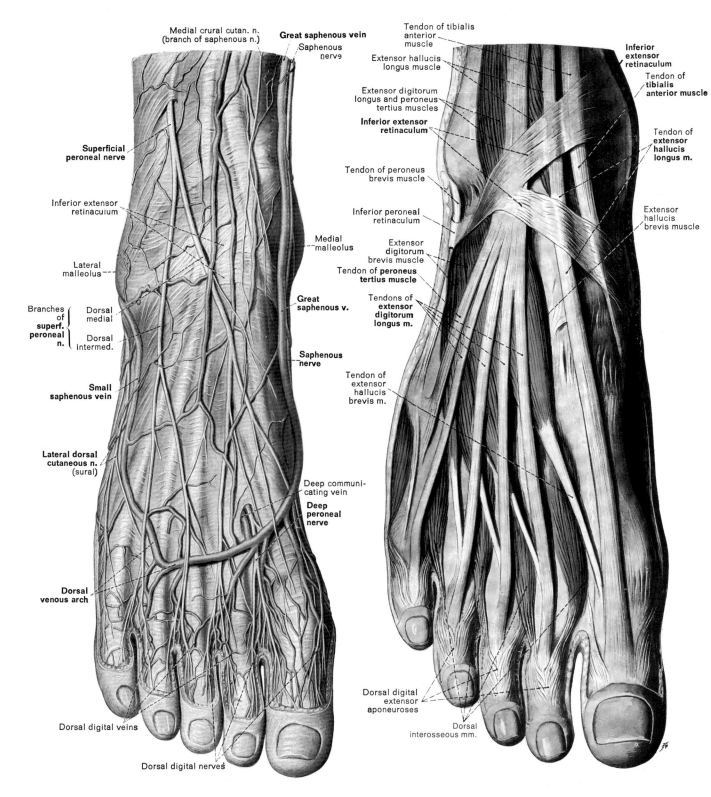

**Fig. 401: Superficial Nerves and Veins of the Dorsal Right Foot**

NOTE: 1) cutaneous innervation of the dorsal foot is supplied principally by the superficial peroneal nerve (L 4, L 5, S 1). Additionally, the deep peroneal nerve (L 4, L 5) supplies the adjacent sides of the 1st and 2nd toes, while the lateral dorsal cutaneous nerve (S 1, S 2; terminal branch of the sural nerve in the foot) supplies the lateral and dorsal aspect of the 5th digit.

2) the digital and metatarsal veins drain back from the toes to form the dorsal venous arch of the foot. From this arch, the great saphenous vein ascends medially and the small saphenous vein laterally on the foot dorsum.

**Fig. 402: Muscles and Tendons of the Dorsal Right Foot (Superficial View)**

NOTE: 1) the tendons of the tibialis anterior, extensor hallucis longus and extensor digitorum longus are bound by the Y-shaped inferior extensor retinaculum as they enter the dorsum of the foot at the level of the ankle joint.

2) the long extensor tendons insert onto the dorsal aspect of the distal phalanx of each toe. In addition, the tendons of the extensor digitorum longus also insert onto the dorsum of the middle phalanx of the lateral four toes.

3) the tendon of the peroneus tertius insert on the base of the 5th metatarsal bone (and at times the 4th also).

Figs. 401, 402

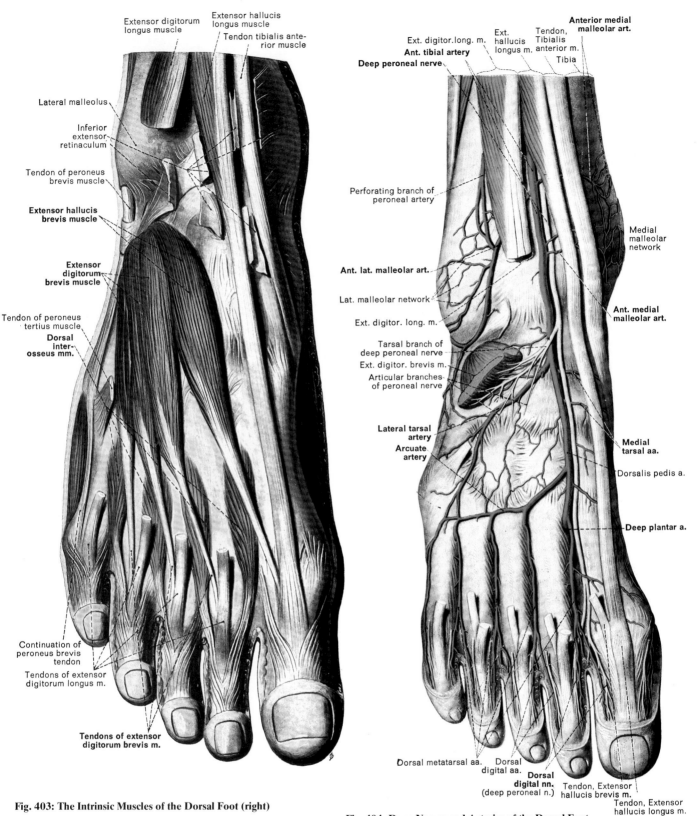

**Fig. 403** (labels):
Extensor digitorum longus muscle
Extensor hallucis longus muscle
Tendon tibialis anterior muscle
Lateral malleolus
Inferior extensor retinaculum
Tendon of peroneus brevis muscle
**Extensor hallucis brevis muscle**
**Extensor digitorum brevis muscle**
Tendon of peroneus tertius muscle
**Dorsal interosseus mm.**
Continuation of peroneus brevis tendon
Tendons of extensor digitorum longus m.
**Tendons of extensor digitorum brevis m.**

**Fig. 404** (labels):
Ext. digitor.long. m.
Ext. hallucis longus m.
Tendon, Tibialis anterior m.
**Anterior medial malleolar art.**
**Ant. tibial artery**
**Deep peroneal nerve**
Tibia
Perforating branch of peroneal artery
Medial malleolar network
**Ant. lat. malleolar art.**
Lat. malleolar network
Ext. digitor. long. m.
**Ant. medial malleolar art.**
Tarsal branch of deep peroneal nerve
Ext. digitor. brevis m.
Articular branches of peroneal nerve
**Lateral tarsal artery**
**Arcuate artery**
**Medial tarsal aa.**
Dorsalis pedis a.
**Deep plantar a.**
Dorsal metatarsal aa.
Dorsal digital aa.
**Dorsal digital nn.** (deep peroneal n.)
Tendon, Extensor hallucis brevis m.
Tendon, Extensor hallucis longus m.

**Fig. 403: The Intrinsic Muscles of the Dorsal Foot (right)**

NOTE: 1) the inferior extensor retinaculum has been opened and the tendons of the extensor digitorum longus and peroneus tertius have been severed.

2) the extensor hallucis brevis and the three small bellies of the extensor digitorum brevis. The delicate tendons of these muscles insert on the proximal phalanx of the medial four toes.

3) the four dorsal interosseous muscles. These muscles abduct the toes from the longitudinal axis of the foot (down the middle of the 2nd toe). The first dorsal interosseous muscle inserts on the medial side of the 2nd toe, while the remaining three insert on the lateral side of the 2nd, 3rd, and 4th toes.

**Fig. 404: Deep Nerves and Arteries of the Dorsal Foot**

NOTE: 1) the deep coursing anterior tibial artery and deep peroneal nerve and their branches have been exposed. They enter the foot between the tendons of the extensor hallucis longus and extensor digitorum.

2) the anterior tibial artery becomes the dorsalis pedis artery below the ankle joint. Observe the malleolar, tarsal, arcuate, dorsal metatarsal and digital arteries.

3) the deep peroneal nerve supplies the extensor brevis muscle in the foot and continues distally to terminate as two dorsal digital nerves supplying the adjacent sides of the 1st and 2nd toes.

Figs. 403, 404    **V**

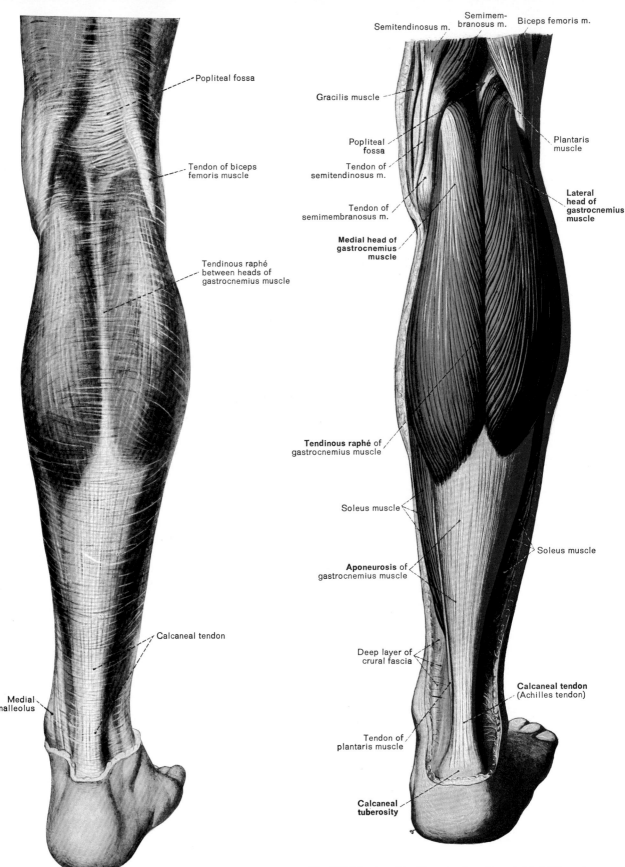

Fig. 405 labels: Popliteal fossa; Tendon of biceps femoris muscle; Tendinous raphé between heads of gastrocnemius muscle; Calcaneal tendon; Medial malleolus

Fig. 406 labels: Semitendinosus m.; Semimembranosus m.; Biceps femoris m.; Gracilis muscle; Popliteal fossa; Tendon of semitendinosus m.; Tendon of semimembranosus m.; **Medial head of gastrocnemius muscle**; Plantaris muscle; **Lateral head of gastrocnemius muscle**; **Tendinous raphé of** gastrocnemius muscle; Soleus muscle; Soleus muscle; **Aponeurosis of** gastrocnemius muscle; Deep layer of crural fascia; **Calcaneal tendon** (Achilles tendon); Tendon of plantaris muscle; **Calcaneal tuberosity**

**Fig. 405: The Deep Fascia of the Leg (the Crural Fascia), Posterior View**

NOTE that the deep fascia of the leg closely invests all of the muscles between the knee and ankle and forms the fascial covering over the popliteal fossa. It is continuous above with the fascia lata of the thigh and inferiorly with the retinacula which bind the tendons close to the bones.

Figs. 405, 406

**Fig. 406: Muscles of the Posterior Leg: Superficial Calf Muscles**

NOTE: 1) the gastrocnemius muscle arises by two heads from the condyles and posterior popliteal surface of the femur and its fibers are oriented inferomedially toward a central tendinous raphe. It inserts by means of the strong calcaneal tendon onto the calcaneal tuberosity.

2) the gastrocnemius is a powerful plantar flexor of the foot and its continued action also tends to flex the leg at the knee joint.

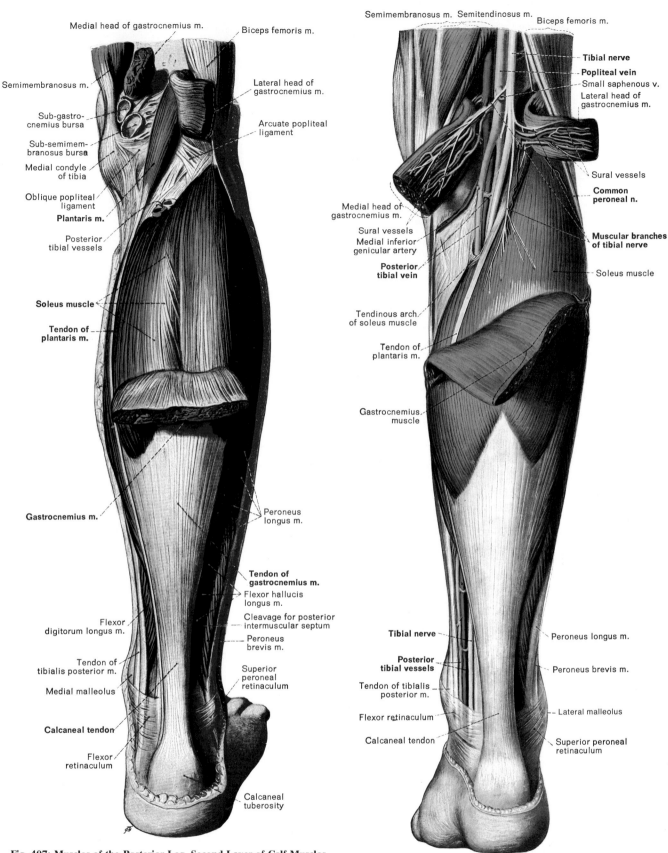

Medial head of gastrocnemius m.

Biceps femoris m.

Semimembranosus m.

Sub-gastro-cnemius bursa

Sub-semimem-branosus bursa

Medial condyle of tibia

Oblique popliteal ligament

**Plantaris m.**

Posterior tibial vessels

**Soleus muscle**

**Tendon of plantaris m.**

Lateral head of gastrocnemius m.

Arcuate popliteal ligament

**Gastrocnemius m.**

Peroneus longus m.

**Tendon of gastrocnemius m.**

Flexor hallucis longus m.

Cleavage for posterior intermuscular septum

Peroneus brevis m.

Superior peroneal retinaculum

Flexor digitorum longus m.

Tendon of tibialis posterior m.

Medial malleolus

**Calcaneal tendon**

Flexor retinaculum

Calcaneal tuberosity

Semimembranosus m. Semitendinosus m.

Biceps femoris m.

**Tibial nerve**

**Popliteal vein**

Small saphenous v.

Lateral head of gastrocnemius m.

Sural vessels

**Common peroneal n.**

**Muscular branches of tibial nerve**

Soleus muscle

Medial head of gastrocnemius m.

Sural vessels

Medial inferior genicular artery

**Posterior tibial vein**

Tendinous arch of soleus muscle

Tendon of plantaris m.

Gastrocnemius muscle

**Tibial nerve**

**Posterior tibial vessels**

Tendon of tibialis posterior m.

Flexor retinaculum

Calcaneal tendon

Peroneus longus m.

Peroneus brevis m.

Lateral malleolus

Superior peroneal retinaculum

**Fig. 407: Muscles of the Posterior Leg, Second Layer of Calf Muscles**

NOTE: 1) both heads of the gastrocnemius have been severed to uncover the underlying soleus and plantaris muscles. The soleus is broad and thick, arising from the posterior surface of the fibula, the intermuscular septum and the dorsal aspect of the tibia. Its fibers join the calcaneal tendon.

2) the plantaris courses between the gastrocnemius and soleus. Both muscles are plantar flexors of the foot.

**Fig. 408: Nerves and Vessels of the Posterior Leg: Superficial Layer**

NOTE that the popliteal vessels and tibial nerve, descending from the popliteal fossa into the posterior compartment of the leg, commence in the middle of the leg and course medially in a gradual fashion so that at the ankle they lie behind the medial malleolus.

Figs. 407, 408    V

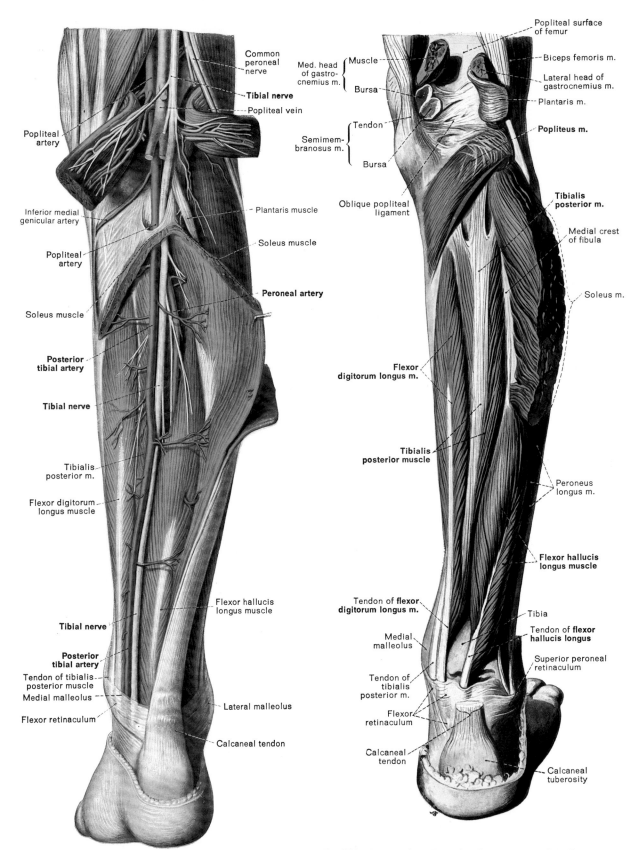

**Fig. 409: Nerves and Vessels of the Right Posterior Leg, Intermediate Layer**

NOTE: 1) the soleus muscle has been severed and reflected laterally, exposing the course of the tibial artery and posterior tibial nerve as far as the medial malleolus.

2) that this vessel and nerve descend in the leg between the flexor hallucis longus and the flexor digitorum longus and dorsal to the tibialis posterior muscle.

**Fig. 410: Muscles of the Posterior Compartment of the Leg: Deep Group: Four Muscles**

NOTE: 1) the four deep posterior compartment muscles are: a) the popliteus, b) the flexor digitorum longus, c) the tibialis posterior and d) the flexor hallucis longus.

2) the popliteus is a femorotibial muscle and tends to rotate the leg medially and flex the leg at the knee joint. The other three muscles are cruropedal muscles and, as a group, they invert the foot, flex the toes and assist in plantarflexion at the ankle joint.

Figs. 409, 410

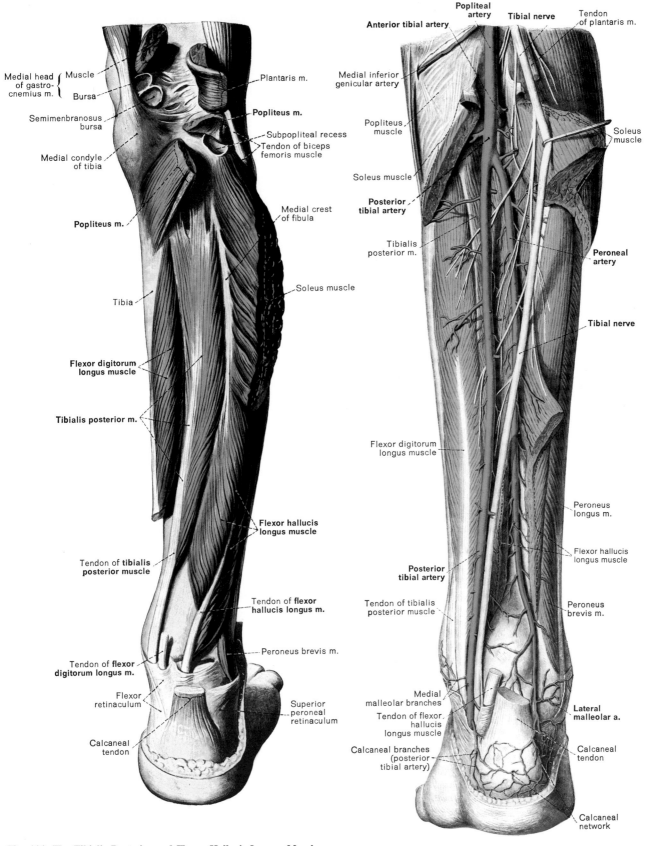

**Medial head of gastro-cnemius m.** { Muscle / Bursa

Semimembranosus bursa

Medial condyle of tibia

**Popliteus m.**

Tibia

**Flexor digitorum longus muscle**

**Tibialis posterior m.**

Tendon of **tibialis posterior muscle**

Tendon of **flexor digitorum longus m.**

Flexor retinaculum

Calcaneal tendon

Plantaris m.

**Popliteus m.**

Subpopliteal recess
Tendon of biceps femoris muscle

Medial crest of fibula

Soleus muscle

**Flexor hallucis longus muscle**

Tendon of **flexor hallucis longus m.**

Peroneus brevis m.

Superior peroneal retinaculum

Popliteal artery

**Anterior tibial artery**

Tibial nerve

Tendon of plantaris m.

Medial inferior genicular artery

Popliteus muscle

Soleus muscle

Soleus muscle

**Posterior tibial artery**

Tibialis posterior m.

**Peroneal artery**

**Tibial nerve**

Flexor digitorum longus muscle

Peroneus longus m.

Flexor hallucis longus muscle

**Posterior tibial artery**

Tendon of tibialis posterior muscle

Peroneus brevis m.

Medial malleolar branches

**Lateral malleolar a.**

Tendon of flexor hallucis longus muscle

Calcaneal branches (posterior tibial artery)

Calcaneal tendon

Calcaneal network

**Fig. 411: The Tibialis Posterior and Flexor Hallucis Longus Muscles**

NOTE: 1) the tendon of the flexor digitorum longus and the popliteus muscle have been severed. The tendon of the tibialis posterior crosses beneath that of the flexor digitorum longus just before entering the foot.

2) the flexor hallucis longus muscle arises from the distal 2/3rds of the fibula and the intermuscular septa. Its tendon lies in a groove on the posterior surface of the talus.

**Fig. 412: Nerves and Muscles of the Deep Posterior Leg**

NOTE: 1) the soleus muscle was resected and the tibial nerve pulled aside. Observe the branching of the peroneal artery from the posterior tibial, and its descending course toward the lateral malleolus.

2) in the popliteal fossa, the tibial nerve courses superficial to the popliteal artery, whereas at the ankle, the posterior tibial artery is superficial to the tibial nerve.

Figs. 411, 412   V

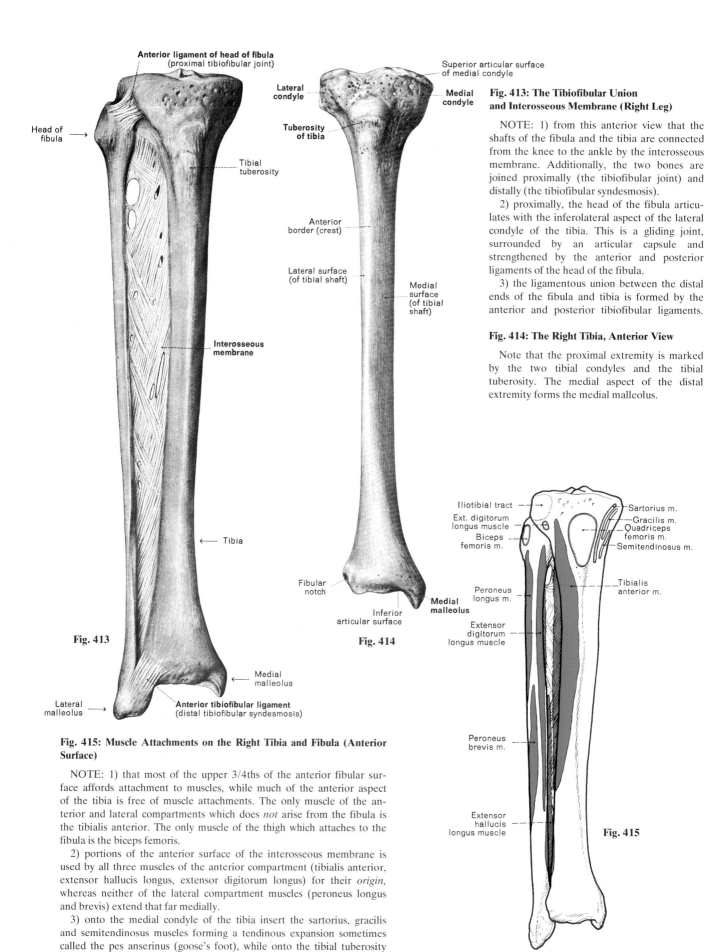

**Anterior ligament of head of fibula**
(proximal tibiofibular joint)

Head of fibula →

Tibial tuberosity

Interosseous membrane

← Tibia

Medial malleolus

Lateral malleolus →

**Anterior tibiofibular ligament**
(distal tibiofibular syndesmosis)

**Fig. 413**

Superior articular surface of medial condyle

Lateral condyle

**Medial condyle**

**Tuberosity of tibia**

Anterior border (crest)

Lateral surface (of tibial shaft)

Medial surface (of tibial shaft)

Fibular notch

**Medial malleolus**

Inferior articular surface

**Fig. 414**

Iliotibial tract

Ext. digitorum longus muscle

Biceps femoris m.

Sartorius m.

Gracilis m.

Quadriceps femoris m.

Semitendinosus m.

Tibialis anterior m.

Peroneus longus m.

Extensor digitorum longus muscle

Peroneus brevis m.

Extensor hallucis longus muscle

**Fig. 415**

## Fig. 413: The Tibiofibular Union and Interosseous Membrane (Right Leg)

NOTE: 1) from this anterior view that the shafts of the fibula and the tibia are connected from the knee to the ankle by the interosseous membrane. Additionally, the two bones are joined proximally (the tibiofibular joint) and distally (the tibiofibular syndesmosis).

2) proximally, the head of the fibula articulates with the inferolateral aspect of the lateral condyle of the tibia. This is a gliding joint, surrounded by an articular capsule and strengthened by the anterior and posterior ligaments of the head of the fibula.

3) the ligamentous union between the distal ends of the fibula and tibia is formed by the anterior and posterior tibiofibular ligaments.

## Fig. 414: The Right Tibia, Anterior View

Note that the proximal extremity is marked by the two tibial condyles and the tibial tuberosity. The medial aspect of the distal extremity forms the medial malleolus.

## Fig. 415: Muscle Attachments on the Right Tibia and Fibula (Anterior Surface)

NOTE: 1) that most of the upper 3/4ths of the anterior fibular surface affords attachment to muscles, while much of the anterior aspect of the tibia is free of muscle attachments. The only muscle of the anterior and lateral compartments which does *not* arise from the fibula is the tibialis anterior. The only muscle of the thigh which attaches to the fibula is the biceps femoris.

2) portions of the anterior surface of the interosseous membrane is used by all three muscles of the anterior compartment (tibialis anterior, extensor hallucis longus, extensor digitorum longus) for their *origin*, whereas neither of the lateral compartment muscles (peroneus longus and brevis) extend that far medially.

3) onto the medial condyle of the tibia insert the sartorius, gracilis and semitendinosus muscles forming a tendinous expansion sometimes called the pes anserinus (goose's foot), while onto the tibial tuberosity inserts the massive quadriceps femoris muscle.

Figs. 413, 414, 415

## Fig. 416: Muscle Attachments on the Right Tibia and Fibula (Posterior Surface)

NOTE: 1) that of the posterior compartment muscles, only the gastrocnemius and plantaris muscles do not attach to the posterior surface of the tibia, fibula or interosseous membrane.

2) that virtually the entire posterior surface of the fibula serves for the origin of muscles. The soleus arises from the upper one-third of the posterior fibular surface and along the soleal line of the tibia. Inferior to the origin of the soleus which spans across both bones, the flexor hallucis longus arises principally from the fibula, while the flexor digitorum longus arises primarily from the tibia.

3) the tibialis posterior is interposed between the flexors hallucis longus and digitorum longus, thereby arising from the posterior surface of the interosseous membrane.

4) the arrows indicating the course of the tendons into the foot from the posterior surface. Observe that the tendon of the tibialis posterior crosses from lateral to medial beneath the tendon of the flexor digitorum longus and enters the foot immediately behind the medial malleolus.

**Fig. 416**

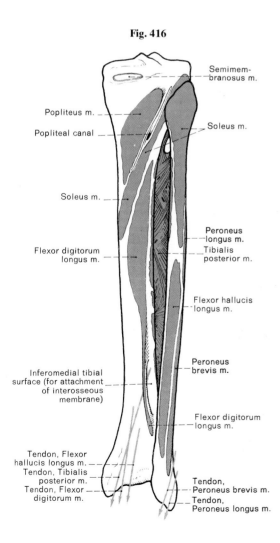

Semimem-branosus m.

Popliteus m.

Popliteal canal

Soleus m.

Soleus m.

Peroneus longus m.

Tibialis posterior m.

Flexor digitorum longus m.

Flexor hallucis longus m.

Peroneus brevis m.

Inferomedial tibial surface (for attachment of interosseous membrane)

Flexor digitorum longus m.

Tendon, Flexor hallucis longus m.
Tendon, Tibialis posterior m.
Tendon, Flexor digitorum m.

Tendon, Peroneus brevis m.
Tendon, Peroneus longus m.

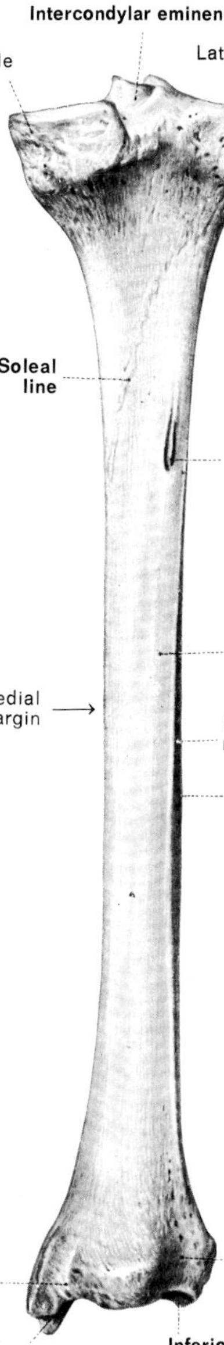

Intercondylar eminence

Medial condyle

Lateral condyle

Apex (styloid process)

Fibular articular surface

Head of fibula

Soleal line

Posterior border

Nutrient foramen

Medial margin

Posterior surface

Interosseous margin

Lateral surface

Anterior border

Lateral surface

Malleolar groove

Distal extremity

Lateral malleolar groove

Lateral malleolus

Malleolar articular surface

Inferior articular surface

**Fig. 417**

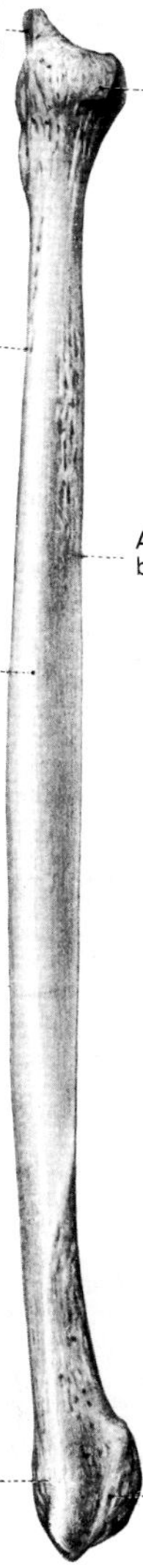

**Fig. 418**

### Fig. 417: The Right Tibia, Posterior View

NOTE: 1) the smooth posterior surface of the shaft of the tibia is marked by a prominent ridge (the soleal line) and a large oblong foramen (the nutrient foramen). The tibial shaft tapers toward a larger proximal extremity and somewhat less pronounced distal extremity.

2) at the proximal extremity the rounded medial and lateral condyles are separated by the intercondylar eminence, anterior and posterior to which attach the cruciate ligaments. At its distal extremity, the tibia articulates with the talus and, on this posterior surface, presents grooves for the passage of the tendons of the tibialis posterior, flexor digitorum longus and flexor hallucis longus.

### Fig. 418: The Right Fibula, Lateral View

NOTE: 1) the fibula is a long slender bone situated lateral to the tibia to which it articulates proximally (see Figure 413). Distally, the fibula expands to form the lateral malleolus. The medial aspect of its inferior articular surface participates with the tibia in forming the talocrural or ankle joint.

2) although the fibula does not bear any weight of the trunk (since it does not participate in the knee joint articulation), it is important because of the numerous muscles which attach to its surfaces (see Figures 415 and 416) and because it assists in the formation of the ankle joint.

Figs. 416, 417, 418    **V**

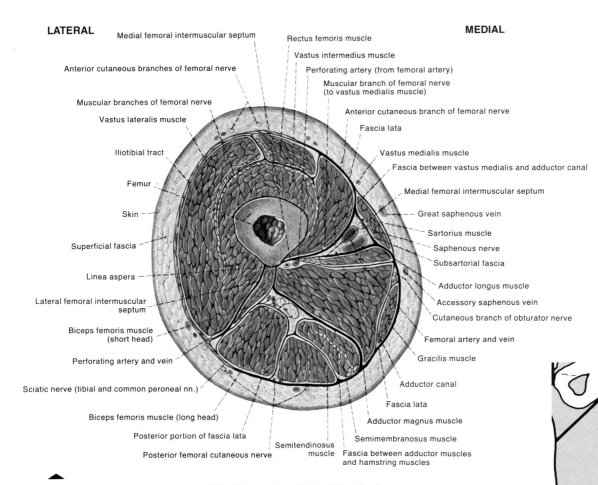

LATERAL        MEDIAL

Medial femoral intermuscular septum

Rectus femoris muscle

Vastus intermedius muscle

Anterior cutaneous branches of femoral nerve

Perforating artery (from femoral artery)

Muscular branch of femoral nerve
(to vastus medialis muscle)

Muscular branches of femoral nerve

Anterior cutaneous branch of femoral nerve

Vastus lateralis muscle

Fascia lata

Iliotibial tract

Vastus medialis muscle

Fascia between vastus medialis and adductor canal

Femur

Medial femoral intermuscular septum

Skin

Great saphenous vein

Superficial fascia

Sartorius muscle

Saphenous nerve

Subsartorial fascia

Linea aspera

Adductor longus muscle

Lateral femoral intermuscular
septum

Accessory saphenous vein

Biceps femoris muscle
(short head)

Cutaneous branch of obturator nerve

Femoral artery and vein

Perforating artery and vein

Gracilis muscle

Adductor canal

Sciatic nerve (tibial and common peroneal nn.)

Fascia lata

Biceps femoris muscle (long head)

Adductor magnus muscle

Posterior portion of fascia lata

Semimembranosus muscle

Semitendinosus
muscle

Posterior femoral cutaneous nerve

Fascia between adductor muscles
and hamstring muscles

▲

**Fig. 419: Cross Section Through Middle Third of Right Thigh (Distal Surface)**

**Fig. 420: Cross Section of Right Thigh Just Above Patella (Distal Surface)**

▼

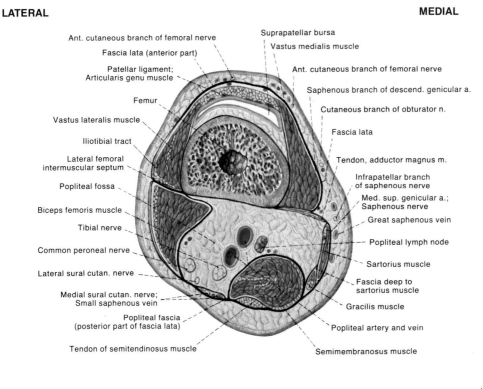

LATERAL        MEDIAL

Suprapatellar bursa

Ant. cutaneous branch of femoral nerve

Vastus medialis muscle

Fascia lata (anterior part)

Ant. cutaneous branch of femoral nerve

Patellar ligament;
Articularis genu muscle

Saphenous branch of descend. genicular a.

Femur

Cutaneous branch of obturator n.

Vastus lateralis muscle

Fascia lata

Iliotibial tract

Tendon, adductor magnus m.

Lateral femoral
intermuscular septum

Infrapatellar branch
of saphenous nerve

Popliteal fossa

Med. sup. genicular a.;
Saphenous nerve

Biceps femoris muscle

Great saphenous vein

Tibial nerve

Popliteal lymph node

Common peroneal nerve

Sartorius muscle

Lateral sural cutan. nerve

Fascia deep to
sartorius muscle

Medial sural cutan. nerve;
Small saphenous vein

Gracilis muscle

Popliteal fascia
(posterior part of fascia lata)

Popliteal artery and vein

Tendon of semitendinosus muscle

Semimembranosus muscle

Fig. 419

Fig. 420

Fig. 422

Fig. 423

Fig. 424

Fig. 448

Fig. 449

**Fig. 421: Cross Sectional Planes of Lower
Extremity Shown in Seven Figures of This Atlas** ▶

Figs. 419, 420, 421

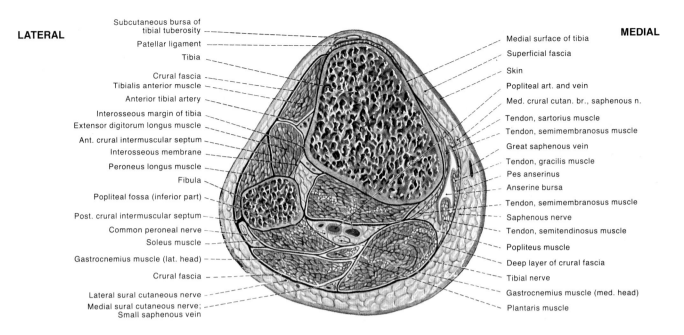

LATERAL | MEDIAL

Subcutaneous bursa of tibial tuberosity
Patellar ligament
Tibia
Crural fascia
Tibialis anterior muscle
Anterior tibial artery
Interosseous margin of tibia
Extensor digitorum longus muscle
Ant. crural intermuscular septum
Interosseous membrane
Peroneus longus muscle
Fibula
Popliteal fossa (inferior part)
Post. crural intermuscular septum
Common peroneal nerve
Soleus muscle
Gastrocnemius muscle (lat. head)
Crural fascia
Lateral sural cutaneous nerve
Medial sural cutaneous nerve; Small saphenous vein

Medial surface of tibia
Superficial fascia
Skin
Popliteal art. and vein
Med. crural cutan. br., saphenous n.
Tendon, sartorius muscle
Tendon, semimembranosus muscle
Great saphenous vein
Tendon, gracilis muscle
Pes anserinus
Anserine bursa
Tendon, semimembranosus muscle
Saphenous nerve
Tendon, semitendinosus muscle
Popliteus muscle
Deep layer of crural fascia
Tibial nerve
Gastrocnemius muscle (med. head)
Plantaris muscle

**Fig. 422: Cross Section Through Upper Third of Right Leg (Distal Surface).**

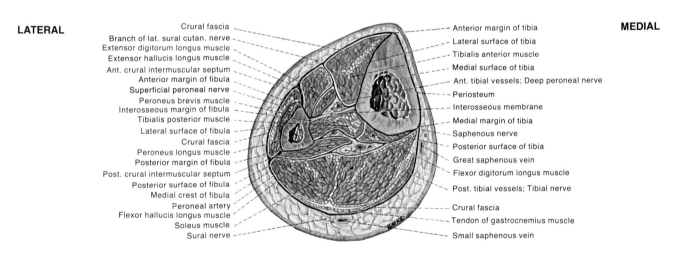

LATERAL | MEDIAL

Crural fascia
Branch of lat. sural cutan. nerve
Extensor digitorum longus muscle
Extensor hallucis longus muscle
Ant. crural intermuscular septum
Anterior margin of fibula
Superficial peroneal nerve
Peroneus brevis muscle
Interosseous margin of fibula
Tibialis posterior muscle
Lateral surface of fibula
Crural fascia
Peroneus longus muscle
Posterior margin of fibula
Post. crural intermuscular septum
Posterior surface of fibula
Medial crest of fibula
Peroneal artery
Flexor hallucis longus muscle
Soleus muscle
Sural nerve

Anterior margin of tibia
Lateral surface of tibia
Tibialis anterior muscle
Medial surface of tibia
Ant. tibial vessels; Deep peroneal nerve
Periosteum
Interosseous membrane
Medial margin of tibia
Saphenous nerve
Posterior surface of tibia
Great saphenous vein
Flexor digitorum longus muscle
Post. tibial vessels; Tibial nerve
Crural fascia
Tendon of gastrocnemius muscle
Small saphenous vein

**Fig. 423: Cross Section Through the Middle of Right Leg (Distal Surface).**

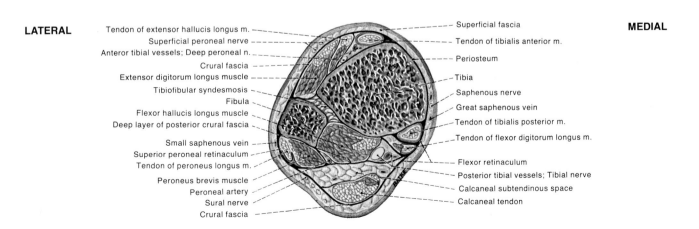

LATERAL | MEDIAL

Tendon of extensor hallucis longus m.
Superficial peroneal nerve
Anteror tibial vessels; Deep peroneal n.
Crural fascia
Extensor digitorum longus muscle
Tibiofibular syndesmosis
Fibula
Flexor hallucis longus muscle
Deep layer of posterior crural fascia
Small saphenous vein
Superior peroneal retinaculum
Tendon of peroneus longus m.
Peroneus brevis muscle
Peroneal artery
Sural nerve
Crural fascia

Superficial fascia
Tendon of tibialis anterior m.
Periosteum
Tibia
Saphenous nerve
Great saphenous vein
Tendon of tibialis posterior m.
Tendon of flexor digitorum longus m.
Flexor retinaculum
Posterior tibial vessels; Tibial nerve
Calcaneal subtendinous space
Calcaneal tendon

**Fig. 424: Cross Section Through the Right Leg Just Above the Malleoli (Distal Surface).**

Figs. 422, 423, 424 **V**

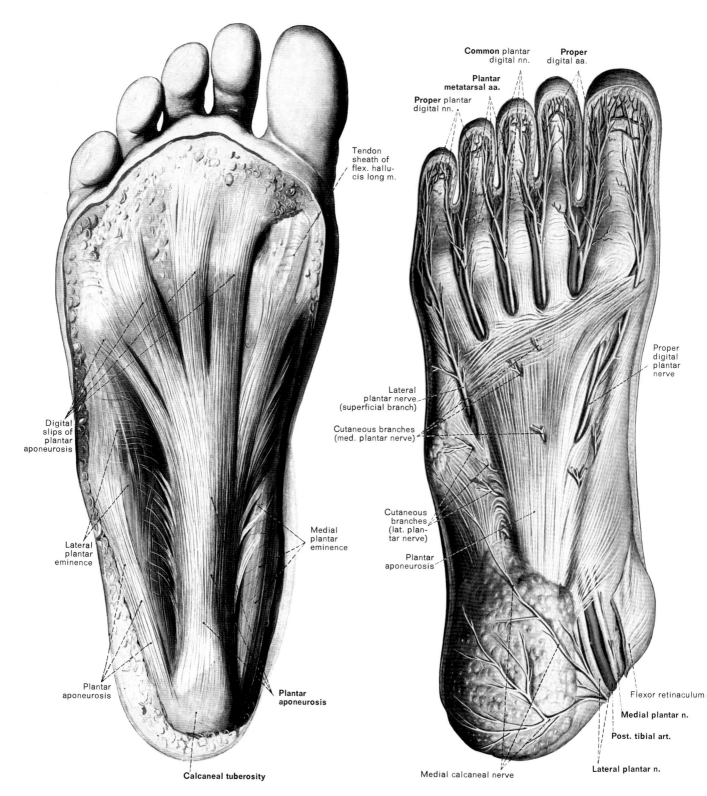

Labels for Fig. 425 (left illustration):

Tendon sheath of flex. hallucis long m.

Digital slips of plantar aponeurosis

Lateral plantar eminence

Medial plantar eminence

Plantar aponeurosis

Plantar aponeurosis

Calcaneal tuberosity

Labels for Fig. 426 (right illustration):

Common plantar digital nn.

Proper digital aa.

Plantar metatarsal aa.

Proper plantar digital nn.

Proper digital plantar nerve

Lateral plantar nerve (superficial branch)

Cutaneous branches (med. plantar nerve)

Cutaneous branches (lat. plantar nerve)

Plantar aponeurosis

Flexor retinaculum

Medial plantar n.

Post. tibial art.

Lateral plantar n.

Medial calcaneal nerve

**Fig. 425: The Sole of the Right Foot: Plantar Aponeurosis**

NOTE: 1) the plantar aponeurosis which stretches across the sole of the foot. Similar to the palmar aponeurosis in the hand, the plantar aponeurosis is a thickened layer of deep fascia which serves both a protective and supportive function to the underlying muscles, vessels and nerves.

2) the longitudinal orientation of the fibers of the plantar aponeurosis and their attachment to the calcaneal tuberosity. Distally, the aponeurosis divides into five digital slips, one of which courses to each toe. Fibers extend from the margins of the aponeurosis to cover partially both the medial and lateral plantar eminences.

**Fig. 426: The Sole of the Right Foot: Superficial Nerves and Arteries**

NOTE: 1) the medial and lateral plantar nerves and posterior tibial artery as they enter the foot behind the medial malleolus and immediately course beneath the plantar aponeurosis toward the digits. Sensory branches of the nerves penetrate the aponeurosis to innervate the overlying skin and superficial fascia.

2) between the digital slips of the plantar aponeurosis, the vessels and the nerves course superficially toward the toes. Metatarsal arteries and common plantar digital nerves divide to supply adjacent portions of the toes as proper plantar digital arteries and nerves.

Figs. 425, 426

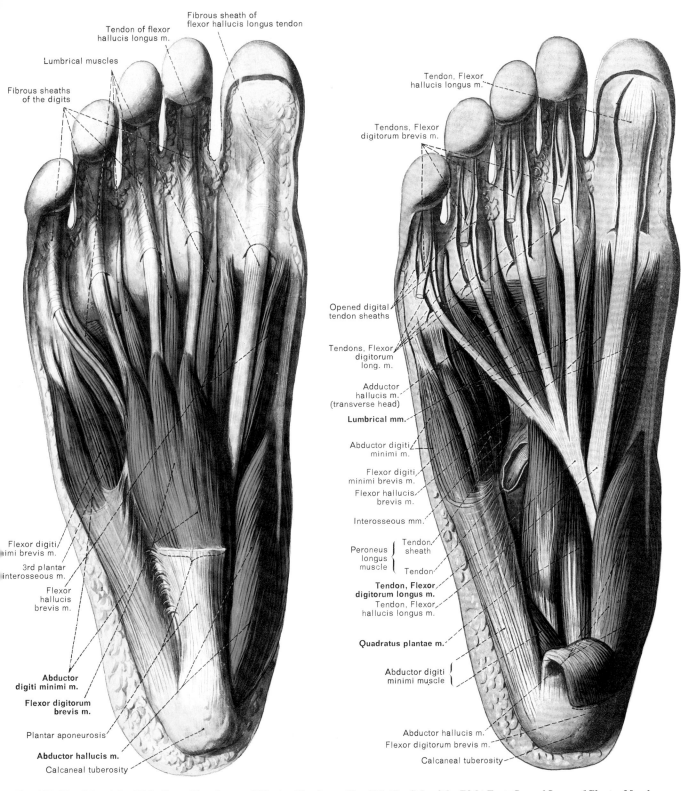

Fibrous sheath of
flexor hallucis longus tendon

Tendon of flexor
hallucis longus m.

Lumbrical muscles

Fibrous sheaths
of the digits

Tendon, Flexor
hallucis longus m.

Tendons, Flexor
digitorum brevis m.

Opened digital
tendon sheaths

Tendons, Flexor
digitorum
long. m.

Adductor
hallucis m.
(transverse head)

Lumbrical mm.

Abductor digiti
minimi m.

Flexor digiti
minimi brevis m.

Flexor hallucis
brevis m.

Interosseous mm.

Peroneus { Tendon
longus sheath
muscle { Tendon

Tendon, Flexor
digitorum longus m.

Tendon, Flexor
hallucis longus m.

Quadratus plantae m.

Abductor digiti {
minimi muscle {

Flexor digiti
imi brevis m.

3rd plantar
interosseous m.

Flexor
hallucis
brevis m.

Abductor
digiti minimi m.

Flexor digitorum
brevis m.

Plantar aponeurosis

Abductor hallucis m.

Calcaneal tuberosity

Abductor hallucis m.
Flexor digitorum brevis m.

Calcaneal tuberosity

**Fig. 427: The Sole of the Right Foot: First Layer of Plantar Muscles**

NOTE: 1) with most of the plantar aponeurosis removed, three muscles comprising the first layer of the sole are exposed. These are the abductor hallucis, the flexor digitorum brevis, and the abductor digiti minimi.

2) all three muscles arise from the tuberosity of the calcaneus. The abductor hallucis inserts on the proximal phalanx of the large toe. The flexor digitorum brevis separates into four tendons which insert onto the middle phalanges of the lateral four toes. The abductor digiti minimi inserts onto the proximal phalanx of the little toe.

**Fig. 428: The Sole of the Right Foot: Second Layer of Plantar Muscles**

NOTE: 1) the tendons of the flexor digitorum brevis muscle were severed and removed, thereby exposing the underlying tendons of the flexor digitorum longus muscle.

2) the muscles of the second layer in the plantar foot include the quadratus plantae muscle and the four lumbrical muscles. The quadratus plantae arises by two heads from the calcaneus and inserts into the tendon of the flexor digitorum longus.

3) the four lumbrical muscles arising from the tendons of the flexor digitorum longus muscle. They insert on the medial aspect of the first phalanx of the lateral four toes as well as on the dorsal extensor hoods.

Figs. 427, 428    V

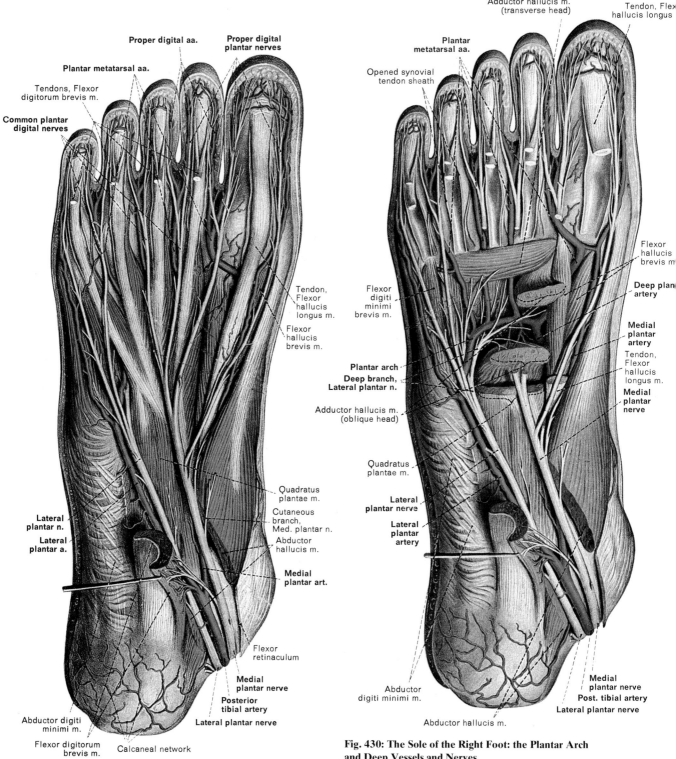

**Fig. 429: The Sole of the Right Foot: the Plantar Nerves and Arteries**

NOTE: 1) whereas the tibial nerve divides into medial and lateral plantar nerves just inferior to the medial malleolus, the posterior tibial artery enters the plantar surface of the foot as a single vessel and divides into medial and lateral plantar arteries beneath or at the medial border of the abductor hallucis muscle.

2) the lateral plantar nerve supplies the lateral 1−1/2 digits while the medial plantar nerve supplies the medial 3−1/2 digits. Observe the formation of the common digital plantar nerves which then divide into the proper digital plantar nerves.

**Fig. 430: The Sole of the Right Foot: the Plantar Arch and Deep Vessels and Nerves**

NOTE: 1) the formation of the deep plantar arch principally from the lateral plantar artery, and the junction of the deep plantar arch with the deep plantar artery from the foot dorsum (see Fig. 404). From the plantar arch branch plantar metatarsal arteries which then divide into proper digital arteries.

2) the muscles of the foot are innervated in the following manner:

|  | *medial plantar nerve* | *lateral plantar nerve* |
| --- | --- | --- |
| 1st layer | abductor hallucis | abductor digiti minimi |
|  | flexor digitorum brevis |  |
| 2nd layer | 1st lumbrical | quadratus plantae |
|  |  | 2nd, 3rd and 4th lumbrical |
| 3rd layer | flexor hallucis brevis | adductor hallucis |
|  |  | flexor digiti minimi brevis |
| 4th layer |  | plantar interossei |
|  |  | dorsal interossei |

Figs. 429, 430

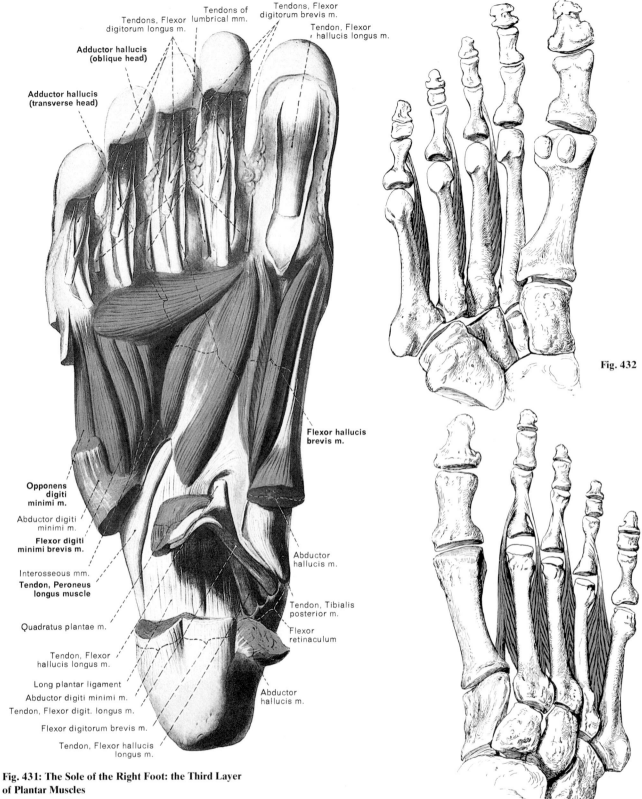

Tendons, Flexor digitorum longus m.

Adductor hallucis (oblique head)

Adductor hallucis (transverse head)

Tendons of lumbrical mm.

Tendons, Flexor digitorum brevis m.

Tendon, Flexor hallucis longus m.

Flexor hallucis brevis m.

Opponens digiti minimi m.

Abductor digiti minimi m.

Flexor digiti minimi brevis m.

Interosseous mm.

Tendon, Peroneus longus muscle

Quadratus plantae m.

Tendon, Flexor hallucis longus m.

Long plantar ligament

Abductor digiti minimi m.

Tendon, Flexor digit. longus m.

Flexor digitorum brevis m.

Tendon, Flexor hallucis longus m.

Abductor hallucis m.

Tendon, Tibialis posterior m.

Flexor retinaculum

Abductor hallucis m.

Fig. 432

Fig. 433

**Fig. 431: The Sole of the Right Foot: the Third Layer of Plantar Muscles**

NOTE: 1) the third layer of plantar muscles consists of two flexors and an adductor, in contrast to the first layer which contains one flexor and two abductors. Thus, the flexor hallucis brevis, flexor digiti minimi brevis and the two heads (oblique and transverse) of the adductor hallucis form the third layer of plantar muscles.

2) at times those fibers of the flexor digiti minimi brevis muscle which insert on the lateral side of the first phalanx of the 5th toe are referred to as a separate muscle, the opponens digiti minimi.

3) the tendon of the peroneus longus muscle which crosses the plantar aspect of the foot obliquely to insert on the lateral side of the base of the first metatarsal and the first (medial) cuneiform bone.

**Fig. 432: The Plantar Interossei**

NOTE that there are three plantar interossei. These muscles adduct the 3rd, 4th and 5th toes toward the 2nd toe which acts as the longitudinal axis of the foot.

**Fig. 433: The Dorsal Interossei**

NOTE that there are four dorsal interossei. These muscles abduct the toes from the reference axis. Both plantar and dorsal interossei flex the metatarsophalangeal joints and extend the interphalangeal joints.

Figs. 431, 432, 433     V

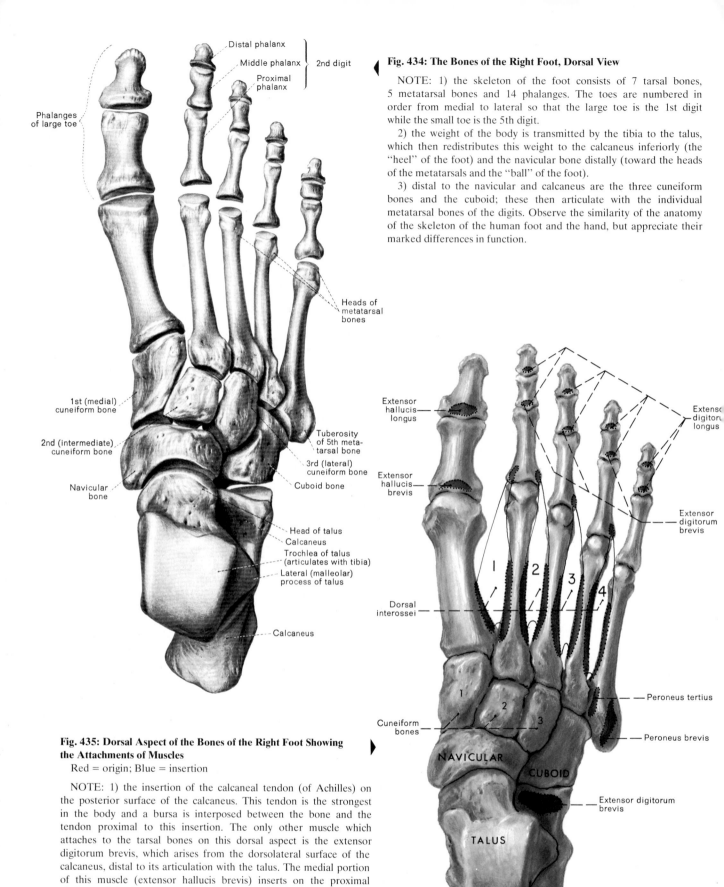

Phalanges of large toe

Distal phalanx
Middle phalanx
Proximal phalanx
} 2nd digit

Heads of metatarsal bones

1st (medial) cuneiform bone

2nd (intermediate) cuneiform bone

Navicular bone

Tuberosity of 5th metatarsal bone

3rd (lateral) cuneiform bone

Cuboid bone

Head of talus
Calcaneus
Trochlea of talus (articulates with tibia)
Lateral (malleolar) process of talus

Calcaneus

### Fig. 434: The Bones of the Right Foot, Dorsal View

NOTE: 1) the skeleton of the foot consists of 7 tarsal bones, 5 metatarsal bones and 14 phalanges. The toes are numbered in order from medial to lateral so that the large toe is the 1st digit while the small toe is the 5th digit.

2) the weight of the body is transmitted by the tibia to the talus, which then redistributes this weight to the calcaneus inferiorly (the "heel" of the foot) and the navicular bone distally (toward the heads of the metatarsals and the "ball" of the foot).

3) distal to the navicular and calcaneus are the three cuneiform bones and the cuboid; these then articulate with the individual metatarsal bones of the digits. Observe the similarity of the anatomy of the skeleton of the human foot and the hand, but appreciate their marked differences in function.

Extensor hallucis longus

Extensor hallucis brevis

Extensor digitorum longus

Extensor digitorum brevis

Dorsal interossei

Cuneiform bones

NAVICULAR

CUBOID

Extensor digitorum brevis

Peroneus tertius

Peroneus brevis

TALUS

CALCANEUS

Calcaneal tendon

### Fig. 435: Dorsal Aspect of the Bones of the Right Foot Showing the Attachments of Muscles

Red = origin; Blue = insertion

NOTE: 1) the insertion of the calcaneal tendon (of Achilles) on the posterior surface of the calcaneus. This tendon is the strongest in the body and a bursa is interposed between the bone and the tendon proximal to this insertion. The only other muscle which attaches to the tarsal bones on this dorsal aspect is the extensor digitorum brevis, which arises from the dorsolateral surface of the calcaneus, distal to its articulation with the talus. The medial portion of this muscle (extensor hallucis brevis) inserts on the proximal phalanx of the large toe, while three other tendons insert onto the middle phalanx of the 2nd, 3rd and 4th toes.

2) the insertions of the peroneus brevis and tertius onto the base of the 5th metatarsal.

3) the 1st and 2nd dorsal interosseus muscles inserting onto the 2nd toe, while the 3rd and 4th insert onto the dorsolateral aspect of the 3rd and 4th digits. These muscles serve as abductors.

Figs. 434, 435

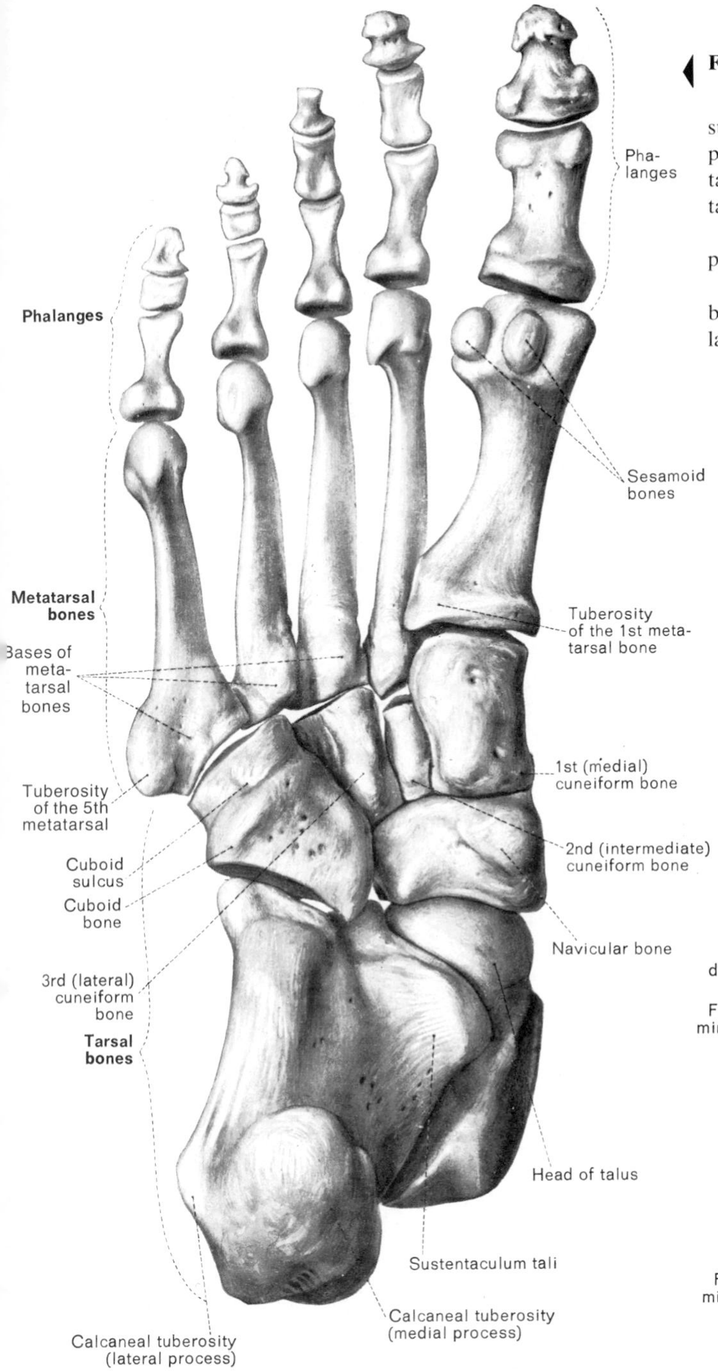

**Phalanges**

Phalanges

Sesamoid bones

**Metatarsal bones**

Bases of metatarsal bones

Tuberosity of the 1st metatarsal bone

Tuberosity of the 5th metatarsal

1st (medial) cuneiform bone

Cuboid sulcus

2nd (intermediate) cuneiform bone

Cuboid bone

Navicular bone

3rd (lateral) cuneiform bone

**Tarsal bones**

Head of talus

Sustentaculum tali

Calcaneal tuberosity (lateral process)

Calcaneal tuberosity (medial process)

### Fig. 436: The Bones of the Right Foot: Plantar View

NOTE: 1) the largest bone in the foot is the calcaneus. From this surface can be seen the prominent calcaneal tuberosity which projects posteriorly and inferiorly (forming the heel) and the sustentaculum tali, the dorsal surface of which contains articular facets for the talus.

2) the cuboid bone and the sulcus on its plantar surface for the passage of the peroneus longus tendon across the sole of the foot.

3) the long, slender metatarsal bones which are curved, such as to be concave on their plantar surface and convex dorsally. Observe the large tuberosity on the lateral side of the base of the 5th metatarsal.

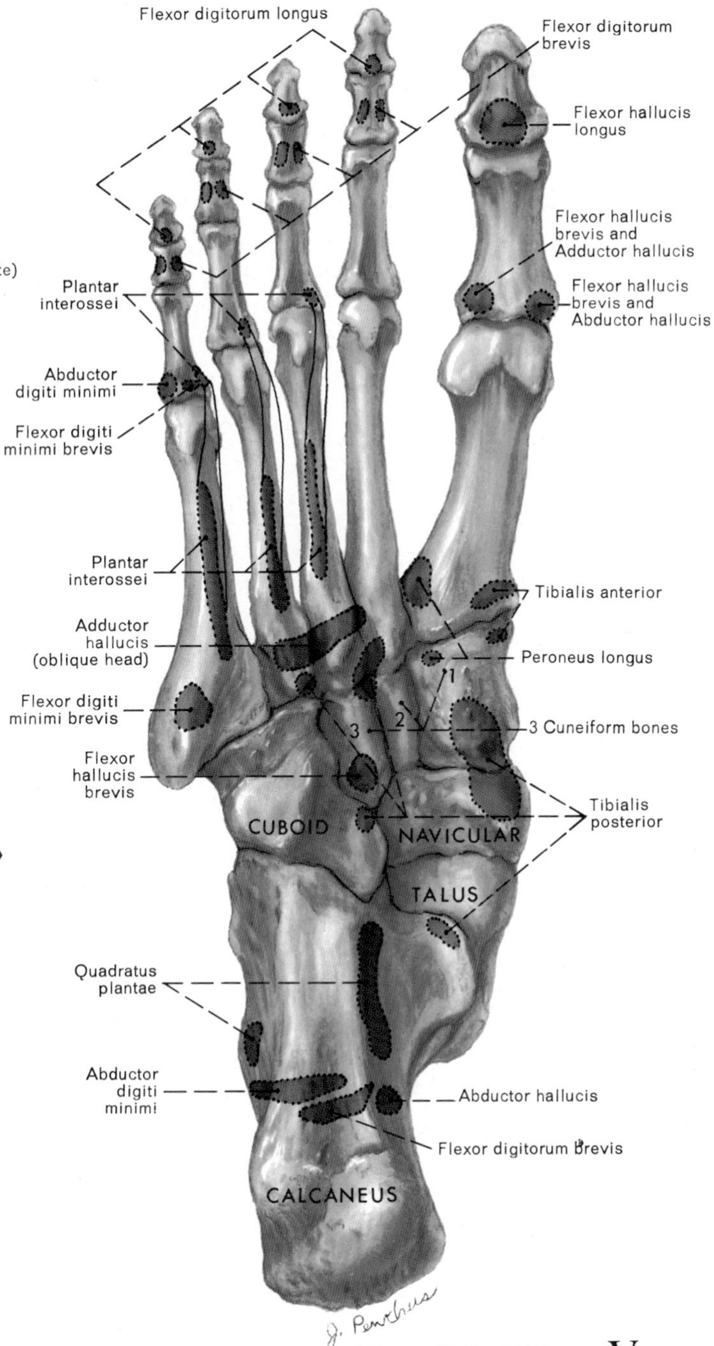

Flexor digitorum longus

Flexor digitorum brevis

Flexor hallucis longus

Flexor hallucis brevis and Adductor hallucis

Flexor hallucis brevis and Abductor hallucis

Plantar interossei

Abductor digiti minimi

Flexor digiti minimi brevis

Plantar interossei

Tibialis anterior

Adductor hallucis (oblique head)

Peroneus longus

Flexor digiti minimi brevis

3 Cuneiform bones

Flexor hallucis brevis

Tibialis posterior

Quadratus plantae

CUBOID

NAVICULAR

TALUS

Abductor digiti minimi

Abductor hallucis

Flexor digitorum brevis

CALCANEUS

### Fig. 437: Plantar Aspect of the Bones of the Right Foot Showing the Attachments of Muscles

NOTE: 1) that the muscles comprising the 1st and 2nd plantar layers (except the lumbricals) all arise from the plantar surface of the calcaneal bone. These four muscles include the abductors hallucis and digiti minimi, the flexor digitorum brevis and the quadratus plantae.

2) the tendons of five extrinsic muscles of the foot (arising in the leg) insert on the plantar aspect. These are the peroneus longus, the tibialis anterior and tibialis posterior and the flexors hallucis longus and digitorum longus. The tendon of the tibialis posterior sends some fibers of insertion onto the plantar surface of six of the seven tarsal bones (only the talus is omitted in its insertion).

3) the three plantar interossei arise from the 3rd, 4th and 5th metatarsals and insert on the proximal phalanges of these same digits. These muscles act as adductors of these three digits, capable of moving them toward the 2nd digit, the center of which is the longitudinal axis of the foot.

Figs. 436, 437     V

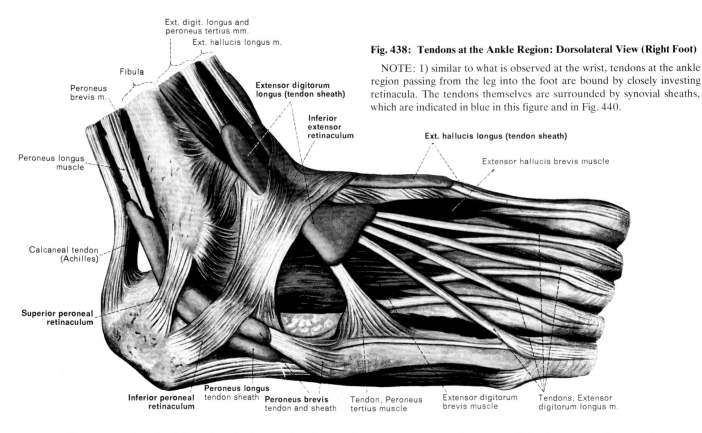

**Fig. 438: Tendons at the Ankle Region: Dorsolateral View (Right Foot)**

NOTE: 1) similar to what is observed at the wrist, tendons at the ankle region passing from the leg into the foot are bound by closely investing retinacula. The tendons themselves are surrounded by synovial sheaths, which are indicated in blue in this figure and in Fig. 440.

Labels (clockwise/around figure):
Ext. digit. longus and peroneus tertius mm.
Ext. hallucis longus m.
Fibula
Peroneus brevis m.
Peroneus longus muscle
Calcaneal tendon (Achilles)
Superior peroneal retinaculum
Inferior peroneal retinaculum
Peroneus longus tendon sheath
Peroneus brevis tendon and sheath
Tendon, Peroneus tertius muscle
Extensor digitorum longus (tendon sheath)
Inferior extensor retinaculum
Ext. hallucis longus (tendon sheath)
Extensor hallucis brevis muscle
Extensor digitorum brevis muscle
Tendons, Extensor digitorum longus m.

2) anterior to the ankle joint and on the dorsum of the foot are three separate synovial sheaths. One is for the extensor digitorum longus and peroneus tertius, a second is for the extensor hallucis longus and the third surrounds the tibialis anterior (see Fig. 440). Behind the lateral malleolus is a single tendon sheath for the peroneus longus and brevis which then splits distally to continue along each individual tendon for some distance.

3) the inferior extensor retinaculum and the superior and inferior peroneal retinacula which bind the tendons and their sheaths close to bone.

**Fig. 439: The Tendons of the Peroneus Longus and Tibialis Anterior Muscles**

NOTE that the tendons of the tibialis anterior and peroneus longus muscles insert on the medial aspect of the plantar surface of the foot. The peroneus longus muscle achieves this insertion by traversing the sole of the foot from lateral to medial. In this manner, the two muscles form a tendinous sling under the foot which serves to support the transverse arch. Also assisting in this support is the tendon of the tibialis posterior muscle.

**Fig. 440: Tendons at the Ankle Region: Medial View (Right Foot)**

NOTE: 1) from this medial view can be seen the synovial sheaths and tendons of the tibialis anterior and extensor hallucis longus on the dorsum of the foot, as well as the three tendons which course beneath the medial malleolus from the posterior compartment of the leg into the plantar foot: tibialis posterior, flexor digitorum longus and flexor hallucis longus.

2) the bifurcating nature of the inferior extensor retinaculum, and the manner in which the flexor retinaculum secures the structures beneath the medial malleolus.

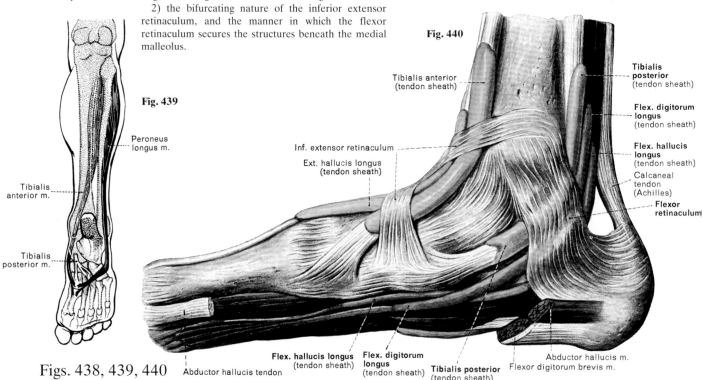

**Fig. 439**
Peroneus longus m.
Tibialis anterior m.
Tibialis posterior m.

**Fig. 440**
Tibialis anterior (tendon sheath)
Inf. extensor retinaculum
Ext. hallucis longus (tendon sheath)
Tibialis posterior (tendon sheath)
Flex. digitorum longus (tendon sheath)
Flex. hallucis longus (tendon sheath)
Calcaneal tendon (Achilles)
Flexor retinaculum
Flex. hallucis longus (tendon sheath)
Flex. digitorum longus (tendon sheath)
Tibialis posterior (tendon sheath)
Abductor hallucis tendon
Abductor hallucis m.
Flexor digitorum brevis m.

Figs. 438, 439, 440

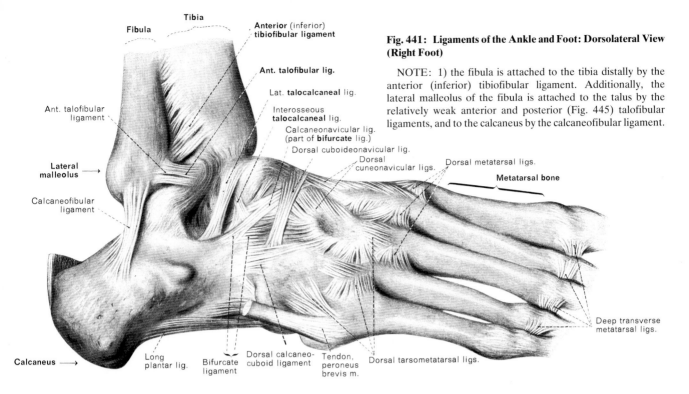

**Fig. 441: Ligaments of the Ankle and Foot: Dorsolateral View (Right Foot)**

NOTE: 1) the fibula is attached to the tibia distally by the anterior (inferior) tibiofibular ligament. Additionally, the lateral malleolus of the fibula is attached to the talus by the relatively weak anterior and posterior (Fig. 445) talofibular ligaments, and to the calcaneus by the calcaneofibular ligament.

2) the joint between the talus and calcaneus (subtalar joint) is principally strenghtened by the interosseous talocalcaneal ligament. The talocalcaneonavicular joint more anteriorly is of important clinical significance since the weight of the body tends to push the head of the talus down between the navicular and calcaneus. The stability of this joint is assisted dorsolaterally by the calcaneonavicular ligament (a part of the bifurcate ligament); however, the thick plantar calcaneonavicular or spring ligament (Figs. 442, 444, 446, 447) is the principal support for this joint in the maintenance of the longitudinal arch of the foot.

3) the bifurcate ligament consists of the calcaneonavicular ligament and the calcaneocuboid ligament.

**Fig. 442: Ligaments of the Ankle and Foot: Medial View (Right Foot)**

NOTE: 1) the medial aspect of the ankle joint is protected by the deltoid ligament, which is triangular in shape and which connects the tibia (medial malleolus) to the navicular, calcaneus and talus. The deltoid ligament consists of 4 parts: a) an anterior part which attaches the medial malleolus to the navicular (tibionavicular part), b) a superficial part attaching the malleolus to the sustentaculum tali of the calcaneus (tibiocalcaneal part), and c) and d) the anterior and posterior tibiotalar parts which lie more deeply and attach the malleolus to the adjacent talus.

2) the insertions of the tendons of the tibialis anterior and tibialis posterior muscles which attach on this medial aspect of the foot. Observe also the long plantar and plantar calcaneonavicular ligaments on the plantar surface. These are shown more clearly in Figures 444, 446 and 447.

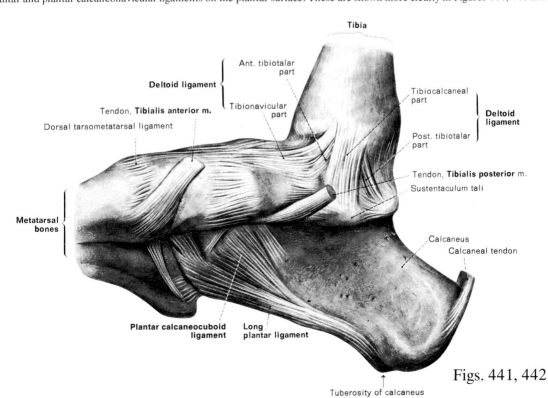

Figs. 441, 442    **V**

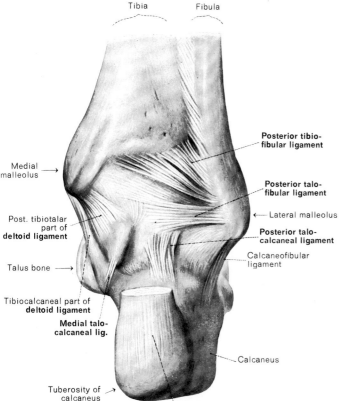

**1st metatarsal (of large toe)**
**2nd metatarsal**
**3rd metatarsal**
**4th metatarsal**
**5th metatarsal**

Tarsometatarsal joint of large toe

Tarsometatarsal joint

1st (med.) cuneiform
2nd (intermed.) cuneiform

Cuneonavicular joint

Navicular bone

**Talonavicular joint**

Talus

Interosseous talocalcaneal lig.

Subtalar joint

Calcaneus

Interosseous metatarsal lig.

Tarsometatarsal joint

Tuberosity of 5th metatarsal

Interosseous tarsal lig.

3rd (lat.) cuneiform

Cuboid bone

**Calcaneocuboid joint**

## Fig. 444: The Talocalcaneonavicular Joint (Viewed from Above), Right

NOTE that the talus has been removed. This reveals the three articulations it makes with the calcaneus and the anterior articulation it makes with the navicular bone. Observe the plantar calcaneonavicular ("spring") ligament stretching across the plantar aspect of the talocalcaneonavicular joint.

Tibia
Fibula

**Posterior tibiofibular ligament**

**Posterior talofibular ligament**

Lateral malleolus

**Posterior talocalcaneal ligament**

Calcaneofibular ligament

Medial malleolus

Post. tibiotalar part of **deltoid ligament**

Talus bone

Tibiocalcaneal part of **deltoid ligament**

**Medial talocalcaneal lig.**

Calcaneus

Tuberosity of calcaneus

Calcaneal tendon

Figs. 443, 444, 445

## Fig. 443: The Intertarsal and Tarsometatarsal Joints (Horizontal Section of the Right Foot)

NOTE: 1) a transverse intertarsal joint, extending across the foot and formed by two separate joint cavities, the calcaneocuboid joint and the talonavicular portion of the talocalcaneonavicular joint. These two joints allow some dorsi and plantarflexion of the anterior part of the foot with respect to the posterior foot.

2) that the joints in the foot form a natural division of the bones into a medial group (talus, navicular, the 3 cuneiform and the medial three metatarsals and phalanges) and a lateral group (calcaneus, cuboid and the lateral two metatarsals and phalanges).

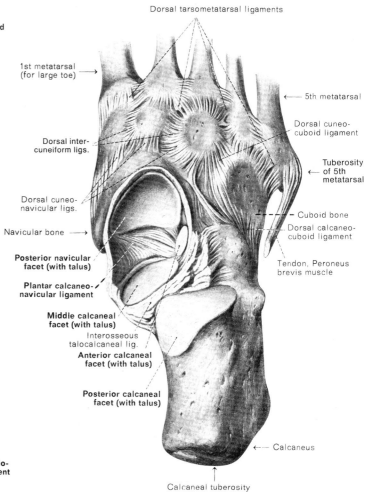

Dorsal tarsometatarsal ligaments

1st metatarsal (for large toe)

5th metatarsal

Dorsal cuneocuboid ligament

Tuberosity of 5th metatarsal

Cuboid bone

Dorsal calcaneocuboid ligament

Tendon, Peroneus brevis muscle

Dorsal intercuneiform ligs.

Dorsal cuneonavicular ligs.

Navicular bone

**Posterior navicular facet (with talus)**

**Plantar calcaneonavicular ligament**

**Middle calcaneal facet (with talus)**

Interosseous talocalcaneal lig.

**Anterior calcaneal facet (with talus)**

**Posterior calcaneal facet (with talus)**

Calcaneus

Calcaneal tuberosity

## Fig. 445: The Ankle Joint (Talocrural) Viewed from Behind (Right Foot)

NOTE: 1) the ankle joint is a ginglymus or hinge joint. The bony structures participating in this joint superiorly are the distal end of the tibia and its medial malleolus, and the distal fibula and its lateral malleolus. Together these structures form a concave receptacle for the convex proximal surface of the talus.

2) the posterior aspect of the articular capsule is somewhat strengthened by the posterior talofibular and posterior tibiofibular ligaments. Laterally, the calcaneofibular ligament and medially, the strong deltoid ligament assist in protecting this joint.

3) the ligamentous bands which help to stabilize the talocalcaneal articulation posteriorly: the posterior and medial talocalcaneal ligaments.

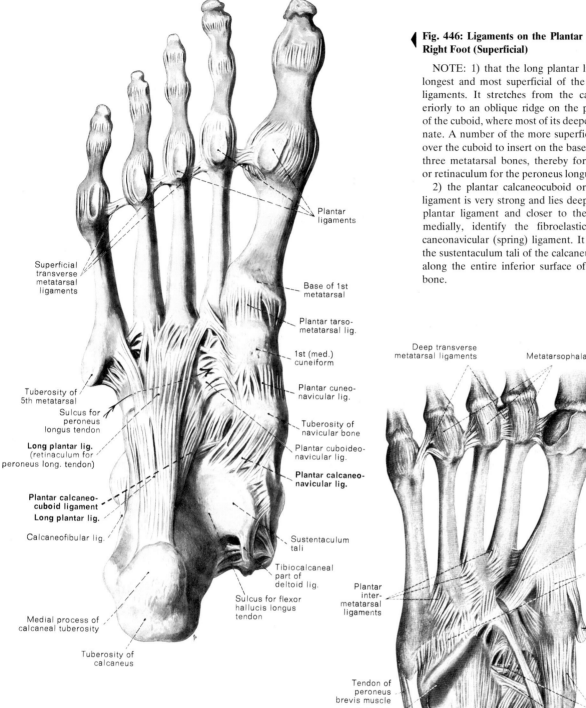

Superficial
transverse
metatarsal
ligaments

Tuberosity of
5th metatarsal

Sulcus for
peroneus
longus tendon

**Long plantar lig.**
(retinaculum for
peroneus long. tendon)

**Plantar calcaneo-
cuboid ligament
Long plantar lig.**

Calcaneofibular lig.

Medial process of
calcaneal tuberosity

Tuberosity of
calcaneus

Plantar
ligaments

Base of 1st
metatarsal

Plantar tarso-
metatarsal lig.

1st (med.)
cuneiform

Plantar cuneo-
navicular lig.

Tuberosity of
navicular bone

Plantar cuboideo-
navicular lig.

**Plantar calcaneo-
navicular lig.**

Sustentaculum
tali

Tibiocalcaneal
part of
deltoid lig.

Sulcus for flexor
hallucis longus
tendon

NOTE: 1) that the long plantar ligament is the
longest and most superficial of the plantar tarsal
ligaments. It stretches from the calcaneus posteriorly to an oblique ridge on the plantar surface
of the cuboid, where most of its deeper fibers terminate. A number of the more superficial fibers pass
over the cuboid to insert on the bases of the lateral
three metatarsal bones, thereby forming a tunnel
or retinaculum for the peroneus longus tendon.

2) the plantar calcaneocuboid or short plantar
ligament is very strong and lies deeper to the long
plantar ligament and closer to the bones. More
medially, identify the fibroelastic plantar calcaneonavicular (spring) ligament. It is attached to
the sustentaculum tali of the calcaneus and extends
along the entire inferior surface of the navicular
bone.

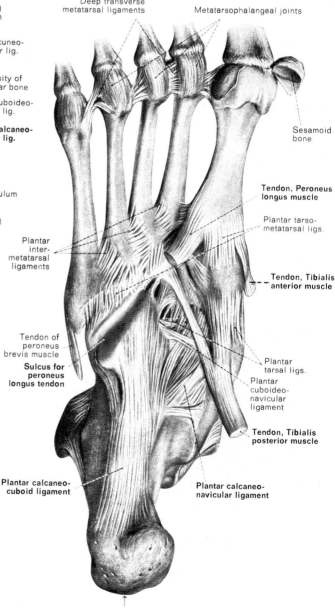

Deep transverse
metatarsal ligaments

Metatarsophalangeal joints

Sesamoid
bone

**Tendon, Peroneus
longus muscle**

Plantar tarso-
metatarsal ligs.

**Tendon, Tibialis
anterior muscle**

Plantar
inter-
metatarsal
ligaments

Plantar
tarsal ligs.

Plantar
cuboideo-
navicular
ligament

**Tendon, Tibialis
posterior muscle**

Tendon of
peroneus
brevis muscle

**Sulcus for
peroneus
longus tendon**

**Plantar calcaneo-
cuboid ligament**

**Plantar calcaneo-
navicular ligament**

Calcaneal tuberosity

**Fig. 447: The Plantar Calcaneonavicular Ligament and the ▶
Insertions of Three Tendons (Right Foot)**

NOTE: 1) the metatarsal extensions of the long plantar
ligament have been cut away to reveal the groove for the
tendon of the peroneus longus muscle. This tendon is seen
inserting onto the base of the 1st metatarsal bone. It also
sends a small slip of insertion to the 1st cuneiform. Two
other long tendons inserting on the medial side of the plantar
surface are those of the tibialis anterior and tibialis posterior
muscles.

2) that the fibers of the calcaneocuboid (short plantar) and
calcaneonavicular (spring) ligaments all stem from the calcaneus and then diverge in a radial manner toward the
medial side of the foot. Observe that the course and insertion
of the tibialis posterior tendon also lends some support to
the short tendon and spring ligaments.

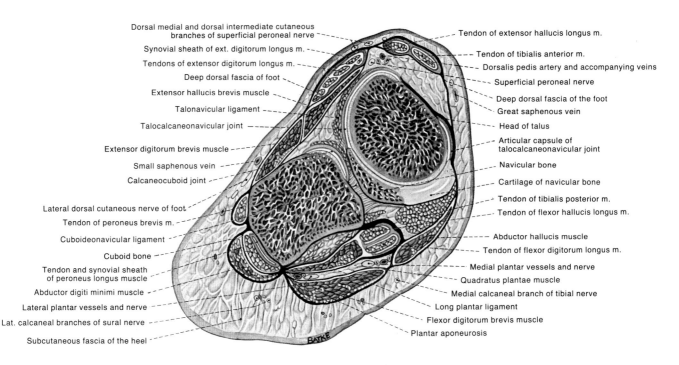

**Fig. 448: Cross Section Through the Right Foot at the Level of the Head of the Talus (Distal Surface)**

NOTE that the tendon sheaths and synovial membranes are shown in light blue. The level of this cross section is shown in the diagram Figure 421.

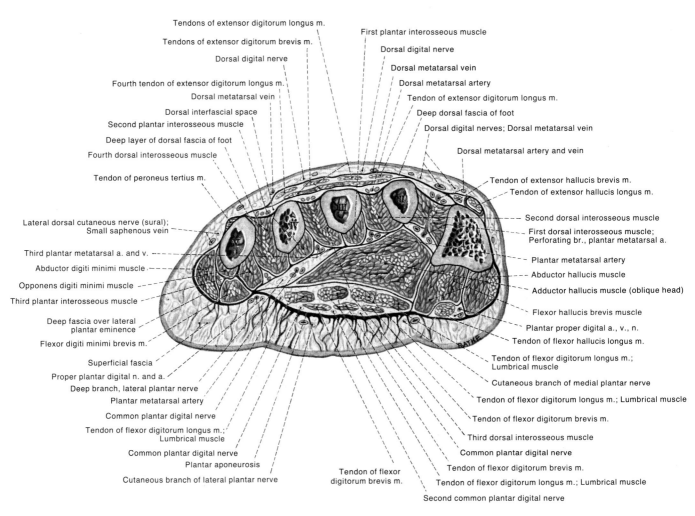

**Fig. 449: Cross Section of the Right Foot Through the Metatarsal Bones (Distal Surface)**

NOTE that the level of this cross section is shown in the diagram Figure 421.

Figs. 448, 449

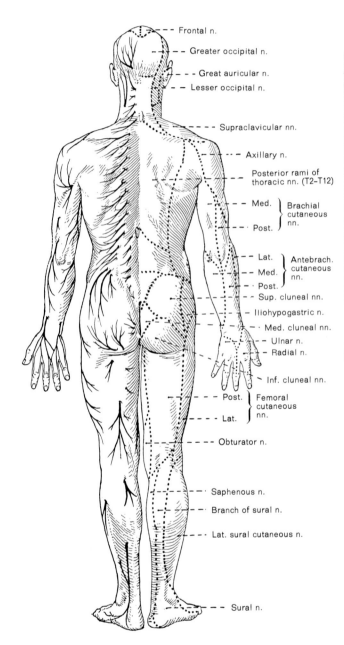

Frontal n.
Greater occipital n.
Great auricular n.
Lesser occipital n.
Supraclavicular nn.
Axillary n.
Posterior rami of thoracic nn. (T2–T12)
Med. } Brachial cutaneous nn.
Post.
Lat. } Antebrach. cutaneous nn.
Med.
Post.
Sup. cluneal nn.
Iliohypogastric n.
Med. cluneal nn.
Ulnar n.
Radial n.
Inf. cluneal nn.
Post. } Femoral cutaneous nn.
Lat.
Obturator n.
Saphenous n.
Branch of sural n.
Lat. sural cutaneous n.
Sural n.

**Fig. 450: The Cutaneous Nerve Surface Areas, Posterior Aspect of the Body**

NOTE that on the left side the position and course of the spinal cutaneous nerves are shown, while on the right side the surface areas of distribution are indicated. Demonstrated are the posterior surface zones for the cervical, thoracic, lumbar and sacral segmental nerves.

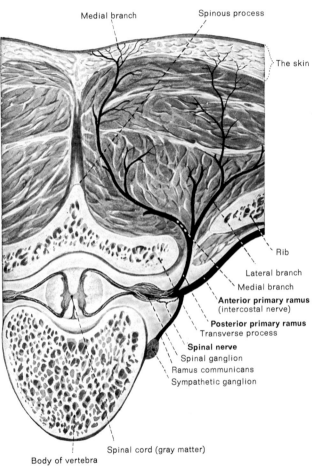

Medial branch
Spinous process
The skin
Rib
Lateral branch
Medial branch
**Anterior primary ramus** (intercostal nerve)
**Posterior primary ramus**
Transverse process
**Spinal nerve**
Spinal ganglion
Ramus communicans
Sympathetic ganglion
Spinal cord (gray matter)
Body of vertebra

**Fig. 451: The Branching of a Typical Spinal Nerve**

NOTE: 1) fibers from both dorsal and motor roots join to form a spinal nerve which soon divides into a posterior and an anterior primary ramus. The posterior primary ramus courses dorsally to innervate the muscles and skin of the back. The anterior primary ramus courses laterally and anteriorly around the body, to innervate the remainder of the segment.

2) the posterior primary divisions of typical spinal nerves are smaller in diameter than the anterior divisions, and each usually divides into medial and lateral branches which contain both motor and sensory fibers innervating structures in the back.

3) unlike the anterior primary divisions of the spinal nerves which join to form the cervical, brachial and lumbosacral plexuses, the peripheral nerves derived from posterior primary divisions, as a rule, do not intercommunicate and form plexuses. There is, however, some segmental overlap of the peripheral sensory fields, as occurs with anterior primary division nerves.

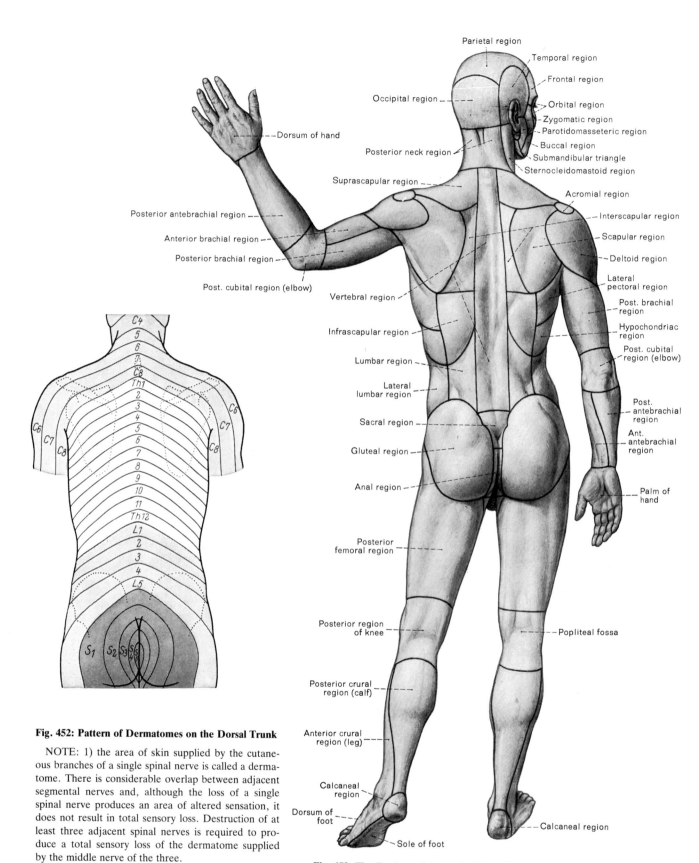

Parietal region
Temporal region
Frontal region
Occipital region
Orbital region
Zygomatic region
Parotidomasseteric region
Buccal region
Posterior neck region
Submandibular triangle
Sternocleidomastoid region
Dorsum of hand
Suprascapular region
Acromial region
Interscapular region
Posterior antebrachial region
Scapular region
Anterior brachial region
Deltoid region
Posterior brachial region
Lateral pectoral region
Post. cubital region (elbow)
Post. brachial region
Vertebral region
Hypochondriac region
Infrascapular region
Post. cubital region (elbow)
Lumbar region
Lateral lumbar region
Post. antebrachial region
Sacral region
Ant. antebrachial region
Gluteal region
Anal region
Palm of hand
Posterior femoral region
Posterior region of knee
Popliteal fossa
Posterior crural region (calf)
Anterior crural region (leg)
Calcaneal region
Dorsum of foot
Calcaneal region
Sole of foot

$C4$
5
6
7
$C8$
$Th1$
2
3
4
5
6
7
8
9
10
11
$Th12$
$L1$
2
3
4
$L5$
$C6$
$C7$
$C8$
$C6$
$C7$
$C8$
$S1$ $S2$ $S3$ $S4$ $S5$

**Fig. 452: Pattern of Dermatomes on the Dorsal Trunk**

NOTE: 1) the area of skin supplied by the cutaneous branches of a single spinal nerve is called a dermatome. There is considerable overlap between adjacent segmental nerves and, although the loss of a single spinal nerve produces an area of altered sensation, it does not result in total sensory loss. Destruction of at least three adjacent spinal nerves is required to produce a total sensory loss of the dermatome supplied by the middle nerve of the three.

2) mapping of skin areas affected by herpes zoster (shingles) has also allowed the mapping of dermatomes. Another method is the method of "remaining sensibility". In the latter, dermatome areas are established after the destruction of several roots above and below the intact root whose dermatome is being studied.

**Fig. 453: The Regions of the Body: Posterior View**

NOTE: the posterior aspect of the head, trunk and limbs is subdivided into many topographic regions to allow more exact anatomical localization and communication. Although the boundaries between the regions are somewhat arbitrary, it can be observed that the regions assume the names of bony structures, muscles, organs, joints and orifices comparable to those observed on the anterior aspect of the body (Figure 7).

Figs. 452, 453

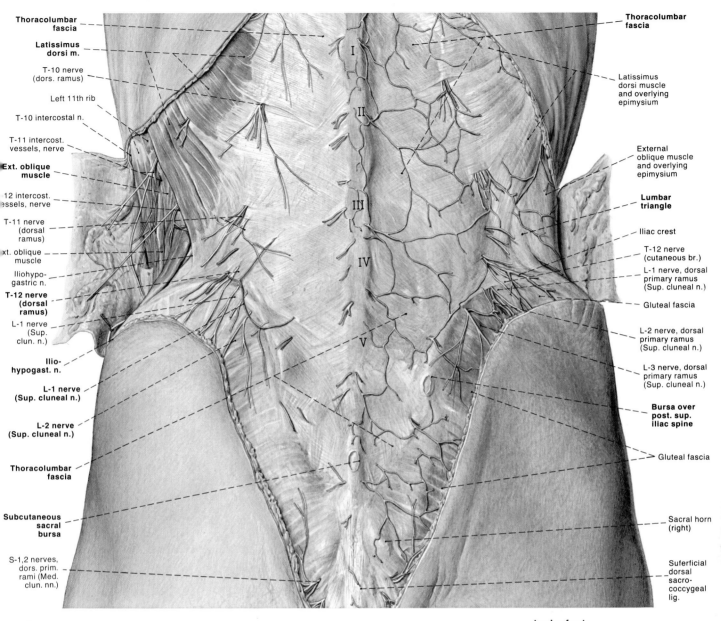

Thoracolumbar fascia
Latissimus dorsi m.
T-10 nerve (dors. ramus)
Left 11th rib
T-10 intercostal n.
T-11 intercost. vessels, nerve
Ext. oblique muscle
12 intercost. essels, nerve
T-11 nerve (dorsal ramus)
xt. oblique muscle
Iliohypo-gastric n.
T-12 nerve (dorsal ramus)
L-1 nerve (Sup. clun. n.)
Ilio-hypogast. n.
L-1 nerve (Sup. cluneal n.)
L-2 nerve (Sup. cluneal n.)
Thoracolumbar fascia
Subcutaneous sacral bursa
S-1,2 nerves, dors. prim. rami (Med. clun. nn.)

Thoracolumbar fascia
Latissimus dorsi muscle and overlying epimysium
External oblique muscle and overlying epimysium
Lumbar triangle
Iliac crest
T-12 nerve (cutaneous br.)
L-1 nerve, dorsal primary ramus (Sup. cluneal n.)
Gluteal fascia
L-2 nerve, dorsal primary ramus (Sup. cluneal n.)
L-3 nerve, dorsal primary ramus (Sup. cluneal n.)
Bursa over post. sup. iliac spine
Gluteal fascia
Sacral horn (right)
Suferficial dorsal sacro-coccygeal lig.

I
II
III
IV
V

Fig. 454: The Lumbosacral Region of the Back, Superficial View

NOTE that the spinous processes of the five lumbar vertebrae are numbered and that the superficial vessels and nerves penetrate the thoracolumbar fascia. Observe the lumbar triangle (labeled on the right) which is bounded by the crest of the ilium and the external oblique and latissimus dorsi muscles (see also Figure 456).

Fig. 455: Cross Section of Back, Lumbar Region

NOTE: the sacrospinalis muscle is ensheathed by the thick lumbar part of the thoracolumbar fascia which attaches medially to the spinous and transverse processes of the lumbar vertebrae, and which becomes continuous laterally with the aponeuroses and fasciae of the latissimus dorsi and anterior abdominal muscles.

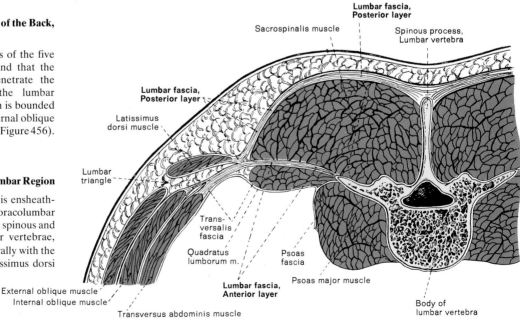

Lumbar fascia, Posterior layer
Sacrospinalis muscle
Spinous process, Lumbar vertebra
Lumbar fascia, Posterior layer
Latissimus dorsi muscle
Lumbar triangle
Trans-versalis fascia
Quadratus lumborum m.
Psoas fascia
Lumbar fascia, Anterior layer
Psoas major muscle
External oblique muscle
Internal oblique muscle
Transversus abdominis muscle
Body of lumbar vertebra

Figs. 454, 455    VI

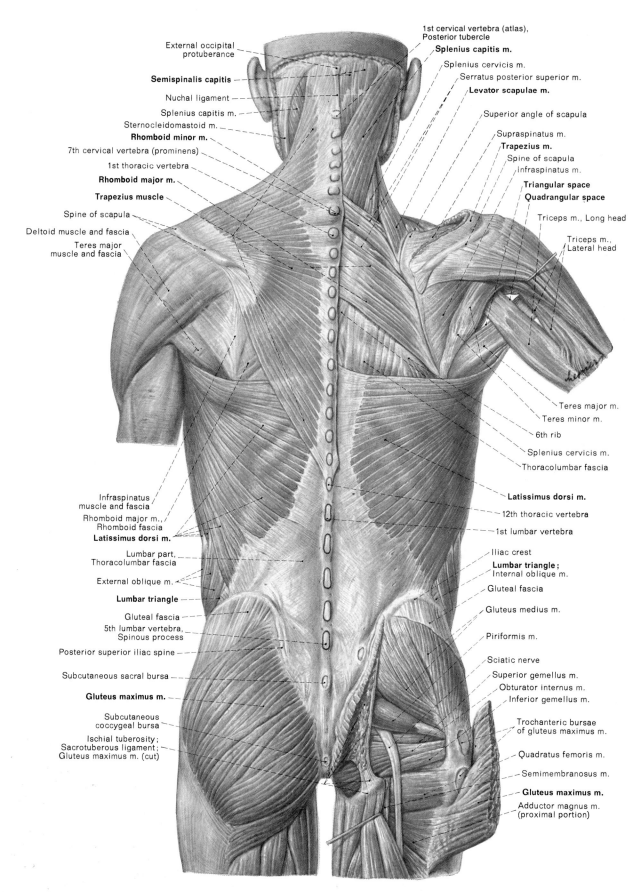

**Fig. 456: Muscles of the Posterior Neck, Shoulder, Back and Gluteal Region**

NOTE that the most superficial layer of back muscles includes the latissimus dorsi and trapezius. Beneath the trapezius, observe the levator scapulae and rhomboid major and minor muscles attaching along the vertebral border of the scapula. In the neck, the splenius capitis and semispinalis capitis muscles lie directly under the trapezius.

Fig. 456

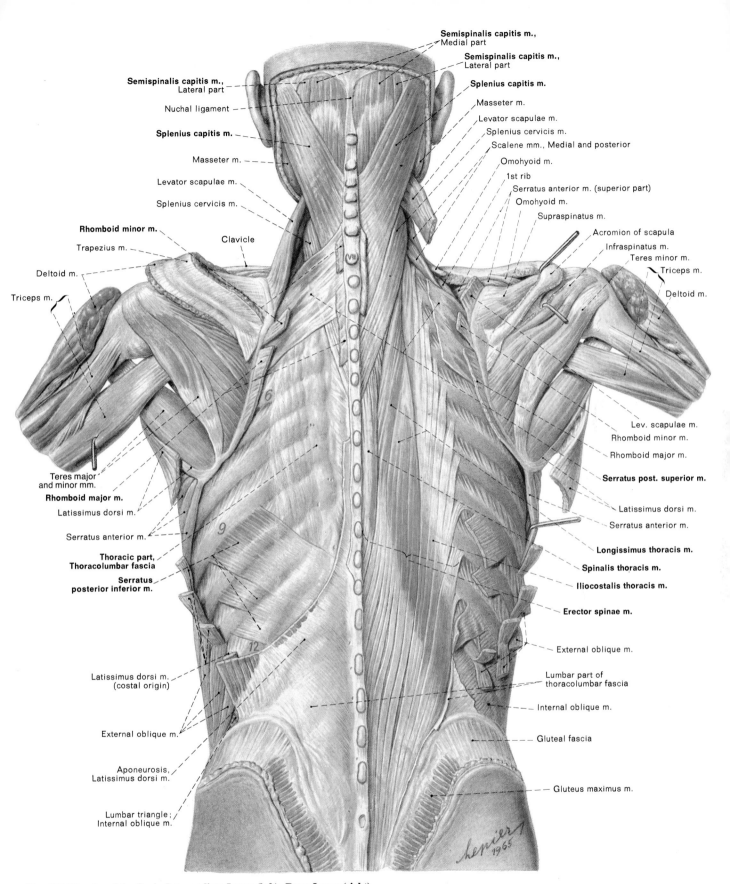

**Semispinalis capitis m.,** Medial part

**Semispinalis capitis m.,** Lateral part

**Splenius capitis m.**

Masseter m.

Levator scapulae m.

Splenius cervicis m.

Scalene mm., Medial and posterior

Omohyoid m.

1st rib

Serratus anterior m. (superior part)

Omohyoid m.

Supraspinatus m.

Acromion of scapula

Infraspinatus m.

Teres minor m.

Triceps m.

Deltoid m.

Lev. scapulae m.

Rhomboid minor m.

Rhomboid major m.

**Serratus post. superior m.**

Latissimus dorsi m.

Serratus anterior m.

**Longissimus thoracis m.**

**Spinalis thoracis m.**

**Iliocostalis thoracis m.**

**Erector spinae m.**

External oblique m.

Lumbar part of thoracolumbar fascia

Internal oblique m.

Gluteal fascia

Gluteus maximus m.

**Semispinalis capitis m.,** Lateral part

Nuchal ligament

**Splenius capitis m.**

Masseter m.

Levator scapulae m.

Splenius cervicis m.

**Rhomboid minor m.**

Trapezius m.

Clavicle

Deltoid m.

Triceps m.

Teres major and minor mm.

**Rhomboid major m.**

Latissimus dorsi m.

Serratus anterior m.

**Thoracic part, Thoracolumbar fascia**

**Serratus posterior inferior m.**

Latissimus dorsi m. (costal origin)

External oblique m.

Aponeurosis, Latissimus dorsi m.

Lumbar triangle; Internal oblique m.

**Fig. 457: Muscles of the Back: Intermediate Layer (left), Deep Layer (right)**

NOTE: 1) *on the left side* the superficial back muscles (trapezius and latissimus dorsi) have been cut, as have the rhomboid major and minor which attach the vertebral border of the scapula to the vertebral column. Observe the underlying serratus posterior superior and serratus posterior inferior muscles.

2) *on the right side* the serratus posterior muscles and the thoracolumbar fascia have been removed, revealing the erector spinae muscle (formerly called the sacrospinalis muscle).

3) *in the neck* the splenius cervicis, splenius capitis and semispinalis capitis underlie the trapezius.

Fig. 457    VI

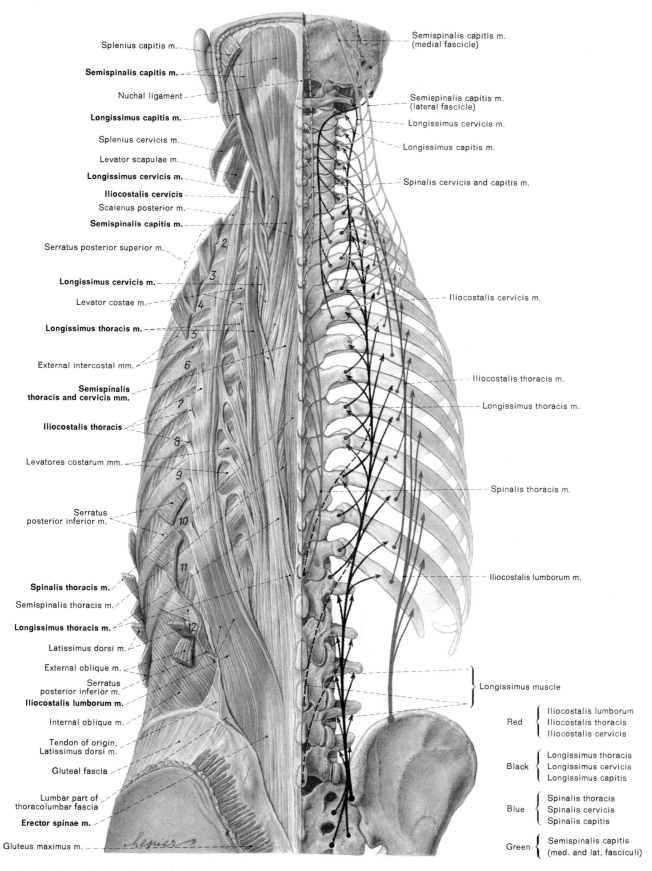

Splenius capitis m.
**Semispinalis capitis m.**
Nuchal ligament
**Longissimus capitis m.**
Splenius cervicis m.
Levator scapulae m.
**Longissimus cervicis m.**
**Iliocostalis cervicis**
Scalenus posterior m.
**Semispinalis capitis m.**
Serratus posterior superior m.
**Longissimus cervicis m.**
Levator costae m.
**Longissimus thoracis m.**
External intercostal mm.
**Semispinalis thoracis and cervicis mm.**
**Iliocostalis thoracis**
Levatores costarum mm.
Serratus posterior inferior m.
**Spinalis thoracis m.**
Semispinalis thoracis m.
**Longissimus thoracis m.**
Latissimus dorsi m.
External oblique m.
Serratus posterior inferior m.
**Iliocostalis lumborum m.**
Internal oblique m.
Tendon of origin, Latissimus dorsi m.
Gluteal fascia
Lumbar part of thoracolumbar fascia
**Erector spinae m.**
Gluteus maximus m.

Semispinalis capitis m. (medial fascicle)
Semispinalis capitis m. (lateral fascicle)
Longissimus cervicis m.
Longissimus capitis m.
Spinalis cervicis and capitis m.
Iliocostalis cervicis m.
Iliocostalis thoracis m.
Longissimus thoracis m.
Spinalis thoracis m.
Iliocostalis lumborum m.
Longissimus muscle

| Red | Iliocostalis lumborum<br>Iliocostalis thoracis<br>Iliocostalis cervicis |
| Black | Longissimus thoracis<br>Longissimus cervicis<br>Longissimus capitis |
| Blue | Spinalis thoracis<br>Spinalis cervicis<br>Spinalis capitis |
| Green | Semispinalis capitis<br>(med. and lat, fasciculi) |

**Fig. 458: Deep Muscles of the Back and Neck: the Erector Spinae Muscle**

NOTE: 1) *on the left,* the erector spinae (sacrospinalis) muscles is separated into its iliocostalis, longissimus and spinalis portions. In the neck observe the semispinalis capitis which has both medial and lateral fascicles. The semispinalis cervicis and thoracis extend inferiorly from above, and lie deep to the sacrospinalis layer of musculature.

2) *on the right,* all of the muscles have been removed and their attachments have been diagrammed by means of colored lines.

Fig. 458

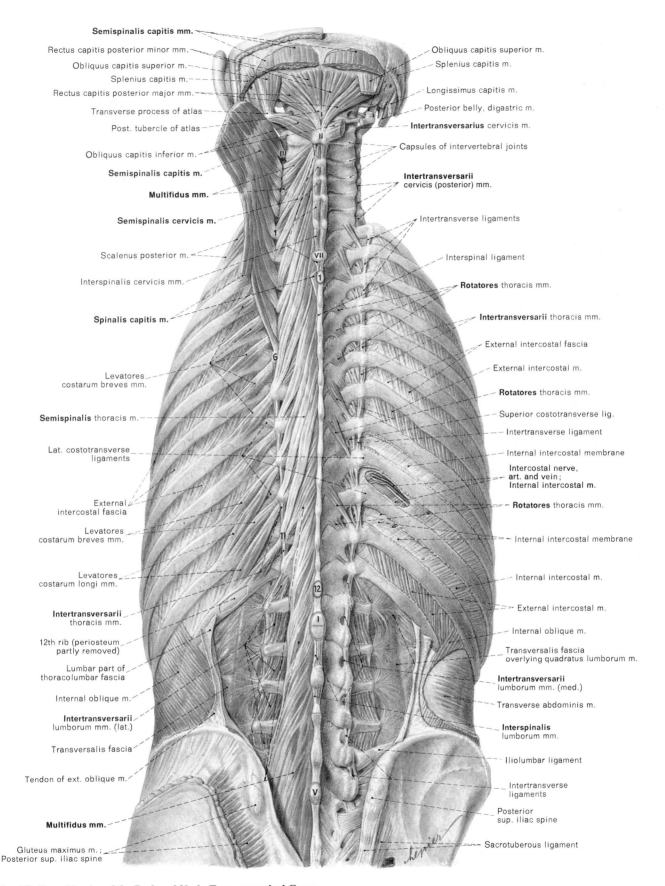

Semispinalis capitis mm.
Rectus capitis posterior minor mm.
Obliquus capitis superior m.
Splenius capitis m.
Rectus capitis posterior major mm.
Transverse process of atlas
Post. tubercle of atlas
Obliquus capitis inferior m.
Semispinalis capitis m.
Multifidus mm.
Semispinalis cervicis m.
Scalenus posterior m.
Interspinalis cervicis mm.
Spinalis capitis m.
Levatores costarum breves mm.
Semispinalis thoracis m.
Lat. costotransverse ligaments
External intercostal fascia
Levatores costarum breves mm.
Levatores costarum longi mm.
Intertransversarii thoracis mm.
12th rib (periosteum partly removed)
Lumbar part of thoracolumbar fascia
Internal oblique m.
Intertransversarii lumborum mm. (lat.)
Transversalis fascia
Tendon of ext. oblique m.
Multifidus mm.
Gluteus maximus m.; Posterior sup. iliac spine

Obliquus capitis superior m.
Splenius capitis m.
Longissimus capitis m.
Posterior belly, digastric m.
Intertransversarius cervicis m.
Capsules of intervertebral joints
Intertransversarii cervicis (posterior) mm.
Intertransverse ligaments
Interspinal ligament
Rotatores thoracis mm.
Intertransversarii thoracis mm.
External intercostal fascia
External intercostal m.
Rotatores thoracis mm.
Superior costotransverse lig.
Intertransverse ligament
Internal intercostal membrane
Intercostal nerve, art. and vein; Internal intercostal m.
Rotatores thoracis mm.
Internal intercostal membrane
Internal intercostal m.
External intercostal m.
Internal oblique m.
Transversalis fascia overlying quadratus lumborum m.
Intertransversarii lumborum mm. (med.)
Transverse abdominis m.
Interspinalis lumborum mm.
Iliolumbar ligament
Intertransverse ligaments
Posterior sup. iliac spine
Sacrotuberous ligament

**Fig. 459: Deep Muscles of the Back and Neck: Transversospinal Group**

NOTE: 1) the transversospinal groups of muscles lie deep to the erector spinae muscles and generally extend between the transverse processes of the vertebrae to the spinous processes of more superior vertebrae. Their actions extend the vertebral column, or upon acting individually and on one side, they bend and rotate the vertebrae.

2) within this group of muscles are the semispinalis (thoracis, cervicis, and capitis), the multifidus, the rotatores (lumborum, thoracis, cervicis), the interspinales (lumborum, thoracis, cervicis) and the intertransversarii.

Fig. 459    **VI**

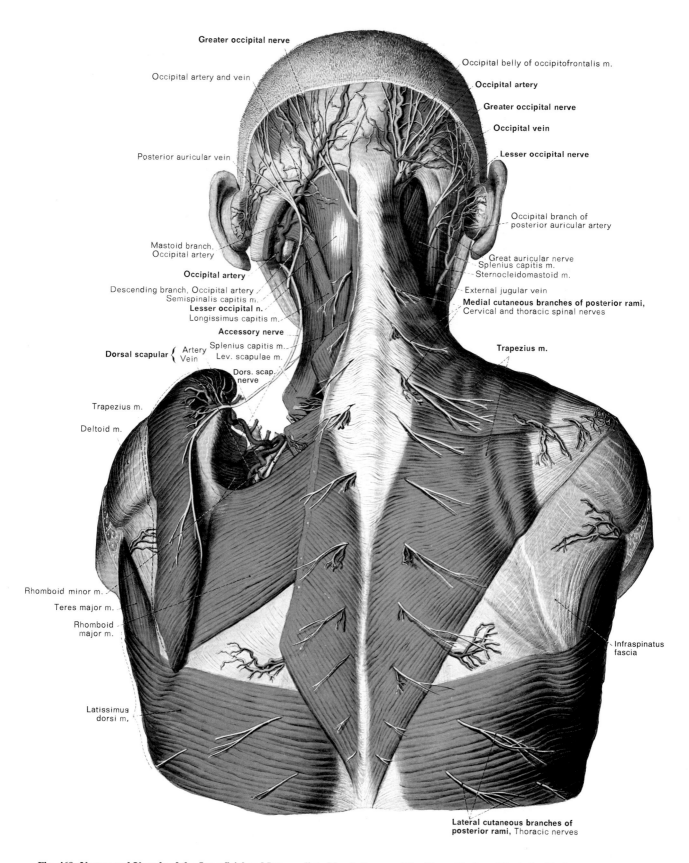

**Greater occipital nerve**

Occipital artery and vein

Posterior auricular vein

Mastoid branch,
Occipital artery

**Occipital artery**

Descending branch, Occipital artery
Semispinalis capitis m.
**Lesser occipital n.**
Longissimus capitis m.

**Accessory nerve**

Splenius capitis m.
**Dorsal scapular** { Artery / Vein } Lev. scapulae m.

Dors. scap.
nerve

Trapezius m.

Deltoid m.

Rhomboid minor m.
Teres major m.
Rhomboid
major m.

Latissimus
dorsi m.

Occipital belly of occipitofrontalis m.

**Occipital artery**

**Greater occipital nerve**

**Occipital vein**

**Lesser occipital nerve**

Occipital branch of
posterior auricular artery

Great auricular nerve
Splenius capitis m.
Sternocleidomastoid m.

External jugular vein
**Medial cutaneous branches of posterior rami,**
Cervical and thoracic spinal nerves

**Trapezius m.**

Infraspinatus
fascia

**Lateral cutaneous branches of
posterior rami, Thoracic nerves**

**Fig. 460: Nerves and Vessels of the Superficial and Intermediate Muscle Layers of the Upper Back and Posterior Neck**

NOTE: 1) the segmental distribution of the cutaneous branches of the posterior primary rami of the cervical and thoracic nerves over the posterior neck and back. Observe the accessory nerve (XI) as it descends to innervate the trapezius and sternocleidomastoid muscles.

2) the greater occipital nerve, which is a sensory nerve, ascending to the posterior scalp. It derives from the posterior primary ramus of the C-2 spinal nerve and is accompanied in its course by the occipital artery and vein. Observe also the lesser occipital nerve which courses to the lateral posterior scalp and which arises from the anterior primary ramus of C-2.

3) the dorsal scapular nerve, artery and vein which course beneath the levator scapulae and the rhomboid muscles.

Fig. 460

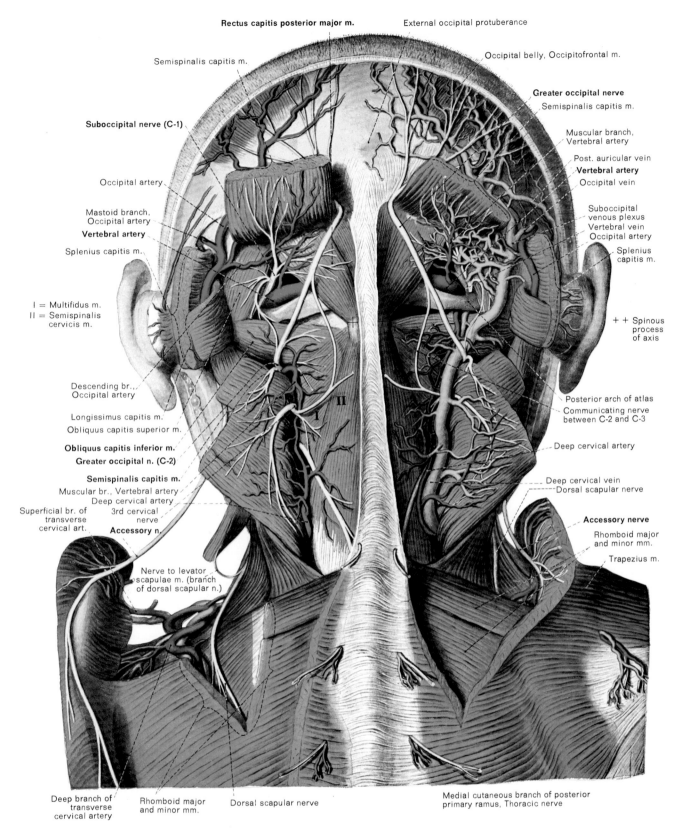

Rectus capitis posterior major m.

External occipital protuberance

Semispinalis capitis m.

Occipital belly, Occipitofrontal m.

Greater occipital nerve

Semispinalis capitis m.

Suboccipital nerve (C-1)

Muscular branch, Vertebral artery

Post. auricular vein

Vertebral artery

Occipital vein

Occipital artery

Suboccipital venous plexus
Vertebral vein
Occipital artery

Mastoid branch, Occipital artery

Vertebral artery

Splenius capitis m.

Splenius capitis m.

I = Multifidus m.
II = Semispinalis cervicis m.

++ Spinous process of axis

Descending br., Occipital artery

Posterior arch of atlas
Communicating nerve between C-2 and C-3

Longissimus capitis m.
Obliquus capitis superior m.

Deep cervical artery

Obliquus capitis inferior m.
Greater occipital n. (C-2)

Semispinalis capitis m.
Muscular br., Vertebral artery
Deep cervical artery
3rd cervical nerve
Accessory n.

Deep cervical vein
Dorsal scapular nerve

Accessory nerve

Superficial br. of transverse cervical art.

Rhomboid major and minor mm.

Trapezius m.

Nerve to levator scapulae m. (branch of dorsal scapular n.)

Deep branch of transverse cervical artery

Rhomboid major and minor mm.

Dorsal scapular nerve

Medial cutaneous branch of posterior primary ramus, Thoracic nerve

**Fig. 461: The Deep Vessels and Nerves of the Suboccipital Region and Upper Back; the Suboccipital Triangle**

NOTE: 1) the suboccipital triangle lies directly beneath the semispinalis capitis muscle and is bounded by the rectus capitis posterior major, obliquus capitis superior and the obliquus capitis inferior.

2) the vertebral artery crosses (from lateral to medial) the suboccipital triangle, while the suboccipital nerve (posterior primary ramus of C-1) emerges through the triangle to distribute motor innervation to the three muscles which bound the triangle, as well as the rectus capitis posterior minor and the overlying semispinalis capitis muscle.

3) the greater occipital nerve (posterior primary ramus of C-2) is a sensory nerve which makes its appearance caudal to the obliquus capitis inferior, and then courses medially and superiorly to become subcutaneous just lateral and below the external occipital protuberance.

Fig. 461    VI

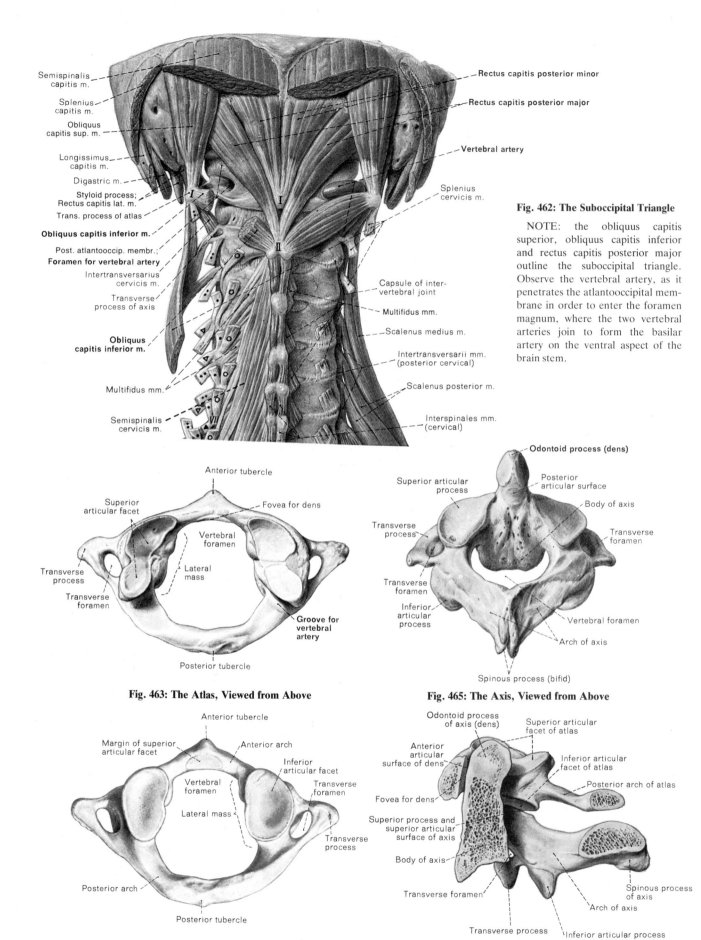

Semispinalis capitis m.
Splenius capitis m.
Obliquus capitis sup. m.
Longissimus capitis m.
Digastric m.
Styloid process; Rectus capitis lat. m.
Trans. process of atlas
**Obliquus capitis inferior m.**
Post. atlantooccip. membr.;
**Foramen for vertebral artery**
Intertransversarius cervicis m.
Transverse process of axis
**Obliquus capitis inferior m.**
Multifidus mm.
Semispinalis cervicis m.

Rectus capitis posterior minor
Rectus capitis posterior major
Vertebral artery
Splenius cervicis m.
Capsule of inter-vertebral joint
Multifidus mm.
Scalenus medius m.
Intertransversarii mm. (posterior cervical)
Scalenus posterior m.
Interspinales mm. (cervical)

**Fig. 462: The Suboccipital Triangle**

NOTE: the obliquus capitis superior, obliquus capitis inferior and rectus capitis posterior major outline the suboccipital triangle. Observe the vertebral artery, as it penetrates the atlantooccipital membrane in order to enter the foramen magnum, where the two vertebral arteries join to form the basilar artery on the ventral aspect of the brain stem.

Anterior tubercle
Superior articular facet
Fovea for dens
Vertebral foramen
Lateral mass
Transverse process
Transverse foramen
Groove for vertebral artery
Posterior tubercle

**Fig. 463: The Atlas, Viewed from Above**

Odontoid process (dens)
Superior articular process
Posterior articular surface
Body of axis
Transverse process
Transverse foramen
Transverse foramen
Inferior articular process
Vertebral foramen
Arch of axis
Spinous process (bifid)

**Fig. 465: The Axis, Viewed from Above**

Anterior tubercle
Margin of superior articular facet
Anterior arch
Inferior articular facet
Transverse foramen
Vertebral foramen
Lateral mass
Transverse process
Posterior arch
Posterior tubercle

**Fig. 464: The Atlas, Caudal View**

Odontoid process of axis (dens)
Superior articular facet of atlas
Anterior articular surface of dens
Inferior articular facet of atlas
Posterior arch of atlas
Fovea for dens
Superior process and superior articular surface of axis
Body of axis
Spinous process of axis
Transverse foramen
Arch of axis
Transverse process
Inferior articular process

**Fig. 466: Articulated Atlas and Axis, Median Sagittal Section**

Figs. 462–466

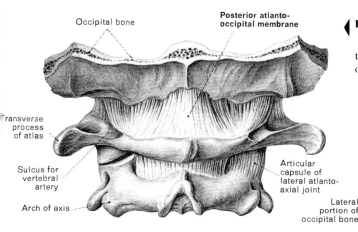

Occipital bone — Posterior atlanto-occipital membrane

Transverse process of atlas

Sulcus for vertebral artery

Arch of axis

Articular capsule of lateral atlanto-axial joint

**Fig. 468: Articulations of Occipital Bone and First Three Cervical Vertebrae (Anterior View)**

NOTE: the anterior atlantooccipital membrane extending between the occipital bone and the anterior arch of the atlas and continuing laterally to join the articular capsules. Also observe the anterior longitudinal ligament.

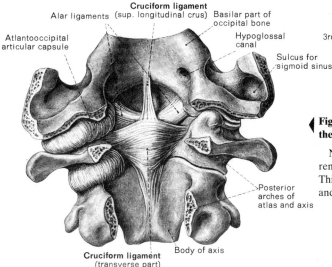

Cruciform ligament (sup. longitudinal crus)

Alar ligaments

Atlantooccipital articular capsule

Basilar part of occipital bone

Hypoglossal canal

Sulcus for sigmoid sinus

Posterior arches of atlas and axis

Cruciform ligament (transverse part)

Body of axis

**Fig. 470: Median Atlantoaxial Joint (from Above)**

NOTE: that the odontoid process (dens) of the axis articulates with the anterior arch of the atlas, thereby forming the median atlantoaxial joint, and that the thick strong transverse ligament (part of the cruciform ligament) of the atlas retains the dens on its posterior surface.

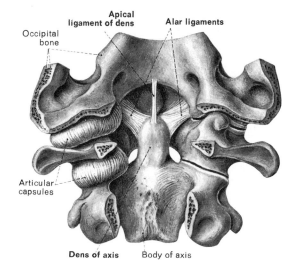

Apical ligament of dens

Alar ligaments

Occipital bone

Articular capsules

Dens of axis    Body of axis

**Fig. 467: Atlantooccipital and Atlantoaxial Joints (Posterior View)**

NOTE: the posterior atlantoccipital membrane extends from the posterior margin of the foramen magnum to the upper border of the posterior arch of the atlas.

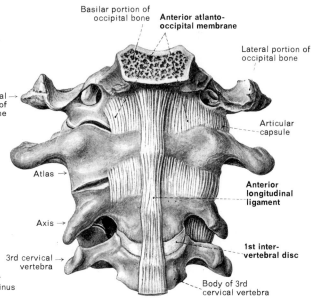

Basilar portion of occipital bone

Anterior atlanto-occipital membrane

Lateral portion of occipital bone

Lateral portion of occipital bone

Articular capsule

Atlas →

Anterior longitudinal ligament

Axis →

1st inter-vertebral disc

3rd cervical vertebra →

Body of 3rd cervical vertebra

**Fig. 469: The Atlantooccipital and Atlantoaxial Joints Showing the Cruciform Ligament (Posterior View)**

NOTE: the posterior arches of the atlas and axis have been removed and the cruciform ligament is seen from this posterior view. This ligament consists of the transverse ligament (see Figure 470) and the longitudinal fascicles extending superiorly and inferiorly.

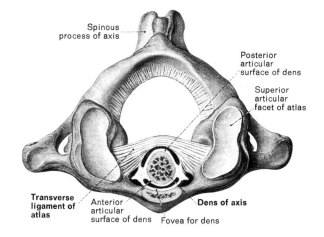

Spinous process of axis

Posterior articular surface of dens

Superior articular facet of atlas

Transverse ligament of atlas

Anterior articular surface of dens

Dens of axis

Fovea for dens

**Fig. 471: The Alar and Apical Ligaments (Posterior View)**

NOTE: this figure's orientation is similar to Figure 469. The posterior arches of the atlas and axis have been removed as well as the cruciform ligament (both transverse and longitudinal parts). This reveals the odontoid process of the axis, which is attached superiorly to the occipital bone by the two alar ligaments and the apical ligament of the dens. These ligaments tend to limit lateral rotation of the skull.

Figs. 467–471   VI

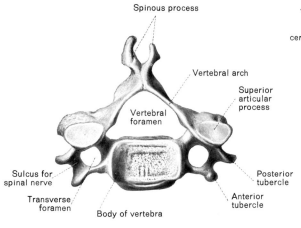

Fig. 473: Median section of Atlantooccipital Region

NOTE: the relationships from anterior to posterior of the following structures: the anterior arch of the atlas, the joint between it and the dens, the dens, the "joint" between the dens and the transverse ligament of the atlas, the tectorial membrane and finally, the dura mater covering the spinal cord.

Fig. 472: The Tectorial Membrane, Dorsal View

NOTE: the tectorial membrane is a broadened upward extension of the posterior longitudinal ligament and attaches the axis to the occipital bone (see also Figure 473). This membrane is seen to cover the posterior surface of the odontoid process and lies dorsal to the cruciform ligament, covering it as well.

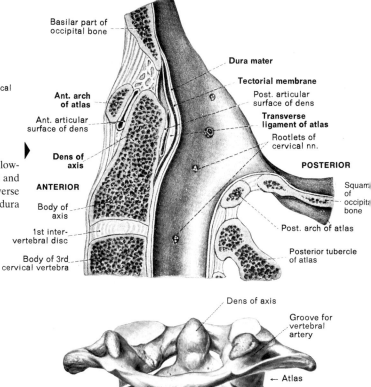

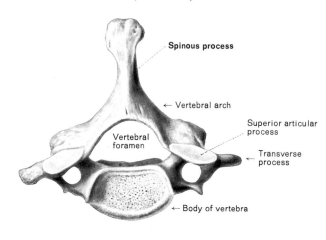

Fig. 474: Fifth Cervical Vertebra (from Above)

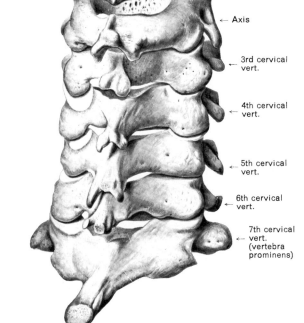

Fig. 476: The Cervical Spinal Column (Dorsal)

NOTE: while flexion and extension of the head are performed at the atlantooccipital joint, rotation of the head is the result of rotation of the atlas on the axis.

Fig. 475: Seventh Cervical Vertebra (from Above)

NOTE: the 7th cervical vertebra, being transitional between the cervical and thoracic vertebrae, has a transverse foramen similar to the cervical and a large spinous process similar to the thoracic. The latter gives it the name vertebra prominens.

Figs. 472–476

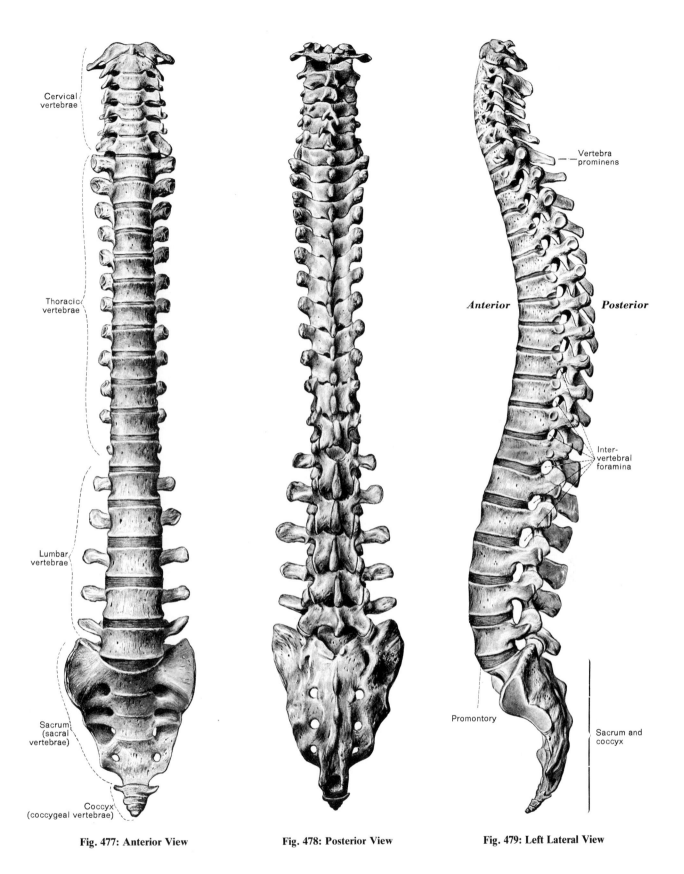

**Fig. 477: Anterior View**  **Fig. 478: Posterior View**  **Fig. 479: Left Lateral View**

**Figs.: 477, 478 and 479: The Vertebral Column, Including the Sacrum and Coccyx**

NOTE: 1) the vertebral column generally consists of 7 cervical, 12 thoracic and 5 lumbar vertebrae and the sacrum and coccyx, thus, 26 bones in all. Its principal functions are to assist in the maintenance of the erect posture in man, to encase and protect the spinal cord and to allow attachments of the musculature important for movements of the head and trunk.

2) from a dorsal or ventral view, the normal spinal column is straight. When viewed from the side, the spinal column presents two ventrally convex curvatures (cervical and lumbar) and two dorsally convex curvatures (thoracic and sacral).

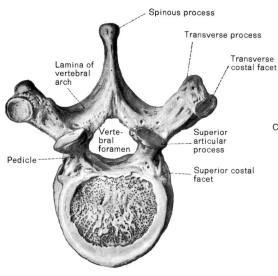

**Fig. 480: Sixth Thoracic Vertebra (from Above)**

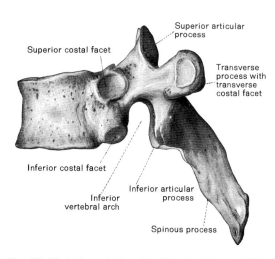

**Fig. 481: Sixth Thoracic Vertebra (from Left Lateral Side)**

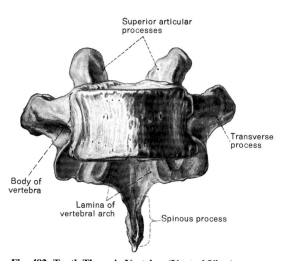

**Fig. 482: Tenth Thoracic Vertebra (Ventral View)**

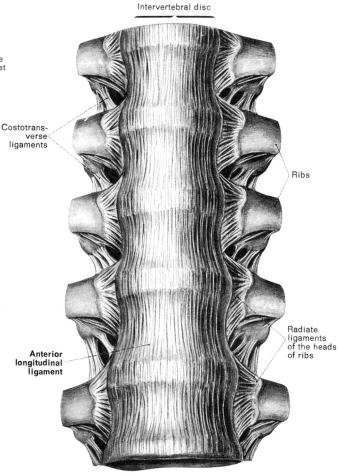

**Fig. 483: Anterior Longitudinal Ligament (Ventral View)**

NOTE: the anterior longitudinal ligament extends from the axis to the sacrum along the anterior aspect of the bodies of the vertebrae and the intervertebral discs to which it is firmly attached. Its longitudinal fibers are white and glistening.

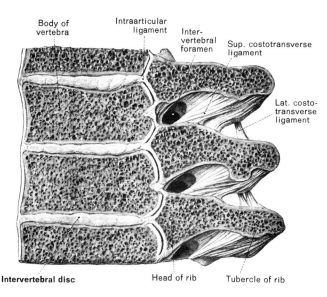

**Fig. 484: Sagittal Section (at an Angle) through Spinal Column Showing Costovertebral Articulations**

NOTE: the intervertebral discs, the intraarticular and costotransverse ligaments, and the intervertebral foramina which transmit the spinal nerves.

Figs. 480–484

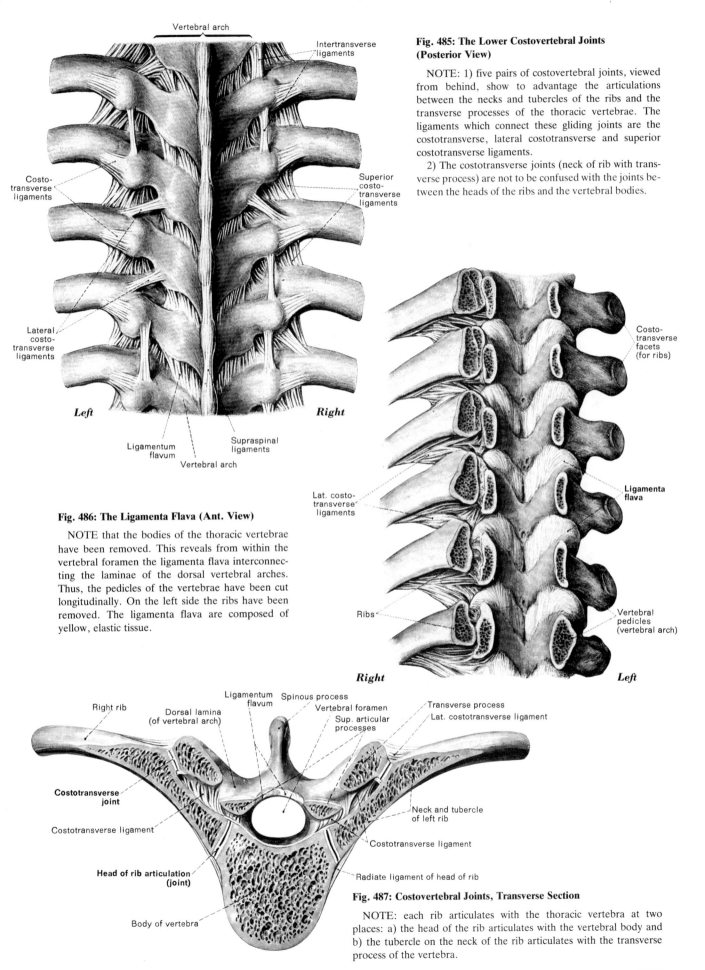

**Fig. 485: The Lower Costovertebral Joints (Posterior View)**

NOTE: 1) five pairs of costovertebral joints, viewed from behind, show to advantage the articulations between the necks and tubercles of the ribs and the transverse processes of the thoracic vertebrae. The ligaments which connect these gliding joints are the costotransverse, lateral costotransverse and superior costotransverse ligaments.

2) The costotransverse joints (neck of rib with transverse process) are not to be confused with the joints between the heads of the ribs and the vertebral bodies.

**Fig. 486: The Ligamenta Flava (Ant. View)**

NOTE that the bodies of the thoracic vertebrae have been removed. This reveals from within the vertebral foramen the ligamenta flava interconnecting the laminae of the dorsal vertebral arches. Thus, the pedicles of the vertebrae have been cut longitudinally. On the left side the ribs have been removed. The ligamenta flava are composed of yellow, elastic tissue.

**Fig. 487: Costovertebral Joints, Transverse Section**

NOTE: each rib articulates with the thoracic vertebra at two places: a) the head of the rib articulates with the vertebral body and b) the tubercle on the neck of the rib articulates with the transverse process of the vertebra.

Figs. 485, 486, 487    VI

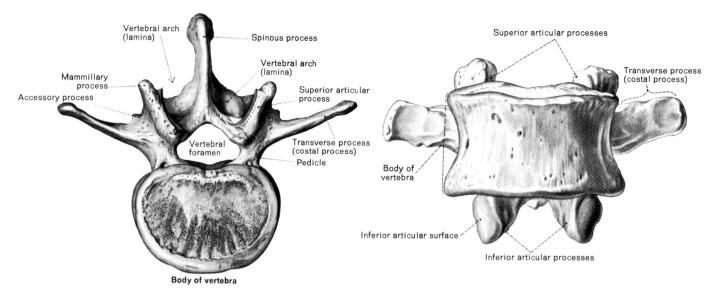

**Fig. 488: Lumbar Vertebra (Cranial View)**

NOTE: the large bodies characteristic of the lumbar vertebrae.

**Fig. 489: Lumbar Vertebra (Anterior View)**

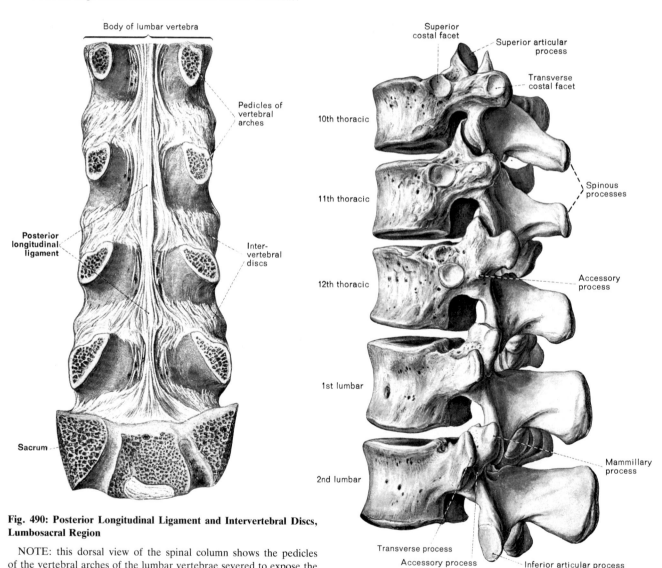

**Fig. 490: Posterior Longitudinal Ligament and Intervertebral Discs, Lumbosacral Region**

NOTE: this dorsal view of the spinal column shows the pedicles of the vertebral arches of the lumbar vertebrae severed to expose the posterior longitudinal ligament coursing along the posterior aspect of the bodies of the lumbar vertebrae within the vertebral canal. This ligament extends from the axis (where it joins the tectorial membrane) to the sacrum, which is shown in this figure.

**Fig. 491: Last Three Thoracic and First Two Lumbar Vertebrae (Lateral View)**

Figs. 488–491

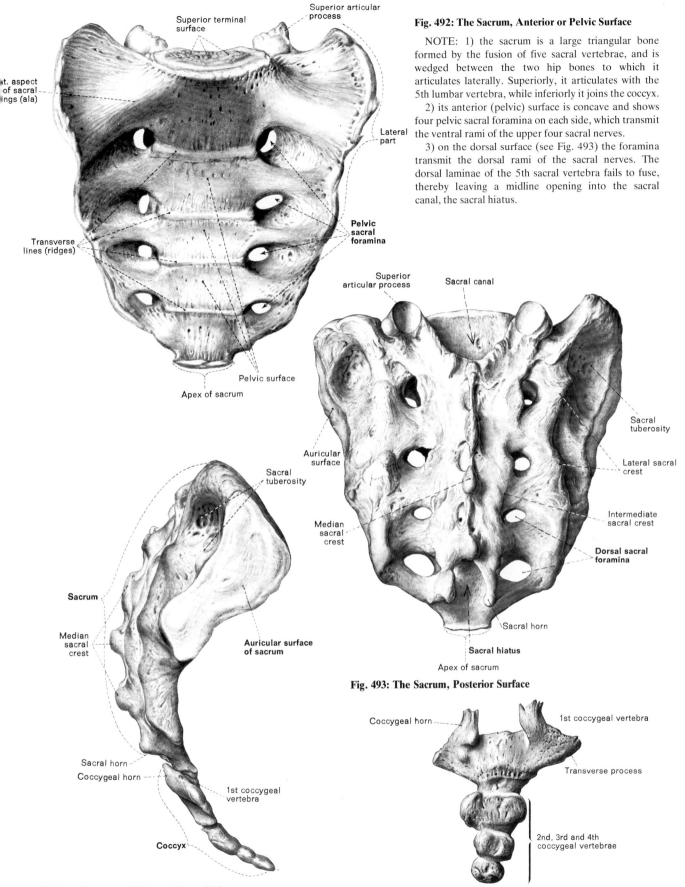

Superior terminal surface

Superior articular process

t. aspect of sacral ings (ala)

Lateral part

Transverse lines (ridges)

Pelvic sacral foramina

Pelvic surface

Apex of sacrum

**Fig. 492: The Sacrum, Anterior or Pelvic Surface**

NOTE: 1) the sacrum is a large triangular bone formed by the fusion of five sacral vertebrae, and is wedged between the two hip bones to which it articulates laterally. Superiorly, it articulates with the 5th lumbar vertebra, while inferiorly it joins the coccyx.

2) its anterior (pelvic) surface is concave and shows four pelvic sacral foramina on each side, which transmit the ventral rami of the upper four sacral nerves.

3) on the dorsal surface (see Fig. 493) the foramina transmit the dorsal rami of the sacral nerves. The dorsal laminae of the 5th sacral vertebra fails to fuse, thereby leaving a midline opening into the sacral canal, the sacral hiatus.

Superior articular process

Sacral canal

Auricular surface

Sacral tuberosity

Median sacral crest

Sacral tuberosity

Lateral sacral crest

Intermediate sacral crest

**Dorsal sacral foramina**

Sacral horn

**Sacral hiatus**

Apex of sacrum

**Fig. 493: The Sacrum, Posterior Surface**

**Sacrum**

Median sacral crest

**Auricular surface of sacrum**

Sacral horn

Coccygeal horn

1st coccygeal vertebra

**Coccyx**

Coccygeal horn

1st coccygeal vertebra

Transverse process

2nd, 3rd and 4th coccygeal vertebrae

**Fig. 494: The Sacrum and Coccyx, Lateral View**

NOTE: the auricular (ear-like) surface of the sacrum articulates with the iliac portion of the pelvis. Inferiorly, the sacral apex joins the coccyx.

**Fig. 495: The Coccyx, Dorsal View**

NOTE: this coccyx has 4 segments, but in many instances there are 3 or 5.

Figs. 492–495    VI

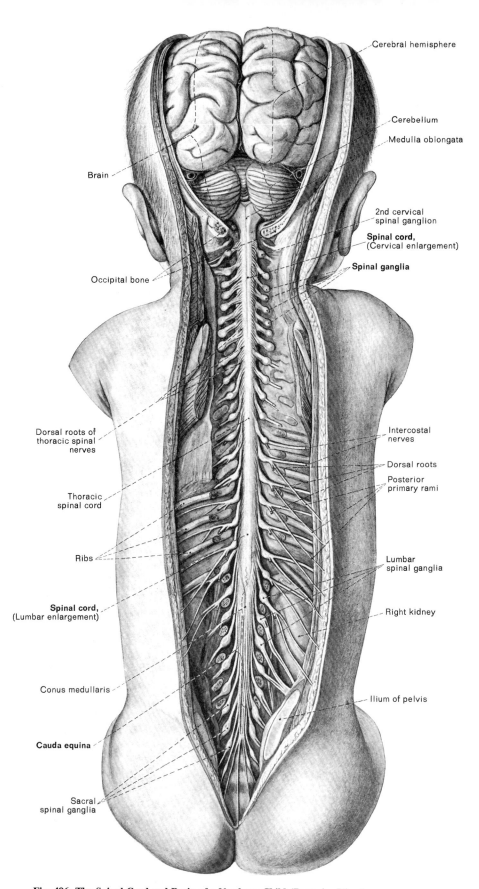

Cerebral hemisphere

Cerebellum

Medulla oblongata

Brain

2nd cervical
spinal ganglion

**Spinal cord,**
(Cervical enlargement)

**Spinal ganglia**

Occipital bone

Dorsal roots of
thoracic spinal
nerves

Intercostal
nerves

Dorsal roots

Posterior
primary rami

Thoracic
spinal cord

Ribs

Lumbar
spinal ganglia

**Spinal cord,**
(Lumbar enlargement)

Right kidney

Conus medullaris

Ilium of pelvis

**Cauda equina**

Sacral
spinal ganglia

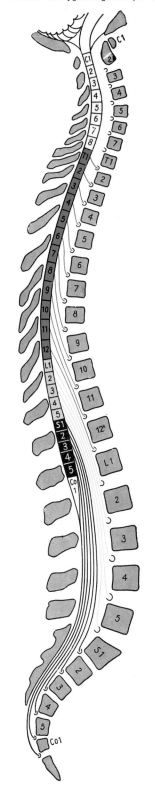

Yellow: Cervical segments (C1–C8)
Red: Thoracic segments (T1–T12)
Blue: Lumbar segments (L1–L5)
Black: Sacral segments (S1–S5)
White: Coccygeal segments (C1–C2)

**Fig. 496: The Spinal Cord and Brain of a Newborn Child (Posterior View)**

NOTE: 1) the central nervous system has been exposed by removal of the spinal column and dorsal cranium. The spinal ganglia have been dissected as well as their corresponding spinal nerves.

2) although in this dissection it appears as though the substance of the spinal cord terminates at about L-1, it is more usual in the newborn for the cord to end at about L-3 or L-4, thereby filling the spinal canal more completely than in the adult.

**Fig. 497: The Emerging Spinal Nerves and their Segments in the Adult**

NOTE: many spinal nerves travel considerable distances before leaving the vertebral canal in the adult.

Figs. 496, 497

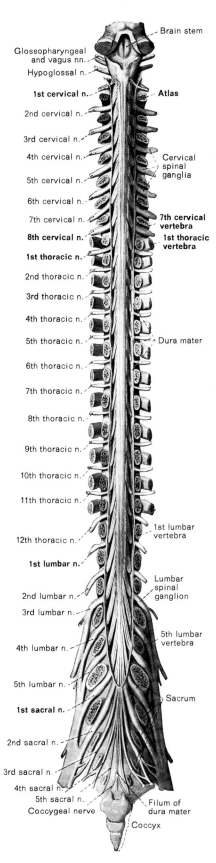

**Fig. 498: The Spinal Cord Within the Vertebral Canal (Dorsal View)**

NOTE: 1) the 1st cervical nerve emerges above the first vertebra and the 8th cervical nerve emerges below the 7th vertebra.

2) the cervical spinal cord is continuous above with the medulla oblongata of the brain stem.

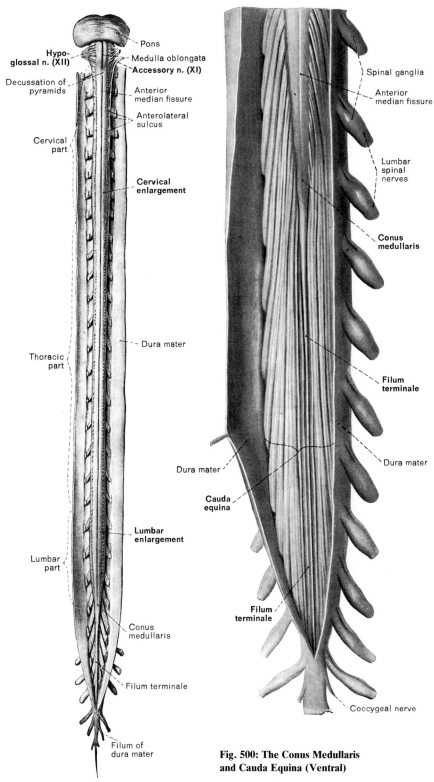

**Fig. 499: The Spinal Cord (Ventral View)**

NOTE: 1) the origin of the spinal portion of the accessory nerve (Cranial XI) arising from the cervical spinal cord and ascending to join the bulbar portion of that nerve.

2) the alignment of the rootlets of the hypoglossal nerve (Cranial XII) with the ventral roots of the spinal cord.

**Fig. 500: The Conus Medullaris and Cauda Equina (Ventral)**

NOTE: 1) the termination of the neural portion of the spinal cord at the conus medullaris, but its membranous continuation as the filum terminale which consists principally of pia mater.

2) the long (approx. 8 inches) cauda equina (horse's tail) consisting of the intravertebral portions of the lower spinal nerves.

3) prolongations of the dura mater continue to cover the spinal nerves for some distance as they enter the intervertebral foramina.

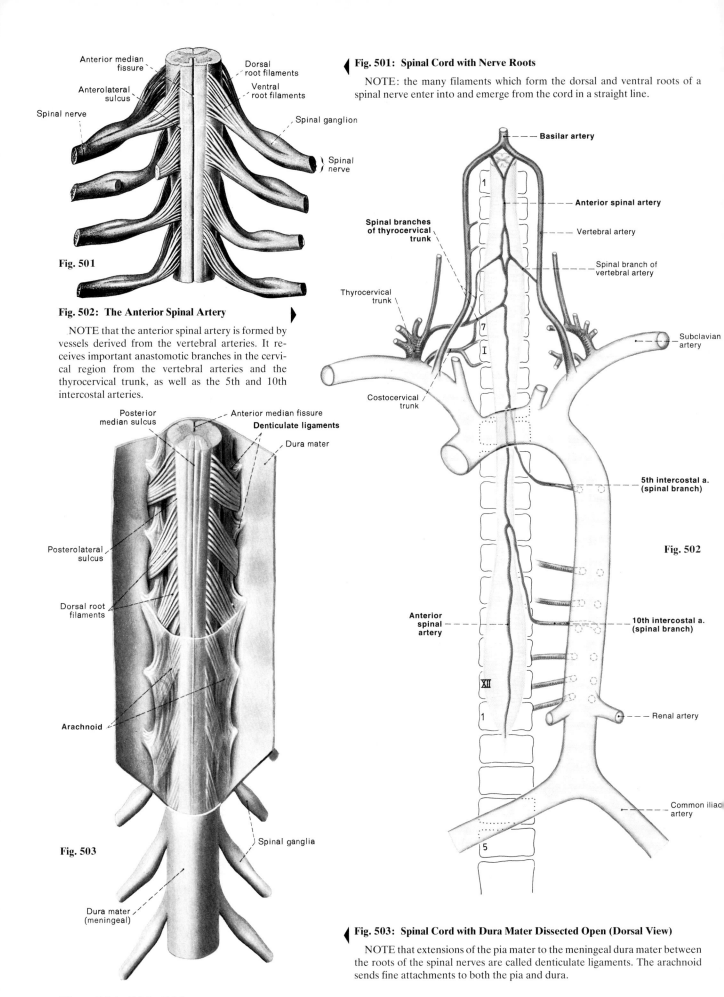

Anterior median fissure

Dorsal root filaments

Anterolateral sulcus

Ventral root filaments

Spinal nerve

Spinal ganglion

Spinal nerve

**Fig. 501**

### Fig. 501: Spinal Cord with Nerve Roots

NOTE: the many filaments which form the dorsal and ventral roots of a spinal nerve enter into and emerge from the cord in a straight line.

### Fig. 502: The Anterior Spinal Artery

NOTE that the anterior spinal artery is formed by vessels derived from the vertebral arteries. It receives important anastomotic branches in the cervical region from the vertebral arteries and the thyrocervical trunk, as well as the 5th and 10th intercostal arteries.

Posterior median sulcus

Anterior median fissure

**Denticulate ligaments**

Dura mater

Posterolateral sulcus

Dorsal root filaments

**Arachnoid**

**Fig. 503**

Spinal ganglia

Dura mater (meningeal)

**Basilar artery**

1

**Anterior spinal artery**

Vertebral artery

**Spinal branches of thyrocervical trunk**

Spinal branch of vertebral artery

7

I

Thyrocervical trunk

Subclavian artery

Costocervical trunk

5th intercostal a. (spinal branch)

**Fig. 502**

Anterior spinal artery

10th intercostal a. (spinal branch)

XII

1

Renal artery

Common iliac artery

5

### Fig. 503: Spinal Cord with Dura Mater Dissected Open (Dorsal View)

NOTE that extensions of the pia mater to the meningeal dura mater between the roots of the spinal nerves are called denticulate ligaments. The arachnoid sends fine attachments to both the pia and dura.

Figs. 501, 502, 503

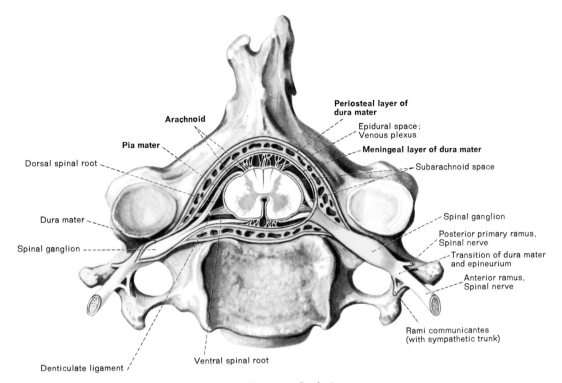

**Fig. 504: Meninges of the Spinal Cord Shown at Cervical Level (Transverse Section)**

NOTE: 1) the meningeal dura mater (inner layer of yellow) surrounds the spinal cord and continues along the spinal nerve through the intervertebral foramen. Its outer periosteal layer (outer layer of yellow) is formed of connective tissue which closely adheres to the bone of the vertebrae forming the vertebral canal.

2) the delicate, film-like arachnoid which lies between the meningeal layer of dura mater, and the vascularized pia mater which is closely applied to the cord.

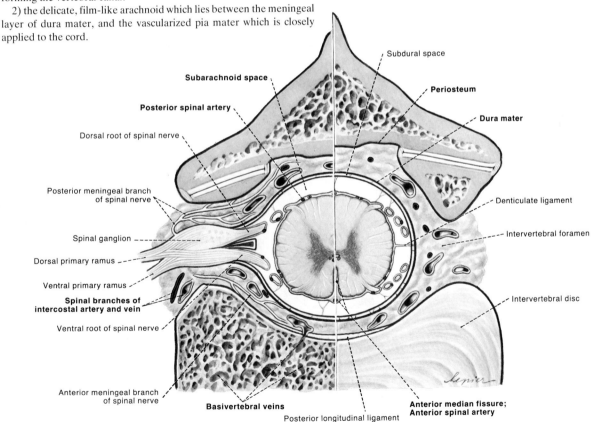

**Fig. 505: The Spinal Cord Within the Vertebral Canal of the Spinal Column (Transverse Section)**

NOTE: 1) that this transverse section is taken through the thoracic region of the spinal cord and shows one level *on the left* through the body of a vertebra and another level *on the right* through an intervertebral disc;

2) that the arachnoid membrane and the arteries are in red; the pia mater and the veins are in blue; the dura mater and the periosteum are in black;

3) the anterior and posterior spinal arteries as well as the intradurally located spinal veins that drain the cord. Observe also the extensive system of extradurally located vertebral veins within the spinal canal which anastomose with the basivertebral veins draining the bodies of the vertebrae.

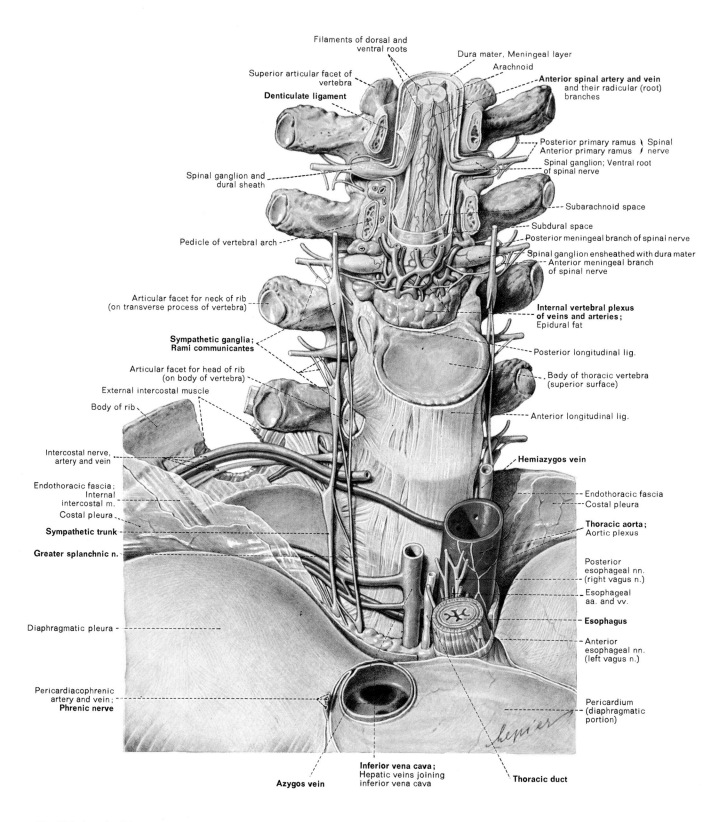

Filaments of dorsal and ventral roots

Dura mater, Meningeal layer
Arachnoid

Superior articular facet of vertebra

**Denticulate ligament**

**Anterior spinal artery and vein**
and their radicular (root) branches

Posterior primary ramus \ Spinal
Anterior primary ramus / nerve

Spinal ganglion; Ventral root of spinal nerve

Spinal ganglion and dural sheath

Subarachnoid space

Subdural space

Pedicle of vertebral arch

Posterior meningeal branch of spinal nerve

Spinal ganglion ensheathed with dura mater
Anterior meningeal branch of spinal nerve

Articular facet for neck of rib (on transverse process of vertebra)

**Internal vertebral plexus of veins and arteries;**
Epidural fat

**Sympathetic ganglia;
Rami communicantes**

Posterior longitudinal lig.

Articular facet for head of rib (on body of vertebra)

Body of thoracic vertebra (superior surface)

External intercostal muscle

Body of rib

Anterior longitudinal lig.

Intercostal nerve, artery and vein

**Hemiazygos vein**

Endothoracic fascia;
Internal intercostal m.

Endothoracic fascia

Costal pleura

Costal pleura

**Sympathetic trunk**

**Thoracic aorta;**
Aortic plexus

**Greater splanchnic n.**

Posterior esophageal nn. (right vagus n.)

Esophageal aa. and vv.

**Esophagus**

Diaphragmatic pleura

Anterior esophageal nn. (left vagus n.)

Pericardiacophrenic artery and vein;
**Phrenic nerve**

Pericardium (diaphragmatic portion)

**Azygos vein**

**Inferior vena cava;**
Hepatic veins joining inferior vena cava

**Thoracic duct**

**Fig. 506: Anterior Dissection of Vertebral Column, Spinal Cord and Prevertebral Structures at a Lower Thoracic Level**

NOTE: 1) the internal vertebral plexus of veins and arteries which lie in the epidural space, where also is found the epidural fat. These should not be confused with the spinal vessels which are situated in the pia mater and which are seen to be intimately applied to the spinal cord tissue.

2) the ganglionated sympathetic chain observable here in the thoracic region receiving and giving communicating rami with the spinal nerves. Note also the formation of the greater splanchnic nerve and its descent prevertebrally into the abdomen.

3) the aorta, inferior vena cava, azygos and hemiazygos veins, esophagus and thoracic duct all lying anterior or somewhat to the left of the vertebral column and passing through the diaphragm.

Fig. 506

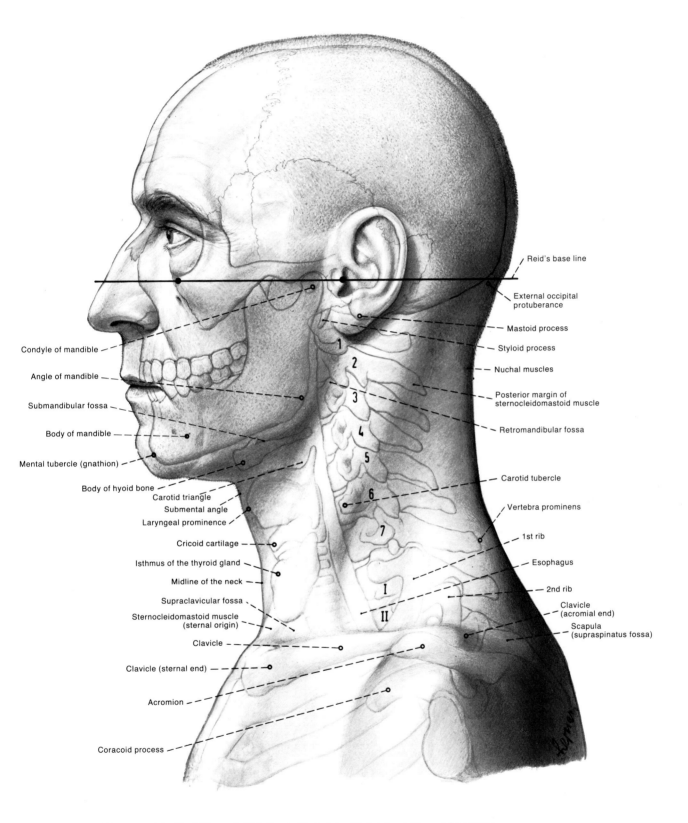

Reid's base line

External occipital protuberance

Mastoid process

Styloid process

Nuchal muscles

Posterior margin of sternocleidomastoid muscle

Retromandibular fossa

Carotid tubercle

Vertebra prominens

1st rib

Esophagus

2nd rib

Clavicle (acromial end)

Scapula (supraspinatus fossa)

Condyle of mandible

Angle of mandible

Submandibular fossa

Body of mandible

Mental tubercle (gnathion)

Body of hyoid bone

Carotid triangle

Submental angle

Laryngeal prominence

Cricoid cartilage

Isthmus of the thyroid gland

Midline of the neck

Supraclavicular fossa

Sternocleidomastoid muscle (sternal origin)

Clavicle

Clavicle (sternal end)

Acromion

Coracoid process

**Fig. 507: External Features of the Neck Shown in Relation to Underlying Skeletal and Visceral Structures**

NOTE: 1) that the palpable bony points are indicated by open circles at the end of certain leader lines;

2) the seven cervical and two upper thoracic vertebrae as well as the prominent skeletal features of the pectoral girdle. Observe the laryngeal cartilages and hyoid bone in the anterior neck and their respective cervical vertebral planes;

3) that a horizontal line (Reid's base line), drawn from the inferior margin of the orbit through the center of the external auditory canal and continuing backward to the center of the occipital bone, is frequently used for cranial topography and cephalometric studies.

Fig. 507    VII

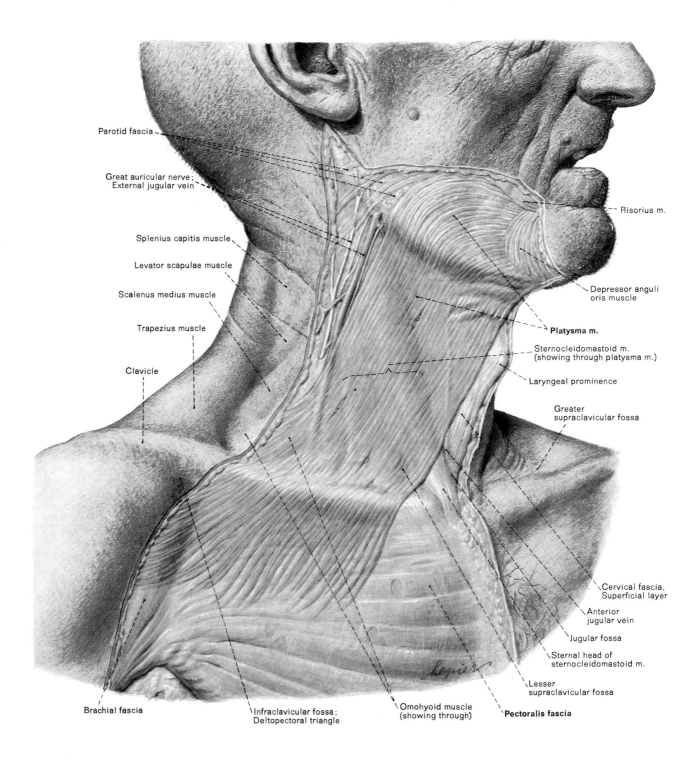

Parotid fascia

Great auricular nerve;
External jugular vein

Splenius capitis muscle

Levator scapulae muscle

Scalenus medius muscle

Trapezius muscle

Clavicle

Brachial fascia

Infraclavicular fossa;
Deltopectoral triangle

Omohyoid muscle
(showing through)

Pectoralis fascia

Risorius m.

Depressor anguli
oris muscle

**Platysma m.**

Sternocleidomastoid m.
(showing through platysma m.)

Laryngeal prominence

Greater
supraclavicular fossa

Cervical fascia,
Superficial layer

Anterior
jugular vein

Jugular fossa

Sternal head of
sternocleidomastoid m.

Lesser
supraclavicular fossa

### Fig. 508: The Right Platysma Muscle and Pectoral Fascia

NOTE: 1) the platysma muscle is a broad, thin quadrangular muscle located in the superficial fascia on the anterolateral aspect of the neck, extending from the angle of the mouth and chin across the clavicle to the upper part of the thorax and anterior shoulder.

2) the platysma muscle can be considered as one of the muscles of facial expression, which characteristically do not arise and insert on bony structures, but within superficial fascia instead. Upon contraction, the platysma tends to depress the angle of the mouth and wrinkle the skin of the neck, thereby participating in the formation of facial expressions of anxiety, sadness, dissatisfaction and suffering.

3) similar to the other muscles of facial expression, the platysma is innervated by the cervical branch of the facial or VIIth cranial nerve.

4) overlying the pectoralis major is the well developed pectoralis fascia which extends from the midline in the thorax laterally to the axilla. Observe the external jugular vein and great auricular nerve exposed in the upper lateral aspect of the neck.

Fig. 508

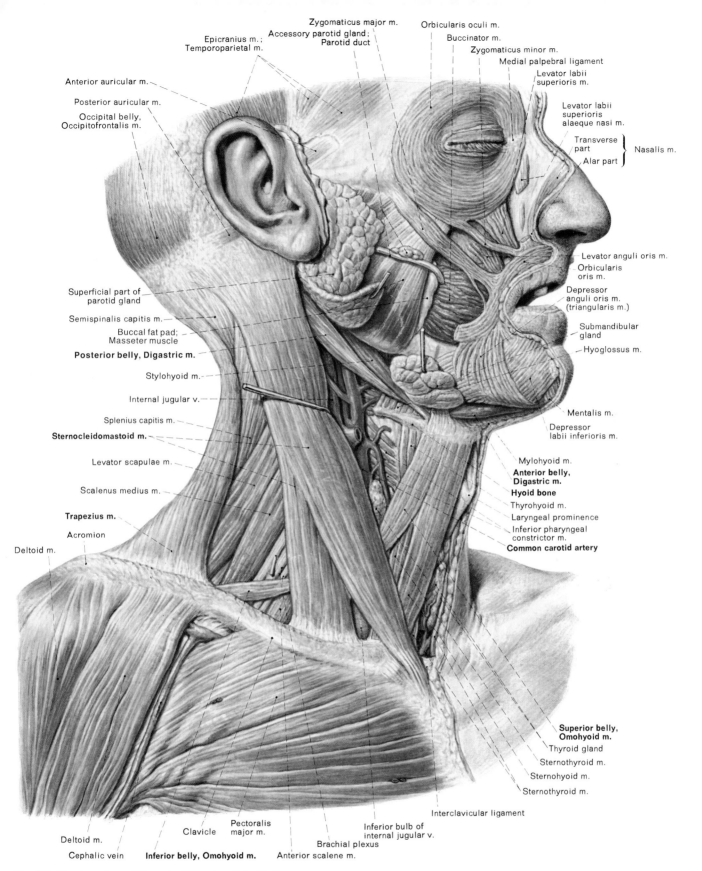

Zygomaticus major m.

Epicranius m.; Temporoparietal m.

Accessory parotid gland; Parotid duct

Orbicularis oculi m.

Buccinator m.

Zygomaticus minor m.

Medial palpebral ligament

Levator labii superioris m.

Anterior auricular m.

Posterior auricular m.

Occipital belly, Occipitofrontalis m.

Levator labii superioris alaeque nasi m.

Transverse part

Alar part

Nasalis m.

Levator anguli oris m.

Orbicularis oris m.

Depressor anguli oris m. (triangularis m.)

Superficial part of parotid gland

Semispinalis capitis m.

Buccal fat pad; Masseter muscle

**Posterior belly, Digastric m.**

Stylohyoid m.

Internal jugular v.

Splenius capitis m.

**Sternocleidomastoid m.**

Levator scapulae m.

Scalenus medius m.

**Trapezius m.**

Acromion

Deltoid m.

Submandibular gland

Hyoglossus m.

Mentalis m.

Depressor labii inferioris m.

Mylohyoid m.

**Anterior belly, Digastric m.**

**Hyoid bone**

Thyrohyoid m.

Laryngeal prominence

Inferior pharyngeal constrictor m.

**Common carotid artery**

**Superior belly, Omohyoid m.**

Thyroid gland

Sternothyroid m.

Sternohyoid m.

Sternothyroid m.

Interclavicular ligament

Deltoid m.

Cephalic vein

Clavicle

Pectoralis major m.

**Inferior belly, Omohyoid m.**

Anterior scalene m.

Brachial plexus

Inferior bulb of internal jugular v.

**Fig. 509: The Anterior and Posterior Triangles of the Neck**

NOTE: 1) the *anterior triangle* of the neck is bounded by the midline of the neck, the anterior border of the sternocleidomastoid and the mandible. This area is further subdivided by the superior belly of the omohyoid and the two bellies of the digastric into the following: a) *muscular triangle* (midline, superior belly of omohyoid, sternocleidomastoid), b) *carotid triangle* (superior belly of omohyoid, sternocleido-mastoid and posterior belly of digastric), c) *submandibular triangle* (anterior and posterior bellies of digastric and the inferior margin of the mandible), and d) *suprahyoid triangle* (midline, anterior belly of digastric and hyoid bone).

2) the *posteror triangle* of the neck is bounded by the posterior border of the sternocleidomastoid, the trapezius and the clavicle. This area is subdivided into the *occipital triangle* above, and *subclavian triangle* below, by the inferior belly of the omohyoid muscle.

Fig. 509    VII

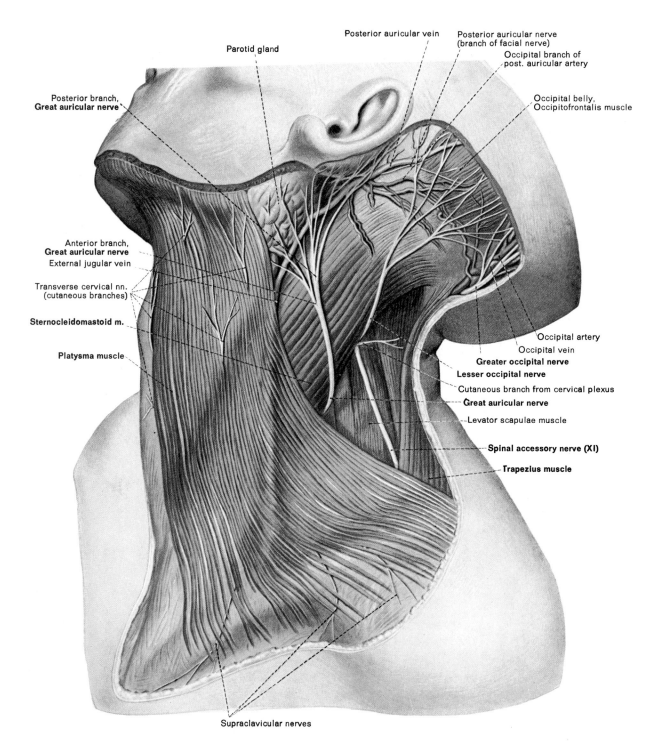

Posterior auricular vein

Parotid gland

Posterior auricular nerve
(branch of facial nerve)

Occipital branch of
post. auricular artery

Posterior branch,
**Great auricular nerve**

Occipital belly,
Occipitofrontalis muscle

Anterior branch,
**Great auricular nerve**

External jugular vein

Transverse cervical nn.
(cutaneous branches)

**Sternocleidomastoid m.**

Platysma muscle

Occipital artery

Occipital vein

**Greater occipital nerve**

**Lesser occipital nerve**

Cutaneous branch from cervical plexus

**Great auricular nerve**

Levator scapulae muscle

**Spinal accessory nerve (XI)**

**Trapezius muscle**

Supraclavicular nerves

**Fig. 510: Nerves and Blood Vessels of the Neck, Stage 1: Platysma Layer**

NOTE: 1) the skin has been removed from both anterior and posterior triangles of the neck to reveal the platysma muscle. Observe the cutaneous branches of the transverse cervical nerves emanating from the cervical plexus and penetrating through the platysma (and superficial fascia) to reach the skin of the anterolateral aspect of the neck.

2) four other nerves: a) the great auricular (C-2, C-3), b) the lesser occipital (C-2), c) the greater occipital (C-2) and d) the spinal accessory (XI).

3) after it has supplied the sternocleidomastoid muscle, the spinal accessory nerve (XI) descends in the posterior triangle to reach the trapezius muscle which it also supplies with motor innervation.

Fig. 510

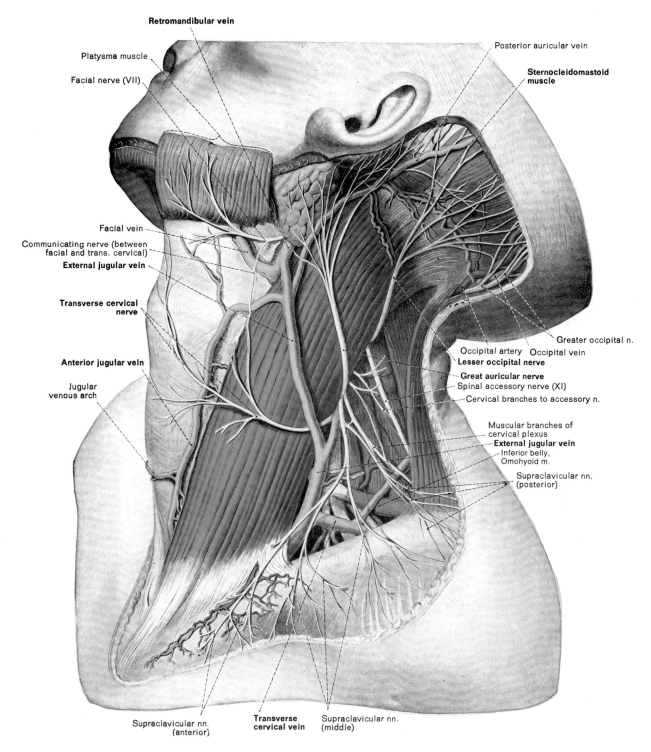

**Retromandibular vein**

Platysma muscle

Facial nerve (VII)

Facial vein

Communicating nerve (between facial and trans. cervical)

**External jugular vein**

**Transverse cervical nerve**

**Anterior jugular vein**

Jugular venous arch

Posterior auricular vein

**Sternocleidomastoid muscle**

Greater occipital n.

Occipital artery    Occipital vein
**Lesser occipital nerve**

**Great auricular nerve**
Spinal accessory nerve (XI)

Cervical branches to accessory n.

Muscular branches of cervical plexus

**External jugular vein**

Inferior belly, Omohyoid m.

Supraclavicular nn. (posterior)

Supraclavicular nn. (anterior)

**Transverse cervical vein**

Supraclavicular nn. (middle)

**Fig. 511: Nerves and Blood Vessels of the Neck, Stage 2: Sternocleidomastoid Layer**

NOTE: 1) with the platysma reflected upward, the full extent of the sternocleidomastoid muscle is exposed. Observe that the nerves of the cervical plexus diverge at the posterior border of the sternocleidomastoid muscle: the great auricular and lesser occipital ascend to the head, the transverse colli course across the neck toward the midline, while the supraclavicular descend over the clavicle.

2) the external jugular vein formed by the junction of the retromandibular and posterior auricular veins. The external jugular crosses the sternocleidomastoid muscle obliquely and receives tributaries from the anterior jugular, posterior external jugular, transverse cervical and suprascapular veins before terminating into the subclavian vein.

3) the cervical branch of the facial (VII) nerve supplying the inner surface of the platysma muscle with motor innervation.

Fig. 511    VII

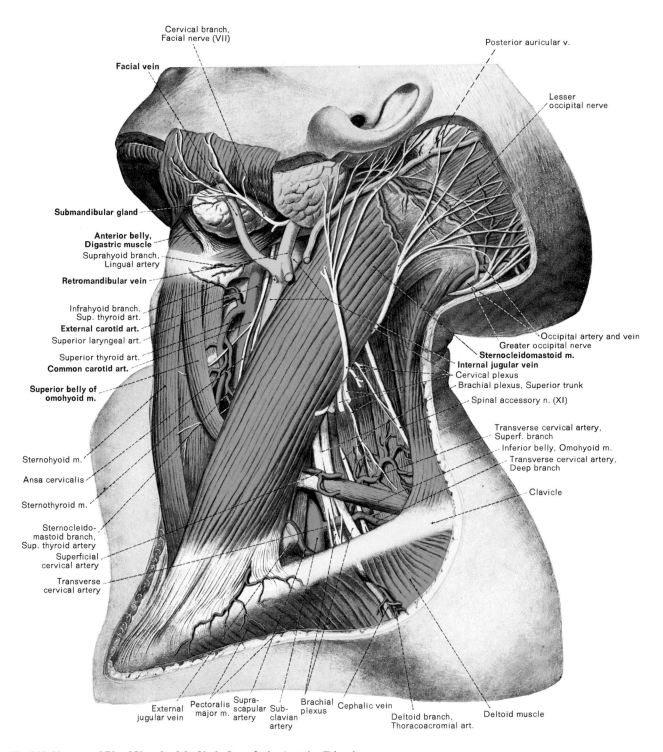

**Fig. 512: Nerves and Blood Vessels of the Neck, Stage 3: the Anterior Triangle**

NOTE: 1) with the investing fascia removed, the outlines of the muscular, carotid and submandibular triangles, which subdivide the anterior neck region, are revealed.

2) the infrahyoid (strap) muscles which cover the thyroid gland in the *muscular triangle* (bounded by sternocleidomastoid, midline and superior belly of omohyoid).

3) the carotid vessels and jugular vein in the *carotid triangle* (bounded by superior belly of omohyoid, posterior belly of digastric and sternocleidomastoid).

4) the submandibular gland in the *submandibular triangle* (bounded by anterior and posterior bellies of digastric and the inferior border of the mandible).

Fig. 512

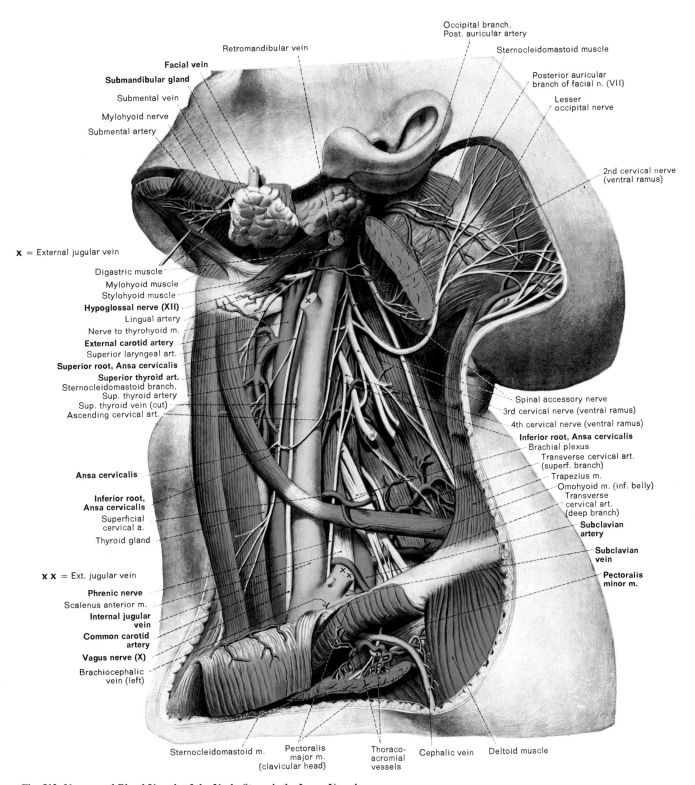

Occipital branch,
Post. auricular artery

Retromandibular vein

Sternocleidomastoid muscle

**Facial vein**

Posterior auricular
branch of facial n. (VII)

**Submandibular gland**

Submental vein

Lesser
occipital nerve

Mylohyoid nerve

Submental artery

2nd cervical nerve
(ventral ramus)

**x** = External jugular vein

Digastric muscle
Mylohyoid muscle
Stylohyoid muscle
**Hypoglossal nerve (XII)**
Lingual artery
Nerve to thyrohyoid m.
**External carotid artery**
Superior laryngeal art.
**Superior root, Ansa cervicalis**
**Superior thyroid art.**
Sternocleidomastoid branch,
Sup. thyroid artery
Sup. thyroid vein (cut)
Ascending cervical art.

Spinal accessory nerve
3rd cervical nerve (ventral ramus)
4th cervical nerve (ventral ramus)
**Inferior root, Ansa cervicalis**
Brachial plexus
Transverse cervical art.
(superf. branch)
Trapezius m.
Omohyoid m. (inf. belly)
Transverse
cervical art.
(deep branch)
**Subclavian
artery**

**Ansa cervicalis**

**Inferior root,
Ansa cervicalis**
Superficial
cervical a.
Thyroid gland

**Subclavian
vein**

**Pectoralis
minor m.**

**x x** = Ext. jugular vein

**Phrenic nerve**
Scalenus anterior m.
**Internal jugular
vein**
**Common carotid
artery**
**Vagus nerve (X)**
Brachiocephalic
vein (left)

Sternocleidomastoid m.   Pectoralis      Thoraco-      Cephalic vein   Deltoid muscle
                        major m.        acromial
                        (clavicular head)  vessels

**Fig. 513: Nerves and Blood Vessels of the Neck, Stage 4: the Large Vessels**

NOTE: 1) the sternocleidomastoid muscle and the superficial veins and nerves have been removed to expose the internal and external carotid arteries, the internal jugular vein, both bellies of the omohyoid muscle, the vagus nerve and the ansa cervicalis.

2) superiorly, the facial vein has been cut and the submandibular gland elevated, thereby exposing the hypoglossal nerve (XII). Observe that nerve fibers (originating from C-1 and travelling for a short distance) leave the hypoglossal nerve to descend in the neck. These form the superior root of the ansa cervicalis and are joined by other descending fibers from C-2 and C-3 which are called the inferior root of the ansa cervicalis. These two roots form the ansa cervicalis, from which innervation for a number of the strap muscles is derived.

Fig. 513   VII

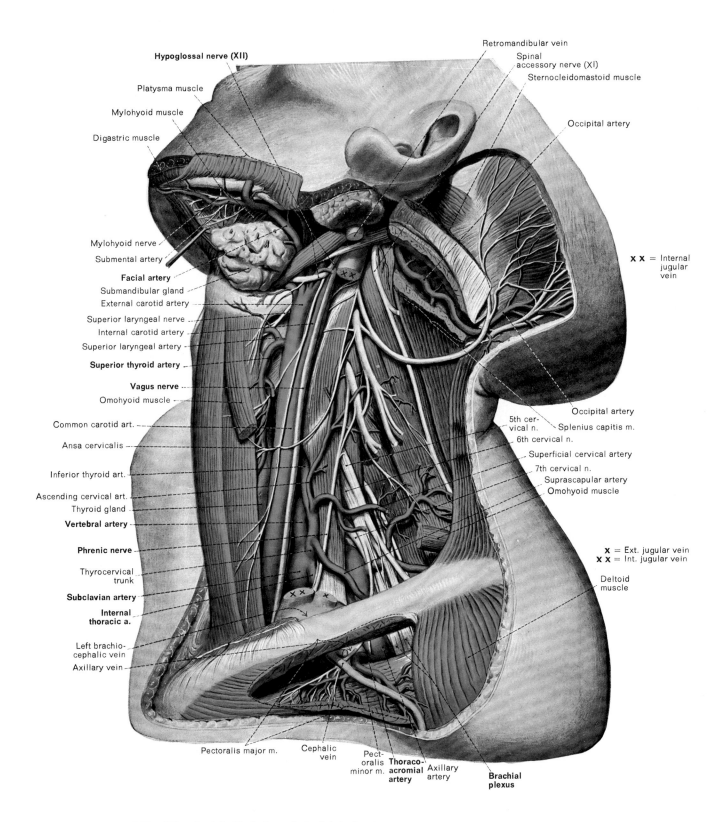

Hypoglossal nerve (XII)

Platysma muscle

Mylohyoid muscle

Digastric muscle

Mylohyoid nerve

Submental artery

**Facial artery**

Submandibular gland

External carotid artery

Superior laryngeal nerve

Internal carotid artery

Superior laryngeal artery

**Superior thyroid artery**

**Vagus nerve**

Omohyoid muscle

Common carotid art.

Ansa cervicalis

Inferior thyroid art.

Ascending cervical art.

Thyroid gland

**Vertebral artery**

**Phrenic nerve**

Thyrocervical trunk

**Subclavian artery**

**Internal thoracic a.**

Left brachio-cephalic vein

Axillary vein

Retromandibular vein

Spinal accessory nerve (XI)

Sternocleidomastoid muscle

Occipital artery

X X = Internal jugular vein

Occipital artery

5th cervical n.

Splenius capitis m.

6th cervical n.

Superficial cervical artery

7th cervical n.

Suprascapular artery

Omohyoid muscle

**X** = Ext. jugular vein
**X X** = Int. jugular vein

Deltoid muscle

Pectoralis major m.

Cephalic vein

Pectoralis minor m.

**Thoraco-acromial artery**

Axillary artery

**Brachial plexus**

**Fig. 514: Nerves and Blood Vessels of the Neck, Stage 5: the Subclavian Artery**

NOTE: 1) with the internal and external jugular veins removed, the subclavian artery becomes exposed as it ascends from the thorax and loops in the subclavian triangle of the neck to descend beneath the clavicle into the axilla. Observe the vertebral, thyrocervical and internal thoracic branches and the transverse cervical artery, which comes off separately in this dissection and which divides into an ascending superficial branch and a descending deep branch (not labelled).

2) the vagus nerve coursing with the internal and common carotid arteries and the phrenic nerve descending in the neck along the surface of the anterior scalene muscle toward the thorax.

Fig. 514

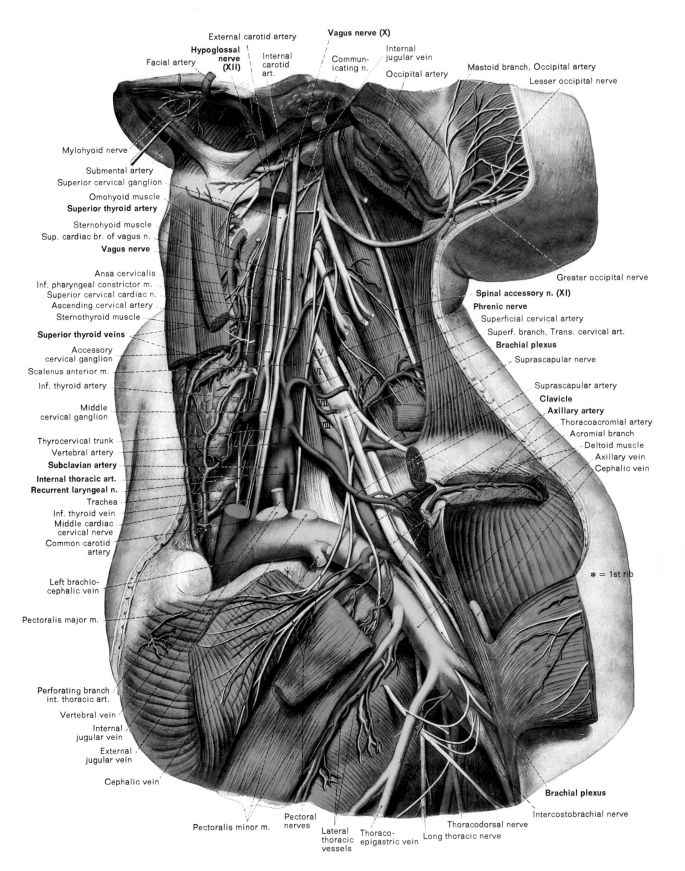

**External carotid artery**

**Vagus nerve (X)**

**Hypoglossal nerve (XII)**

Facial artery

Internal carotid art.

Communicating n.

Internal jugular vein

Occipital artery

Mastoid branch, Occipital artery

Lesser occipital nerve

Mylohyoid nerve

Submental artery

Superior cervical ganglion

Omohyoid muscle

**Superior thyroid artery**

Sternohyoid muscle

Sup. cardiac br. of vagus n.

**Vagus nerve**

Ansa cervicalis

Inf. pharyngeal constrictor m.

Superior cervical cardiac n.

Ascending cervical artery

Sternothyroid muscle

**Superior thyroid veins**

Accessory cervical ganglion

Scalenus anterior m.

Inf. thyroid artery

Middle cervical ganglion

Thyrocervical trunk

Vertebral artery

**Subclavian artery**

**Internal thoracic art.**

**Recurrent laryngeal n.**

Trachea

Inf. thyroid vein

Middle cardiac cervical nerve

Common carotid artery

Left brachio-cephalic vein

Pectoralis major m.

Perforating branch int. thoracic art.

Vertebral vein

Internal jugular vein

External jugular vein

Cephalic vein

Greater occipital nerve

**Spinal accessory n. (XI)**

**Phrenic nerve**

Superficial cervical artery

Superf. branch, Trans. cervical art.

**Brachial plexus**

Suprascapular nerve

Suprascapular artery

**Clavicle**

**Axillary artery**

Thoracoacromial artery

Acromial branch

Deltoid muscle

Axillary vein

Cephalic vein

* = 1st rib

**Brachial plexus**

Intercostobrachial nerve

Pectoralis minor m.

Pectoral nerves

Lateral thoracic vessels

Thoraco-epigastric vein

Long thoracic nerve

Thoracodorsal nerve

**Fig. 515: Nerves and Blood Vessels of the Neck, Stage 6: the Brachial Plexus**

NOTE: 1) with the carotid arteries, jugular vein and clavicle removed, the roots forming the trunks of the brachial plexus are exposed as they divide and descend into the axilla to surround the axillary artery.

2) the sympathetic trunk lying deep to the carotid arteries and coursing with the vagus nerve and the superior cardiac branch of the vagus nerve.

3) the thyroid gland receiving the superior and inferior thyroid arteries and being drained by the thyroid veins. Observe also the proximity of the recurrent laryngeal nerve to the thyroid gland.

Fig. 515    VII

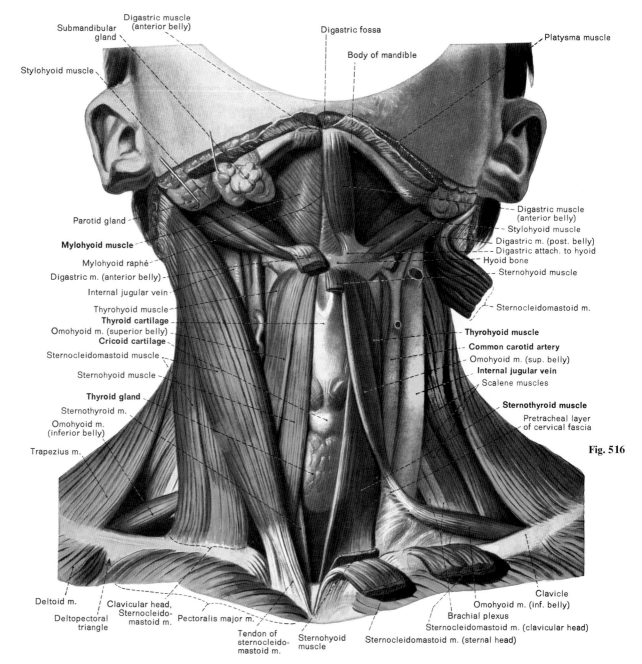

Submandibular gland
Digastric muscle (anterior belly)
Digastric fossa
Body of mandible
Platysma muscle
Stylohyoid muscle

Parotid gland
Digastric muscle (anterior belly)
Stylohyoid muscle
Digastric m. (post. belly)
Digastric attach. to hyoid
Hyoid bone
Sternohyoid muscle

**Mylohyoid muscle**
Mylohyoid raphé
Digastric m. (anterior belly)
Internal jugular vein
Thyrohyoid muscle
**Thyroid cartilage**
Omohyoid m. (superior belly)
**Cricoid cartilage**
Sternocleidomastoid muscle
Sternohyoid muscle

**Thyroid gland**
Sternothyroid m.
Omohyoid m. (inferior belly)
Trapezius m.

Sternocleidomastoid m.

**Thyrohyoid muscle**
**Common carotid artery**
Omohyoid m. (sup. belly)
**Internal jugular vein**
Scalene muscles

**Sternothyroid muscle**
Pretracheal layer of cervical fascia

**Fig. 516**

Deltoid m.
Clavicular head, Sternocleido-mastoid m.
Deltopectoral triangle
Pectoralis major m.
Tendon of sternocleido-mastoid m.
Sternohyoid muscle
Sternocleidomastoid m. (sternal head)
Brachial plexus
Sternocleidomastoid m. (clavicular head)
Omohyoid m. (inf. belly)
Clavicle

**Fig. 517**

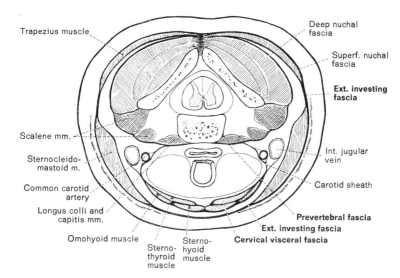

Trapezius muscle
Deep nuchal fascia
Superf. nuchal fascia
**Ext. investing fascia**
Scalene mm.
Sternocleido-mastoid m.
Common carotid artery
Longus colli and capitis mm.
Omohyoid muscle
Sterno-thyroid muscle
Sterno-hyoid muscle
Int. jugular vein
Carotid sheath
**Prevertebral fascia**
Ext. investing fascia
**Cervical visceral fascia**

**Fig. 516: Anterior View of the Musculature in the Neck**

NOTE: 1) the right superior belly of the digastric muscle was removed and submandibular gland elevated in order to show the mylohyoid muscle. On the left side, the sternocleidomastoid and sternohyoid muscles have been transected and the submandibular gland removed.

2) the relationship of the strap muscles to the thyroid gland and realize that inferior to the thyroid gland and above the suprasternal notch, the trachea lies immediately under the skin.

**Fig. 517: Fascial Planes of the Neck in a Newborn Child (Cross Section)**

NOTE: the external investing fascia splits to encase the sternocleidomastoid and trapezius muscles. The prevertebral fascia encloses the vertebral column and its muscles, while the cervical visceral fascia encloses the esophagus, trachea, thyroid gland and strap muscles.

Figs. 516, 517

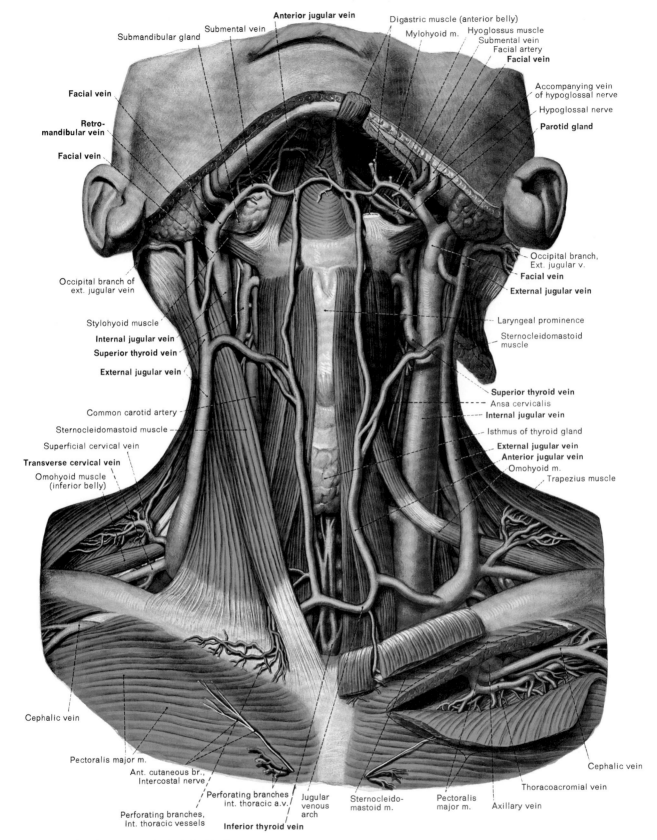

Submandibular gland
Submental vein
**Anterior jugular vein**
Digastric muscle (anterior belly)
Mylohyoid m.
Hyoglossus muscle
Submental vein
Facial artery
**Facial vein**

**Facial vein**

Accompanying vein of hypoglossal nerve
Hypoglossal nerve
**Parotid gland**

**Retro-mandibular vein**

**Facial vein**

Occipital branch, Ext. jugular v.
**Facial vein**
**External jugular vein**

Occipital branch of ext. jugular vein

Laryngeal prominence
Sternocleidomastoid muscle

Stylohyoid muscle
**Internal jugular vein**
**Superior thyroid vein**

**External jugular vein**

**Superior thyroid vein**
Ansa cervicalis
**Internal jugular vein**

Common carotid artery
Sternocleidomastoid muscle
Superficial cervical vein
**Transverse cervical vein**
Omohyoid muscle (inferior belly)

Isthmus of thyroid gland
**External jugular vein**
**Anterior jugular vein**
Omohyoid m.
Trapezius muscle

Cephalic vein

Cephalic vein

Pectoralis major m.

Thoracoacromial vein

Ant. cutaneous br., Intercostal nerve
Perforating branches int. thoracic a.v.
Jugular venous arch
Sternocleido-mastoid m.
Pectoralis major m.
Axillary vein

Perforating branches, Int. thoracic vessels
**Inferior thyroid vein**

## Fig. 518: Veins of the Neck and Infraclavicular Region

NOTE: 1) the jugular system of veins, although somewhat variable, generally consists of an anterior jugular, external jugular and internal jugular vein, all of which are shown on the left side where the sternocleidomastoid muscle has been removed.

2) the anterior jugular descends close to the midline, is frequently small and drains laterally through several tributaries into the external jugular vein. The external jugular courses along the surface of the sternocleidomastoid muscle. It commences usually within the parotid gland and enlarges through the junction of occipital, retromandibular and facial branches. It flows into the subclavian vein with the internal jugular after it receives branches from the shoulder and clavicular regions.

3) the internal jugular is large and collects blood from the brain, face and neck. At its junction with the subclavian, the brachiocephalic vein is formed.

Fig. 518    VII

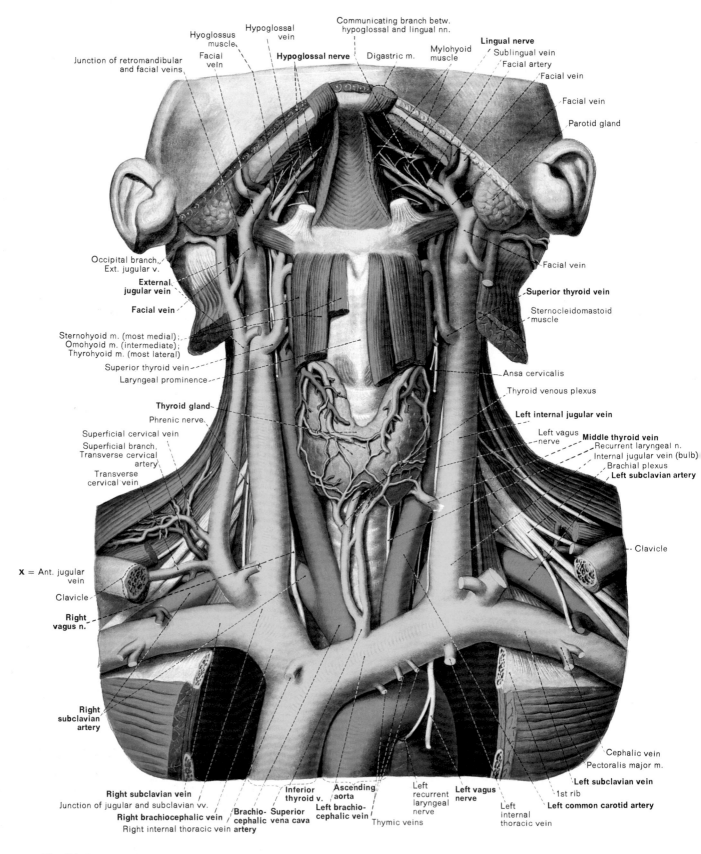

**Fig. 519: Deep Arteries and Veins of the Neck and Great Vessels of the Thorax**

NOTE: 1) in the neck, the sternocleidomastoid and strap muscles have been removed, thereby exposing the carotid arteries, internal jugular veins and thyroid gland.

2) the middle portion of the anterior thoracic wall has been resected in order to show the aortic arch and its branches, the brachiocephalic veins, the superior vena cava and the vagus nerves.

3) in the submandibular region, the mylohyoid and anterior digastric muscles have been cut, revealing the lingual and hypoglossal nerves.

Fig. 519

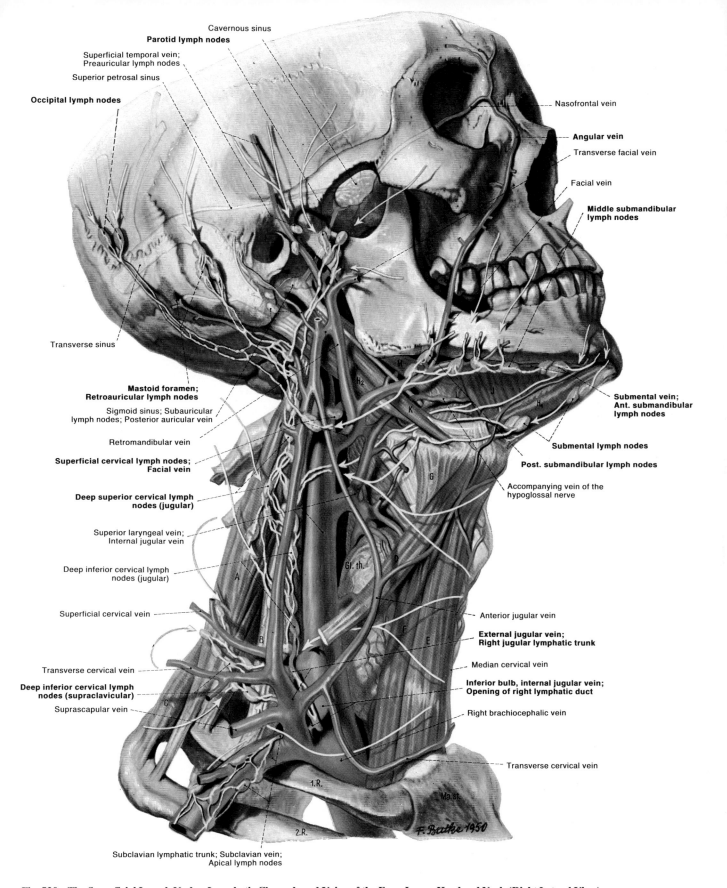

Cavernous sinus
Parotid lymph nodes
Superficial temporal vein;
Preauricular lymph nodes
Superior petrosal sinus
Occipital lymph nodes

Nasofrontal vein
Angular vein
Transverse facial vein
Facial vein
Middle submandibular
lymph nodes

Transverse sinus

Mastoid foramen;
Retroauricular lymph nodes
Sigmoid sinus; Subauricular
lymph nodes; Posterior auricular vein
Retromandibular vein
Superficial cervical lymph nodes;
Facial vein
Deep superior cervical lymph
nodes (jugular)
Superior laryngeal vein;
Internal jugular vein
Deep inferior cervical lymph
nodes (jugular)
Superficial cervical vein
Transverse cervical vein
Deep inferior cervical lymph
nodes (supraclavicular)
Suprascapular vein

Submental vein;
Ant. submandibular
lymph nodes
Submental lymph nodes
Post. submandibular lymph nodes
Accompanying vein of the
hypoglossal nerve

Anterior jugular vein
External jugular vein;
Right jugular lymphatic trunk
Median cervical vein
Inferior bulb, internal jugular vein;
Opening of right lymphatic duct
Right brachiocephalic vein

Transverse cervical vein

Subclavian lymphatic trunk; Subclavian vein;
Apical lymph nodes

**Fig. 520: The Superficial Lymph Nodes, Lymphatic Channels and Veins of the Face, Lower Head and Neck (Right Lateral View)**

NOTE that the superficial lymphatic channels of the face and the temporal and occipital regions of the head drain inferiorly and posteriorly to the superficial and deeper cervical nodes accompanying the internal jugular vein. These in turn drain into the right jugular lymphatic trunk.

A = Middle scalene m.
B = Ant. scalene m.
C = Post. scalene m.
D = Omohyoid m.

E = Sternohyoid m.
F = Sternothyroid m.
G = Thyrohyoid m.
Gl. th. = Thyroid gland

$H_1$ = Digastric m. (ant. belly)
$H_2$ = Digastric m. (post belly)
J = Mylohyoid m.
K = Stylohyoid m.

L = Hyoglossus m.
M = Styloglossus m.
Ma. st. = Manubrium sterni
1., 2. R = 1st and 2nd ribs

Fig. 520    VII

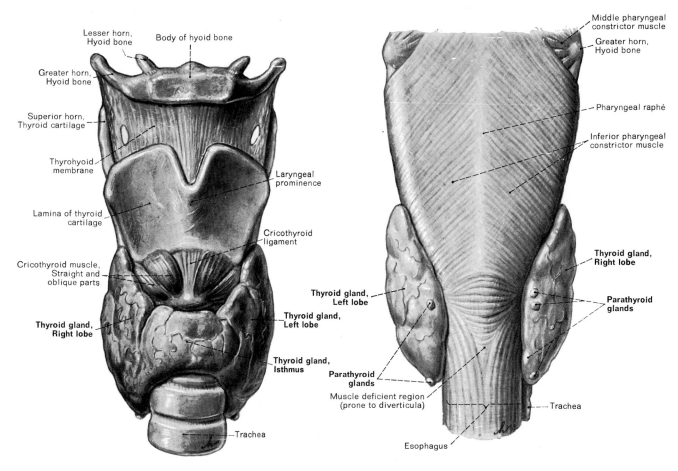

**Fig. 521: Ventral View of Thyroid Gland Showing Relation to Larynx and Trachea**

**Fig. 522: Dorsal View of Thyroid Gland Showing Relation to Pharynx and Parathyroids**

**Fig. 523: Cross Section of Cervical Viscera Showing Relation of Thyroid Gland to Trachea, Esophagus, Parathyroid Glands and Cervical Vessels and Nerves**

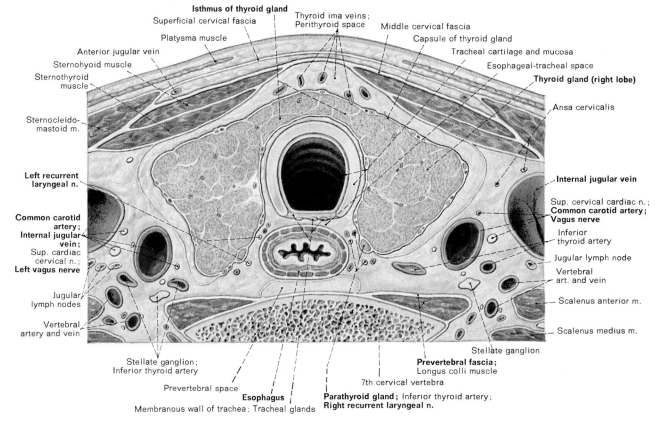

Figs. 521, 522, 523

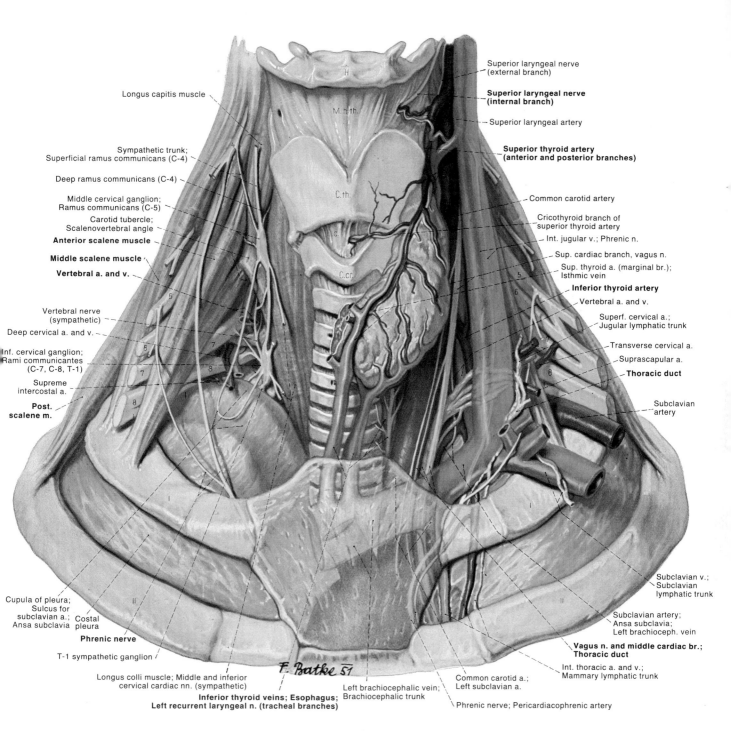

Longus capitis muscle

Sympathetic trunk;
Superficial ramus communicans (C-4)

Deep ramus communicans (C-4)

Middle cervical ganglion;
Ramus communicans (C-5)

Carotid tubercle;
Scalenovertebral angle

**Anterior scalene muscle**

**Middle scalene muscle**

**Vertebral a. and v.**

Vertebral nerve
(sympathetic)

Deep cervical a. and v.

Inf. cervical ganglion;
Rami communicantes
(C-7, C-8, T-1)

Supreme
intercostal a.

**Post.
scalene m.**

Cupula of pleura;
Sulcus for
subclavian a.; Costal
Ansa subclavia pleura

**Phrenic nerve**

T-1 sympathetic ganglion

Longus colli muscle; Middle and inferior
cervical cardiac nn. (sympathetic)

**Inferior thyroid veins; Esophagus;
Left recurrent laryngeal n. (tracheal branches)**

Superior laryngeal nerve
(external branch)

**Superior laryngeal nerve
(internal branch)**

Superior laryngeal artery

**Superior thyroid artery
(anterior and posterior branches)**

Common carotid artery

Cricothyroid branch of
superior thyroid artery

Int. jugular v.; Phrenic n.

Sup. cardiac branch, vagus n.

Sup. thyroid a. (marginal br.);
Isthmic vein

**Inferior thyroid artery**

Vertebral a. and v.

Superf. cervical a.;
Jugular lymphatic trunk

Transverse cervical a.

Suprascapular a.

**Thoracic duct**

Subclavian
artery

Subclavian v.;
Subclavian
lymphatic trunk

Subclavian artery;
Ansa subclavia;
Left brachioceph. vein

**Vagus n. and middle cardiac br.;
Thoracic duct**

Int. thoracic a. and v.;
Mammary lymphatic trunk

Common carotid a.;
Left subclavian a.

Left brachiocephalic vein;
Brachiocephalic trunk

Phrenic nerve; Pericardiacophrenic artery

F. Batke 51

**Fig. 524: The Root of the Neck and the Thoracic Inlet, Anterior View.**

NOTE: 1) that the sternocleidomastoid and strap muscles have been removed. Additionally, *on the right side* (reader's left), the large vessels, vagus nerve, and right lobe of the thyroid gland have been resected to reveal the scalene muscles, the roots of the brachial plexus, the inferior and middle cervical ganglia and cupula of the right pleura.

2) *on the left side*, the course of the vagus nerve and its recurrent laryngeal branch. Observe also the thoracic duct as it ascends into the root of the neck to open into the venous system at the angle of junction between the left internal jugular and left subclavian veins.

3) the descending course of the phrenic nerves. These nerves are derived from the 3rd, 4th, and 5th cervical segments, lie along the ventral surface of the anterior scalene muscle, and enter the thorax deep to the sternocostal joints of the first rib.

4) the cupula of the pleura overlying the apex of the lung. On each side these project 3 to 5 cm above the sternal end of the first rib and, therefore, are unprotected by bone.

5) the superior thyroid vessels and their superior laryngeal and cricothyroid branches. Observe the rich vascularity of the thyroid gland and the veins (of considerable size) which course anterior to the trachea at the site where tracheostomy is frequently performed.

| | | |
|---|---|---|
| C. cr. = Cricoid cartilage | L. c. = Cricothyroid ligament | 4–8 = Ventral rami of C-4 to C-8 nerves |
| C. th. = Thyroid cartilage | M. h. th. = Thyrohyoid membrane | I = Ventral ramus of T-1 nerve |
| H = Hyoid bone | I, II = 1st and 2nd ribs | |

Fig. 524    VII

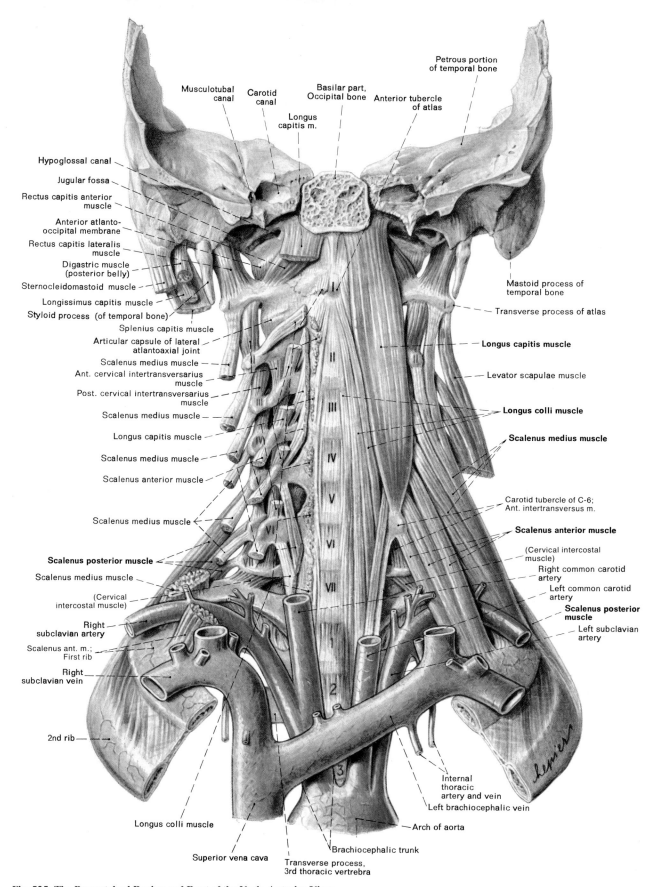

**Fig. 525: The Prevertebral Region and Root of the Neck, Anterior View**

NOTE: 1) on the specimen's right side, the longus capitis, longus colli and scalene muscles have been removed, exposing the transverse processes of the cervical vertebrae onto which these muscles are seen to attach.

2) the scalenus posterior muscle inserts of the 2nd rib, whereas both the scalenus anterior and medius insert onto the 1st rib. Thus, when these muscles are fixed superiorly, they would act as inspiratory muscles by elevating the first two ribs. Fixed inferiorly, they assist in bending the cervical vertebral column to one or the other side. Between the scalenus anterior and medius emerge the roots which form the trunks of the brachial plexus (see Figs. 524 and 527).

Fig. 525

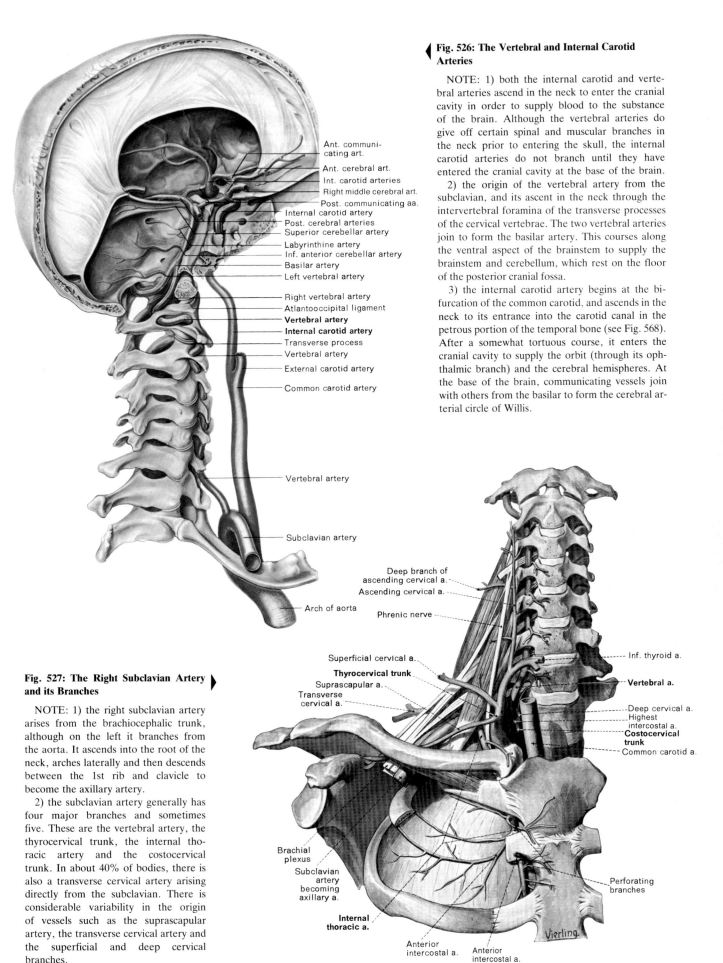

### Fig. 526: The Vertebral and Internal Carotid Arteries

NOTE: 1) both the internal carotid and vertebral arteries ascend in the neck to enter the cranial cavity in order to supply blood to the substance of the brain. Although the vertebral arteries do give off certain spinal and muscular branches in the neck prior to entering the skull, the internal carotid arteries do not branch until they have entered the cranial cavity at the base of the brain.

2) the origin of the vertebral artery from the subclavian, and its ascent in the neck through the intervertebral foramina of the transverse processes of the cervical vertebrae. The two vertebral arteries join to form the basilar artery. This courses along the ventral aspect of the brainstem to supply the brainstem and cerebellum, which rest on the floor of the posterior cranial fossa.

3) the internal carotid artery begins at the bifurcation of the common carotid, and ascends in the neck to its entrance into the carotid canal in the petrous portion of the temporal bone (see Fig. 568). After a somewhat tortuous course, it enters the cranial cavity to supply the orbit (through its ophthalmic branch) and the cerebral hemispheres. At the base of the brain, communicating vessels join with others from the basilar to form the cerebral arterial circle of Willis.

Labels (Fig. 526):
- Ant. communicating art.
- Ant. cerebral art.
- Int. carotid arteries
- Right middle cerebral art.
- Post. communicating aa.
- Internal carotid artery
- Post. cerebral arteries
- Superior cerebellar artery
- Labyrinthine artery
- Inf. anterior cerebellar artery
- Basilar artery
- Left vertebral artery
- Right vertebral artery
- Atlantooccipital ligament
- **Vertebral artery**
- **Internal carotid artery**
- Transverse process
- Vertebral artery
- External carotid artery
- Common carotid artery
- Vertebral artery
- Subclavian artery
- Arch of aorta

### Fig. 527: The Right Subclavian Artery and its Branches

NOTE: 1) the right subclavian artery arises from the brachiocephalic trunk, although on the left it branches from the aorta. It ascends into the root of the neck, arches laterally and then descends between the 1st rib and clavicle to become the axillary artery.

2) the subclavian artery generally has four major branches and sometimes five. These are the vertebral artery, the thyrocervical trunk, the internal thoracic artery and the costocervical trunk. In about 40% of bodies, there is also a transverse cervical artery arising directly from the subclavian. There is considerable variability in the origin of vessels such as the suprascapular artery, the transverse cervical artery and the superficial and deep cervical branches.

Labels (Fig. 527):
- Deep branch of ascending cervical a.
- Ascending cervical a.
- Phrenic nerve
- Superficial cervical a.
- **Thyrocervical trunk**
- Suprascapular a.
- Transverse cervical a.
- Inf. thyroid a.
- **Vertebral a.**
- Deep cervical a.
- Highest intercostal a.
- **Costocervical trunk**
- Common carotid a.
- Brachial plexus
- Subclavian artery becoming axillary a.
- **Internal thoracic a.**
- Anterior intercostal a.
- Anterior intercostal a.
- Perforating branches
- Vierling.

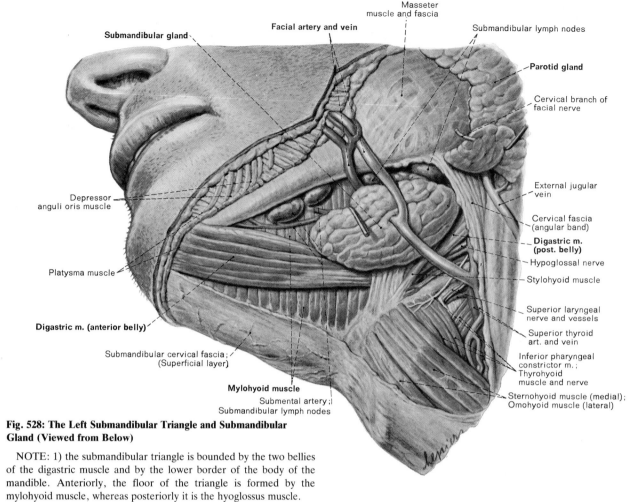

**Fig. 528: The Left Submandibular Triangle and Submandibular Gland (Viewed from Below)**

NOTE: 1) the submandibular triangle is bounded by the two bellies of the digastric muscle and by the lower border of the body of the mandible. Anteriorly, the floor of the triangle is formed by the mylohyoid muscle, whereas posteriorly it is the hyoglossus muscle.

2) the submandibular gland is situated in the anterior part of the triangle. Crossing obliquely are the anterior facial vein and facial artery. Overlying the posterior part of the triangle is the inferior extension of the parotid gland. Likewise, arranged along the lower border of the body of the mandible are a number of submandibular lymph nodes.

**Fig. 529: The Suprahyoid Muscles and Hyoid Bone (Viewed from Below)**

NOTE that indicated on the mandible are the inner attachments of the mylohyoid muscle (broken line) and the anterior belly of the digastric muscle (circle). Observe the attachments of the mylohyoid, digastric and stylohyoid muscles as well as the stylohyoid ligament onto the hyoid bone.

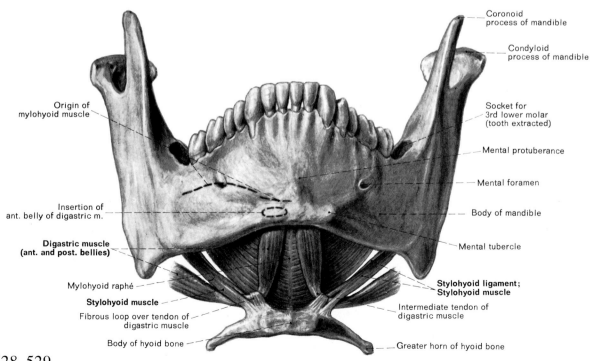

Figs. 528, 529

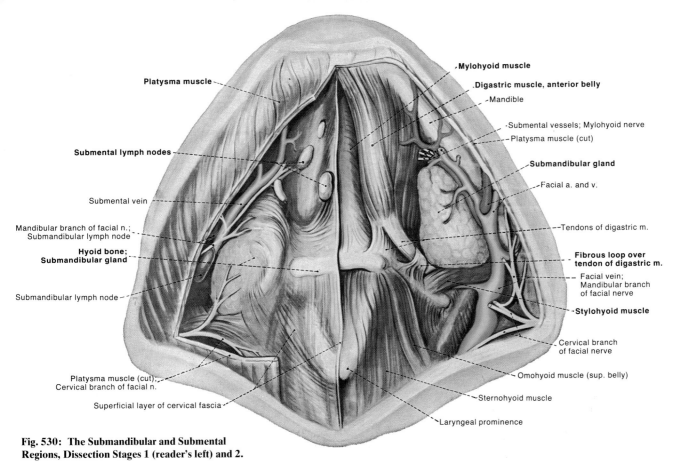

Platysma muscle

Submental lymph nodes

Submental vein

Mandibular branch of facial n.;
Submandibular lymph node

**Hyoid bone;
Submandibular gland**

Submandibular lymph node

Platysma muscle (cut);
Cervical branch of facial n.

Superficial layer of cervical fascia

**Mylohyoid muscle**

Digastric muscle, anterior belly

Mandible

Submental vessels; Mylohyoid nerve

Platysma muscle (cut)

**Submandibular gland**

Facial a. and v.

Tendons of digastric m.

**Fibrous loop over
tendon of digastric m.**

Facial vein;
Mandibular branch
of facial nerve

**Stylohyoid muscle**

Cervical branch
of facial nerve

Omohyoid muscle (sup. belly)

Sternohyoid muscle

Laryngeal prominence

**Fig. 530: The Submandibular and Submental
Regions, Dissection Stages 1 (reader's left) and 2.**

NOTE that in Dissection Stage 1 the superficial fascia containing the platysma has been opened, revealing the submandibular gland and the superficial lymph nodes. In Stage 2 (reader's right), the superficial layer of cervical fascia has been removed, thereby exposing the substance of the submandibular gland and the digastric (anterior belly), mylohyoid and stylohyoid muscles.

**Fig. 531: The Submandibular and Submental Regions, Dissection Stages 3 (reader's left) and 4.**

NOTE that in Dissection Stage 3 much of the submandibular gland has been removed, revealing the posterior border of the mylohyoid muscle and the submental vessels and mylohyoid nerve. In Stage 4, the anterior belly of the digastric and the mylohyoid muscles have been partially removed, exposing the hypoglossal nerve and its accompanying vein.

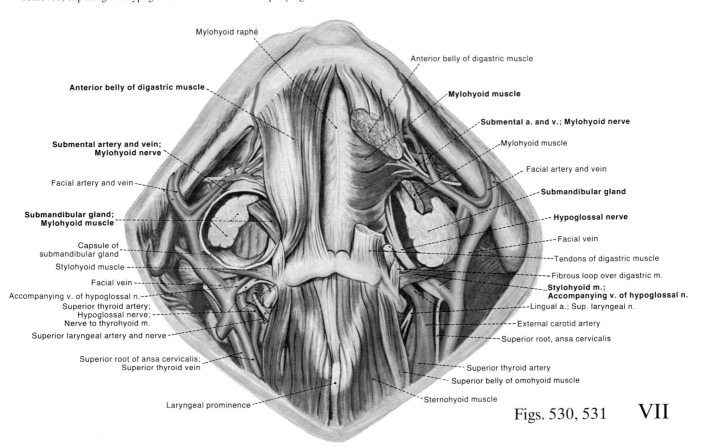

Mylohyoid raphé

Anterior belly of digastric muscle

**Anterior belly of digastric muscle**

**Submental artery and vein;
Mylohyoid nerve**

Facial artery and vein

**Submandibular gland;
Mylohyoid muscle**

Capsule of
submandibular gland

Stylohyoid muscle

Facial vein

Accompanying v. of hypoglossal n.
Superior thyroid artery;
Hypoglossal nerve;
Nerve to thyrohyoid m.

Superior laryngeal artery and nerve

Superior root of ansa cervicalis;
Superior thyroid vein

Laryngeal prominence

**Mylohyoid muscle**

**Submental a. and v.; Mylohyoid nerve**

Mylohyoid muscle

Facial artery and vein

**Submandibular gland**

**Hypoglossal nerve**

Facial vein

Tendons of digastric muscle

Fibrous loop over digastric m.

**Stylohyoid m.;
Accompanying v. of hypoglossal n.**

Lingual a.; Sup. laryngeal n.

External carotid artery

Superior root, ansa cervicalis

Superior thyroid artery

Superior belly of omohyoid muscle

Sternohyoid muscle

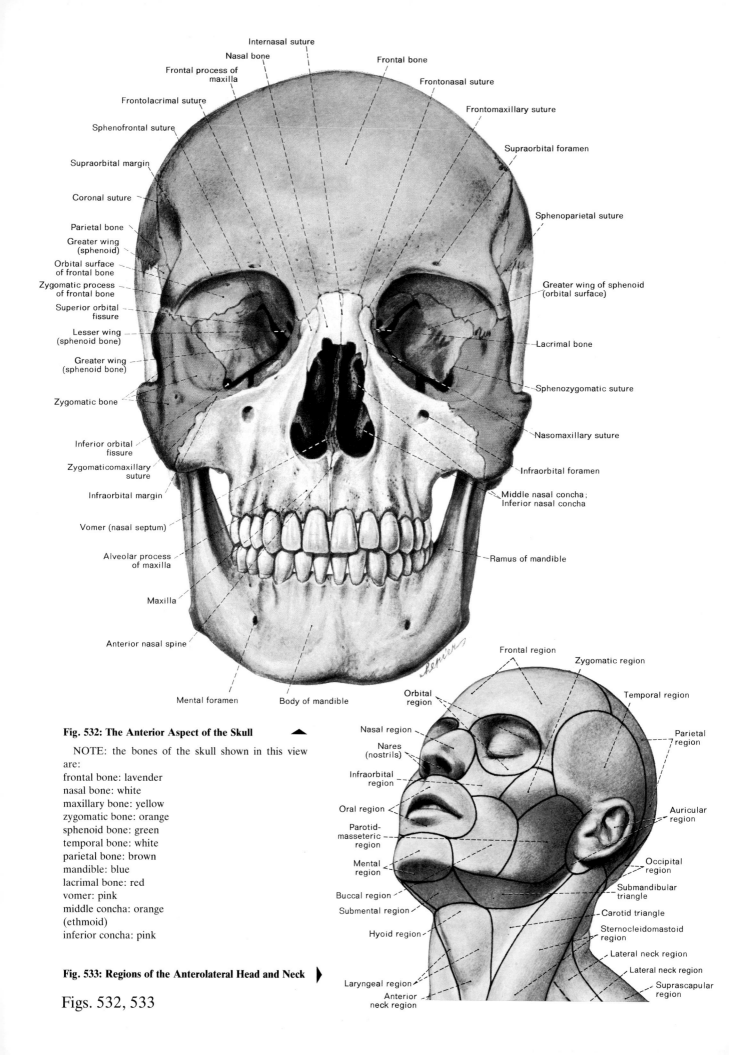

Internasal suture

Nasal bone

Frontal process of
maxilla

Frontolacrimal suture

Sphenofrontal suture

Supraorbital margin

Coronal suture

Parietal bone

Greater wing
(sphenoid)

Orbital surface
of frontal bone

Zygomatic process
of frontal bone

Superior orbital
fissure

Lesser wing
(sphenoid bone)

Greater wing
(sphenoid bone)

Zygomatic bone

Inferior orbital
fissure

Zygomaticomaxillary
suture

Infraorbital margin

Vomer (nasal septum)

Alveolar process
of maxilla

Maxilla

Anterior nasal spine

Mental foramen

Frontal bone

Frontonasal suture

Frontomaxillary suture

Supraorbital foramen

Sphenoparietal suture

Greater wing of sphenoid
(orbital surface)

Lacrimal bone

Sphenozygomatic suture

Nasomaxillary suture

Infraorbital foramen

Middle nasal concha;
Inferior nasal concha

Ramus of mandible

Body of mandible

**Fig. 532: The Anterior Aspect of the Skull** ▲

NOTE: the bones of the skull shown in this view
are:
frontal bone: lavender
nasal bone: white
maxillary bone: yellow
zygomatic bone: orange
sphenoid bone: green
temporal bone: white
parietal bone: brown
mandible: blue
lacrimal bone: red
vomer: pink
middle concha: orange
(ethmoid)
inferior concha: pink

**Fig. 533: Regions of the Anterolateral Head and Neck** ▶

Figs. 532, 533

Frontal region

Zygomatic region

Temporal region

Orbital
region

Parietal
region

Nasal region

Nares
(nostrils)

Infraorbital
region

Oral region

Parotid-
masseteric
region

Auricular
region

Mental
region

Occipital
region

Buccal region

Submental region

Submandibular
triangle

Carotid triangle

Sternocleidomastoid
region

Lateral neck region

Hyoid region

Lateral neck region

Laryngeal region

Suprascapular
region

Anterior
neck region

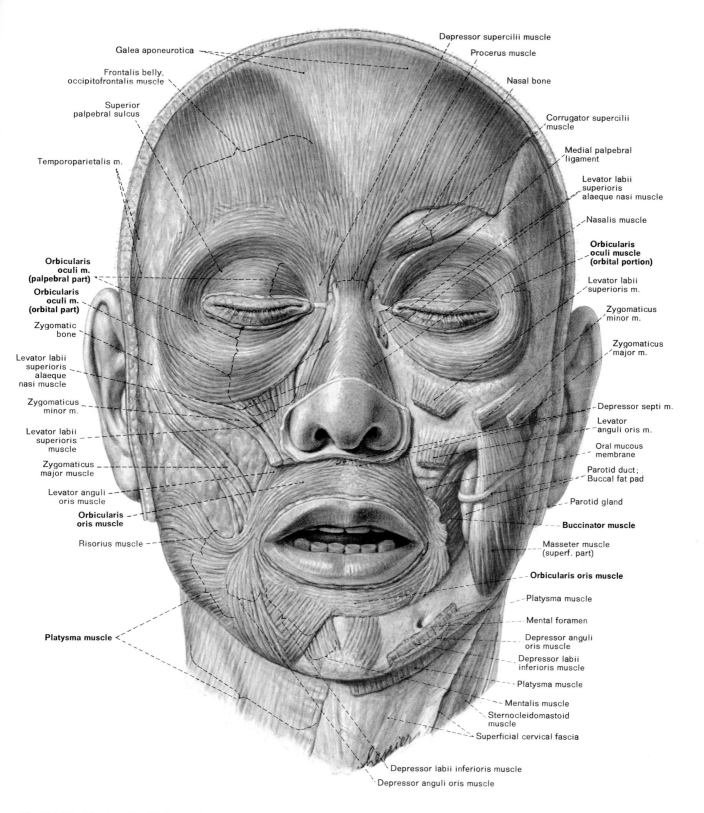

**Fig. 534: The Muscles of Facial Expression (Anterior View)**

NOTE: 1) the muscles of facial expression are superficial muscles located within the layers of subcutaneous fascia. Having developed from the mesoderm of the 2nd branchial arch, they are all innervated by the nerve of that arch, the seventh cranial or facial nerve.

2) the facial muscles may be grouped into: a) the muscles of the scalp, b) the muscles of external ear, c) the muscles of the eyelid, d) the nasal muscles and e) the oral muscles. Frequently, the limits of the facial muscles are not easily defined and there is a tendency for them to merge. The platysma muscle also belongs in the facial group, even though it extends over the neck.

3) the circular muscles surrounding the eyes (orbicularis oculi) and the mouth (orbicularis oris) assist in closure of the orbital and oral apertures, and thus contribute to functions such as blinking of the eyelids and the oral ingestion of liquids and food.

4) since facial muscles can respond to thoughts and emotions, they are of assistance in communicative functions. The buccinator muscles are flat and are situated on the lateral aspects of the oral cavity. They assist in mastication by pressing the cheeks against the teeth, and thus, prevent food from accumulating in the oral vestibule.

Fig. 534  **VII**

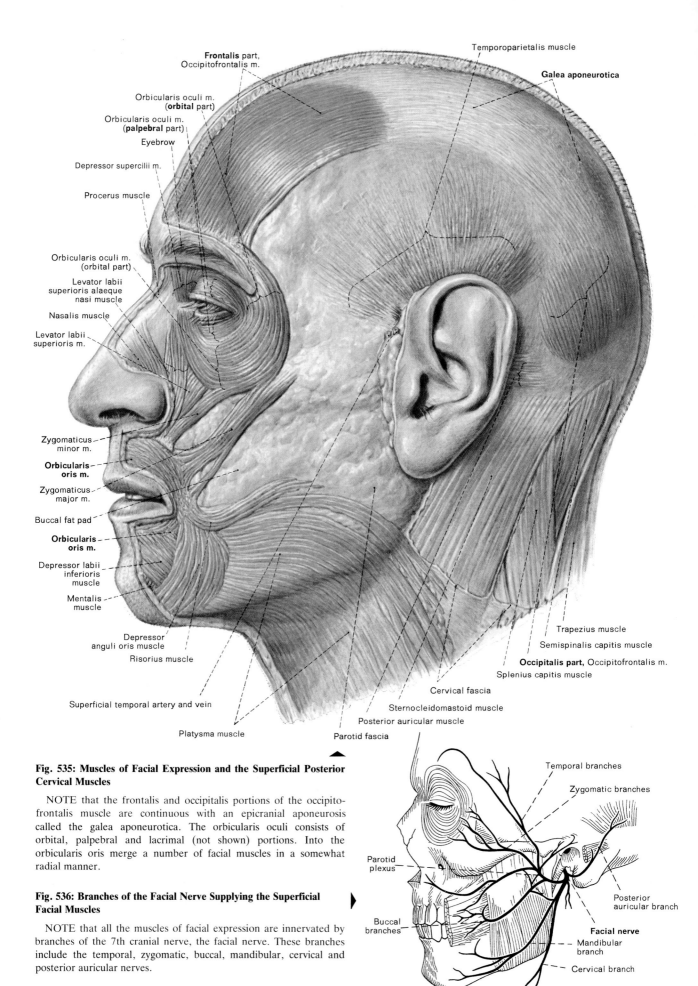

Frontalis part,
Occipitofrontalis m.

Temporoparietalis muscle

Galea aponeurotica

Orbicularis oculi m.
(orbital part)

Orbicularis oculi m.
(palpebral part)

Eyebrow

Depressor supercilii m.

Procerus muscle

Orbicularis oculi m.
(orbital part)

Levator labii
superioris alaeque
nasi muscle

Nasalis muscle

Levator labii
superioris m.

Zygomaticus
minor m.

Orbicularis
oris m.

Zygomaticus
major m.

Buccal fat pad

Orbicularis
oris m.

Depressor labii
inferioris
muscle

Mentalis
muscle

Depressor
anguli oris muscle

Risorius muscle

Superficial temporal artery and vein

Platysma muscle

Parotid fascia

Trapezius muscle

Semispinalis capitis muscle

Occipitalis part, Occipitofrontalis m.

Splenius capitis muscle

Cervical fascia

Sternocleidomastoid muscle

Posterior auricular muscle

**Fig. 535: Muscles of Facial Expression and the Superficial Posterior Cervical Muscles**

NOTE that the frontalis and occipitalis portions of the occipito-frontalis muscle are continuous with an epicranial aponeurosis called the galea aponeurotica. The orbicularis oculi consists of orbital, palpebral and lacrimal (not shown) portions. Into the orbicularis oris merge a number of facial muscles in a somewhat radial manner.

**Fig. 536: Branches of the Facial Nerve Supplying the Superficial Facial Muscles**

NOTE that all the muscles of facial expression are innervated by branches of the 7th cranial nerve, the facial nerve. These branches include the temporal, zygomatic, buccal, mandibular, cervical and posterior auricular nerves.

Temporal branches

Zygomatic branches

Parotid
plexus

Posterior
auricular branch

Buccal
branches

**Facial nerve**

Mandibular
branch

Cervical branch

Figs. 535, 536

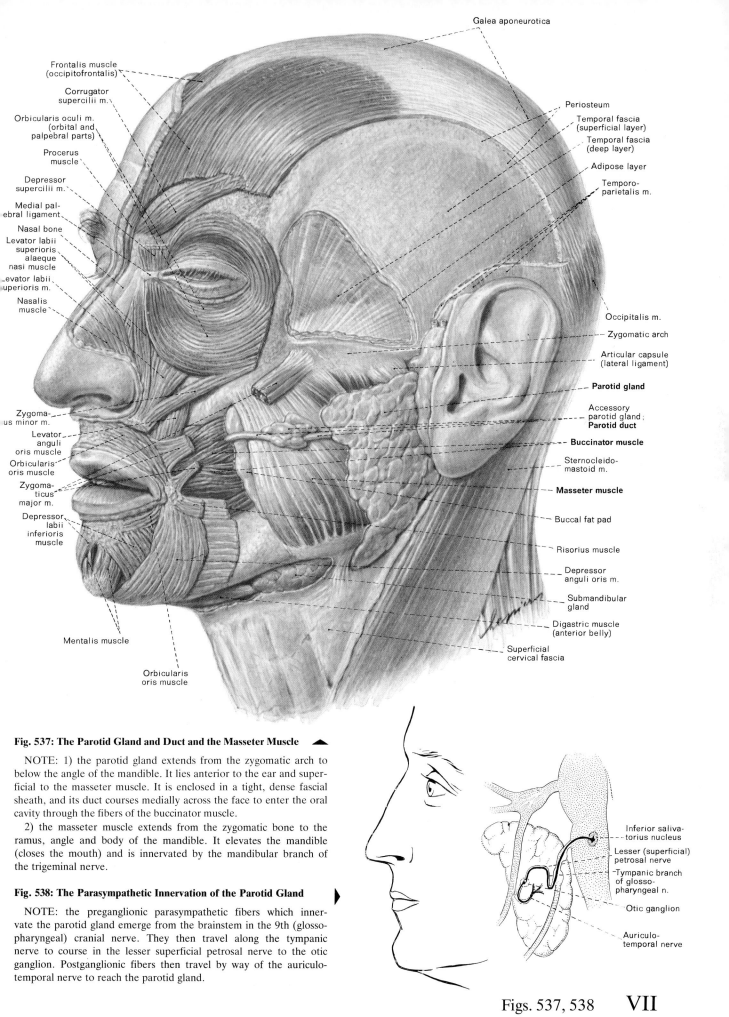

Galea aponeurotica

Frontalis muscle
(occipitofrontalis)

Corrugator
supercilii m.

Orbicularis oculi m.
(orbital and
palpebral parts)

Procerus
muscle

Depressor
supercilii m.

Medial pal-
ebral ligament

Nasal bone

Levator labii
superioris
alaeque
nasi muscle

Levator labii
superioris m.

Nasalis
muscle

Zygoma-
us minor m.

Levator
anguli
oris muscle

Orbicularis
oris muscle

Zygoma-
ticus
major m.

Depressor
labii
inferioris
muscle

Mentalis muscle

Orbicularis
oris muscle

Periosteum

Temporal fascia
(superficial layer)

Temporal fascia
(deep layer)

Adipose layer

Temporo-
parietalis m.

Occipitalis m.

Zygomatic arch

Articular capsule
(lateral ligament)

**Parotid gland**

Accessory
parotid gland;
**Parotid duct**

**Buccinator muscle**

Sternocleido-
mastoid m.

**Masseter muscle**

Buccal fat pad

Risorius muscle

Depressor
anguli oris m.

Submandibular
gland

Digastric muscle
(anterior belly)

Superficial
cervical fascia

**Fig. 537: The Parotid Gland and Duct and the Masseter Muscle** ▲

NOTE: 1) the parotid gland extends from the zygomatic arch to below the angle of the mandible. It lies anterior to the ear and superficial to the masseter muscle. It is enclosed in a tight, dense fascial sheath, and its duct courses medially across the face to enter the oral cavity through the fibers of the buccinator muscle.

2) the masseter muscle extends from the zygomatic bone to the ramus, angle and body of the mandible. It elevates the mandible (closes the mouth) and is innervated by the mandibular branch of the trigeminal nerve.

**Fig. 538: The Parasympathetic Innervation of the Parotid Gland** ▶

NOTE: the preganglionic parasympathetic fibers which innervate the parotid gland emerge from the brainstem in the 9th (glossopharyngeal) cranial nerve. They then travel along the tympanic nerve to course in the lesser superficial petrosal nerve to the otic ganglion. Postganglionic fibers then travel by way of the auriculotemporal nerve to reach the parotid gland.

Inferior saliva-
torius nucleus

Lesser (superficial)
petrosal nerve

Tympanic branch
of glosso-
pharyngeal n.

Otic ganglion

Auriculo-
temporal nerve

Figs. 537, 538     VII

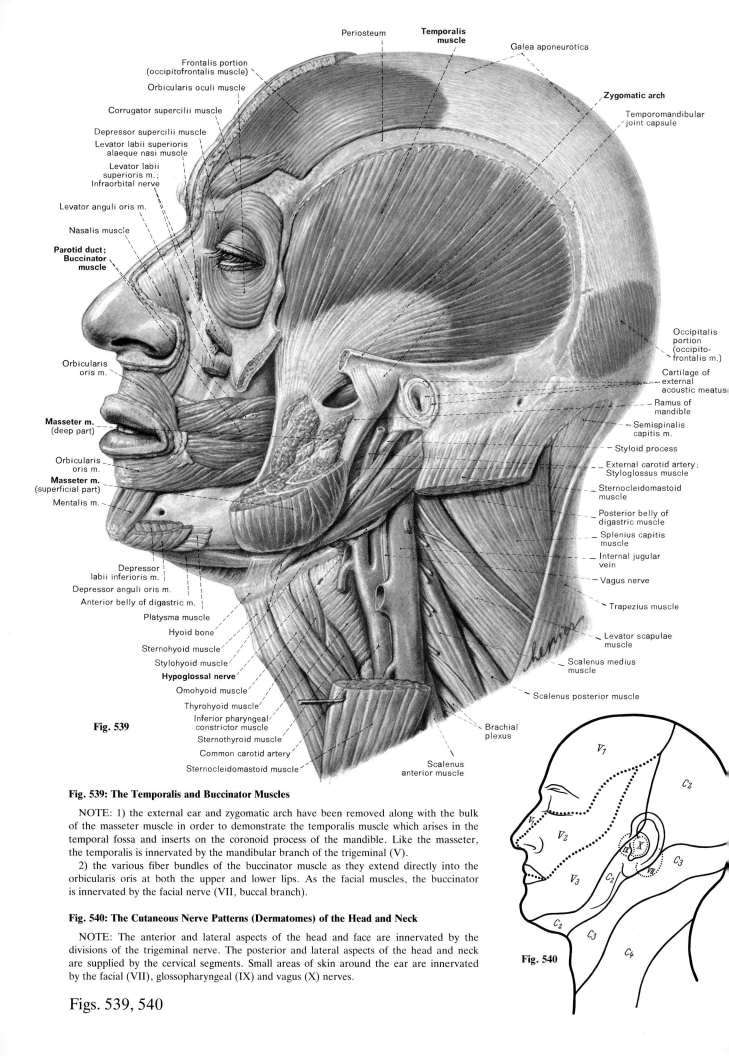

**Fig. 539**

Periosteum

Frontalis portion
(occipitofrontalis muscle)

Orbicularis oculi muscle

Corrugator supercilii muscle

Depressor supercilii muscle

Levator labii superioris
alaeque nasi muscle

Levator labii
superioris m. ;
Infraorbital nerve

Levator anguli oris m.

Nasalis muscle

**Parotid duct ;
Buccinator
muscle**

Orbicularis
oris m.

**Masseter m.
(deep part)**

Orbicularis
oris m.

**Masseter m.
(superficial part)**

Mentalis m.

Depressor
labii inferioris m.

Depressor anguli oris m.

Anterior belly of digastric m.

Platysma muscle

Hyoid bone

Sternohyoid muscle

Stylohyoid muscle

**Hypoglossal nerve**

Omohyoid muscle

Thyrohyoid muscle

Inferior pharyngeal
constrictor muscle

Sternothyroid muscle

Common carotid artery

Sternocleidomastoid muscle

**Temporalis
muscle**

Galea aponeurotica

**Zygomatic arch**

Temporomandibular
joint capsule

Occipitalis
portion
(occipito-
frontalis m.)

Cartilage of
external
acoustic meatus

Ramus of
mandible

Semispinalis
capitis m.

Styloid process

External carotid artery ;
Styloglossus muscle

Sternocleidomastoid
muscle

Posterior belly of
digastric muscle

Splenius capitis
muscle

Internal jugular
vein

Vagus nerve

Trapezius muscle

Levator scapulae
muscle

Scalenus medius
muscle

Scalenus posterior muscle

Brachial
plexus

Scalenus
anterior muscle

**Fig. 539: The Temporalis and Buccinator Muscles**

NOTE: 1) the external ear and zygomatic arch have been removed along with the bulk of the masseter muscle in order to demonstrate the temporalis muscle which arises in the temporal fossa and inserts on the coronoid process of the mandible. Like the masseter, the temporalis is innervated by the mandibular branch of the trigeminal (V).

2) the various fiber bundles of the buccinator muscle as they extend directly into the orbicularis oris at both the upper and lower lips. As the facial muscles, the buccinator is innervated by the facial nerve (VII, buccal branch).

**Fig. 540: The Cutaneous Nerve Patterns (Dermatomes) of the Head and Neck**

NOTE: The anterior and lateral aspects of the head and face are innervated by the divisions of the trigeminal nerve. The posterior and lateral aspects of the head and neck are supplied by the cervical segments. Small areas of skin around the ear are innervated by the facial (VII), glossopharyngeal (IX) and vagus (X) nerves.

$V_1$   $C_2$

$V_2$

$V_3$   $C_2$   $C_3$

$C_2$   $C_3$

$C_4$

**Fig. 540**

Figs. 539, 540

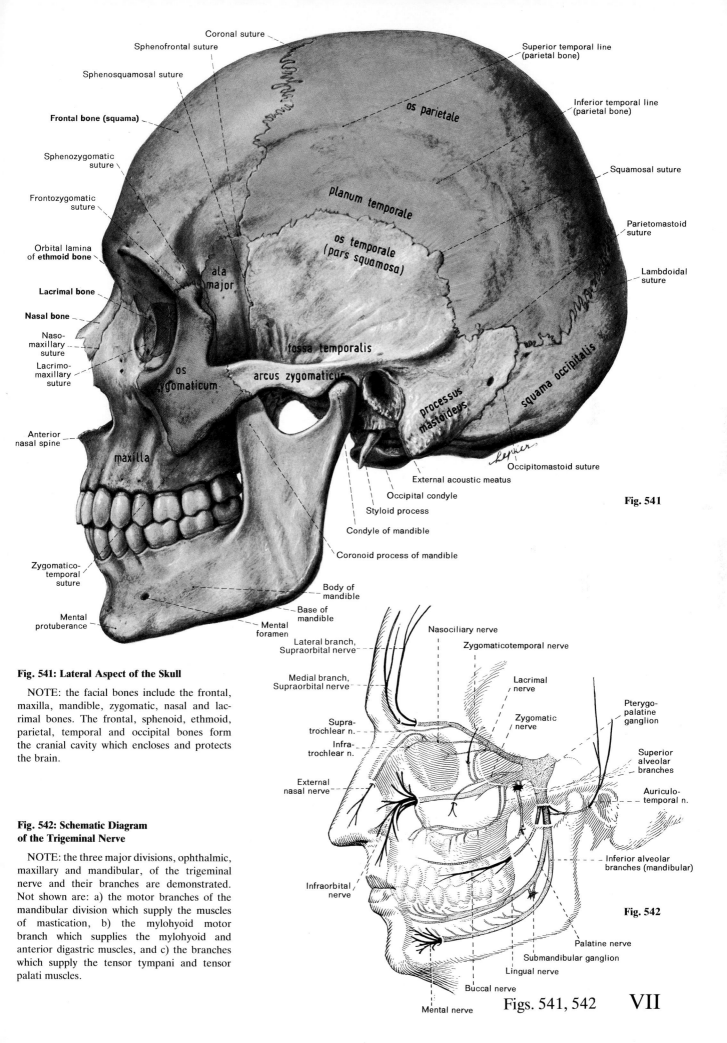

**Fig. 541: Lateral Aspect of the Skull**

NOTE: the facial bones include the frontal, maxilla, mandible, zygomatic, nasal and lacrimal bones. The frontal, sphenoid, ethmoid, parietal, temporal and occipital bones form the cranial cavity which encloses and protects the brain.

**Fig. 542: Schematic Diagram of the Trigeminal Nerve**

NOTE: the three major divisions, ophthalmic, maxillary and mandibular, of the trigeminal nerve and their branches are demonstrated. Not shown are: a) the motor branches of the mandibular division which supply the muscles of mastication, b) the mylohyoid motor branch which supplies the mylohyoid and anterior digastric muscles, and c) the branches which supply the tensor tympani and tensor palati muscles.

Figs. 541, 542     VII

## Fig. 543: The Right Temporomandibular Joint (Lateral View)

NOTE: 1) the articular capsule and the lateral (temporomandibular) ligaments which extend between the zygomatic process of the temporal bone above to the neck of the condylar process of the mandibular ramus below;

2) that the articular capsule is a loose sac which is fused anteriorly and laterally with the lateral (temporomandibular) ligament. Note also the stylomandibular ligament extending from the tip of the styloid process to the angle and posterior border of the mandible.

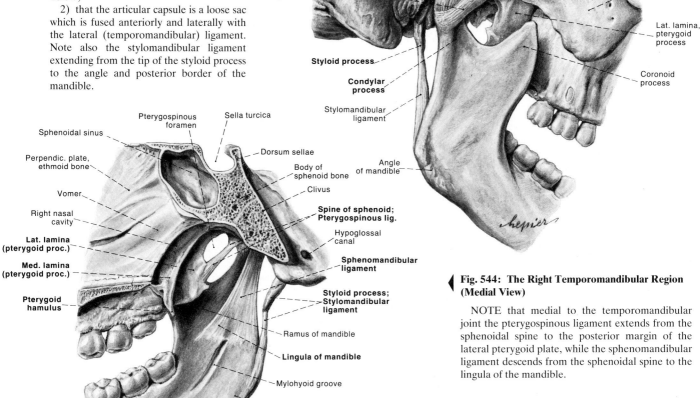

**Articular capsule** — **Zygomatic process of temporal bone**

**External acoustic meatus**

**Lateral (temporo- mandibular) ligament** — Zygomatic bone

**Styloid process** — Lat. lamina, pterygoid process

**Condylar process** — Coronoid process

Stylomandibular ligament

Angle of mandible

Sphenoidal sinus

Pterygospinous foramen — Sella turcica

Perpendic. plate, ethmoid bone — Dorsum sellae

Vomer — Body of sphenoid bone

Right nasal cavity — Clivus

**Lat. lamina (pterygoid proc.)** — **Spine of sphenoid; Pterygospinous lig.**

**Med. lamina (pterygoid proc.)** — Hypoglossal canal

**Pterygoid hamulus** — **Sphenomandibular ligament**

**Styloid process; Stylomandibular ligament**

Ramus of mandible

**Lingula of mandible**

Mylohyoid groove

Angle of mandible

Mylohyoid line

## Fig. 544: The Right Temporomandibular Region (Medial View)

NOTE that medial to the temporomandibular joint the pterygospinous ligament extends from the sphenoidal spine to the posterior margin of the lateral pterygoid plate, while the sphenomandibular ligament descends from the sphenoidal spine to the lingula of the mandible.

## Fig. 545  The Medial and Lateral Pterygoid Muscles (Lateral View)

NOTE: 1) the left zygomatic arch has been removed. Posteriorly, the bone has been cut through the temporomandibular joint, revealing the articular disc. The location of the medial pterygoid muscle and part of the lateral pterygoid muscle on the inner aspect of the ramus of the mandible is represented as though the bone were transparent.

2) the lateral pterygoid muscle arises by two heads, a superior from the great wing of the sphenoid bone and an inferior from the lateral surface of the lateral pterygoid plate of the sphenoid. The two heads insert posteriorly on the neck of the condyle of the mandible. The lateral pterygoid muscle opens and protracts the mandible and also moves it from side to side.

3) the medial pterygoid muscle arises from the medial surface of the lateral pterygoid plate of the sphenoid as well as from the palatine bone, and inserts on the medial surface of the ramus and angle of the mandible. It assists the masseter and temporalis in closing the jaw.

Figs. 543, 544, 545

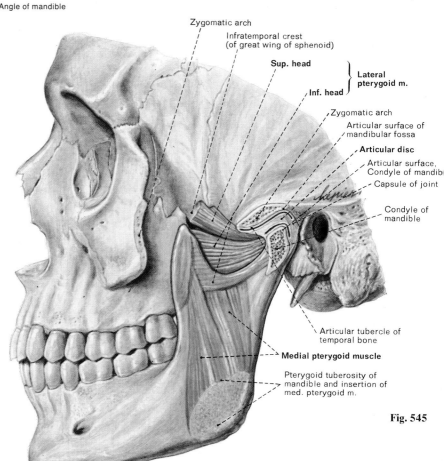

Zygomatic arch

Infratemporal crest (of great wing of sphenoid)

**Sup. head** — } **Lateral pterygoid m.**

**Inf. head** — }

Zygomatic arch

Articular surface of mandibular fossa

**Articular disc**

Articular surface, Condyle of mandib

Capsule of joint

Condyle of mandible

Articular tubercle of temporal bone

**Medial pterygoid muscle**

Pterygoid tuberosity of mandible and insertion of med. pterygoid m.

Fig. 545

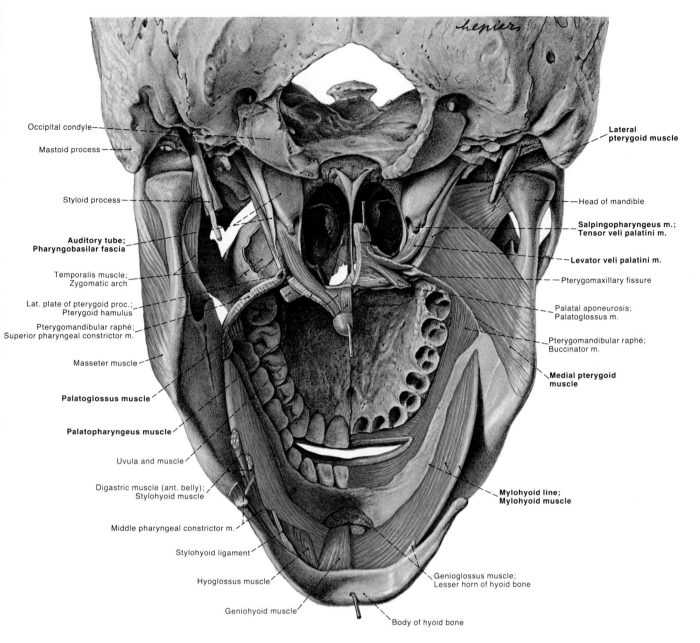

Occipital condyle—

Mastoid process—

Styloid process—

**Auditory tube;**
**Pharyngobasilar fascia**

Temporalis muscle;
Zygomatic arch

Lat. plate of pterygoid proc.;
Pterygoid hamulus

Pterygomandibular raphé;
Superior pharyngeal constrictor m.

Masseter muscle—

**Palatoglossus muscle**—

**Palatopharyngeus muscle**—

Uvula and muscle—

Digastric muscle (ant. belly);
Stylohyoid muscle

Middle pharyngeal constrictor m.—

Stylohyoid ligament—

Hyoglossus muscle—

Geniohyoid muscle—

**Lateral**
**pterygoid muscle**

—Head of mandible

**Salpingopharyngeus m.;**
**Tensor veli palatini m.**

—**Levator veli palatini m.**

—Pterygomaxillary fissure

—Palatal aponeurosis;
Palatoglossus m.

—Pterygomandibular raphé;
Buccinator m.

\—**Medial pterygoid**
**muscle**

**Mylohyoid line;**
**Mylohyoid muscle**

Genioglossus muscle;
Lesser horn of hyoid bone

Body of hyoid bone

**Fig. 546:  The Pterygoid, Buccinator and Mylohyoid Muscles as Seen from Below and Behind.**

NOTE: 1)  that a muscular sling is formed around the posterior border of the ramus of the mandible as far as its angle by the insertions of the medial pterygoid muscle (seen on the right) and the masseter muscle (seen on the left). The medial pterygoid muscle descends to attach along the medial aspect of the mandible, while the fibers of the masseter course downward to insert on the outer aspect of the jaw.

2)  that the fibers of the lateral pterygoid muscle (right side) course principally in the horizontal plane. Observe that the mylohyoid and geniohyoid muscles attach the mandible to the hyoid bone. Other muscles shown to advantage in this figure are the tensor and levator veli palatini muscles.

3)  the right pterygomandibular raphé extending between the pterygoid hamulus and the mylohyoid line. This raphé gives attachment to the buccinator muscle which forms the soft lateral wall of the oral cavity on each side.

**Figs. 547 and 548:  Sagittal Sections of Temporomandibular Joint**

NOTE: 1) the articular disc (stippled structure) is an oval plate interposed between the mandibular fossa of the temporal bone and the condyle of the mandible. Thus, there exists a joint cavity between the disc and the mandibular fossa and another between the disc and the condyle.

2) with the jaw closed (547), the head of the condyle of the mandible and the articular disc lie totally within the mandibular fossa. When the jaw is opened (548), the condyle turns in a hinge-fashion on the disc, and both bone and disc glide forward within the joint capsule to lie opposite the articular tubercle of the temporal bone.

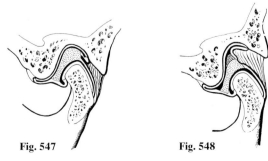

**Fig. 547**          **Fig. 548**

Figs. 546, 547, 548    VII

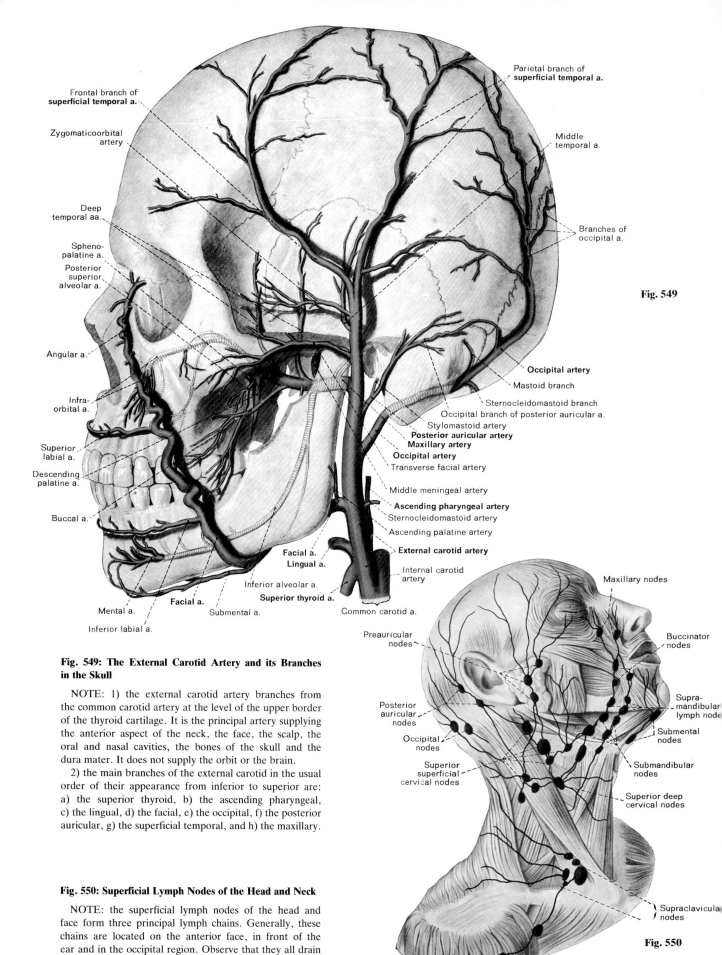

Frontal branch of **superficial temporal a.**

Zygomaticoorbital artery

Deep temporal aa.

Spheno-palatine a.

Posterior superior alveolar a.

Angular a.

Infra-orbital a.

Superior labial a.

Descending palatine a.

Buccal a.

Mental a.

Inferior labial a.

**Facial a.**

Submental a.

**Facial a.**
**Lingual a.**

Inferior alveolar a.

**Superior thyroid a.**

Common carotid a.

Internal carotid artery

**External carotid artery**

Ascending palatine artery

Sternocleidomastoid artery

**Ascending pharyngeal artery**

Middle meningeal artery

Transverse facial artery

**Occipital artery**
**Maxillary artery**
**Posterior auricular artery**

Stylomastoid artery

Occipital branch of posterior auricular a.

Sternocleidomastoid branch

Mastoid branch

**Occipital artery**

Branches of occipital a.

Middle temporal a.

Parietal branch of **superficial temporal a.**

**Fig. 549**

**Fig. 549: The External Carotid Artery and its Branches in the Skull**

NOTE: 1) the external carotid artery branches from the common carotid artery at the level of the upper border of the thyroid cartilage. It is the principal artery supplying the anterior aspect of the neck, the face, the scalp, the oral and nasal cavities, the bones of the skull and the dura mater. It does not supply the orbit or the brain.

2) the main branches of the external carotid in the usual order of their appearance from inferior to superior are: a) the superior thyroid, b) the ascending pharyngeal, c) the lingual, d) the facial, e) the occipital, f) the posterior auricular, g) the superficial temporal, and h) the maxillary.

**Fig. 550: Superficial Lymph Nodes of the Head and Neck**

NOTE: the superficial lymph nodes of the head and face form three principal lymph chains. Generally, these chains are located on the anterior face, in front of the ear and in the occipital region. Observe that they all drain inferiorly and posteriorly to the superficial and deeper nodes of the neck.

Maxillary nodes

Buccinator nodes

Supra-mandibular lymph node

Submental nodes

Submandibular nodes

Superior deep cervical nodes

Supraclavicular nodes

Superior superficial cervical nodes

Occipital nodes

Posterior auricular nodes

Preauricular nodes

**Fig. 550**

Figs. 549, 550

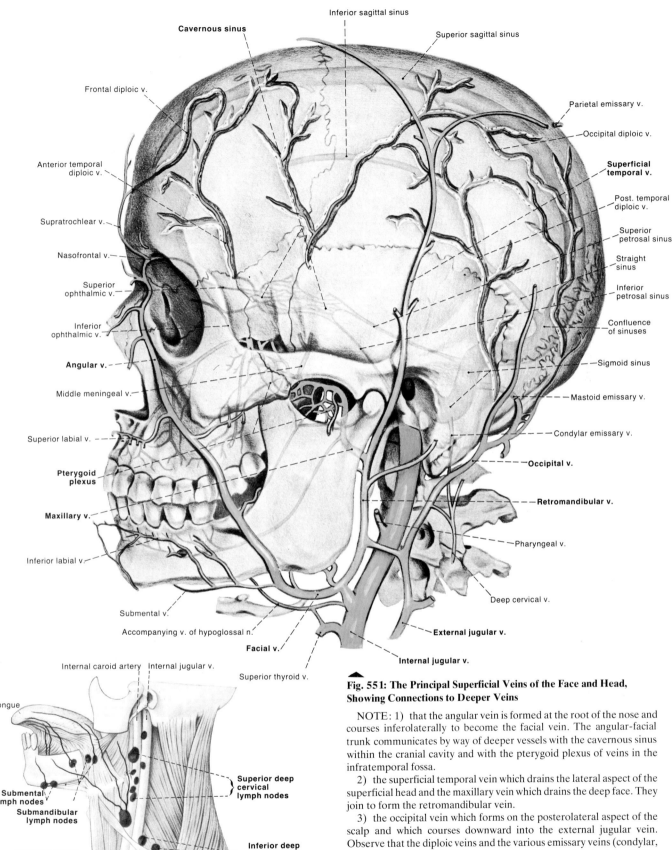

**Fig. 551: The Principal Superficial Veins of the Face and Head, Showing Connections to Deeper Veins**

NOTE: 1) that the angular vein is formed at the root of the nose and courses inferolaterally to become the facial vein. The angular-facial trunk communicates by way of deeper vessels with the cavernous sinus within the cranial cavity and with the pterygoid plexus of veins in the infratemporal fossa.

2) the superficial temporal vein which drains the lateral aspect of the superficial head and the maxillary vein which drains the deep face. They join to form the retromandibular vein.

3) the occipital vein which forms on the posterolateral aspect of the scalp and which courses downward into the external jugular vein. Observe that the diploic veins and the various emissary veins (condylar, mastoid and parietal) which interconnect the superficial veins with the dural sinuses.

**Fig. 552: Lymphatic Drainage from the Tongue and Lower Oral Cavity**

NOTE that lymph from the tongue and lower oral cavity drains downward and posteriorly into submandibular and superior deep cervical nodes along the internal jugular vein.

Figs. 551, 552    VII

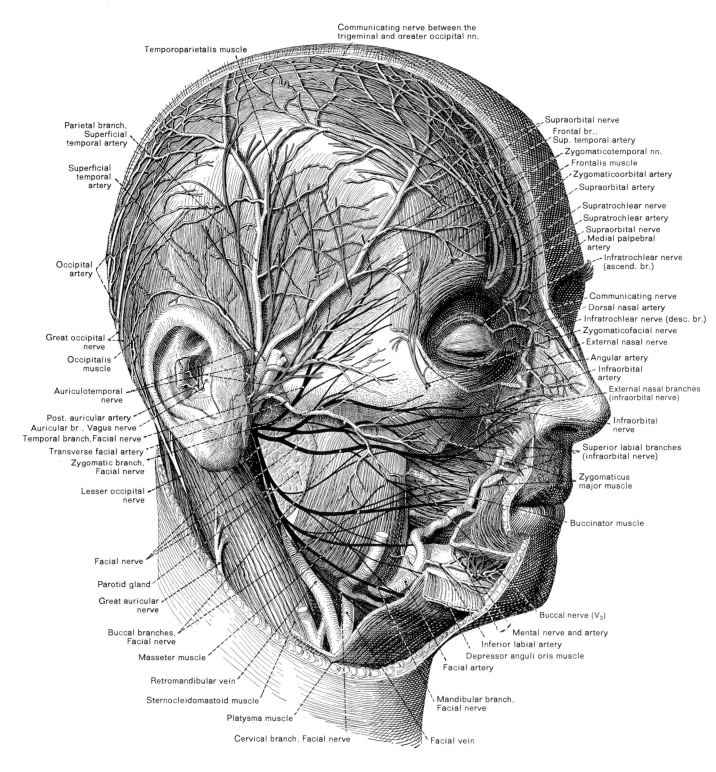

**Fig. 553: Superficial Nerves and Vessels of the Face and Head**

NOTE: 1) a portion of the parotid gland has been removed in order to reveal the branches of the facial nerve (black) which emerge from within the substance of the gland to supply the superficial muscles of facial expression. Identify the temporal, zygomatic, buccal, mandibular, and cervical branches. The posterior auricular branch is not shown.

2) the superficial branches of the trigeminal nerve are indicated in various colors; ophthlamic (yellow), maxillary (blue) and mandibular (green). The trigeminal nerve serves as the cutaneous nerve of the anterior and lateral face, but is also the motor nerve to the muscles of mastication. The cervical sensory nerves (white, not colored) supply the occipital region and much of the ear and neck.

3) the general distribution of the superficial temporal artery and its branches, the zygomaticoorbital and transverse facial arteries. Follow the course of the facial artery across the face to become the angular artery. Among other structures, the facial supplies the chin and the upper and lower lips and anastomoses with vessels emerging from the orbit.

Fig. 553

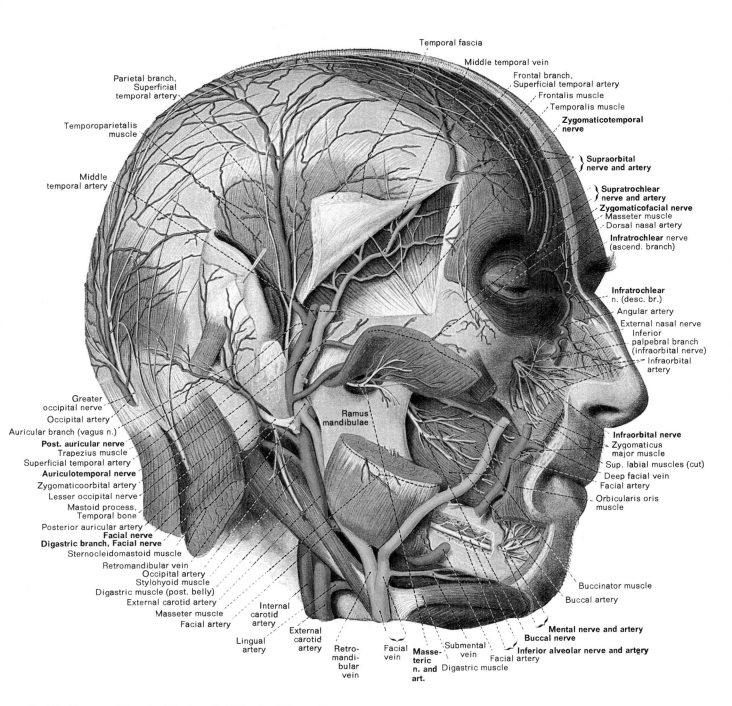

Temporal fascia
Middle temporal vein
Frontal branch, Superficial temporal artery
Frontalis muscle
Temporalis muscle
**Zygomaticotemporal nerve**
**Supraorbital nerve and artery**
**Supratrochlear nerve and artery**
**Zygomaticofacial nerve**
Masseter muscle
Dorsal nasal artery
**Infratrochlear** nerve (ascend. branch)
**Infratrochlear** n. (desc. br.)
Angular artery
External nasal nerve
Inferior palpebral branch (infraorbital nerve)
Infraorbital artery
**Infraorbital nerve**
Zygomaticus major muscle
Sup. labial muscles (cut)
Deep facial vein
Facial artery
Orbicularis oris muscle
Buccinator muscle
Buccal artery
**Mental nerve and artery**
**Buccal nerve**
**Inferior alveolar nerve and artery**

Parietal branch, Superficial temporal artery
Temporoparietalis muscle
Middle temporal artery
Greater occipital nerve
Occipital artery
Auricular branch (vagus n.)
**Post. auricular nerve**
Trapezius muscle
Superficial temporal artery
**Auriculotemporal nerve**
Zygomaticoorbital artery
Lesser occipital nerve
Mastoid process, Temporal bone
Posterior auricular artery
**Facial nerve**
**Digastric branch, Facial nerve**
Sternocleidomastoid muscle
Retromandibular vein
Occipital artery
Stylohyoid muscle
Digastric muscle (post. belly)
External carotid artery
Masseter muscle
Facial artery
Lingual artery
Internal carotid artery
External carotid artery
Retromandibular vein
Facial vein
**Masseteric n. and art.**
Submental vein
Digastric muscle
Facial artery

Ramus mandibulae

## Fig. 554: Nerves and Vessels of the Superficial Head and Deeper Face

NOTE: 1) in this dissection, the temporal fascia has been cut and partially reflected. The superficial muscles on the side of the face have been removed along with the parotid gland. The main trunk of the facial nerve has been cut and its branches across the face removed. The masseter muscle has been severed and its upper half reflected upward.

2a) the supraorbital, supratrochlear, infratrochlear and external nasal branches of the ophthalmic division of the trigeminal nerve.

b) zygomaticotemporal, zygomaticofacial and infraorbital branches of the maxillary division of the trigeminal nerve.

c) auriculotemporal, masseteric, buccal, inferior alveolar and mental branches of the mandibular division of the trigeminal nerve.

3) the posterior auricular, digastric and stylohyoid branches of the facial nerve which arise from the main nerve trunk prior to its division within the parotid gland.

4) the anastomosis of arteries above and at the medial aspect of the orbit. The vessels involved include the frontal branch of the superficial temporal, the supraorbital, supratrochlear, dorsal nasal and angular arteries. Observe the palpebral branches (not labelled) supplying the upper and lower eyelids.

Fig. 554     VII

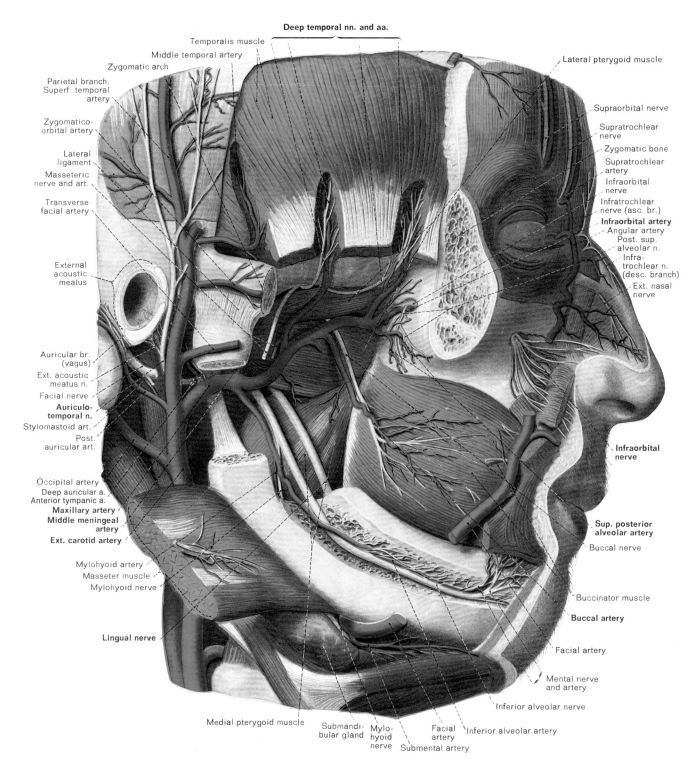

**Deep temporal nn. and aa.**

Temporalis muscle
Middle temporal artery
Zygomatic arch
Parietal branch,
Superf. temporal
artery
Zygomatico-
orbital artery
Lateral
ligament
Masseteric
nerve and art.
Transverse
facial artery
External
acoustic
meatus
Auricular br.
(vagus)
Ext. acoustic
meatus n.
Facial nerve
**Auriculo-
temporal n.**
Stylomastoid art.
Post.
auricular art.
Occipital artery
Deep auricular a.
Anterior tympanic a.
**Maxillary artery**
**Middle meningeal
artery**
**Ext. carotid artery**
Mylohyoid artery
Masseter muscle
Mylohyoid nerve
**Lingual nerve**

Lateral pterygoid muscle
Supraorbital nerve
Supratrochlear
nerve
Zygomatic bone
Supratrochlear
artery
Infraorbital
nerve
Infratrochlear
nerve (asc. br.)
**Infraorbital artery**
Angular artery
Post. sup.
alveolar n.
Infra-
trochlear n.
(desc. branch)
Ext. nasal
nerve
**Infraorbital
nerve**
**Sup. posterior
alveolar artery**
Buccal nerve
Buccinator muscle
**Buccal artery**
Facial artery
Mental nerve
and artery
Inferior alveolar nerve

Medial pterygoid muscle
Submandi-
bular gland
Mylo-
hyoid
nerve
Facial
artery
Submental artery
Inferior alveolar artery

**Fig. 555: The Infratemporal Region and the Maxillary Artery**

NOTE: 1) the zygomatic arch and a portion of the ramus of the mandible have been removed and the temporalis and masseter muscles have been cut and partially reflected. The pterygoid venous plexus has been removed revealing the maxillary artery and its branches.

2) the infratemporal fossa lies deep to the zygomatic arch and posterior to the maxilla. It contains the medial and lateral pterygoid muscles, the inferior part of the temporalis muscle, the maxillary artery, the pterygoid plexus of veins (not shown) and the mandibular division of the trigeminal nerve.

3) the maxillary artery and a number of its branches. Seen in this dissection are the following branches of the maxillary artery: a) deep auricular, b) anterior tympanic, c) inferior alveolar, d) middle meningeal, e) masseteric (cut), f) deep temporal, g) pterygoid (not labelled), h) buccal, i) posterior superior alveolar, j) infraorbital. Branches of the maxillary artery not seen from this view are the greater palatine, the artery of the pterygoid canal, pharyngeal and the sphenopalatine.

4) the auriculotemporal, lingual, inferior alveolar, mylohyoid, masseteric and deep temporal branches of the mandibular division of the trigeminal nerve. Observe the course of the inferior alveolar nerve, accompanied by the inferior alveolar artery within the mandible.

Fig. 555

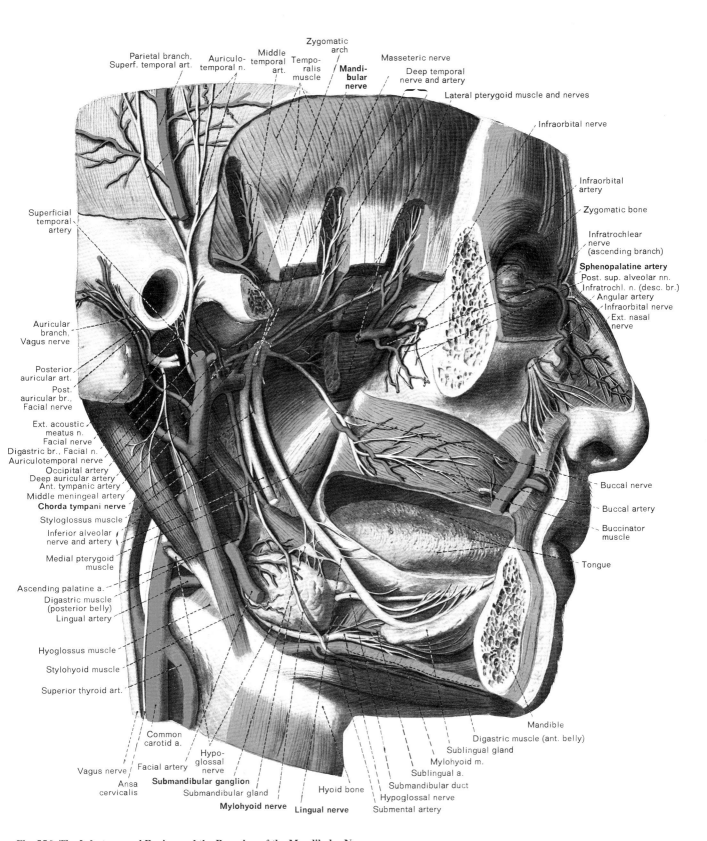

**Fig. 556: The Infratemporal Region and the Branches of the Mandibular Nerve**

NOTE: 1) this dissection of the deep face has removed the zygomatic arch, much of the right mandible and the lateral pterygoid muscle. A portion of the maxillary artery has been cut away along with the distal part of the inferior alveolar nerve beyond the point where the mylohyoid nerve branches.

2) the lingual nerve as it courses to the tongue. High in the infratemporal fossa, the chorda tympani nerve (which is a branch of the facial) joins the lingual. The chorda tympani not only carries special sensory fibers for taste for the anterior two-thirds of the tongue, but additionally carries the preganglionic parasympathetic fibers from the facial nerve to the submandibular ganglion.

3) the distal portion of the maxillary artery as it courses toward the sphenopalatine foramen. After giving off the infraorbital artery, the vessel passes through the foramen and enters the nasal cavity as the sphenopalatine artery, becoming the principal vessel supplying the mucosa overlying the conchae.

Fig. 556    VII

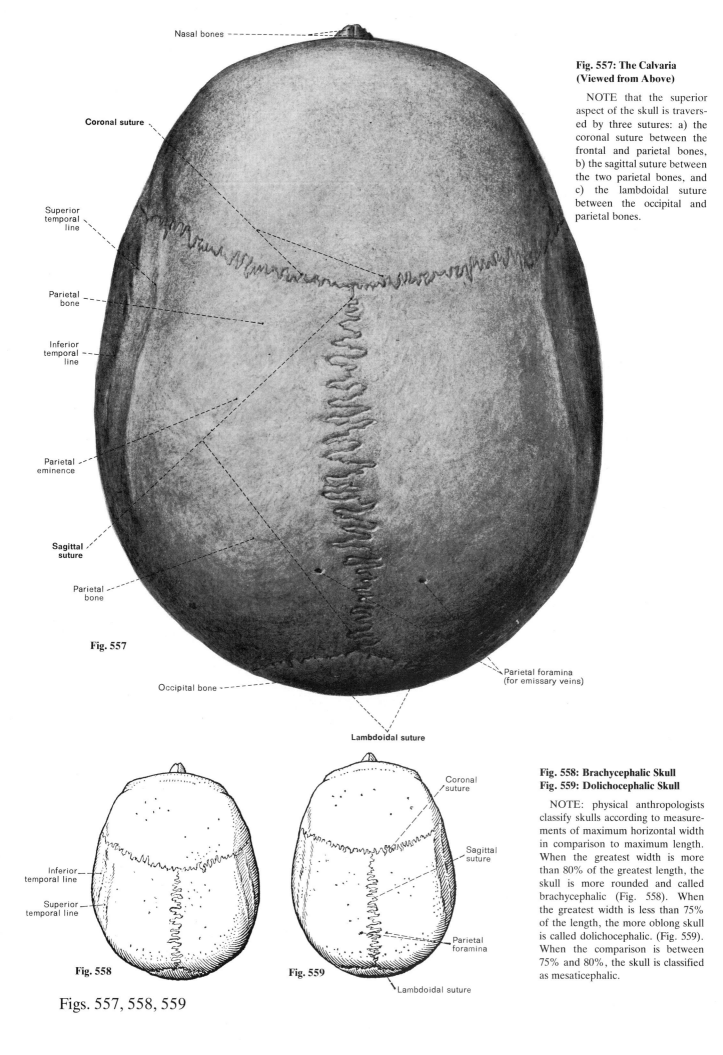

Nasal bones

**Coronal suture**

Superior temporal line

Parietal bone

Inferior temporal line

Parietal eminence

**Sagittal suture**

Parietal bone

**Fig. 557**

Occipital bone

Lambdoidal suture

Parietal foramina (for emissary veins)

**Fig. 557: The Calvaria (Viewed from Above)**

NOTE that the superior aspect of the skull is traversed by three sutures: a) the coronal suture between the frontal and parietal bones, b) the sagittal suture between the two parietal bones, and c) the lambdoidal suture between the occipital and parietal bones.

Coronal suture

Sagittal suture

Parietal foramina

Inferior temporal line

Superior temporal line

**Fig. 558**

**Fig. 559**

Lambdoidal suture

**Fig. 558: Brachycephalic Skull**
**Fig. 559: Dolichocephalic Skull**

NOTE: physical anthropologists classify skulls according to measurements of maximum horizontal width in comparison to maximum length. When the greatest width is more than 80% of the greatest length, the skull is more rounded and called brachycephalic (Fig. 558). When the greatest width is less than 75% of the length, the more oblong skull is called dolichocephalic. (Fig. 559). When the comparison is between 75% and 80%, the skull is classified as mesaticephalic.

Figs. 557, 558, 559

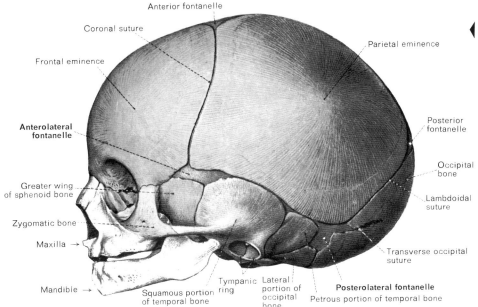

Anterior fontanelle

Coronal suture

Frontal eminence

Parietal eminence

**Anterolateral fontanelle**

Posterior fontanelle

Occipital bone

Greater wing of sphenoid bone

Zygomatic bone

Lambdoidal suture

Maxilla →

Mandible →

Squamous portion of temporal bone

Tympanic ring

Lateral portion of occipital bone

Transverse occipital suture

**Posterolateral fontanelle**

Petrous portion of temporal bone

**Fig. 560: The Skull at Birth (Lateral View)**

NOTE: 1) ossification of the maturing flat bones of the skull is accomplished by the intramembranous process of bone formation. At birth this process is incomplete, thereby leaving softened membranous sites between the growing bones.

2) the nature of the skull just prior to birth is of some benefit, however, since the mobility of the bones permits some changes in its shape, as might be required during the birth process.

3) the soft sites on the skull of the newborn infant are called fontanelles. From this lateral view can be seen at least two such fontanelles, the antero-lateral (or sphenoid) which is at the pterion, and the posterolateral (or mastoid) at the asterion.

**Fig. 561: The Skull at Birth (Seen from Above)**

NOTE: 1) the largest of the fontanelles at birth is the anterior fontanelle located at the bregma and interconnecting the frontal and parietal bones. It is approximately diamond-shaped and is situated at the junction of the coronal and sagittal sutures.

2) following the sagittal suture to its junction with the occipital bone will locate the posterior fontanelle (at the lambda). This is generally triangular in shape and is relatively small at birth.

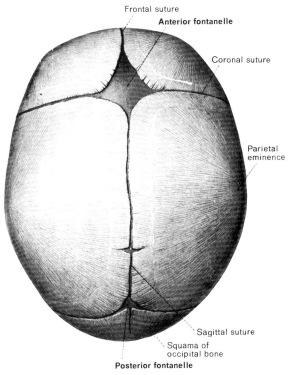

Frontal suture

**Anterior fontanelle**

Coronal suture

Parietal eminence

Sagittal suture

Squama of occipital bone

**Posterior fontanelle**

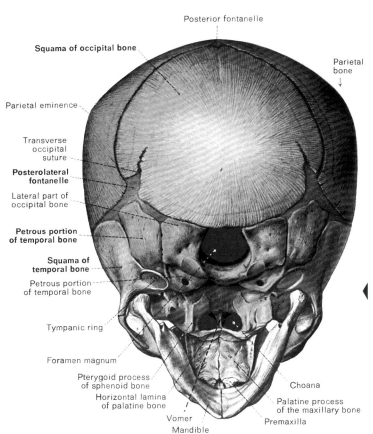

Posterior fontanelle

**Squama of occipital bone**

Parietal bone ↓

Parietal eminence

Transverse occipital suture

**Posterolateral fontanelle**

Lateral part of occipital bone

**Petrous portion of temporal bone**

**Squama of temporal bone**

Petrous portion of temporal bone

Tympanic ring

Foramen magnum

Pterygoid process of sphenoid bone

Horizontal lamina of palatine bone

Vomer

Mandible

Choana

Palatine process of the maxillary bone

Premaxilla

**Fig. 562: The Skull at Birth (Posterior-Inferior View)**

NOTE: 1) the separate ossification of the petrous and squamous portions of the temporal bone as well as the basilar and squamous portions of the occipital bone. The posterolateral fontanelles are found at the articulation of the occipital, temporal and parietal bones.

2) the skull is large at birth in comparison to the size of the rest of the body, however, the facial bones (see Fig. 560) are still rudimentary and not well developed. The teeth have yet to erupt, and the sinuses and nasal cavity are small.

Figs. 560, 561, 562    VII

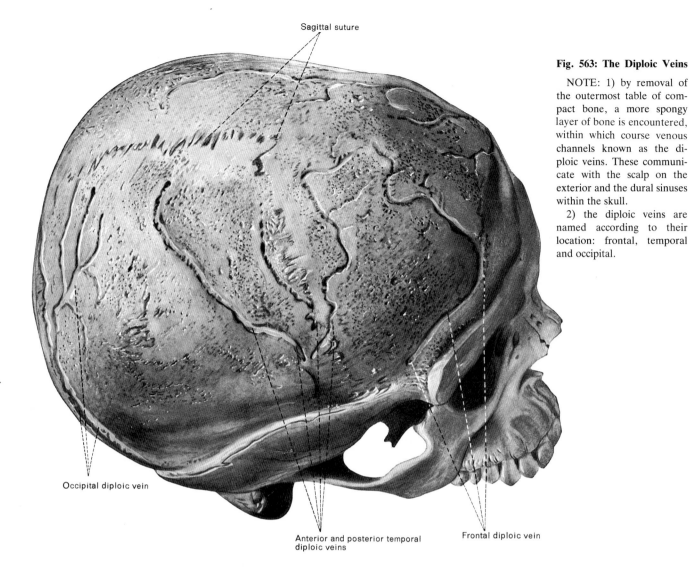

Sagittal suture

Occipital diploic vein

Anterior and posterior temporal diploic veins

Frontal diploic vein

**Fig. 563: The Diploic Veins**

NOTE: 1) by removal of the outermost table of compact bone, a more spongy layer of bone is encountered, within which course venous channels known as the diploic veins. These communicate with the scalp on the exterior and the dural sinuses within the skull.

2) the diploic veins are named according to their location: frontal, temporal and occipital.

**Fig. 564: The Scalp, Skull, Meninges and Brain**

NOTE: 1) this frontal section through the cranium and upper cerebrum depicts the bony and soft coverings of the brain. The veins and dural sinuses are shown in blue. The layers of the scalp and the bony tissue of the skull lie superficial to the dura mater, arachnoid and pia mater coverings of the neural tissue of the brain.

2) the arachnoid granulations which project into the dural sinuses. These tufts of arachnoid lie next to the endothelium of the sinuses and allow the passage of cerebrospinal fluid from the subarachnoid space into the venous system.

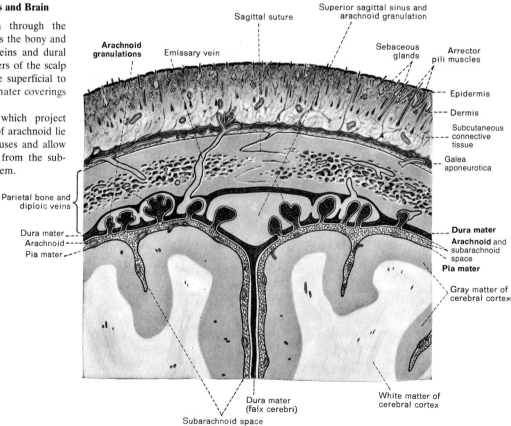

Sagittal suture

Superior sagittal sinus and arachnoid granulation

**Arachnoid granulations**

Emissary vein

Sebaceous glands

Arrector pili muscles

Epidermis

Dermis

Subcutaneous connective tissue

Galea aponeurotica

Parietal bone and diploic veins

Dura mater
Arachnoid
Pia mater

**Dura mater**
**Arachnoid** and subarachnoid space
**Pia mater**

Gray matter of cerebral cortex

Dura mater (falx cerebri)

Subarachnoid space

White matter of cerebral cortex

Figs. 563, 564

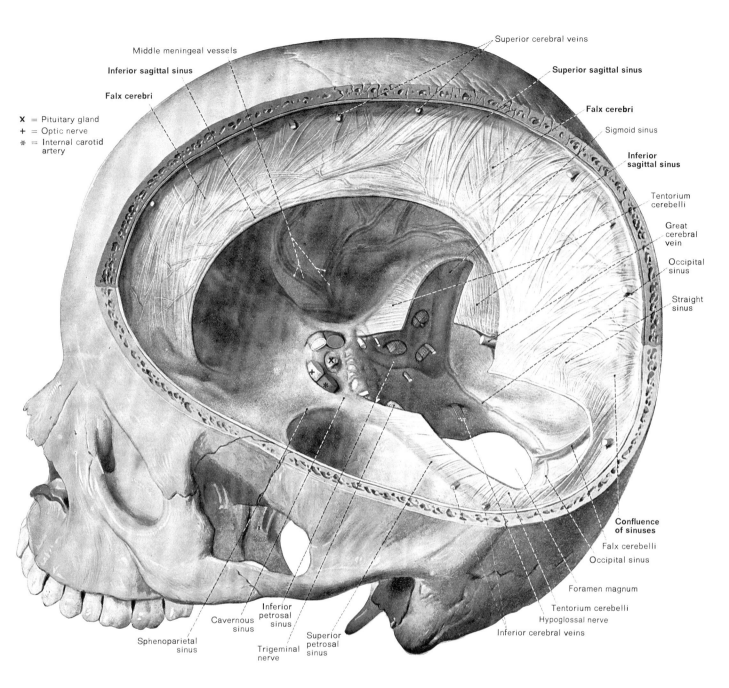

Middle meningeal vessels

Inferior sagittal sinus

Falx cerebri

Superior cerebral veins

Superior sagittal sinus

Falx cerebri

Sigmoid sinus

Inferior sagittal sinus

Tentorium cerebelli

Great cerebral vein

Occipital sinus

Straight sinus

**X** = Pituitary gland
**+** = Optic nerve
**✳** = Internal carotid artery

Confluence of sinuses

Falx cerebelli

Occipital sinus

Foramen magnum

Tentorium cerebelli

Hypoglossal nerve

Inferior cerebral veins

Sphenoparietal sinus

Cavernous sinus

Trigeminal nerve

Inferior petrosal sinus

Superior petrosal sinus

### Fig. 565: The Intracranial Dura Mater and the Dural Sinuses

NOTE: 1) with the left skull opened and the brain removed, the reflections of the dura mater and its venous sinuses are exposed. The sinuses are colored blue while the arteries are red. Most of the left tentorium cerebelli and a portion of the right were cut away to open the posterior cranial fossa.

2) the five *unpaired* dural sinuses: the superior sagittal sinus, the inferior sagittal sinus, the straight sinus. Two other unpaired sinuses (not labelled) at the base of the skull include the intercavernous sinus and the basilar sinus. These can be seen in Fig. 566.

3) that the sphenoparietal sinuses course near the posterior margin of the lesser wings of the sphenoid bone and help to form the boundary between the anterior and middle cranial fossae. Similarly, the superior petrosal sinuses course along the superior margins of the petrous portions of the temporal bones at the boundary between the middle and posterior cranial fossae.

4) the seven *paired* dural sinuses: transverse sinus, sigmoid sinus, occipital sinus, superior petrosal sinus, inferior petrosal sinus, cavernous sinus and sphenoparietal sinus. The dural sinuses consist of spaces between the two layers of dura mater which drain the cerebral blood, returning it to the internal jugular veins.

5) the sickle-shaped falx cerebri. This double layer, midline reflection of dura mater extends from the crista galli anteriorly to the tentorium cerebelli posteriorly. It also extends vertically between the two cerebral hemispheres. Within the layers of the falx, observe the superior and inferior sagittal sinuses and the straight sinus which meet at the confluence of sinuses.

6) the tentorium cerebelli is a tent-like reflection of dura mater which forms a partition separating the occipital lobes of the cerebral cortex and the surface of the cerebellum. The falx cerebelli extends vertically between the two cerebellar hemispheres.

Fig. 565    VII

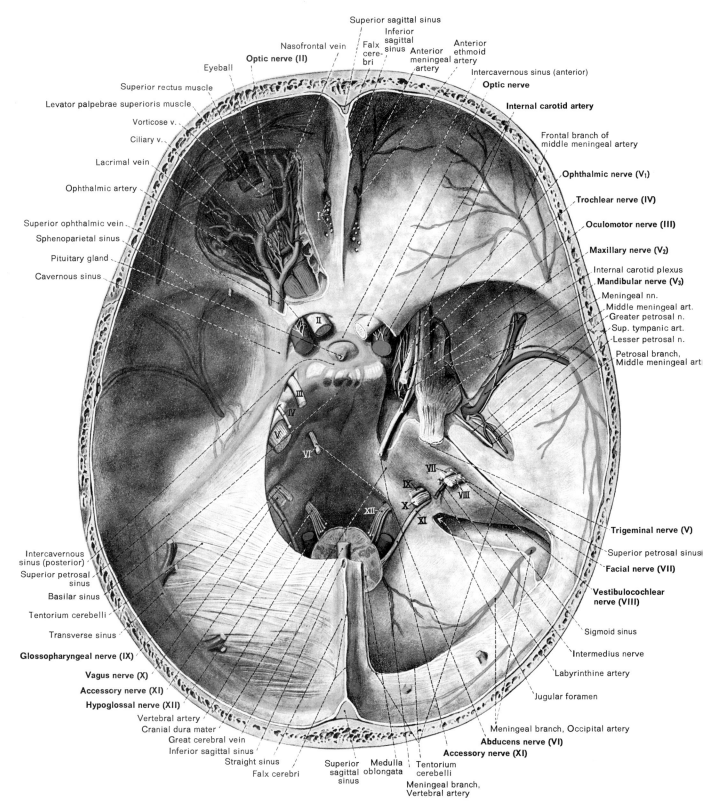

**Fig. 566: The Base of the Cranial Cavity: Vessels, Nerves and Dura Mater**

NOTE: 1) the base of the cranial cavity displays anterior, middle and posterior cranial fossae. The anterior fossa sustains the frontal lobes while the temporal lobes of the brain rest in the middle fossa. Posteriorly, the brain stem and the overlying cerebellum rest in the posterior fossa.

2) the dura mater and the orbital plate of the left frontal bone have been chipped away to expose the structures in the left orbit. The superior ophthalmic vein drains posteriorly and the optic nerve is seen to course from the orbit through the optic canal. Caudal to the optic foramina, observe the pituitary gland within the sella turcica.

3) the medial aspect of the middle cranial fossa shows the internal carotid artery, the 3rd, 4th, 5th and 6th cranial nerves coursing anteriorly or inferiorly toward the orbit or face and the middle meningeal artery traversing the foramen spinosum.

4) the posterior cranial fossa is marked by foramina for the last six pairs of cranial nerves. The 7th and 8th nerves pass through the internal acoustic meatus while the 9th, 10th and 11th nerves emerge through the jugular foramen. The 12th nerve courses through the hypoglossal canal in the occipital bone.

Fig. 566

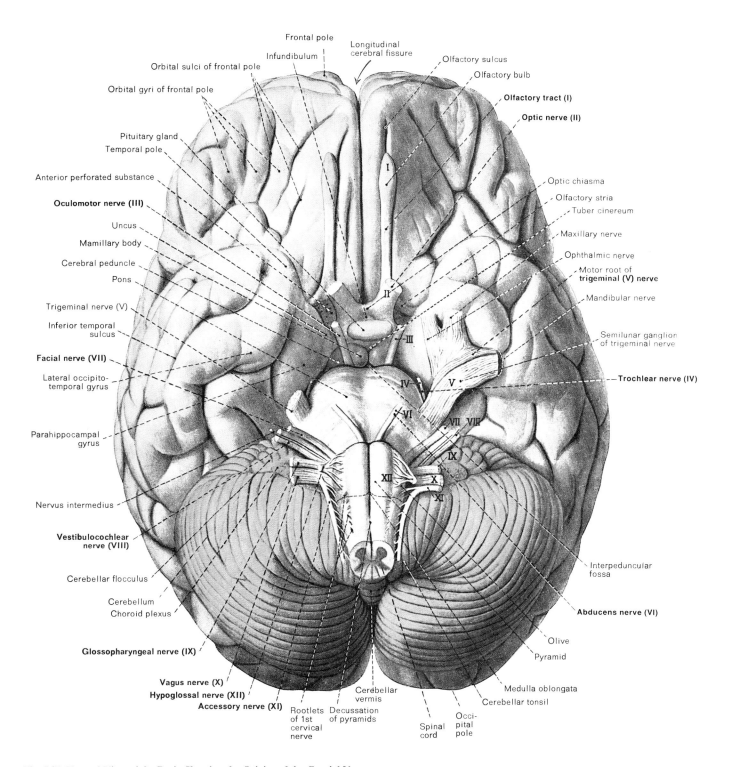

**Fig. 567: Ventral View of the Brain Showing the Origins of the Cranial Nerves**

NOTE: 1) the cranial nerves are numbered sequentially with Roman numerals. The olfactory tracts and optic nerves (I and II) subserve receptors of special sense in the nose and eye and, as cranial nerve trunks, they attach to the base of the forebrain in contrast to all the other cranial nerves which attach at midbrain, pontine or medullary levels.

2) the oculomotor (III), trochlear (IV) and abducens (VI) nerves are motor nerves to the extraocular muscles. While the trigeminal nerve (V) is the largest of all the cranial nerves, the trochlear is the smallest. The abducens nerve emerges from the brainstem at the pontomedullary junction at about the same level, but somewhat more laterally, as the attachments of the facial (VII) and vestibulocochlear (VIII) nerves.

3) the glossopharyngeal (IX) and vagus (X) nerves emerge from the medulla laterally, in a line roughly comparable to the spinal and medullary portions of the accessory nerve (XI). In contrast, the hypoglossal (XII) nerve rootlets emerge from the ventral medulla in a line consistent with the motor ventral rootlets of the cervical segments of the spinal cord.

Fig. 567    VII

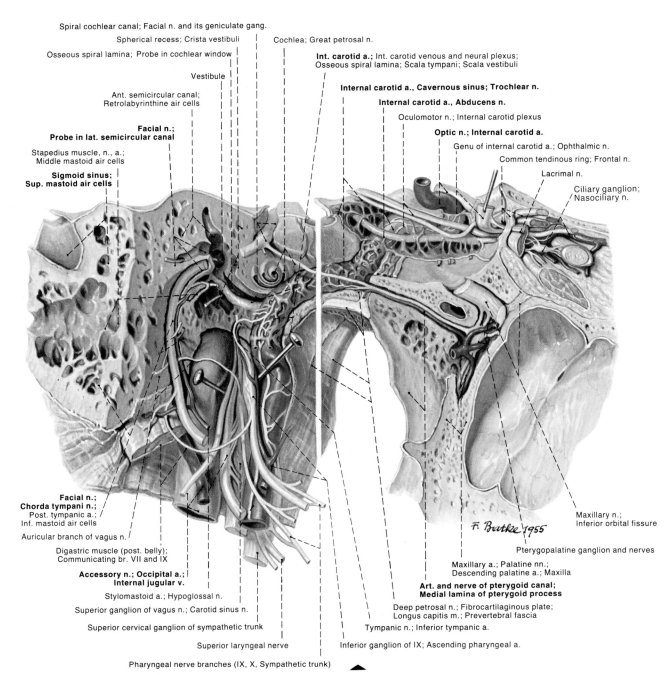

Spiral cochlear canal; Facial n. and its geniculate gang.

Spherical recess; Crista vestibuli

Cochlea; Great petrosal n.

Osseous spiral lamina; Probe in cochlear window

Vestibule

**Int. carotid a.;** Int. carotid venous and neural plexus;
Osseous spiral lamina; Scala tympani; Scala vestibuli

Ant. semicircular canal;
Retrolabyrinthine air cells

**Internal carotid a., Cavernous sinus; Trochlear n.**

**Internal carotid a., Abducens n.**

**Facial n.;**
**Probe in lat. semicircular canal**

Oculomotor n.; Internal carotid plexus

**Optic n.; Internal carotid a.**

Stapedius muscle, n., a.;
Middle mastoid air cells

Genu of internal carotid a.; Ophthalmic n.

Common tendinous ring; Frontal n.

**Sigmoid sinus;**
**Sup. mastoid air cells**

Lacrimal n.

Ciliary ganglion;
Nasociliary n.

**Facial n.;**
**Chorda tympani n.;**
Post. tympanic a.;
Inf. mastoid air cells

Maxillary n.;
Inferior orbital fissure

Auricular branch of vagus n.

Pterygopalatine ganglion and nerves

Digastric muscle (post. belly);
Communicating br. VII and IX

Maxillary a.; Palatine nn.;
Descending palatine a.; Maxilla

**Accessory n.; Occipital a.;**
**Internal jugular v.**

**Art. and nerve of pterygoid canal;**
**Medial lamina of pterygoid process**

Stylomastoid a.; Hypoglossal n.

Deep petrosal n.; Fibrocartilaginous plate;
Longus capitis m.; Prevertebral fascia

Superior ganglion of vagus n.; Carotid sinus n.

Tympanic n.; Inferior tympanic a.

Superior cervical ganglion of sympathetic trunk

Inferior ganglion of IX; Ascending pharyngeal a.

Superior laryngeal nerve

Pharyngeal nerve branches (IX, X, Sympathetic trunk)

F. Batke 1955

**Fig. 568: The Petrous, Cavernous and Cerebral Portions of the Internal Carotid Artery**

NOTE: 1) a vertical section oriented along the superior margin of the petrous portion of the right temporal bone has been made, thereby opening the carotid and facial canals and the inner ear. More anteriorly, the section goes through the sphenoid bone, opening its pterygoid canal and meeting the petrous section in a V-shaped manner.

2) that the *petrous portion* of the internal carotid ascends vertically in the carotid canal and then curves medially and anteriorly. Surrounded by a plexus of small veins and sympathetic nerve fibers, the *cavernous portion* of the artery ascends into the cavernous sinus and curves forward in the carotid sulcus along the side of the body of the sphenoid bone. It then, once again, curves upward to perforate the dura mater just lateral to the optic nerve. This *cerebral portion* immediately passes backward between the optic and oculomotor nerves, where it divides into its terminal branches.

Internal carotid a.

Dura mater

Optic nerve

Oculomotor n.

Trochlear n.

Pituitary gland

Abducens n.

**Internal carotid a.**

Ophthalmic n.

Mucosal lining of the sphenoid sinus

Maxillary n.

Trabeculae in the cavernous sinus

Dura mater

Body of sphenoid bone

**Fig. 569: Frontal Section Through the Left Cavernous Sinus**

NOTE that the internal carotid artery (which is seen to have turned back on itself above) and the oculomotor, trochlear, $V_1$, $V_2$, and abducens nerves pass through the cavernous sinus.

Figs. 568, 569

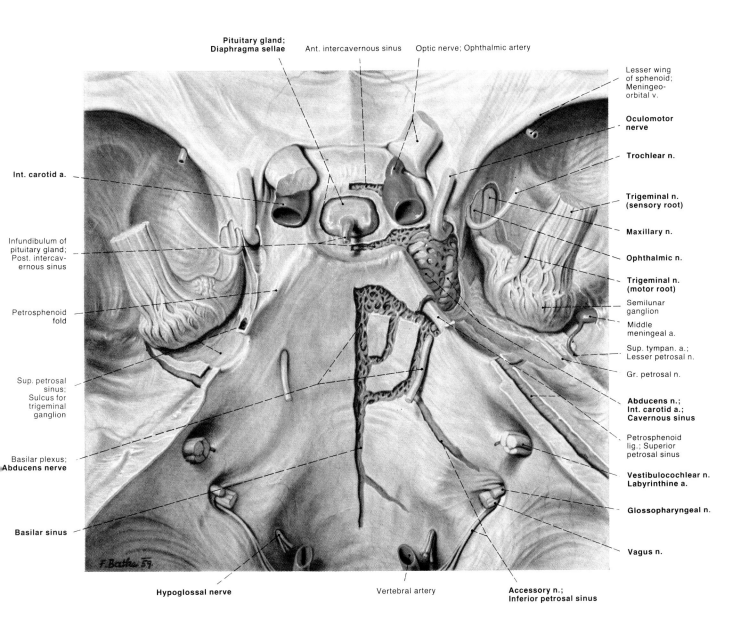

**Pituitary gland;**
**Diaphragma sellae**

Ant. intercavernous sinus

Optic nerve; Ophthalmic artery

Lesser wing
of sphenoid;
Meningeo-
orbital v.

**Oculomotor
nerve**

**Trochlear n.**

Int. carotid a.

**Trigeminal n.
(sensory root)**

**Maxillary n.**

**Ophthalmic n.**

Infundibulum of
pituitary gland;
Post. intercav-
ernous sinus

**Trigeminal n.
(motor root)**

Semilunar
ganglion

Petrosphenoid
fold

Middle
meningeal a.

Sup. tympan. a.;
Lesser petrosal n.

Gr. petrosal n.

Sup. petrosal
sinus;
Sulcus for
trigeminal
ganglion

**Abducens n.;
Int. carotid a.;
Cavernous sinus**

Petrosphenoid
lig.; Superior
petrosal sinus

**Vestibulocochlear n.
Labyrinthine a.**

Basilar plexus;
**Abducens nerve**

**Glossopharyngeal n.**

Basilar sinus

**Vagus n.**

F. Batke 59.

**Hypoglossal nerve**

Vertebral artery

**Accessory n.;
Inferior petrosal sinus**

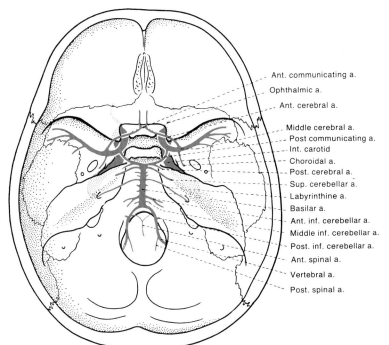

Ant. communicating a.

Ophthalmic a.

Ant. cerebral a.

Middle cerebral a.

Post communicating a.

Int. carotid

Choroidal a.

Post. cerebral a.

Sup. cerebellar a.

Labyrinthine a.

Basilar a.

Ant. inf. cerebellar a.

Middle inf. cerebellar a.

Post. inf. cerebellar a.

Ant. spinal a.

Vertebral a.

Post. spinal a.

**Fig. 570: Blood Vessels and Nerves in the Region of the Sella
Turcica Viewed from Above**

NOTE: 1) that portions of the dura mater have been opened
to expose the right cavernous sinus, the anterior and posterior
intercavernous sinuses, the basilar plexus of veins and basilar
sinus, as well as the right superior and inferior petrosal sinuses.

2) that the stumps of the oculomotor, trochlear and trigeminal nerves have been pulled forward or laterally, and the right
optic nerve has been elevated to reveal the origin of the ophthalmic artery from the cerebral portion of the internal carotid
artery.

3) the infundibulum, or stalk, of the pituitary gland by which
the gland was attached to the hypothalamus of the brain. Also
observe the stumps of all the cranial nerves, (except the olfactory
tracts), traversing their respective foramina.

**Fig. 571: The Relationship of the Arteries Supplying the Brain
to the Bones at the Base of the Cranial Cavity**

From the two vertebral arteries which form the basilar artery
and from the two internal carotid arteries branch all of the
named vessels shown in this diagram. For more details, see
Figure 572.

Fig. 570, 571    **VII**

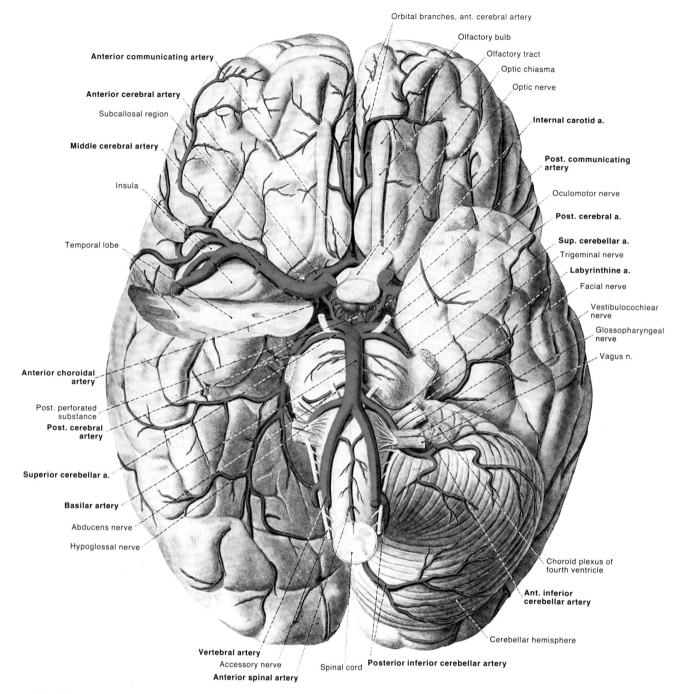

**Fig. 572: The Arteries at the Base of the Brain**

NOTE: 1) that branches of the vertebral arteries form the anterior spinal artery medially and the posterior inferior cerebellar arteries laterally.

2) the basilar artery is formed near the pontomedullary junction and successively gives off the anterior inferior cerebellar, labyrinthine, pontine (not labelled), superior cerebellar and posterior cerebral arteries.

3) the internal carotid arteries interconnect with the posterior cerebral by way of the posterior communicating arteries, and then give off the middle and anterior cerebral arteries. The anterior cerebral arteries are joined by the anterior communicating artery.

4) the circle of Willis surrounds the optic chiasma and is formed by the posterior cerebral, posterior communicating, internal carotid, anterior cerebral and anterior communicating arteries.

**Fig. 573 con't.**

**Middle Cranial Fossa:** a) *optic foramen:* optic nerve and ophthalmic artery. – b) *superior orbital fissure:* oculomotor nerve, trochlear nerve, ophthalmic nerve, abducens nerve, sympathetic fibers, superior ophthalmic vein, orbital branches of the middle meningeal artery and a dural recurrent branch from the lacrimal artery. – c) *foramen rotundum:* maxillary nerve. – d) *foramen ovale:* mandibular nerve, accessory meningeal artery. – e) *foramen spinosum:* middle meningeal artery, recurrent branch from mandibular nerve. – f) *foramen lacerum:* internal carotid artery passes across the superior part of the foramen but does not traverse it; nerve of pterygoid canal and meningeal branch of ascending pharyngeal artery traverse foramen lacerum.

**Posterior Cranial Fossa:** a) *internal acoustic meatus:* facial nerve, vestibulocochlear nerve, labyrinthine artery. – b) *jugular foramen:* inferior petrosal sinus and transverse sinus which together form the jugular vein; meningeal branches of occipital and ascending pharyngeal arteries; glosso-pharyngeal, vagus and accessory nerves. – c) *hypoglossal canal:* hypoglossal nerve. – d) *foramen magnum:* spinal cord; accessory nerve; anterior and posterior spinal arteries; vertebral arteries; tectorial membrane.

Fig. 572

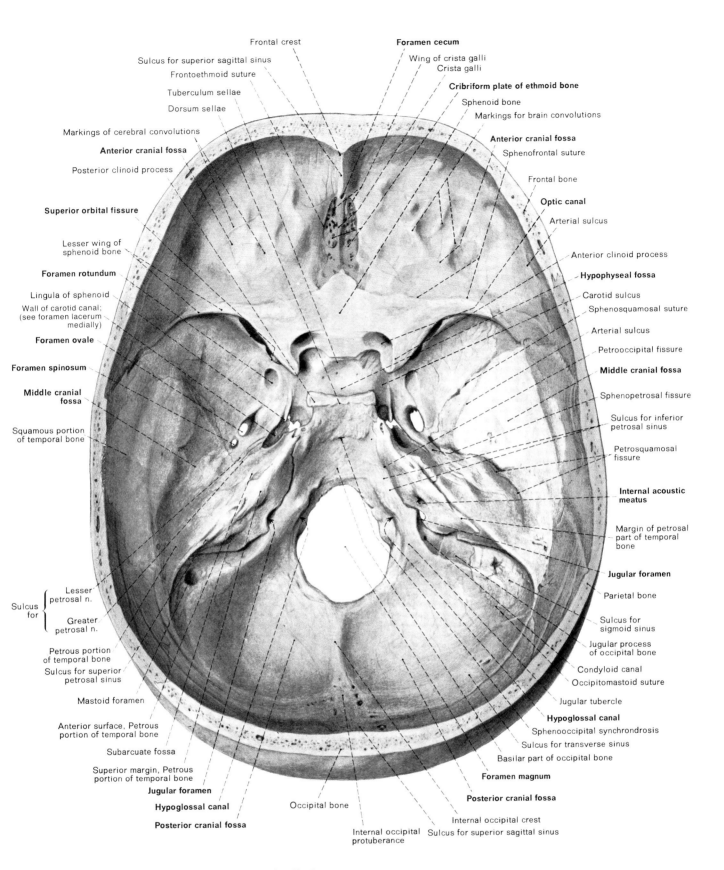

Frontal crest

Foramen Cecum

Wing of crista galli

Crista galli

Sulcus for superior sagittal sinus

Frontoethmoid suture

Cribriform plate of ethmoid bone

Tuberculum sellae

Sphenoid bone

Dorsum sellae

Markings for brain convolutions

Markings of cerebral convolutions

Anterior cranial fossa

Anterior cranial fossa

Sphenofrontal suture

Posterior clinoid process

Frontal bone

Superior orbital fissure

Optic canal

Arterial sulcus

Lesser wing of sphenoid bone

Anterior clinoid process

Foramen rotundum

Hypophyseal fossa

Lingula of sphenoid

Carotid sulcus

Wall of carotid canal; (see foramen lacerum medially)

Sphenosquamosal suture

Arterial sulcus

Foramen ovale

Petrooccipital fissure

Foramen spinosum

Middle cranial fossa

Middle cranial fossa

Sphenopetrosal fissure

Squamous portion of temporal bone

Sulcus for inferior petrosal sinus

Petrosquamosal fissure

Internal acoustic meatus

Margin of petrosal part of temporal bone

Sulcus for Lesser petrosal n.

Greater petrosal n.

Jugular foramen

Parietal bone

Sulcus for sigmoid sinus

Jugular process of occipital bone

Petrous portion of temporal bone

Sulcus for superior petrosal sinus

Condyloid canal

Occipitomastoid suture

Mastoid foramen

Jugular tubercle

Anterior surface, Petrous portion of temporal bone

Hypoglossal canal

Sphenooccipital synchrondrosis

Subarcuate fossa

Sulcus for transverse sinus

Superior margin, Petrous portion of temporal bone

Basilar part of occipital bone

Jugular foramen

Foramen magnum

Hypoglossal canal

Posterior cranial fossa

Posterior cranial fossa

Occipital bone

Internal occipital crest

Internal occipital protuberance

Sulcus for superior sagittal sinus

## Fig. 573: The Base of the Skull: Internal Aspect (Superior View)

NOTE: 1) the base of the cranial cavity is composed principally of the frontal (lavender) bones, the ethmoid (orange) bone, the sphenoid (green) bone, the temporal (gray) bones and the occipital (blue) bone. Additionally, the sphenoidal angle of each parietal (tan) bone is interposed between the frontal and temporal bones.

2) Important structures traverse the various foramina through the base of the skull:

**Anterior Cranial Fossa:** a) *foramen cecum:* a small vein. b) *foramina of cribriform plate:* filaments of olfactory receptor neurons to olfactory bulb. c) *anterior ethmoid foramen:* anterior ethmoidal vessels and nasociliary nerve. d) *posterior ethmoid foramen:* posterior ethmoidal vessels and nerve.

Fig. 573   VII

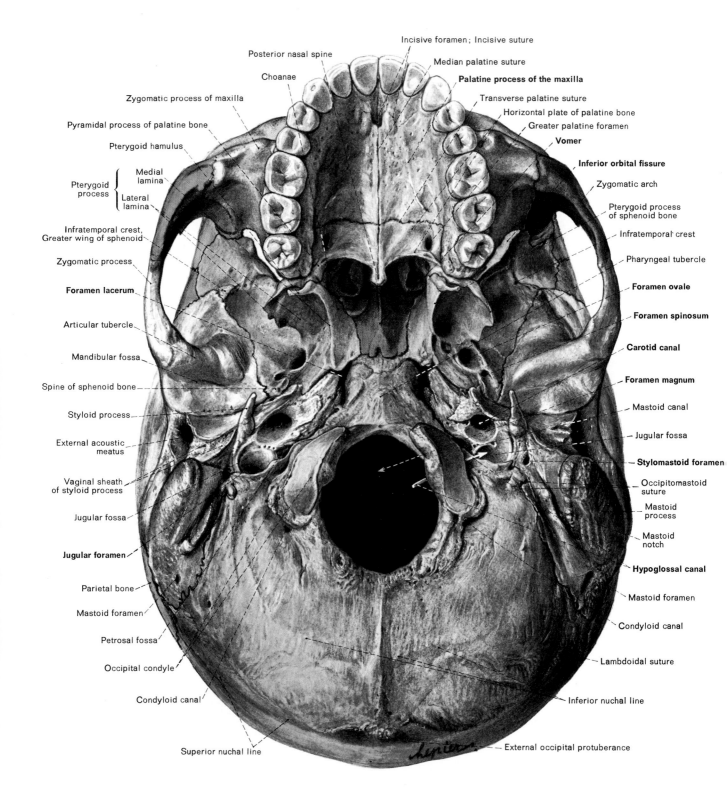

**Fig. 574: The Base of the Skull: External Aspect (Inferior View)**

NOTE: 1) the base of the skull reveals a posterior region comprised of the occipital and temporal bones which are attached by muscles to the thoracic and vertebral skeleton. More anteriorly are the facial bones consisting of the maxilla, palatine, zygomatic and vomer. Interposed between these two groups of bones is the sphenoid bone.

2) the bony palate and the cruciform suture where the transverse processes of the maxillary bones meet the horizontal plates of the palatine bones. Observe the incisive and greater palatine foramina. The lesser palatine foramina are shown but not labelled.

3) The posterior aspect of the vomer (in red) bounding the posterior nasal apertures, or choanae. Observe the medial and lateral laminae of the pterygoid process of the sphenoid bone (in green), behind which are the foramen ovale and foramen spinosum in the greater wings of that bone.

4) The petrous and mastoid parts of the temporal bone. Identify the foramen lacerum interposed between the sphenoid and temporal bones, as well as the carotid canal and jugular foramen located medial to the styloid process of the temporal bone.

5) That the foramen magnum lies completely within the occipital bone. An arrow has been placed through the hypoglossal canal located just above the occipital condyles.

Fig. 574

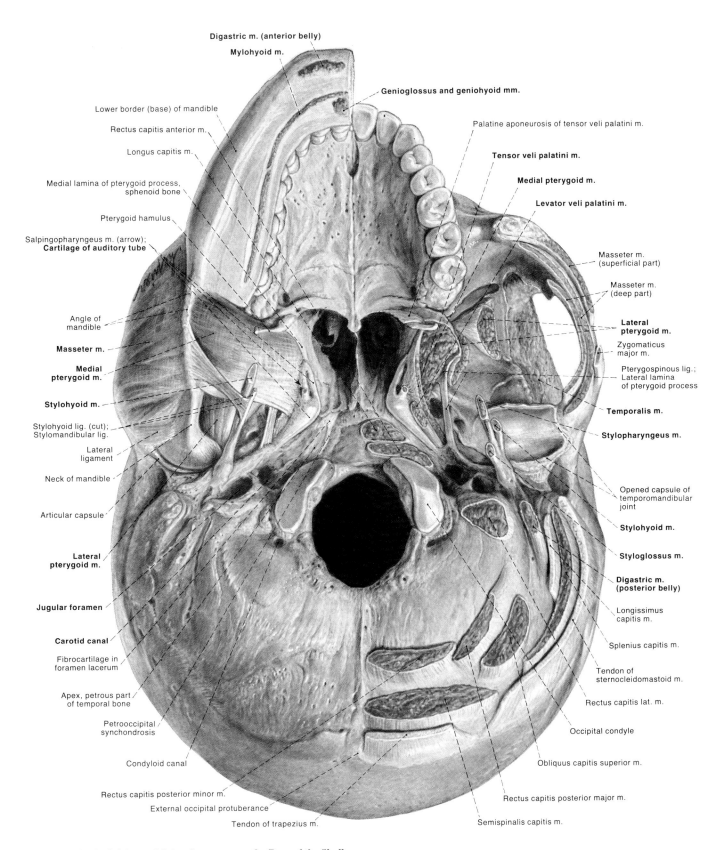

Digastric m. (anterior belly)

Mylohyoid m.

Genioglossus and geniohyoid mm.

Lower border (base) of mandible

Palatine aponeurosis of tensor veli palatini m.

Rectus capitis anterior m.

Tensor veli palatini m.

Longus capitis m.

Medial pterygoid m.

Medial lamina of pterygoid process, sphenoid bone

Levator veli palatini m.

Pterygoid hamulus

Masseter m. (superficial part)

Salpingopharyngeus m. (arrow); Cartilage of auditory tube

Masseter m. (deep part)

Lateral pterygoid m.

Angle of mandible

Zygomaticus major m.

Masseter m.

Pterygospinous lig.; Lateral lamina of pterygoid process

Medial pterygoid m.

Temporalis m.

Stylohyoid m.

Stylopharyngeus m.

Stylohyoid lig. (cut); Stylomandibular lig.

Lateral ligament

Neck of mandible

Opened capsule of temporomandibular joint

Articular capsule

Stylohyoid m.

Styloglossus m.

Lateral pterygoid m.

Digastric m. (posterior belly)

Jugular foramen

Longissimus capitis m.

Carotid canal

Splenius capitis m.

Fibrocartilage in foramen lacerum

Tendon of sternocleidomastoid m.

Apex, petrous part of temporal bone

Rectus capitis lat. m.

Petrooccipital synchondrosis

Occipital condyle

Condyloid canal

Obliquus capitis superior m.

Rectus capitis posterior minor m.

External occipital protuberance

Rectus capitis posterior major m.

Tendon of trapezius m.

Semispinalis capitis m.

**Fig. 575: Muscle Origins and Other Structures on the Base of the Skull**

NOTE: 1) that the left mandible (reader's right) has been removed while the right muscles of mastication (reader's left), covered by their fascial sheaths, have been retained. Observe the attachments of the superficial and deep parts of the *masseter* muscle, the *temporalis,* the two heads of the *lateral pterygoid* and the *medial pterygoid* muscles.

2) that the cartilage of the auditory tube as it opens inferomedially in the lateral wall of the nasopharynx, and the origins of the *tensor* and *levator veli palatini* muscles. The levator arises from the inferior surface of the apex of the petrous temporal bone, anterior to the opening of the carotid canal. The tensor veli palatini lies lateral and anterior to the levator, and it arises from the scaphoid fossa at the base of the medial pterygoid plate, the sphenoidal spine and the lateral aspect of the cartilaginous auditory tube.

3) that the muscles which pass from the skull to cervical and back structures arise from the occipital bone and the mastoid and styloid processes of the temporal bone.

Fig. 575    VII

## Fig. 576: The Left Bony Orbital Cavity (Anterior View)

NOTE: 1) the bony structure of the orbit is comprised of parts of seven bones: the maxilla, zygomatic, frontal, lacrimal, palatine, ethmoid and sphenoid.

2) the *roof* of the orbit is formed by the orbital plate of the frontal bone; the *floor* consists of the orbital plate of the maxilla, the palatine (blue, not labelled) and zygomatic bones; the *medial wall* is thin and delicate and is formed by the frontal process of the maxilla, the orbital lamina of the ethmoid and the lacrimal bone; the strong *lateral wall* consists of the orbital processes of the sphenoid and zygomatic bones.

3) the optic foramen and the superior and inferior orbital fissures.

Fig. 576 labels:
- Frontal notch
- Anterior and posterior ethmoid foramina
- Optic foramen
- Superior orbital fissure
- Orbital lamina of ethmoid bone
- Frontomaxillary suture
- Nasal bone
- Anterior lacrimal crest
- Orbital surface, greater wing of sphenoid bone
- Zygomatic bone
- Orbital surface, Zygomatic bone
- Zygomaticofacial foramen
- Posterior lacrimal crest
- Suture
- Canal
- Infraorbital
- Infra-orbital sulcus
- Zygomatico-maxillary suture
- Inferior orbital fissure

## Fig. 577: The Right Eye and Eyelids

NOTE: 1) the eyeball, protected anteriorly by two thin, movable eyelids or palpebrae, is covered by a transparent mucous membrane, the conjunctiva, which is continuous along the inner surface of both eyelids as the palpebral conjunctiva.

2) at the medial angle of the eye is located a small, reddish island of skin called the caruncula lacrimalis. It contains sebaceous and sweat glands which secrete a whitish substance.

3) the pubil is the opening in the iris. Constriction and dilatation of the pupil is controlled autonomically. Parasympathetic fibers in the oculomotor nerve innervate the constrictor muscle of the pupil, while sympathetic fibers from the superior cervical ganglion supply the pupillary dilator muscle.

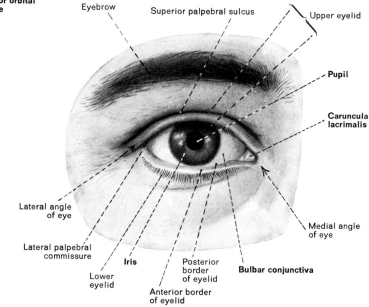

Fig. 577 labels:
- Eyebrow
- Superior palpebral sulcus
- Upper eyelid
- Pupil
- Caruncula lacrimalis
- Lateral angle of eye
- Medial angle of eye
- Lateral palpebral commissure
- Iris
- Bulbar conjunctiva
- Lower eyelid
- Posterior border of eyelid
- Anterior border of eyelid

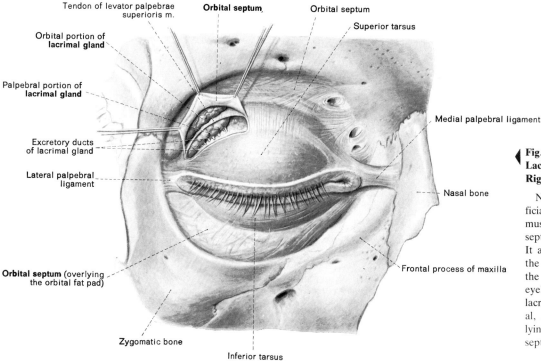

Fig. 578 labels:
- Tendon of levator palpebrae superioris m.
- Orbital septum
- Orbital septum
- Superior tarsus
- Orbital portion of lacrimal gland
- Palpebral portion of lacrimal gland
- Medial palpebral ligament
- Excretory ducts of lacrimal gland
- Lateral palpebral ligament
- Nasal bone
- Orbital septum (overlying the orbital fat pad)
- Frontal process of maxilla
- Zygomatic bone
- Inferior tarsus

## Fig. 578: The Orbital Septum, Lacrimal Gland and Tarsi of the Right Eye

NOTE: With the skin, superficial fascia and orbicularis oculi muscle removed, the orbital septum is exposed anteriorly. It attaches to the periosteum of the bone peripherally around the orbit and to the tarsi of the eyelids centrally. Observe the lacrimal gland in the upper lateral, aspect of the anterior orbit, lying just beneath the orbital septum.

Figs. 576, 577, 578

## Fig. 579: The Palpebral Ligaments and Tarsal Plates ▶

NOTE: 1) the superficial structures of the anterior orbit have been removed along with the orbital septum and the tendon of the levator palpebrae superioris muscle.

2) the lateral and medial margins of the tarsal plates are attached to the lateral and medial palpebral ligaments which in turn are attached to bone. Observe that the medial ligament is located just anterior to the lacrimal sac.

3) from this anterior view, both the tendon of the superior oblique muscle and the inferior oblique muscle can be visualized. Note also the location of the orbital portion of the lacrimal gland. Its secretions course from lateral to medial across the surface of the eye.

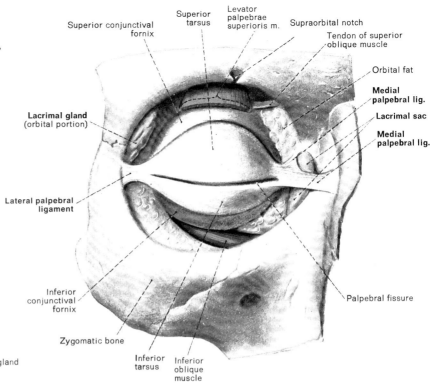

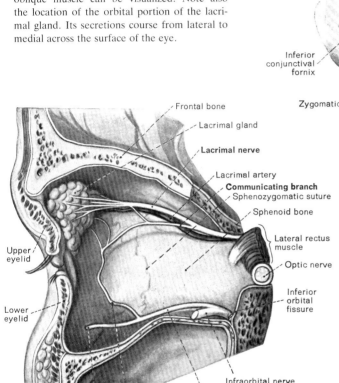

## Fig. 580: The Innervation of the Lacrimal Gland ◀

NOTE: 1) the lacrimal gland receives postganglionic parasympathetic nerve fibers which are secretomotor in nature. The preganglionic fibers are generally said to emerge from the brain with the facial nerve (VII). The synapse between pre and postganglionic fibers occurs in the pterygopalatine ganglion.

2) the preganglionic parasympathetic fibers reach the pterygopalatine ganglion by way of the greater petrosal nerve which becomes the nerve of the pterygoid canal. The postganglionic fibers leave the ganglion and travel for a short distance with the zygomatic branch of the infraorbital nerve. From this point in the inferior aspect of the orbit, the parasympathetic fibers travel by way of a communicating branch to the lacrimal nerve by which they achieve the lacrimal gland.

## Fig. 581: The Lacrimal Canaliculi, Lacrimal Sac and Nasolacrimal Duct ▶

NOTE: 1) at the medial edge of both the upper and lower eyelids are found single minute orifices (puncta lacrimalia) of small ducts, the lacrimal canaliculi, which lead from the eyelids to the lacrimal sac. The sac forms the upper dilated end of the nasolacrimal duct, which then extends a distance of about 3½ inches into the inferior meatus of the nasal cavity.

2) secretions from the lacrimal gland pass medially across the surface of the eye toward the canaliculi and then are transported to the nasal cavity by way of the nasolacrimal duct. Excessive secretions (such as during crying) cannot be handled in this manner and, thus, roll over the edge of the lower eyelid as tears.

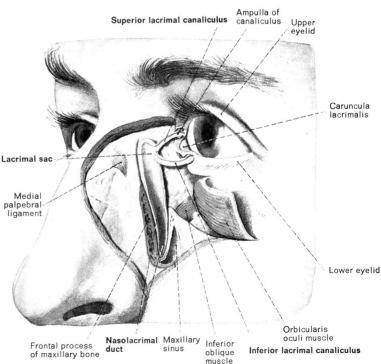

Figs. 579, 580, 581    VII

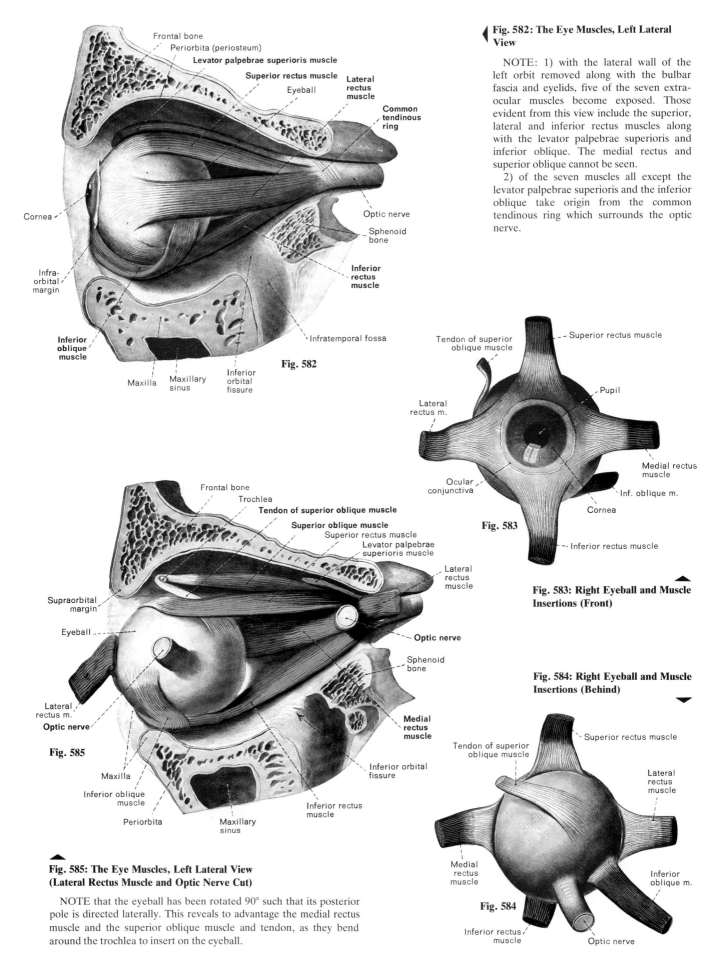

### Fig. 582: The Eye Muscles, Left Lateral View

NOTE: 1) with the lateral wall of the left orbit removed along with the bulbar fascia and eyelids, five of the seven extra-ocular muscles become exposed. Those evident from this view include the superior, lateral and inferior rectus muscles along with the levator palpebrae superioris and inferior oblique. The medial rectus and superior oblique cannot be seen.

2) of the seven muscles all except the levator palpebrae superioris and the inferior oblique take origin from the common tendinous ring which surrounds the optic nerve.

**Fig. 582**

Frontal bone
Periorbita (periosteum)
**Levator palpebrae superioris muscle**
**Superior rectus muscle**
Eyeball
Lateral rectus muscle
**Common tendinous ring**
Optic nerve
Sphenoid bone
**Inferior rectus muscle**
Cornea
Infra-orbital margin
**Inferior oblique muscle**
Maxilla
Maxillary sinus
Inferior orbital fissure
Infratemporal fossa

**Fig. 583: Right Eyeball and Muscle Insertions (Front)**

Tendon of superior oblique muscle
Superior rectus muscle
Lateral rectus m.
Pupil
Medial rectus muscle
Inf. oblique m.
Ocular conjunctiva
Cornea
**Fig. 583**
Inferior rectus muscle

**Fig. 584: Right Eyeball and Muscle Insertions (Behind)**

Frontal bone
Trochlea
**Tendon of superior oblique muscle**
**Superior oblique muscle**
Superior rectus muscle
Levator palpebrae superioris muscle
Lateral rectus muscle
Supraorbital margin
**Optic nerve**
Sphenoid bone
Eyeball
**Medial rectus muscle**
Lateral rectus m.
**Optic nerve**
**Fig. 585**
Inferior orbital fissure
Maxilla
Inferior oblique muscle
Periorbita
Maxillary sinus
Inferior rectus muscle

Tendon of superior oblique muscle
Superior rectus muscle
Lateral rectus muscle
Medial rectus muscle
Inferior oblique m.
**Fig. 584**
Inferior rectus muscle
Optic nerve

**Fig. 585: The Eye Muscles, Left Lateral View (Lateral Rectus Muscle and Optic Nerve Cut)**

NOTE that the eyeball has been rotated 90° such that its posterior pole is directed laterally. This reveals to advantage the medial rectus muscle and the superior oblique muscle and tendon, as they bend around the trochlea to insert on the eyeball.

Figs. 582–585

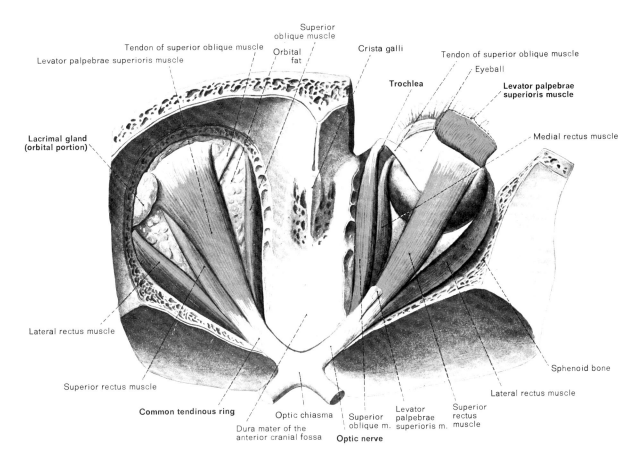

Fig. 586: **The Muscles of the Orbital Cavity as seen from above**

NOTE: 1) the orbital plates of the frontal bone have been removed from within the cranium. On the left side, only the bony roof of the orbit has been opened and the muscles, orbital fat and lacrimal gland have been left intact.

2) on the right side, the levator palpebrae superioris muscle has been resected and the orbital fat removed in order to expose the ocular muscles.

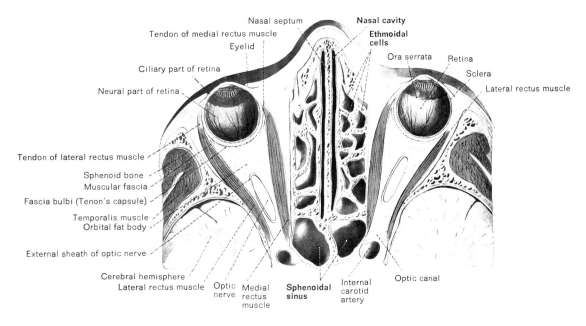

Fig. 587: **A Horizontal Section Through Both Orbits at the Level of the Sphenoid Sinus**

NOTE: 1) between the orbital cavities is situated the ethmoid bone containing the ethmoidal air sinuses (air cells). The vertically oriented perpendicular plate of the ethmoid serves as the nasal septum, which subdivides the nasal cavity into two symmetrical chambers.

2) the posterior portion of the orbits are separated by the sphenoidal sinuses, located within the body of the sphenoid bone. These sinuses usually are not symmetrical.

Figs. 586, 587    VII

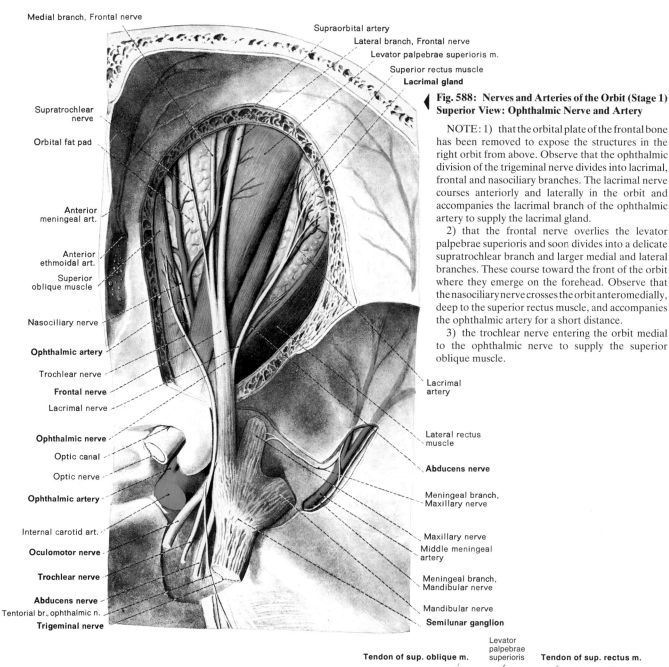

Medial branch, Frontal nerve

Supratrochlear nerve

Orbital fat pad

Anterior meningeal art.

Anterior ethmoidal art.

Superior oblique muscle

Nasociliary nerve

**Ophthalmic artery**

Trochlear nerve

**Frontal nerve**

Lacrimal nerve

**Ophthalmic nerve**

Optic canal

Optic nerve

**Ophthalmic artery**

Internal carotid art.

**Oculomotor nerve**

**Trochlear nerve**

**Abducens nerve**

Tentorial br., ophthalmic n.

**Trigeminal nerve**

Supraorbital artery

Lateral branch, Frontal nerve

Levator palpebrae superioris m.

Superior rectus muscle

**Lacrimal gland**

Lacrimal artery

Lateral rectus muscle

**Abducens nerve**

Meningeal branch, Maxillary nerve

Maxillary nerve

Middle meningeal artery

Meningeal branch, Mandibular nerve

Mandibular nerve

**Semilunar ganglion**

**Fig. 588: Nerves and Arteries of the Orbit (Stage 1) Superior View: Ophthalmic Nerve and Artery**

NOTE: 1) that the orbital plate of the frontal bone has been removed to expose the structures in the right orbit from above. Observe that the ophthalmic division of the trigeminal nerve divides into lacrimal, frontal and nasociliary branches. The lacrimal nerve courses anteriorly and laterally in the orbit and accompanies the lacrimal branch of the ophthalmic artery to supply the lacrimal gland.

2) that the frontal nerve overlies the levator palpebrae superioris and soon divides into a delicate supratrochlear branch and larger medial and lateral branches. These course toward the front of the orbit where they emerge on the forehead. Observe that the nasociliary nerve crosses the orbit anteromedially, deep to the superior rectus muscle, and accompanies the ophthalmic artery for a short distance.

3) the trochlear nerve entering the orbit medial to the ophthalmic nerve to supply the superior oblique muscle.

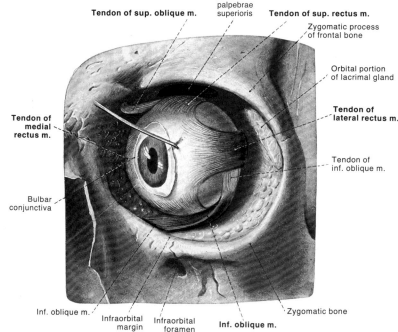

Tendon of sup. oblique m.

Levator palpebrae superioris

**Tendon of sup. rectus m.**

Zygomatic process of frontal bone

Orbital portion of lacrimal gland

**Tendon of lateral rectus m.**

Tendon of inf. oblique m.

Tendon of medial rectus m.

Bulbar conjunctiva

Inf. oblique m.

Infraorbital margin

Infraorbital foramen

**Inf. oblique m.**

Zygomatic bone

**Fig. 589: The Extrinsic Muscles of the Left Eyeball, Anterolateral View**

NOTE that the skin, eyelids and fascia have been removed. Observe that the tendon of the inferior oblique muscle inserts onto the lateral part of the eyeball, behind its equator and between the insertions of the superior and lateral recti muscles.

Figs. 588, 589

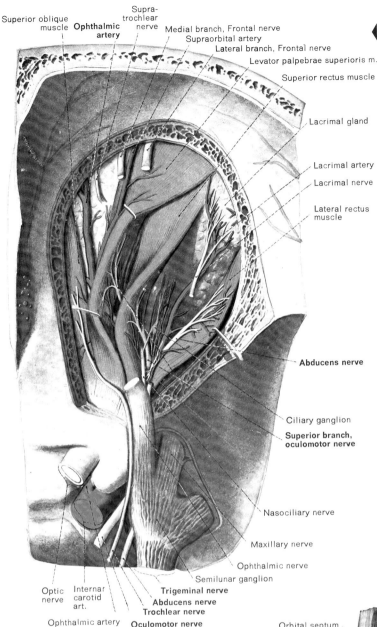

Superior oblique muscle · **Ophthalmic artery** · Supra-trochlear nerve · Medial branch, Frontal nerve · Supraorbital artery · Lateral branch, Frontal nerve · Levator palpebrae superioris m. · Superior rectus muscle · Lacrimal gland · Lacrimal artery · Lacrimal nerve · Lateral rectus muscle · **Abducens nerve** · Ciliary ganglion · **Superior branch, oculomotor nerve** · Nasociliary nerve · Maxillary nerve · Ophthalmic nerve · Semilunar ganglion · **Trigeminal nerve** · **Abducens nerve** · **Trochlear nerve** · **Oculomotor nerve** · Ophthalmic artery · Internal carotid art. · Optic nerve

### Fig. 591: Sagittal View of the Orbital Cavity and Eyeball

NOTE: 1) the bulbar fascia (also seen in Figure 595) is a thin membrane which encloses the posterior 3/4ths of the eyeball, separating the eyeball from the orbital fat and other contents of the orbital cavity. This fascia is pierced by the tendons of the ocular muscles, over which the fascia is prolonged like a tubular sheath.

2) the insertion of the levator palpebrae superioris is trilaminar. The superficial layer inserts into the upper eyelid, the middle into the superior tarsus and the deep layer inserts into the superior fornix of the conjunctiva.

3) the palpebral conjunctive is a thin transparent mucous membrane on the innermost aspect of the eyelid. At the conjunctival angle (fornix), it reflects over the eyeball as far as the sclerocorneal junction.

### Fig. 590: Nerves and Arteries of the Orbit (Stage 2) Superior View: The Trochlear and Abducens Nerves

NOTE: 1) that with the right orbit opened from above, the ophthalmic division of the trigeminal nerve and its lacrimal, supratrochlear and frontal branches have been cut. The levator palpebrae superioris and superior rectus muscles have been pulled medially to reveal their inferior surface where filaments from the *superior branch of the oculomotor nerve* innervate the two muscles.

2) that the *nasociliary branch* of the ophthalmic nerve is still intact, and it is seen turning medially deep to the superior rectus muscle. Observe that a fine communicating filament containing sensory fibers interconnects the ciliary ganglion with the nasociliary nerve.

3) the *trochlear nerve* as it supplies the superior oblique muscle along its upper surface. If this nerve is injured, the patient has difficulty turning the eyeball laterally and downward. When asked to look inferolaterally, the affected eye rotates medially, resulting in double vision or diplopia.

4) the *abducens nerve* as it supplies the lateral rectus muscle along its inner or medial surface. After emerging from the brain stem at the pontomedullary junction, the abducens nerve follows a long course in the floor of the cranial cavity to achieve the orbit by way of the superior orbital fissure. Injury to this nerve produces a diminished ability to move the eyeball laterally. From the resulting medial or convergent gaze of the affected eyeball, the patient complains of diplopia (double vision).

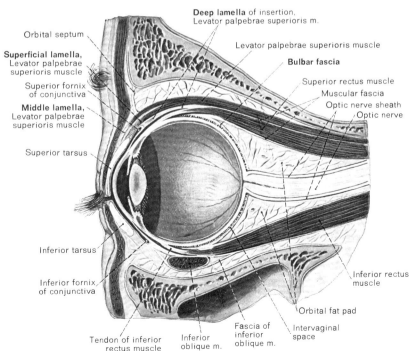

Orbital septum · **Superficial lamella,** Levator palpebrae superioris muscle · Superior fornix of conjunctiva · **Middle lamella,** Levator palpebrae superioris muscle · Superior tarsus · Inferior tarsus · Inferior fornix of conjunctiva · Tendon of inferior rectus muscle · Inferior oblique m. · Fascia of inferior oblique m. · Intervaginal space · Orbital fat pad · Inferior rectus muscle · Optic nerve · Optic nerve sheath · Muscular fascia · Superior rectus muscle · **Bulbar fascia** · Levator palpebrae superioris muscle · **Deep lamella** of insertion, Levator palpebrae superioris m.

## Fig. 592: Nerves and Arteries of the Orbit (Stage 3) Superior View: The Optic Nerve and Ciliary Ganglion

NOTE: 1) that with the levator palpebrae superioris, superior rectus and superior oblique muscles cut and reflected, the nasociliary nerve and ophthalmic artery are seen crossing over the optic nerve from lateral to medial.

2) the optic nerve and the longitudinally oriented long ciliary arteries (from the ophthalmic) and long ciliary nerves (usually 2 or 3 branches of the nasociliary nerve).

3) the ciliary ganglion lateral to the optic nerve. Its *parasymphathetic root* comes from the oculomotor nerve and its *sensory root* from the nasociliary nerve. Postganglionic parasymphathetic fibers reach the eyeball by way of the short ciliary nerves.

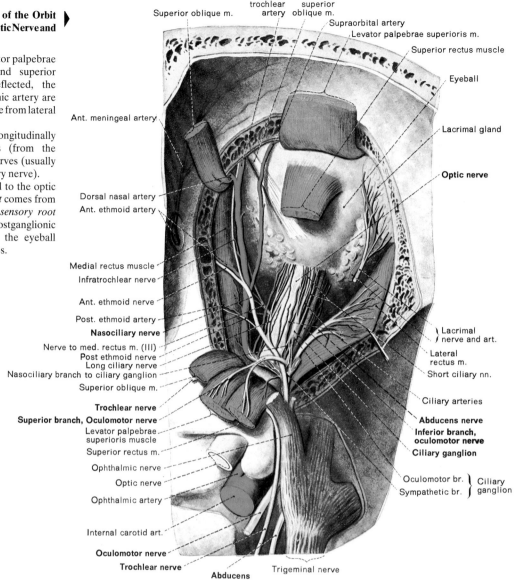

## Fig. 593: Origins of the Ocular Muscles, Apex of Left Orbit

NOTE: 1) this anterior view of the apex of the left orbit shows the stumps of the ocular muscles which have been cut close to their origins.

2) the four rectus muscles arise from a common tendinous ring surrounding the optic canal. The levator palpebrae superioris and superior oblique muscles arise from the sphenoid bone close to the tendinous ring, while the inferior oblique (not shown) arises from the orbital surface of the maxilla.

3)  a. The **lateral rectus** *abducts* the eyeball;
   b. the **superior oblique** *abducts, depresses and medially rotates* the eyeball;
   c. the **inferior oblique** *abducts, elevates* and *laterally rotates* the eyeball;
   d. the **medial rectus** *adducts* the eyeball;
   e. the **inferior rectus** *adducts, depresses* and *laterally rotates* the eyeball;
   f. the **superior rectus** *adducts, elevates* and *medially rotates* the eyeball.

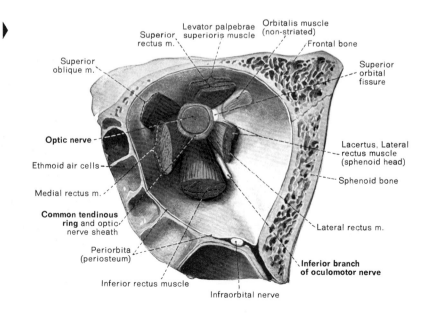

Figs. 592, 593

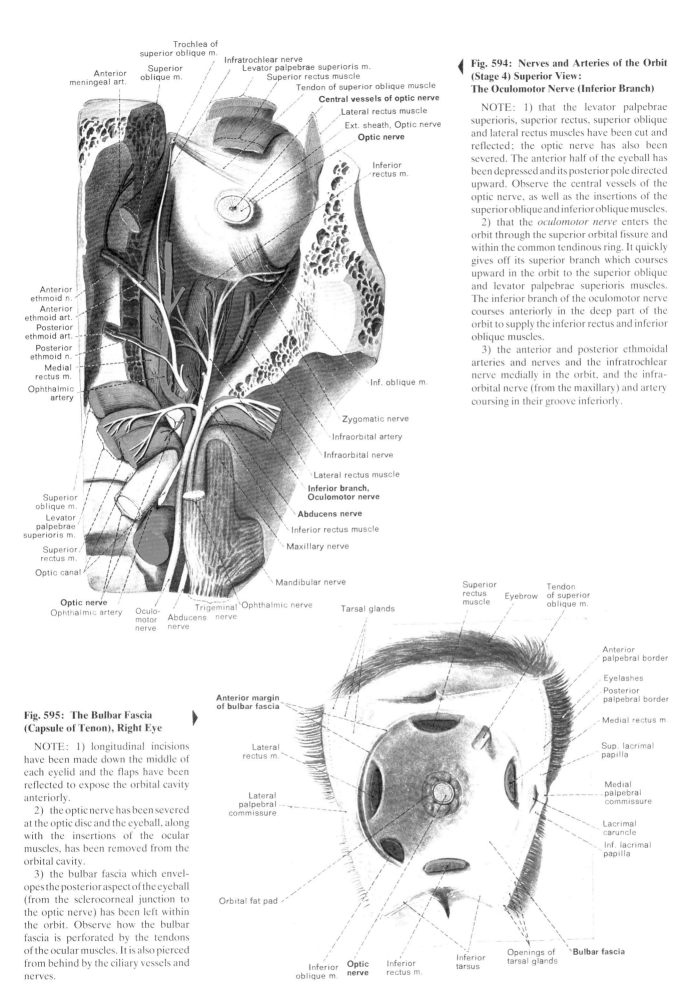

Trochlea of
superior oblique m.
Anterior
meningeal art.
Superior
oblique m.
Infratrochlear nerve
Levator palpebrae superioris m.
Superior rectus muscle
Tendon of superior oblique muscle
**Central vessels of optic nerve**
Lateral rectus muscle
Ext. sheath, Optic nerve
**Optic nerve**
Inferior
rectus m.
Anterior
ethmoid n.
Anterior
ethmoid art.
Posterior
ethmoid art.
Posterior
ethmoid n.
Medial
rectus m.
Ophthalmic
artery
Inf. oblique m.
Zygomatic nerve
Infraorbital artery
Infraorbital nerve
Lateral rectus muscle
**Inferior branch,
Oculomotor nerve**
**Abducens nerve**
Inferior rectus muscle
Maxillary nerve
Superior
oblique m.
Levator
palpebrae
superioris m.
Superior
rectus m.
Optic canal
**Optic nerve**
Ophthalmic artery
Oculo-
motor
nerve
Abducens
nerve
Trigeminal
nerve
Ophthalmic nerve
Mandibular nerve

### Fig. 594: Nerves and Arteries of the Orbit (Stage 4) Superior View: The Oculomotor Nerve (Inferior Branch)

NOTE: 1) that the levator palpebrae superioris, superior rectus, superior oblique and lateral rectus muscles have been cut and reflected; the optic nerve has also been severed. The anterior half of the eyeball has been depressed and its posterior pole directed upward. Observe the central vessels of the optic nerve, as well as the insertions of the superior oblique and inferior oblique muscles.

2) that the *oculomotor nerve* enters the orbit through the superior orbital fissure and within the common tendinous ring. It quickly gives off its superior branch which courses upward in the orbit to the superior oblique and levator palpebrae superioris muscles. The inferior branch of the oculomotor nerve courses anteriorly in the deep part of the orbit to supply the inferior rectus and inferior oblique muscles.

3) the anterior and posterior ethmoidal arteries and nerves and the infratrochlear nerve medially in the orbit, and the infraorbital nerve (from the maxillary) and artery coursing in their groove inferiorly.

### Fig. 595: The Bulbar Fascia (Capsule of Tenon), Right Eye

NOTE: 1) longitudinal incisions have been made down the middle of each eyelid and the flaps have been reflected to expose the orbital cavity anteriorly.

2) the optic nerve has been severed at the optic disc and the eyeball, along with the insertions of the ocular muscles, has been removed from the orbital cavity.

3) the bulbar fascia which envelopes the posterior aspect of the eyeball (from the sclerocorneal junction to the optic nerve) has been left within the orbit. Observe how the bulbar fascia is perforated by the tendons of the ocular muscles. It is also pierced from behind by the ciliary vessels and nerves.

Tarsal glands
**Anterior margin
of bulbar fascia**
Lateral
rectus m.
Lateral
palpebral
commissure
Orbital fat pad
Inferior
oblique m.
**Optic
nerve**
Inferior
rectus m.
Inferior
tarsus
Openings of
tarsal glands
**Bulbar fascia**
Superior
rectus
muscle
Eyebrow
Tendon
of superior
oblique m.
Anterior
palpebral border
Eyelashes
Posterior
palpebral border
Medial rectus m.
Sup. lacrimal
papilla
Medial
palpebral
commissure
Lacrimal
caruncle
Inf. lacrimal
papilla

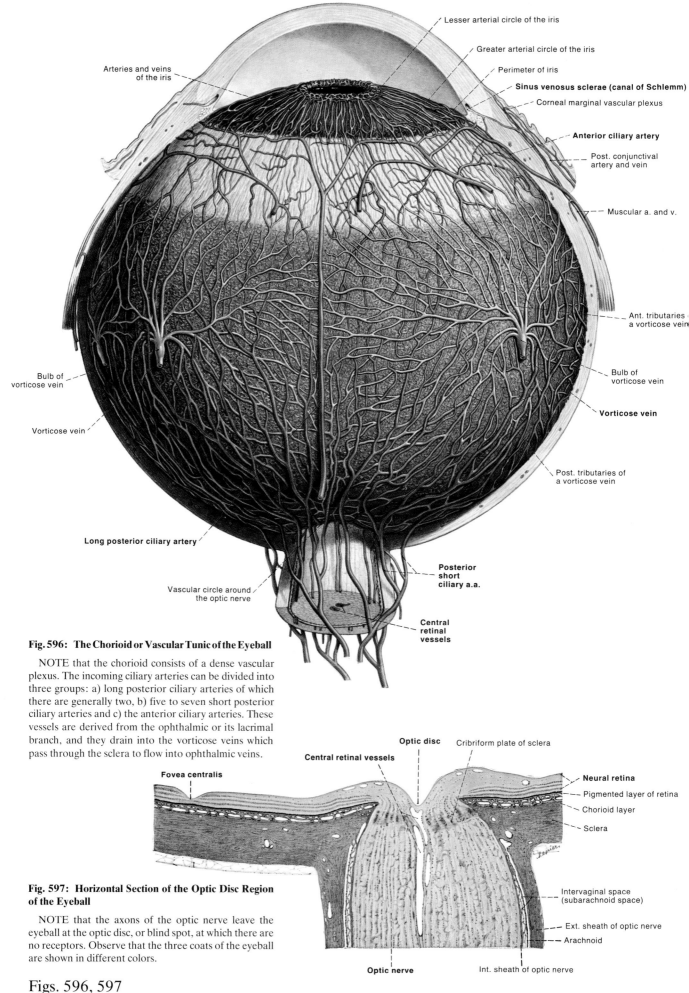

**Fig. 596: The Chorioid or Vascular Tunic of the Eyeball**

NOTE that the chorioid consists of a dense vascular plexus. The incoming ciliary arteries can be divided into three groups: a) long posterior ciliary arteries of which there are generally two, b) five to seven short posterior ciliary arteries and c) the anterior ciliary arteries. These vessels are derived from the ophthalmic or its lacrimal branch, and they drain into the vorticose veins which pass through the sclera to flow into ophthalmic veins.

**Fig. 597: Horizontal Section of the Optic Disc Region of the Eyeball**

NOTE that the axons of the optic nerve leave the eyeball at the optic disc, or blind spot, at which there are no receptors. Observe that the three coats of the eyeball are shown in different colors.

Figs. 596, 597

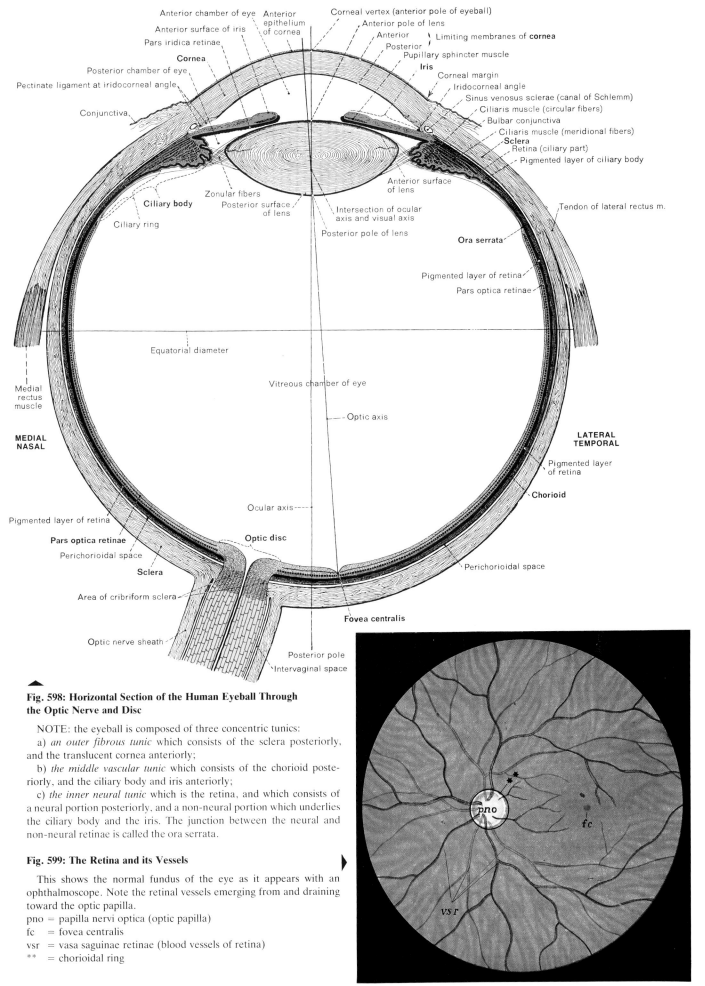

Anterior chamber of eye
Anterior epithelium of cornea
Anterior surface of iris
Pars iridica retinae
**Cornea**
Posterior chamber of eye
Pectinate ligament at iridocorneal angle
Conjunctiva
Corneal vertex (anterior pole of eyeball)
Anterior pole of lens
Anterior
Posterior
Pupillary sphincter muscle
**Iris**
Corneal margin
Iridocorneal angle
Sinus venosus sclerae (canal of Schlemm)
Ciliaris muscle (circular fibers)
Bulbar conjunctiva
Ciliaris muscle (meridional fibers)
**Sclera**
Retina (ciliary part)
Pigmented layer of ciliary body
Limiting membranes of **cornea**
Zonular fibers
**Ciliary body**
Posterior surface of lens
Ciliary ring
Anterior surface of lens
Intersection of ocular axis and visual axis
Posterior pole of lens
**Ora serrata**
Tendon of lateral rectus m.
Pigmented layer of retina
Pars optica retinae
Equatorial diameter
Vitreous chamber of eye
Optic axis
**Medial rectus muscle**
**MEDIAL NASAL**
**LATERAL TEMPORAL**
Pigmented layer of retina
**Chorioid**
Ocular axis
Pigmented layer of retina
**Pars optica retinae**
Perichorioidal space
**Sclera**
**Optic disc**
Area of cribriform sclera
Perichorioidal space
Optic nerve sheath
**Fovea centralis**
Posterior pole
Intervaginal space

**Fig. 598: Horizontal Section of the Human Eyeball Through the Optic Nerve and Disc**

NOTE: the eyeball is composed of three concentric tunics:

a) *an outer fibrous tunic* which consists of the sclera posteriorly, and the translucent cornea anteriorly;

b) *the middle vascular tunic* which consists of the chorioid posteriorly, and the ciliary body and iris anteriorly;

c) *the inner neural tunic* which is the retina, and which consists of a neural portion posteriorly, and a non-neural portion which underlies the ciliary body and the iris. The junction between the neural and non-neural retinae is called the ora serrata.

**Fig. 599: The Retina and its Vessels**

This shows the normal fundus of the eye as it appears with an ophthalmoscope. Note the retinal vessels emerging from and draining toward the optic papilla.

pno = papilla nervi optica (optic papilla)
fc  = fovea centralis
vsr = vasa saguinae retinae (blood vessels of retina)
**  = chorioidal ring

Figs. 598, 599    **VII**

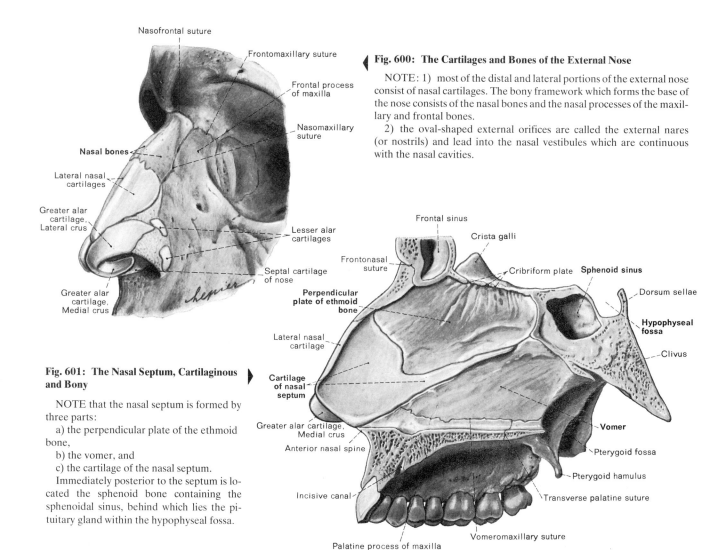

**Fig. 600: The Cartilages and Bones of the External Nose**

NOTE: 1) most of the distal and lateral portions of the external nose consist of nasal cartilages. The bony framework which forms the base of the nose consists of the nasal bones and the nasal processes of the maxillary and frontal bones.

2) the oval-shaped external orifices are called the external nares (or nostrils) and lead into the nasal vestibules which are continuous with the nasal cavities.

**Fig. 601: The Nasal Septum, Cartilaginous and Bony**

NOTE that the nasal septum is formed by three parts:

a) the perpendicular plate of the ethmoid bone,

b) the vomer, and

c) the cartilage of the nasal septum.

Immediately posterior to the septum is located the sphenoid bone containing the sphenoidal sinus, behind which lies the pituitary gland within the hypophyseal fossa.

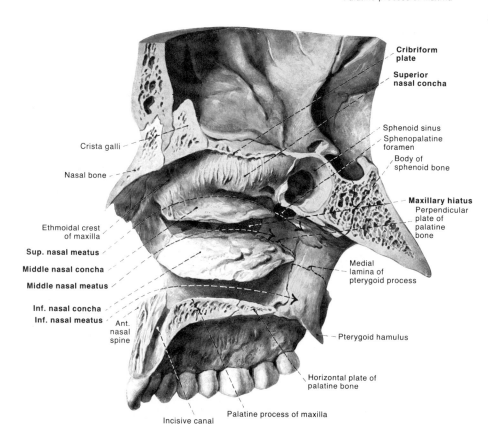

**Fig. 602: The Bony Lateral Wall of the Right Nasal Cavity**

NOTE: 1) that the nasal septum has been removed and the mucosa stripped from the bones that form the irregular lateral wall of the nasal cavity and the hard palate. Observe that the crista galli, cribriform plate, superior nasal concha and middle nasal concha are all parts of the ethmoid bone (light orange). Below these is the thin, slightly curved inferior nasal concha (gray), which is a separate bone.

2) that in front of the nasal conchae are the nasal bone (gray), the small lacrimal bone (red, not labelled), and the maxilla (yellow), while behind is the perpendicular plate of the palatine bone (blue). The bony floor of the nasal cavity is the hard palate, which is formed by the palatine process of the maxilla and the horizontal plate of the palatine bone.

3) the three posteriorly directed curved arrows. These follow the courses of the superior, middle and inferior meatuses, each of which underlies its respective nasal concha, and is oriented posteroinferiorly to that part of the nasal cavity which becomes the nasopharynx.

4) the sphenoidal sinus in the body of the sphenoid bone, the sphenopalatine foramen and the opening of the maxillary sinus (maxillary hiatus).

Figs. 600, 601, 602

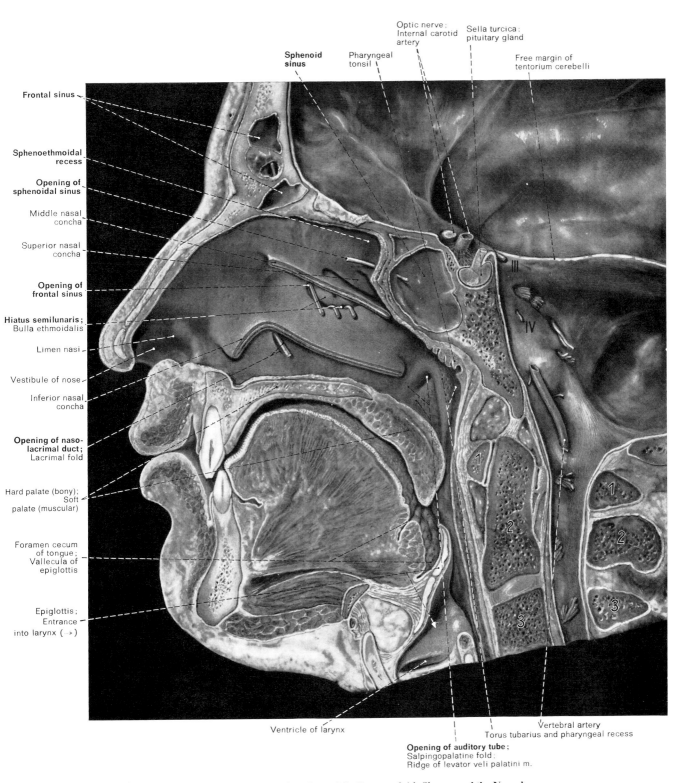

Frontal sinus

Sphenoethmoidal recess

**Opening of sphenoidal sinus**

Middle nasal concha

Superior nasal concha

**Opening of frontal sinus**

**Hiatus semilunaris;** Bulla ethmoidalis

Limen nasi

Vestibule of nose

Inferior nasal concha

**Opening of naso-lacrimal duct;** Lacrimal fold

Hard palate (bony); Soft palate (muscular)

Foramen cecum of tongue; Vallecula of epiglottis

Epiglottis; Entrance into larynx (→)

**Sphenoid sinus**

Pharyngeal tonsil

Optic nerve; Internal carotid artery

Sella turcica; pituitary gland

Free margin of tentorium cerebelli

Ventricle of larynx

Vertebral artery

Torus tubarius and pharyngeal recess

**Opening of auditory tube;** Salpingopalatine fold; Ridge of levator veli palatini m.

**Fig. 603: Lateral Wall of the Right Nasal Cavity Showing Openings of the Paranasal Air Sinuses and the Nasopharynx**

NOTE: 1) this median sagittal section of the adult head displays the right nasal cavity with the middle and inferior nasal conchae removed. The nasal cavity communicates anteriorly with the environment through the vestibule and nostril, and posteriorly with the pharynx (nasopharynx).

2) opening of the various paranasal sinuses and other structures. These include:

a) the *sphenoid sinus* which opens into the sphenoethmoidal recess above the superior concha.

b) the *frontal sinus* and *maxillary sinus* both of which open into a groove called the hiatus semilunaris in the middle meatus below the middle concha.

c) the *nasolacrimal duct* which opens into the inferior meatus below the inferior concha.

d) the *auditory tube* which opens into the nasopharynx just behind the inferior concha. This tube stretches between the cavity of the middle ear (tympanic cavity) and the nasopharynx, thereby allowing the cavity of the middle ear to alter its air pressure consistent with the environment. This mechanism equalizes the air pressure on both sides of the tympanic membrane.

3) the nasal cavity, oral cavity and laryngeal cavity all communicate with the pharynx, forming, in turn, the nasopharynx, oral pharynx and laryngeal pharynx.

Fig. 603    VII

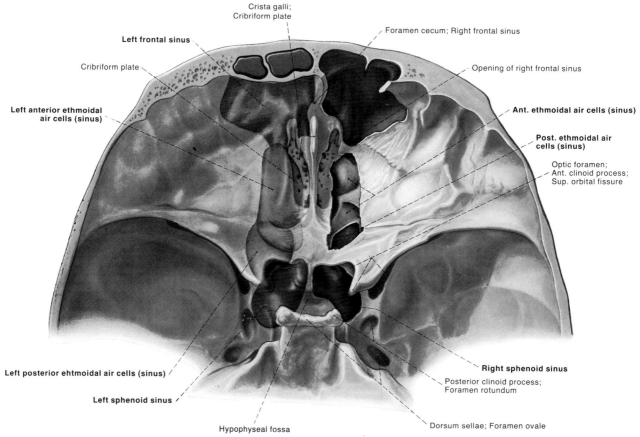

**Fig. 604: The Paranasal Sinuses Viewed from Above**

NOTE: 1) that on the left side the frontal (reddish brown), anterior ethmoid (green), posterior ethmoid (lavender) and sphenoid (brown) sinuses are projected onto the bones of the base of the skull. On the right side portions of the frontal, ethmoid and sphenoid bones have been removed to bring the sinuses into view from above.

2) each of these sinuses drain into the nasal cavity, as indicated in Fig. 603. There is some variation in size and considerable variation in the geometry of the sinuses, but all are lined by a delicate mucosa formed by pseudostratified columnar epithelium with many goblet cells, and an underlying connective tissue layer containing many mucous glands.

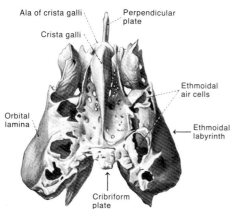

**Fig. 605: Ethmoid Bone: Superior Surface, Viewed from Above**

NOTE the same orientation as Fig. 604.

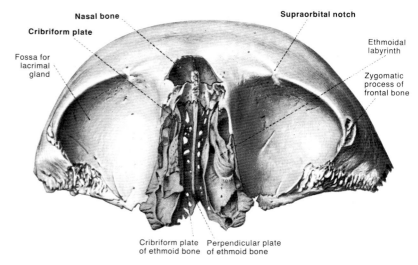

**Fig. 607: The Frontal, Ethmoid and Nasal Bones Viewed from Below**

NOTE that the cribriform plate of the ethmoid bone (orange), which extends laterally from the midline on each side, is perforated by many foramina. Through the foramina course the nerve fibers of the primary olfactory receptor cells. These first order special sense afferent fibers enter the cranial cavity and synapse with second order neurons in the overlying olfactory bulbs of the brain (see Figs. 608 and 609).

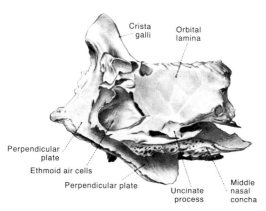

**Fig. 606: Ethmoid Bone, Left Lateral View**

Figs. 604–607

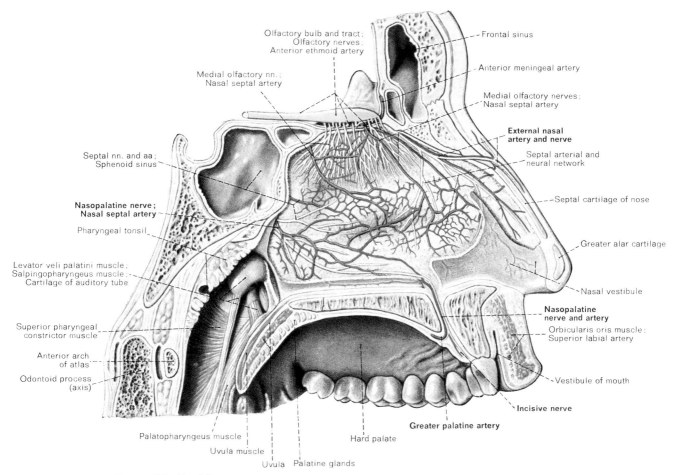

Olfactory bulb and tract;
Olfactory nerves;
Anterior ethmoid artery

Frontal sinus

Anterior meningeal artery

Medial olfactory nn.;
Nasal septal artery

Medial olfactory nerves;
Nasal septal artery

**External nasal
artery and nerve**

Septal arterial and
neural network

Septal nn. and aa;
Sphenoid sinus

Septal cartilage of nose

**Nasopalatine nerve;
Nasal septal artery**

Pharyngeal tonsil

Greater alar cartilage

Levator veli palatini muscle;
Salpingopharyngeus muscle;
Cartilage of auditory tube

Nasal vestibule

**Nasopalatine
nerve and artery**

Orbicularis oris muscle;
Superior labial artery

Superior pharyngeal
constrictor muscle

Anterior arch
of atlas

Vestibule of mouth

Odontoid process
(axis)

**Incisive nerve**

**Greater palatine artery**

Palatopharyngeus muscle

Uvula muscle

Hard palate

Uvula    Palatine glands

**Fig. 608: Arteries and Nerves of the Nasal Septum**

NOTE that the mucous membrane has been removed from the nasal septum and nasopharynx revealing the spetal vessels and nerves and the nasopharyngeal muscles.

**Fig. 609: The Lateral Wall of the Left Nasal Cavity**

NOTE: the mucous membrane overlying the lateral olfactory nerves has been removed. The lateral wall of the nasal cavity is marked by the superior, middle and inferior nasal conchae. Beneath each concha courses its corresponding nasal passage or meatus.

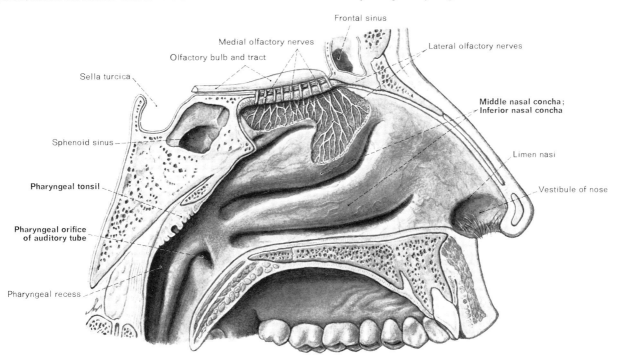

Frontal sinus

Medial olfactory nerves

Lateral olfactory nerves

Olfactory bulb and tract

Sella turcica

**Middle nasal concha;
Inferior nasal concha**

Sphenoid sinus

Limen nasi

**Pharyngeal tonsil**

Vestibule of nose

**Pharyngeal orifice
of auditory tube**

Pharyngeal recess

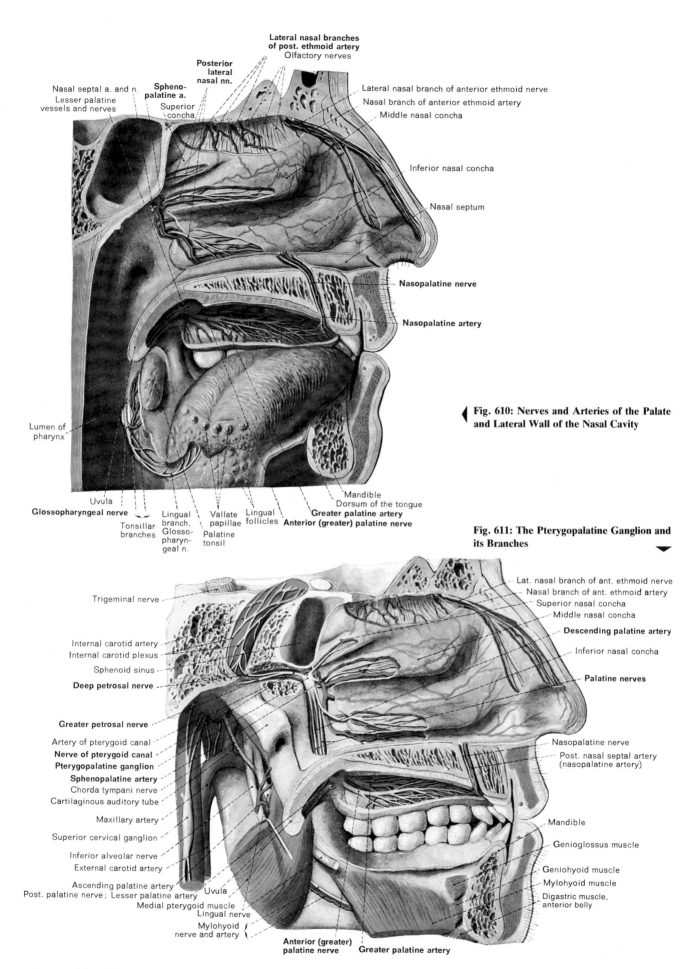

Lateral nasal branches
of post. ethmoid artery
Olfactory nerves

Nasal septal a. and n.
Lesser palatine
vessels and nerves

Spheno-
palatine a.

Posterior
lateral
nasal nn.

Superior
concha

Lateral nasal branch of anterior ethmoid nerve
Nasal branch of anterior ethmoid artery
Middle nasal concha

Inferior nasal concha

Nasal septum

Nasopalatine nerve

Nasopalatine artery

**Fig. 610: Nerves and Arteries of the Palate
and Lateral Wall of the Nasal Cavity**

Lumen of
pharynx

Uvula
**Glossopharyngeal nerve**
Tonsillar
branches

Lingual
branch,
Glosso-
pharyn-
geal n.

Vallate
papillae
Palatine
tonsil

Lingual
follicles

Mandible
Dorsum of the tongue
**Greater palatine artery**
**Anterior (greater) palatine nerve**

**Fig. 611: The Pterygopalatine Ganglion and
its Branches**

Trigeminal nerve

Internal carotid artery
Internal carotid plexus
Sphenoid sinus
**Deep petrosal nerve**

**Greater petrosal nerve**

Artery of pterygoid canal
**Nerve of pterygoid canal**
**Pterygopalatine ganglion**
**Sphenopalatine artery**
Chorda tympani nerve
Cartilaginous auditory tube

Maxillary artery
Superior cervical ganglion
Inferior alveolar nerve
External carotid artery

Ascending palatine artery
Post. palatine nerve; Lesser palatine artery
Medial pterygoid muscle
Lingual nerve
Mylohyoid
nerve and artery

Uvula

**Anterior (greater)
palatine nerve**

**Greater palatine artery**

Lat. nasal branch of ant. ethmoid nerve
Nasal branch of ant. ethmoid artery
Superior nasal concha
Middle nasal concha
**Descending palatine artery**
Inferior nasal concha
**Palatine nerves**

Nasopalatine nerve
Post. nasal septal artery
(nasopalatine artery)

Mandible
Genioglossus muscle
Geniohyoid muscle
Mylohyoid muscle
Digastric muscle,
anterior belly

Figs. 610, 611

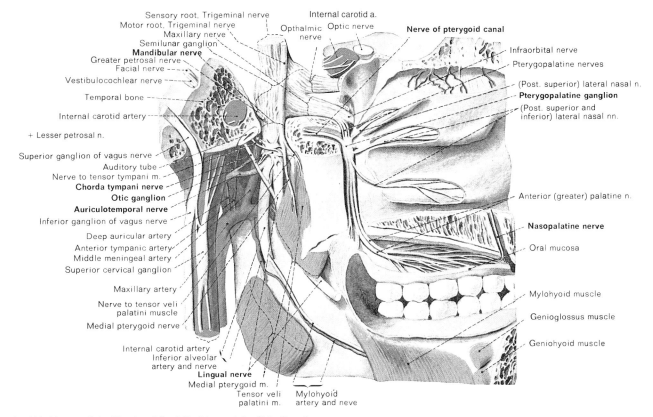

Sensory root, Trigeminal nerve
Motor root, Trigeminal nerve
Maxillary nerve
Semilunar ganglion
**Mandibular nerve**
Greater petrosal nerve
Facial nerve
Vestibulocochlear nerve
Temporal bone
Internal carotid artery
+ Lesser petrosal n.
Superior ganglion of vagus nerve
Auditory tube
Nerve to tensor tympani m.
**Chorda tympani nerve**
**Otic ganglion**
**Auriculotemporal nerve**
Inferior ganglion of vagus nerve
Deep auricular artery
Anterior tympanic artery
Middle meningeal artery
Superior cervical ganglion
Maxillary artery
Nerve to tensor veli palatini muscle
Medial pterygoid nerve
Internal carotid artery
Inferior alveolar artery and nerve
**Lingual nerve**
Medial pterygoid m.
Tensor veli palatini m.
Mylohyoid artery and neve

Internal carotid a.
Opthalmic nerve
Optic nerve
**Nerve of pterygoid canal**
Infraorbital nerve
Pterygopalatine nerves
(Post. superior) lateral nasal n.
**Pterygopalatine ganglion**
(Post. superior and inferior) lateral nasal nn.
Anterior (greater) palatine n.
**Nasopalatine nerve**
Oral mucosa
Mylohyoid muscle
Genioglossus muscle
Geniohyoid muscle

**Fig. 612: Nerves of the Nasal and Oral Cavities and the Otic Ganglion**

NOTE the junction of the chorda tympani nerve with the lingual nerve and the position of the otic ganglion in relation to the mandibular branch of the trigeminal. This ganglion receives preganglionic parasympathetic fibers by way of the tympanic branch of the glossopharyngeal nerve. Its postganglionic fibers supply the parotid gland.

**Fig. 613: The Maxillary Nerve, the Petrosal Nerves and the Facial Nerve**

NOTE that the nerve of the pterygoid canal is formed by the union of the deep petrosal and greater petrosal nerves. The deep petrosal nerve transmits postganglionic sympathetic fibers, while the greater petrosal nerve contains sensory fibers from the geniculate ganglion of the facial nerve and preganglionic parasympathetic fibers from the nervus intermedius portion of the facial nerve. The lesser petrosal nerve carries preganglionic fibers of the glossopharyngeal nerve to the otic ganglion (see Fig. 612).

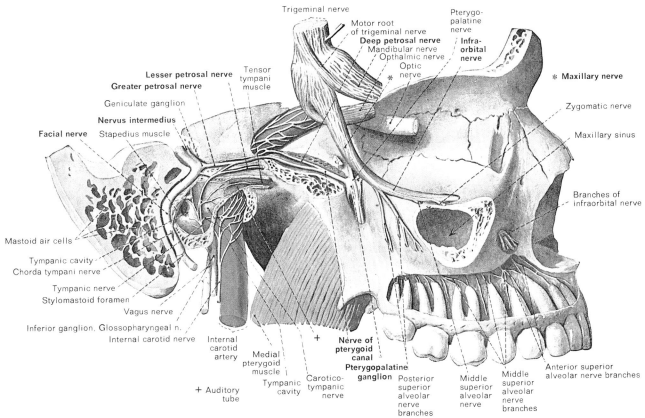

Trigeminal nerve
Motor root of trigeminal nerve
Pterygopalatine nerve
**Deep petrosal nerve**
Mandibular nerve
Opthalmic nerve
Optic nerve
Infraorbital nerve
**Lesser petrosal nerve**
**Greater petrosal nerve**
Tensor tympani muscle
Geniculate ganglion
**Nervus intermedius**
**Facial nerve**
Stapedius muscle
Mastoid air cells
Tympanic cavity
Chorda tympani nerve
Tympanic nerve
Stylomastoid foramen
Vagus nerve
Inferior ganglion, Glossopharyngeal n.
Internal carotid nerve
+ Auditory tube
Internal carotid artery
Medial pterygoid muscle
Tympanic cavity
Caroticotympanic nerve
+ Nerve of pterygoid canal
**Pterygopalatine ganglion**
Posterior superior alveolar nerve branches
Middle superior alveolar nerve
Middle superior alveolar nerve branches
Anterior superior alveolar nerve branches
* **Maxillary nerve**
Zygomatic nerve
Maxillary sinus
Branches of infraorbital nerve

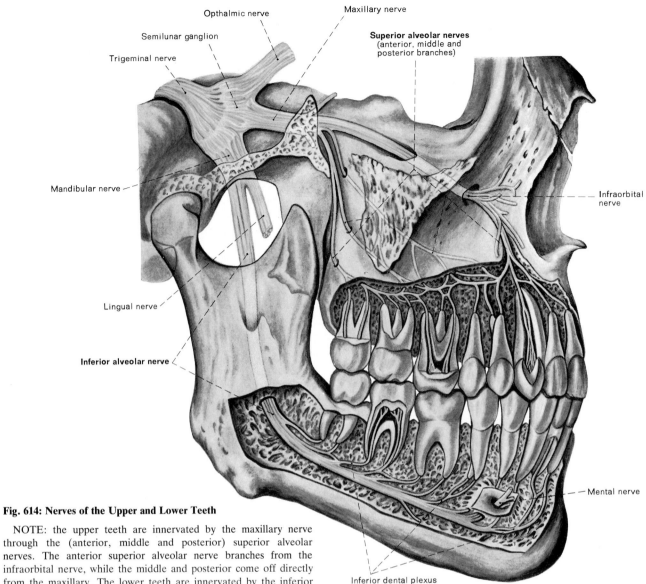

Opthalmic nerve

Maxillary nerve

Semilunar ganglion

**Superior alveolar nerves**
(anterior, middle and
posterior branches)

Trigeminal nerve

Mandibular nerve

Infraorbital
nerve

Lingual nerve

Inferior alveolar nerve

Mental nerve

**Fig. 614: Nerves of the Upper and Lower Teeth**

NOTE: the upper teeth are innervated by the maxillary nerve through the (anterior, middle and posterior) superior alveolar nerves. The anterior superior alveolar nerve branches from the infraorbital nerve, while the middle and posterior come off directly from the maxillary. The lower teeth are innervated by the inferior alveolar branch of the mandibular nerve after it enters the mandibular foramen.

Inferior dental plexus

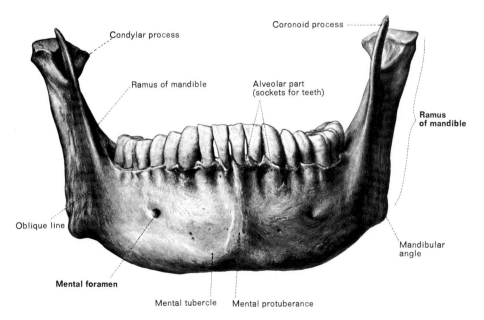

Condylar process

Coronoid process

Ramus of mandible

Alveolar part
(sockets for teeth)

Ramus
of mandible

Oblique line

Mandibular
angle

**Mental foramen**

Mental tubercle    Mental protuberance

**Fig. 615: The Mandible as seen from the Front**

NOTE: 1) th anterior aspect of the mandible forms the bony substructure of the mentum or chin. The two vertical rami of the mandible are continuous with the body of the mandible at the mandibular angle.

2) the mental foramen transmits the mental branch of the inferior alveolar nerve to the skin of the chin and lower lip on each side. The mental branch of the inferior alveolar artery accompanies the mental nerve and participates in the vascular supply of the lower lip.

Figs. 614, 615

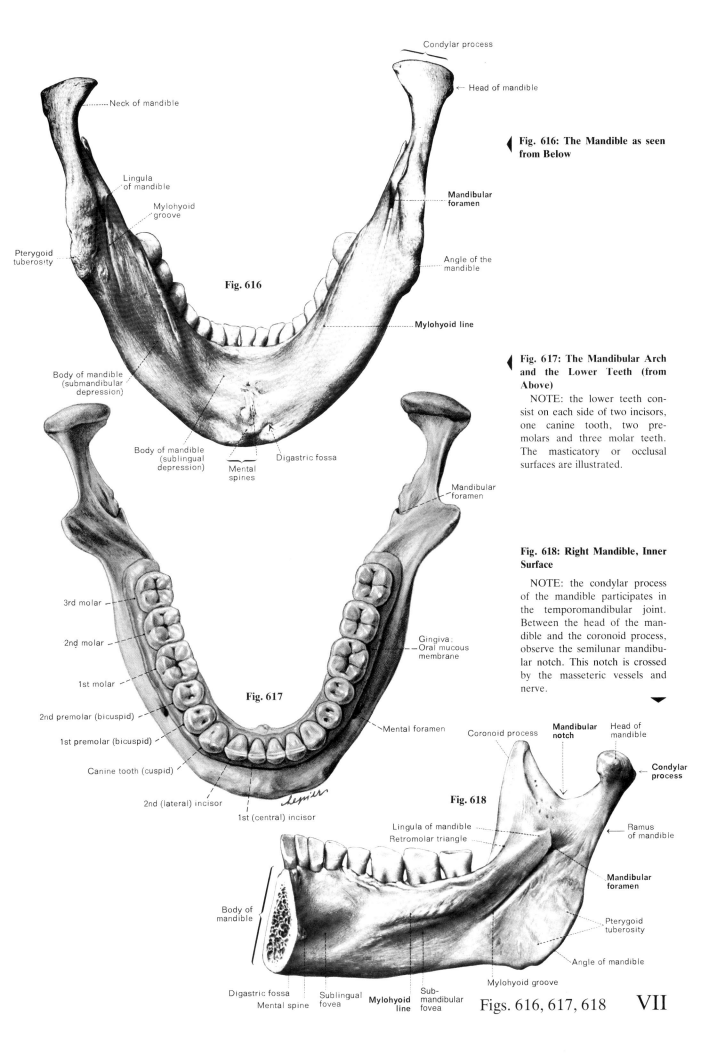

Neck of mandible

Condylar process

Head of mandible

**Fig. 616: The Mandible as seen from Below**

Lingula of mandible

Mylohyoid groove

**Mandibular foramen**

Pterygoid tuberosity

Angle of the mandible

**Fig. 616**

**Mylohyoid line**

Body of mandible (submandibular depression)

**Fig. 617: The Mandibular Arch and the Lower Teeth (from Above)**

NOTE: the lower teeth consist on each side of two incisors, one canine tooth, two premolars and three molar teeth. The masticatory or occlusal surfaces are illustrated.

Body of mandible (sublingual depression)

Digastric fossa

Mental spines

Mandibular foramen

**Fig. 618: Right Mandible, Inner Surface**

NOTE: the condylar process of the mandible participates in the temporomandibular joint. Between the head of the mandible and the coronoid process, observe the semilunar mandibular notch. This notch is crossed by the masseteric vessels and nerve.

3rd molar

2nd molar

1st molar

2nd premolar (bicuspid)

1st premolar (bicuspid)

Gingiva; Oral mucous membrane

**Fig. 617**

Canine tooth (cuspid)

Mental foramen

2nd (lateral) incisor

1st (central) incisor

Coronoid process

**Mandibular notch**

Head of mandible

**Condylar process**

**Fig. 618**

Lingula of mandible

Retromolar triangle

Ramus of mandible

**Mandibular foramen**

Body of mandible

Pterygoid tuberosity

Angle of mandible

Digastric fossa

Mental spine

Sublingual fovea

**Mylohyoid line**

Submandibular fovea

Mylohyoid groove

Figs. 616, 617, 618 VII

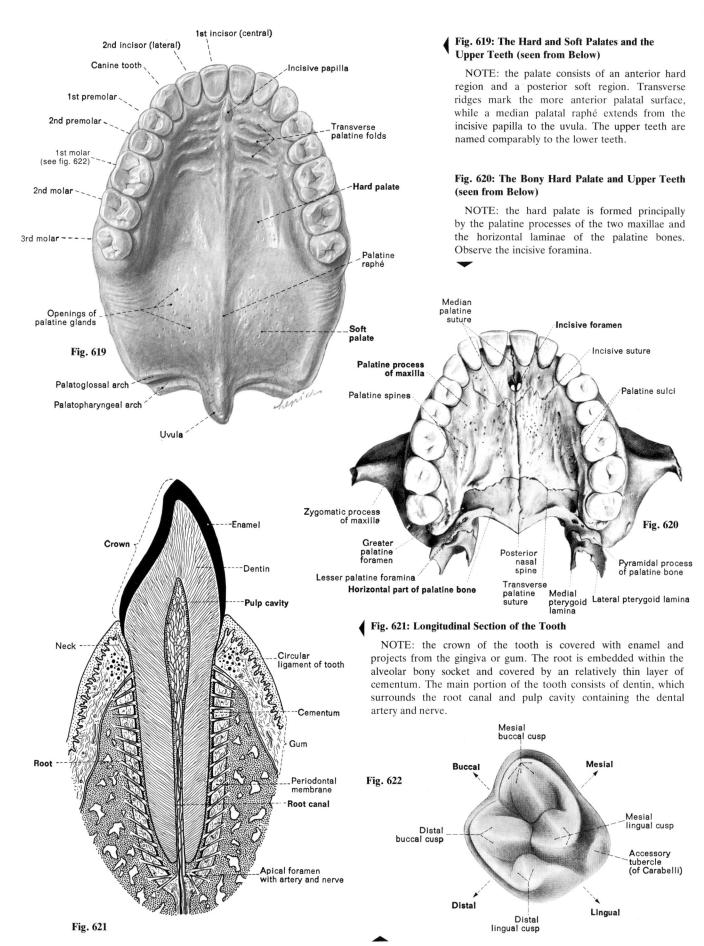

1st incisor (central)

2nd incisor (lateral)

Canine tooth

1st premolar

2nd premolar

1st molar
(see fig. 622)

2nd molar

3rd molar

Openings of
palatine glands

Fig. 619

Incisive papilla

Transverse
palatine folds

Hard palate

Palatine
raphé

Soft
palate

Palatoglossal arch

Palatopharyngeal arch

Uvula

◀ **Fig. 619: The Hard and Soft Palates and the
Upper Teeth (seen from Below)**

NOTE: the palate consists of an anterior hard
region and a posterior soft region. Transverse
ridges mark the more anterior palatal surface,
while a median palatal raphé extends from the
incisive papilla to the uvula. The upper teeth are
named comparably to the lower teeth.

**Fig. 620: The Bony Hard Palate and Upper Teeth
(seen from Below)**

NOTE: the hard palate is formed principally
by the palatine processes of the two maxillae and
the horizontal laminae of the palatine bones.
Observe the incisive foramina. ▼

Median
palatine
suture

Palatine process
of maxilla

Palatine spines

Zygomatic process
of maxilla

Greater
palatine
foramen

Lesser palatine foramina

**Horizontal part of palatine bone**

**Incisive foramen**

Incisive suture

Palatine sulci

Posterior
nasal
spine

Transverse
palatine
suture

Medial
pterygoid
lamina

Lateral pterygoid lamina

Pyramidal process
of palatine bone

**Fig. 620**

Crown

Neck

Root

Fig. 621

Enamel

Dentin

**Pulp cavity**

Circular
ligament of tooth

Cementum

Gum

Periodontal
membrane

**Root canal**

Apical foramen
with artery and nerve

◀ **Fig. 621: Longitudinal Section of the Tooth**

NOTE: the crown of the tooth is covered with enamel and
projects from the gingiva or gum. The root is embedded within the
alveolar bony socket and covered by an relatively thin layer of
cementum. The main portion of the tooth consists of dentin, which
surrounds the root canal and pulp cavity containing the dental
artery and nerve.

Mesial
buccal cusp

**Buccal**

**Mesial**

**Fig. 622**

Distal
buccal cusp

Mesial
lingual cusp

Accessory
tubercle
(of Carabelli)

**Distal**

Distal
lingual cusp

**Lingual**

▲ **Fig. 622: The Occlusal Surface of the Right Upper First Molar**

Figs. 619–622

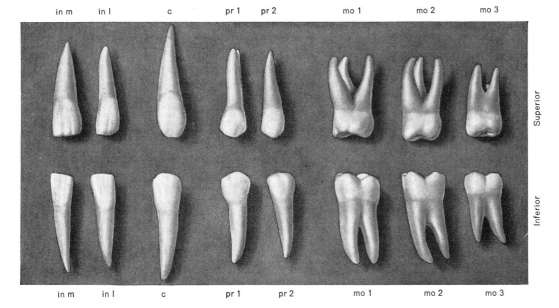

| in m | in l | c | pr 1 | pr 2 | mo 1 | mo 2 | mo 3 |

Superior

Inferior

| in m | in l | c | pr 1 | pr 2 | mo 1 | mo 2 | mo 3 |

in m = Medial incisor
in l = Lateral incisor
c = Canine
pr 1 = 1st premolar
pr 2 = 2nd premolar
mo 1 = 1st molar
mo 2 = 2nd molar
mo 3 = 3rd molar

Fig. 623

**Fig. 623: The Maxillary and Mandibular Permanent Teeth (Buccal Surfaces)**

6 to 9 M.
8 to 12 M.
16 to 20 M.
12 to 16 M.
20 to 30 M.

Fig. 625

**Fig. 625: Diagram Showing Eruption Times of Deciduous Upper Teeth**

NOTE: on the left side of the illustration the times of eruption are shown in *months* for each tooth, while the sequential order of appearance of the erupted *deciduous* teeth is indicated on the right side by numbers.

**Fig. 624: Diagram Showing Eruption Times of Permanent Upper Teeth**

NOTE: on the left side of the illustration the times of eruption are shown in *years* for each tooth while the sequential order of appearance of the erupted *permanent* teeth is indicated on the right side by numbers.

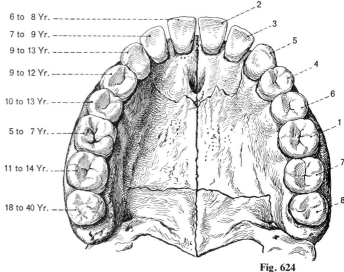

6 to 8 Yr.
7 to 9 Yr.
9 to 13 Yr.
9 to 12 Yr.
10 to 13 Yr.
5 to 7 Yr.
11 to 14 Yr.
18 to 40 Yr.

Fig. 624

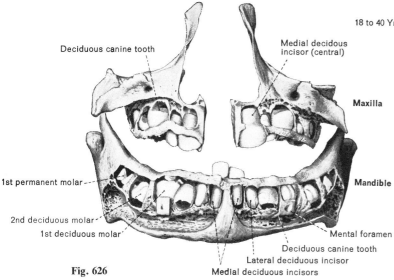

Deciduous canine tooth

Medial decidous incisor (central)

Maxilla

Mandible

1st permanent molar

2nd deciduous molar

1st deciduous molar

Mental foramen

Deciduous canine tooth

Lateral deciduous incisor

Medial deciduous incisors

Fig. 626

**Fig. 626: Dentition of a Child of Nearly One Year of Age**

NOTE: 1) the deciduous or "milk teeth" number 20 in all, including two incisors, one canine and two molars in each jaw quadrant. The earliest of these teeth to erupt are the incisors, which generally penetrate through the gum line before the end of the first year.

2) generally speaking:
a 1 year old child has 6 teeth,
a 1½ year old child has 12 teeth,
a 2 year old child has 16 teeth, and
a 2½ year old child has 20 teeth.

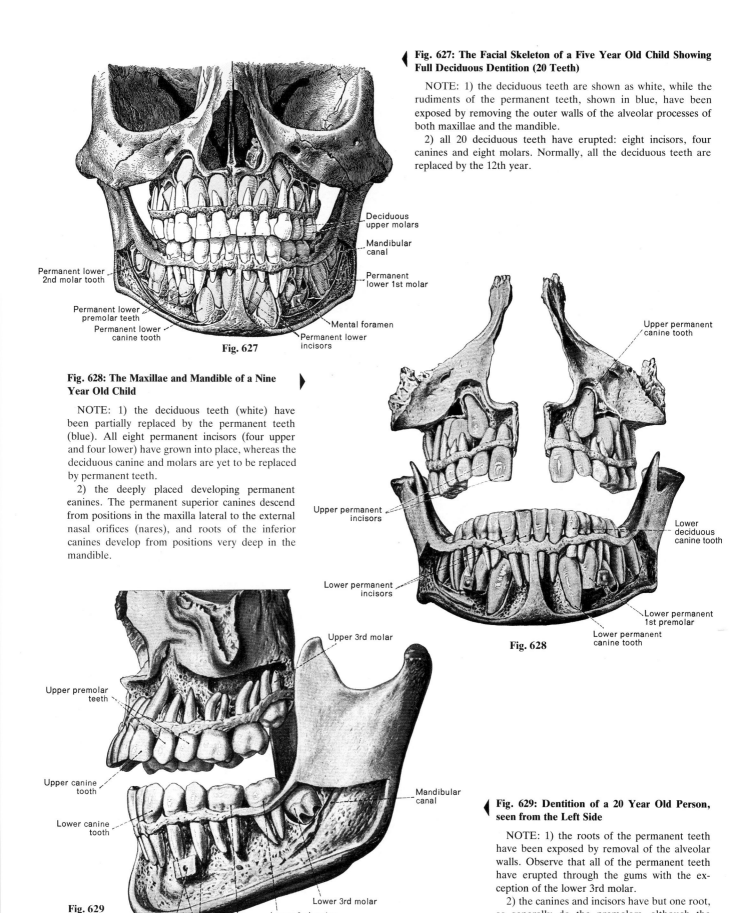

**Fig. 627: The Facial Skeleton of a Five Year Old Child Showing Full Deciduous Dentition (20 Teeth)**

NOTE: 1) the deciduous teeth are shown as white, while the rudiments of the permanent teeth, shown in blue, have been exposed by removing the outer walls of the alveolar processes of both maxillae and the mandible.

2) all 20 deciduous teeth have erupted: eight incisors, four canines and eight molars. Normally, all the deciduous teeth are replaced by the 12th year.

*Labels on Fig. 627:*
Deciduous upper molars
Mandibular canal
Permanent lower 1st molar
Permanent lower 2nd molar tooth
Permanent lower premolar teeth
Permanent lower canine tooth
Mental foramen
Permanent lower incisors

**Fig. 627**

**Fig. 628: The Maxillae and Mandible of a Nine Year Old Child**

NOTE: 1) the deciduous teeth (white) have been partially replaced by the permanent teeth (blue). All eight permanent incisors (four upper and four lower) have grown into place, whereas the deciduous canine and molars are yet to be replaced by permanent teeth.

2) the deeply placed developing permanent canines. The permanent superior canines descend from positions in the maxilla lateral to the external nasal orifices (nares), and roots of the inferior canines develop from positions very deep in the mandible.

*Labels on Fig. 628:*
Upper permanent canine tooth
Upper permanent incisors
Lower deciduous canine tooth
Lower permanent incisors
Lower permanent 1st premolar
Lower permanent canine tooth

**Fig. 628**

*Labels on Fig. 629:*
Upper 3rd molar
Upper premolar teeth
Upper canine tooth
Lower canine tooth
Mandibular canal
Mental foramen
Lower premolars
Lower 1st molar
Lower 2nd molar
Lower 3rd molar

**Fig. 629**

**Fig. 629: Dentition of a 20 Year Old Person, seen from the Left Side**

NOTE: 1) the roots of the permanent teeth have been exposed by removal of the alveolar walls. Observe that all of the permanent teeth have erupted through the gums with the exception of the lower 3rd molar.

2) the canines and incisors have but one root, as generally do the premolars, although the latter teeth may have two roots. The 1st and 2nd molars usually have three roots, whereas the smaller 3rd molar may have less than three and may even be single rooted.

Figs. 627, 628, 629

UPPER TEETH

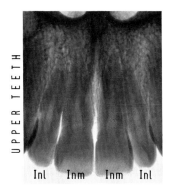

Inl  Inm  Inm  Inl

**Fig. 630: The Four Incisors**

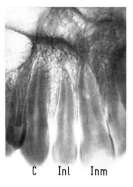

C  Inl  Inm

**Fig. 631: The Two Right Incisors and Canine Teeth**

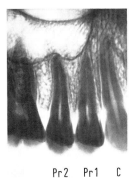

Pr2  Pr1  C

**Fig. 632: The Right Canine Tooth and Two Premolars**

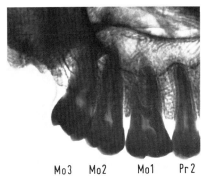

Mo3  Mo2  Mo1  Pr2

**Fig. 633: The Right Second Premolar and Three Molars**

LOWER TEETH

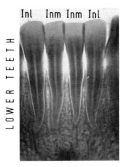

Inl  Inm  Inm  Inl

**Fig. 634: The Four Incisors**

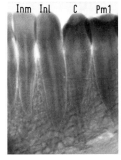

Inm  Inl  C  Pm1

**Fig. 635: The Two Incisors, Canine and First Premolar**

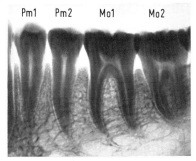

Pm1  Pm2  Mo1  Mo2

**Fig. 636: The Two Premolars and First Two Molar Teeth**

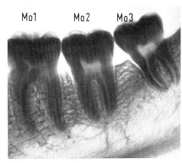

Mo1  Mo2  Mo3

**Fig. 637: The Three Molar Teeth.**

**Fig. 638: The Right Upper and Lower Teeth, Lateral View**

NOTE: 1) that the right upper eight and right lower eight teeth have been completely exposed by removal of the outer bony layers of the alveolar processes from both the maxilla and mandible. Each tooth has been cut along its longitudinal axis to reveal the pulp cavity and root canal.

2) the fine canaliculi leading to the root canals along which course the delicate vessels and nerves supplying the individual teeth.

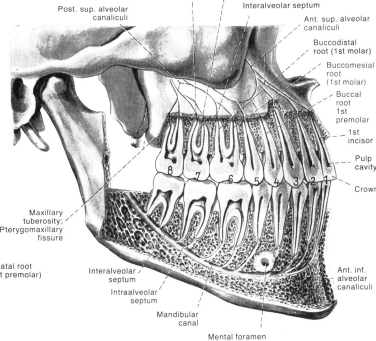

Alveolar foramen
Intraalveolar septum
Interalveolar septum
Post. sup. alveolar canaliculi
Ant. sup. alveolar canaliculi
Buccodistal root (1st molar)
Buccomesial root (1st molar)
Buccal root 1st premolar
1st incisor
Pulp cavity
Crown
Maxillary tuberosity; Pterygomaxillary fissure
Interalveolar septum
Intraalveolar septum
Ant. inf. alveolar canaliculi
Mandibular canal
Mental foramen

**Fig. 639: The Left Upper and Lower Teeth, Medial View**

NOTE that the inner aspect of the roots of the teeth on the left side have been exposed. Observe that the sockets for the canine teeth are the deepest, while those for the molar teeth are the widest. Interalveolar bony septa separate the sockets of individual teeth, and in the case of the multiple rooted molar teeth, intraalveolar septa separate each root.

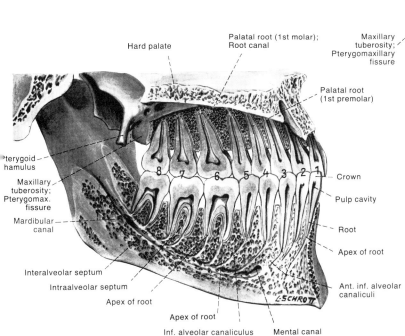

Hard palate
Palatal root (1st molar); Root canal
Palatal root (1st premolar)
Pterygoid hamulus
Maxillary tuberosity; Pterygomax. fissure
Mandibular canal
Interalveolar septum
Intraalveolar septum
Apex of root
Apex of root
Inf. alveolar canaliculus
Mental canal
Crown
Pulp cavity
Root
Apex of root
Ant. inf. alveolar canaliculi
L. SCHROTT

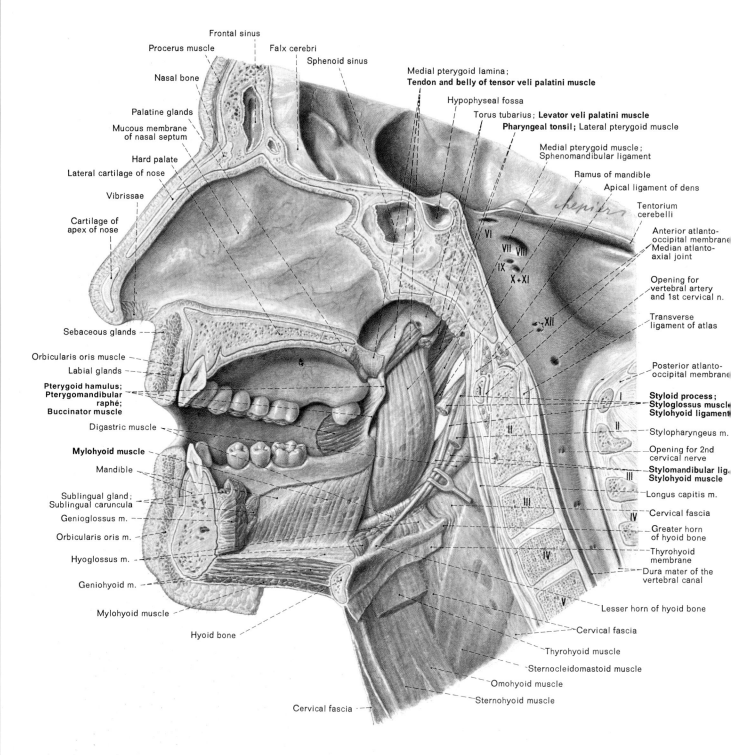

Frontal sinus

Procerus muscle

Falx cerebri

Sphenoid sinus

Nasal bone

Medial pterygoid lamina;
**Tendon and belly of tensor veli palatini muscle**

Palatine glands

Hypophyseal fossa

Mucous membrane
of nasal septum

Torus tubarius; **Levator veli palatini muscle**

Hard palate

**Pharyngeal tonsil;** Lateral pterygoid muscle

Lateral cartilage of nose

Medial pterygoid muscle;
Sphenomandibular ligament

Vibrissae

Ramus of mandible
Apical ligament of dens

Cartilage of
apex of nose

Tentorium
cerebelli

Anterior atlanto-
occipital membrane
Median atlanto-
axial joint

VI

VII VIII

IX

X + XI

Opening for
vertebral artery
and 1st cervical n.

Transverse
ligament of atlas

XII

Sebaceous glands

Posterior atlanto-
occipital membrane

Orbicularis oris muscle

Labial glands

**Pterygoid hamulus;**
**Pterygomandibular**
**raphé;**
**Buccinator muscle**

**Styloid process;**
**Styloglossus muscle**
**Stylohyoid ligament**

Stylopharyngeus m.

Digastric muscle

Opening for 2nd
cervical nerve

**Mylohyoid muscle**

**Stylomandibular lig.**
**Stylohyoid muscle**

Mandible

Longus capitis m.

Sublingual gland;
Sublingual caruncula

Cervical fascia

Genioglossus m.

Greater horn
of hyoid bone

Orbicularis oris m.

Thyrohyoid
membrane

Hyoglossus m.

Dura mater of the
vertebral canal

Geniohyoid m.

Mylohyoid muscle

Lesser horn of hyoid bone

Hyoid bone

Cervical fascia

Thyrohyoid muscle

Sternocleidomastoid muscle

Omohyoid muscle

Sternohyoid muscle

Cervical fascia

**Fig. 640: Paramedian Sagittal View of the Face and Neck**

NOTE: 1) this dissection has exposed the right half of the oral cavity and the nasal septum. The mucous membrane has been removed from the floor of the mouth exposing the mylohyoid muscle; the pharyngeal constrictors have been removed. Observe the pterygomandibular raphé and the buccinator muscle.

2) the tendon of the tensor veli palatini muscle as it turns medially around the pterygoid hamulus. The tendon has been severed at its insertion into the palatine aponeurosis. This muscle tightens the soft palate and, being derived from the first or mandibular branchial arch, it is innervated by the trigeminal nerve.

3) the stylohyoid ligament and the styloglossus and stylopharyngeus muscles which have been cut. These three structures all attach to the styloid process, as do the stylomandibular ligament and the stylohyoid muscles which have not been cut.

4) that the hyoid bone lies at the level of the third cervical vertebra and that the atlas (1st vertebra) and axis (2nd vertebra), which surround the uppermost part of the cervical spinal cord, lie directly behind the oral cavity and oropharynx. The spinomedullary junction and the lower medulla oblongata lie posterior to the palate and nasopharynx.

5) that the genioglossus and hyoglossus muscles have been cut. These attach the base and sides of the tongue to the mandible and hyoid bone.

Fig. 640

2) the *trigeminal field* (nerve of 1st branchial arch). The *dark blue* zones are supplied by the ophthalmic division of the trigeminal nerve through its anterior and posterior ethmoidal branches. This includes the mucosa of the anterior nasal cavity and the frontal sinus. At times the posterior ethmoidal branch reaches the sphenoid sinus.

The *blue-gray* zones, which include the posterior part of the nasal cavity, the upper nasopharynx, most of the palate and the upper gums of the oral cavity, are supplied by the maxillary division of the trigeminal nerve. This is achieved by branches from the greater and lesser palatine nerves and mucosal branches from the superior alveolar and superior labial nerves. Observe the *white dots* outlining the superior part of the nasal cavity. The mucosa at this site contains olfactory receptor cells for the special sense of smell.

The *blue-green* zones are supplied by the mandibular division of the trigeminal nerve. These include the anterior two-thirds of the tongue, the lower gums and lateral walls of the oral cavity by way of the lingual, buccal and inferior alveolar nerves. Note the *red dots* on the anterior tongue. These represent the field of the chorda tympani nerve which supplies the region with special sensory taste fibers.

3) the *glossopharyngeal field* (nerve of 3rd branchial arch). The *yellow* zones indicate the general sensory supply of the lingual and pharyngeal branches of the glossopharyngeal nerve. These include the posterior one-third of the tongue, part of the soft palate, the oropharynx and the lower part of the nasopharynx. The *white dots* indicate that this nerve also supplies the posterior one-third of the tongue with special sensory fibers of taste.

4) the *vagal field* (nerve of 4th and 6th branchial arches). The green zones represent fields supplied by fibers of general sensation from pharyngeal and laryngeal branches of the vagus nerve. These zones include the laryngopharynx, the larynx and trachea, as well as the esophagus.

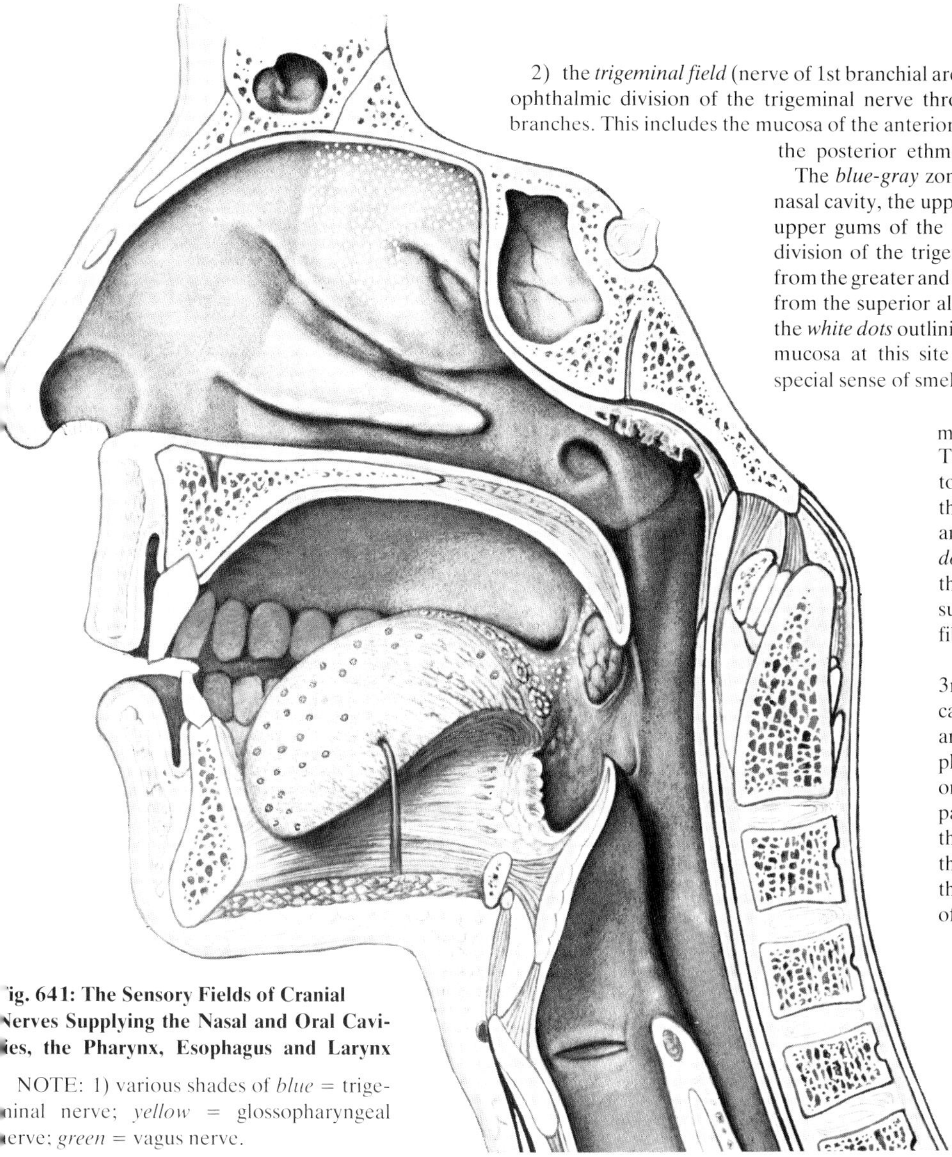

**Fig. 641: The Sensory Fields of Cranial Nerves Supplying the Nasal and Oral Cavities, the Pharynx, Esophagus and Larynx**

NOTE: 1) various shades of *blue* = trigeminal nerve; *yellow* = glossopharyngeal nerve; *green* = vagus nerve.

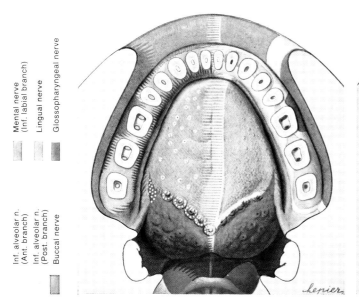

Mental nerve (Inf. labial branch)

Lingual nerve

Glossopharyngeal nerve

Inf. alveolar n. (Ant. branch)

Inf. alveolar n. (Post. branch)

Buccal nerve

**Fig. 642: Sensory Innervation of the Tongue. Cheeks and Floor of the Oral Cavity**

NOTE that on the right side are specific areas of distribution; on the left side, the overlapping fields. *White circles:* taste zone of chorda tympani nerve; *white dots:* taste zone of glossopharyngeal nerve.

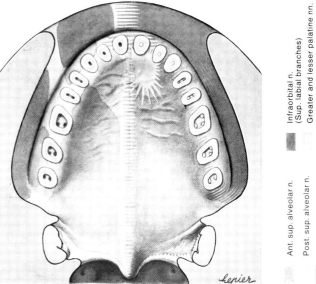

Infraorbital n. (Sup. labial branches)

Greater and lesser palatine nn.

Nasopalatine nerve

Ant. sup. alveolar n.

Post. sup. alveolar n.

Buccal nerve

**Fig. 643: Sensory Innervation of the Palate, Cheeks and Upper Gums of the Oral Cavity**

NOTE that on the (reader's) left side are shown specific fields of distribution of the individual sensory nerves, while on the right side the overlapping fields of innervation are shown.

Figs. 641, 642, 643    VII

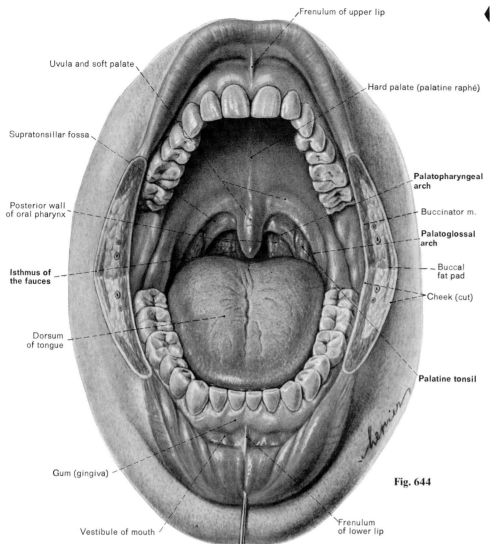

Frenulum of upper lip

Uvula and soft palate

Supratonsillar fossa

Posterior wall
of oral pharynx

**Isthmus of
the fauces**

Dorsum
of tongue

Gum (gingiva)

Vestibule of mouth

Hard palate (palatine raphé)

**Palatopharyngeal
arch**

Buccinator m.

**Palatoglossal
arch**

Buccal
fat pad

Cheek (cut)

**Palatine tonsil**

Frenulum
of lower lip

**Fig. 644**

### Fig. 644: The Oral Cavity

NOTE: 1) the position of the palatine tonsils located on each side of the oral cavity within fossae between the palatoglossal and palatopharyngeal arches. These soft folds are formed by correspondingly named muscles covered by oral mucous membrane (see Figure 646).

2) the passage between the oral cavity and the oral pharynx is called the fauces. This aperture or isthmus commences anteriorly at the palatoglossal arches on each side and is also bounded by the soft palate superiorly and the dorsum of the tongue inferiorly.

3) that portion of the oral cavity between the teeth and the lips anteriorly, and between the teeth and cheeks laterally, is called the vestibule. The vestibule communicates with the larger oral cavity proper behind the 3rd molar teeth.

### Fig. 646: The Palate: Muscular Folds and Glands

NOTE: the oral mucosa has been removed from both the hard and soft palate revealing the palatal musculature, vessels and glands. Observe the palatoglossus and palatopharyngeus muscles along with the greater and lesser palatine nerves and vessels. A branch of the lesser palatine artery contributes to the tonsillar blood supply.

### Fig. 645: The Lips Viewed from Within the Oral Cavity

NOTE: 1) this dissection demonstrates the muscles of the mouth from within the oral cavity after the oral mucous membrane has been removed. Observe the numerous small labial glands.

2) the contour of the lips as they surround the oral orifice depends on the arrangement of the muscular bundles which interlace at the labial margins. These include the elevators and depressors of the lips and their angles, along with the orbicularis oris and buccinator muscles.

3) the fibers of the buccinator muscle converging at the angle of the mouth. Many of these fibers decussate, becoming continuous with the fibers of the orbicularis oris muscle of both the upper and lower lips.

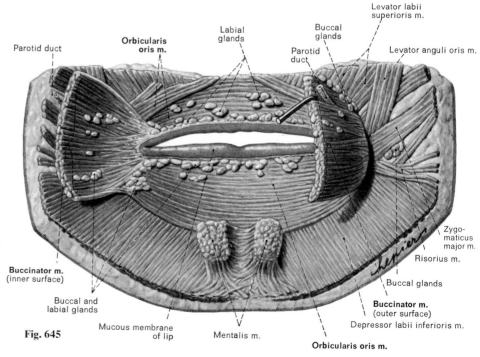

Parotid duct

**Orbicularis
oris m.**

Labial
glands

Buccal
glands

Parotid
duct

Levator labii
superioris m.

Levator anguli oris m.

Zygo-
maticus
major m.

Risorius m.

Buccal glands

**Buccinator m.**
(outer surface)

Depressor labii inferioris m.

**Orbicularis oris m.**

Mentalis m.

Mucous membrane
of lip

Buccal and
labial glands

**Buccinator m.**
(inner surface)

**Fig. 645**

Figs. 644, 645

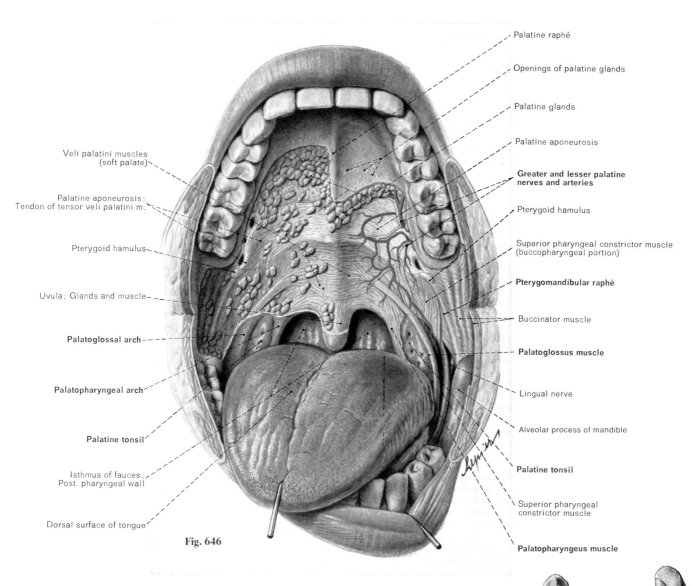

Veli palatini muscles (soft palate)

Palatine aponeurosis; Tendon of tensor veli palatini m.

Pterygoid hamulus

Uvula; Glands and muscle

**Palatoglossal arch**

**Palatopharyngeal arch**

**Palatine tonsil**

Isthmus of fauces; Post. pharyngeal wall

Dorsal surface of tongue

Palatine raphé

Openings of palatine glands

Palatine glands

Palatine aponeurosis

**Greater and lesser palatine nerves and arteries**

Pterygoid hamulus

Superior pharyngeal constrictor muscle (buccopharyngeal portion)

**Pterygomandibular raphé**

Buccinator muscle

**Palatoglossus muscle**

Lingual nerve

Alveolar process of mandible

**Palatine tonsil**

Superior pharyngeal constrictor muscle

**Palatopharyngeus muscle**

**Fig. 646**

## Fig. 647: The Submandibular and Sublingual Glands

NOTE: 1) with the tongue removed, and the genioglossus and geniohyoid muscles cut anteriorly, the submandibular and sublingual glands have been exposed and their relationship to the inner aspect of the right mandible demonstrated.

2) the submandibular duct which measures about 2 inches in length and which courses anteriorly between the sublingual gland and the genioglossus muscle (which is cut). This duct opens into the floor of the mouth on each side of the frenulum of the tongue (sublingual caruncle).

3) the sublingual gland lies along the lingual surface of the body of the mandible and its 10 to 20 small ducts open along the sublingual fold. The most anterior duct frequently joins the submandibular duct at its orifice.

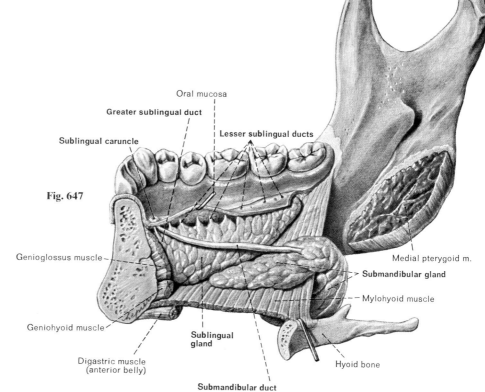

Oral mucosa

**Greater sublingual duct**

**Sublingual caruncle**

**Lesser sublingual ducts**

**Fig. 647**

Genioglossus muscle

Geniohyoid muscle

Digastric muscle (anterior belly)

**Sublingual gland**

Medial pterygoid m.

**Submandibular gland**

Mylohyoid muscle

Hyoid bone

**Submandibular duct**

Figs. 646, 647   VII

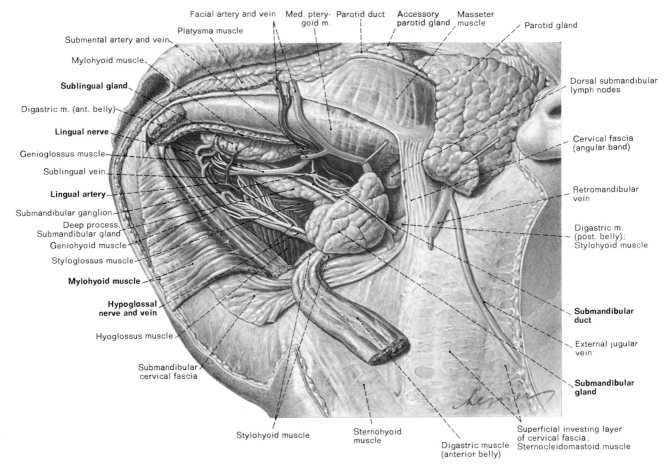

Submental artery and vein

Facial artery and vein

Platysma muscle

Med. ptery-goid m.

Parotid duct

Accessory parotid gland

Masseter muscle

Parotid gland

Mylohyoid muscle

**Sublingual gland**

Digastric m. (ant. belly)

**Lingual nerve**

Genioglossus muscle

Sublingual vein

**Lingual artery**

Submandibular ganglion

Deep process, Submandibular gland

Geniohyoid muscle

Styloglossus muscle

**Mylohyoid muscle**

**Hypoglossal nerve and vein**

Hyoglossus muscle

Submandibular cervical fascia

Dorsal submandibular lymph nodes

Cervical fascia (angular band)

Retromandibular vein

Digastric m. (post. belly); Stylohyoid muscle

**Submandibular duct**

External jugular vein

**Submandibular gland**

Stylohyoid muscle

Sternohyoid muscle

Digastric muscle (anterior belly)

Superficial investing layer of cervical fascia; Sternocleidomastoid muscle

### Fig. 648: The Floor of the Oral Cavity Opened from the Submandibular Triangle, Viewed from Below

NOTE: 1) the anterior belly of the digastric muscle and the mylohyoid muscle have been reflected in order to reveal the following structures: the sublingual gland, the lingual nerve, the submandibular ganglion and duct, the hypoglossal nerve and vein and the lingual artery.

2) presynaptic parasympathetic fibers (VII) accompany the lingual nerve (V) to reach the submandibular ganglion, where they synapse with postganglionic neurons whose fibers innervate both the submandibular and sublingual glands.

3) the hypoglossal (XII) nerve is the motor nerve to all tongue muscles, except the palatoglossus, while the lingual nerve (V) supplies the anterior 2/3rds of the tongue with general sensation.

### Fig. 649: The Mylohyoid and Geniohyoid Muscles (Viewed from Above)

NOTE that the mylohyoid muscles along with the geniohyoid muscles form the muscular floor of the oral cavity. The mylohyoids arise along the mylohyoid lines of the mandible and insert into the median fibrous raphé which extends from the hyoid bone to the symphysis menti. Observe that the genioglossal muscles have been severed near their origin.

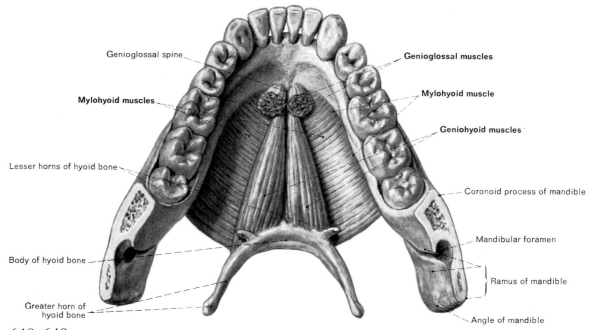

Genioglossal spine

**Genioglossal muscles**

**Mylohyoid muscles**

**Mylohyoid muscle**

**Geniohyoid muscles**

Lesser horns of hyoid bone

Coronoid process of mandible

Mandibular foramen

Body of hyoid bone

Ramus of mandible

Greater horn of hyoid bone

Angle of mandible

Figs. 648, 649

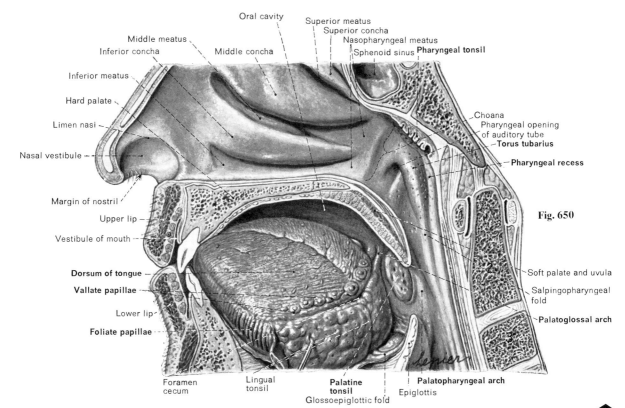

Oral cavity
Middle meatus
Inferior concha
Middle concha
Inferior meatus
Hard palate
Limen nasi
Nasal vestibule
Margin of nostril
Upper lip
Vestibule of mouth
**Dorsum of tongue**
**Vallate papillae**
Lower lip
**Foliate papillae**
Foramen cecum
Lingual tonsil
Superior meatus
Superior concha
Nasopharyngeal meatus
Sphenoid sinus **Pharyngeal tonsil**
Choana
Pharyngeal opening of auditory tube
**Torus tubarius**
**Pharyngeal recess**
**Fig. 650**
Soft palate and uvula
Salpingopharyngeal fold
**Palatoglossal arch**
**Palatine tonsil**
Glossoepiglottic fold
**Palatopharyngeal arch**
Epiglottis

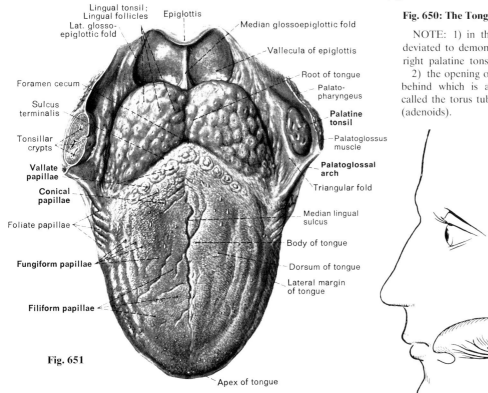

Lingual tonsil; Lingual follicles
Lat. glosso-epiglottic fold
Epiglottis
Median glossoepiglottic fold
Vallecula of epiglottis
Foramen cecum
Sulcus terminalis
Tonsillar crypts
**Vallate papillae**
**Conical papillae**
Foliate papillae
**Fungiform papillae**
**Filiform papillae**
Root of tongue
Palato-pharyngeus
**Palatine tonsil**
Palatoglossus muscle
**Palatoglossal arch**
Triangular fold
Median lingual sulcus
Body of tongue
Dorsum of tongue
Lateral margin of tongue
**Fig. 651**
Apex of tongue

## Fig. 650: The Tongue, Palatine Tonsil and the Oropharynx

NOTE: 1) in this sagittal view, the tongue has been deviated to demonstrate the right palatoglossal arch and right palatine tonsil. Observe the large vallate papillae.

2) the opening of the auditory tube in the nasopharynx behind which is a cartilaginous elevation of the tube called the torus tubarius. Note also the pharyngeal tonsil (adenoids).

Geniculate ganglion
Chorda tympani n.
Nucleus of tractus solitarius
Lingual n.
Glossopharyngeal n.
**Fig. 652**

## Fig. 651: Dorsal Surface of the Tongue

NOTE:1) the dorsum of the tongue is marked by numerous elevations called papillae. These serve as receptor sites for the special sense of taste. Observe the inverted V-shaped group of large vallate papillae.

2) the fungiform papillae which are found principally at the sides and apex of the tongue. These are relatively large and round and have a deep red color.

3) the filiform (conical) papillae. These are very small and generally arranged in rows which course parallel to the vallate papillae.

## Fig. 652: The Principal Pathways for Taste

NOTE: 1) that the two principal pathways for taste are by means of the chorda tympani nerve for the anterior two-thirds of the tongue and the glossopharyngeal nerve for the posterior one-third of the tongue;

2) that two lesser pathways also exist (not shown in this figure). From the epiglottis, taste fibers enter the brain by way of the internal laryngeal branch of the vagus, and taste fibers from the palate course through the palatine nerves and nerve of the pterygoid canal to the greater petrosal nerve and nervus intermedius of the facial nerve.

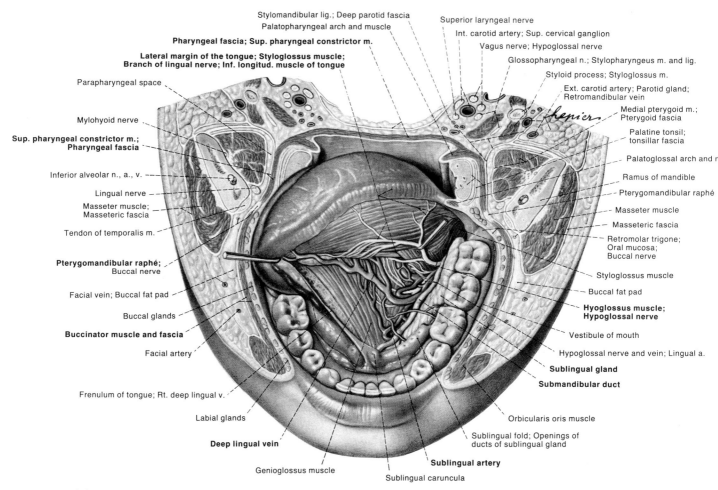

**Fig. 653: Vessels and Nerves in the Floor of the Oral Cavity, Viewed from Above and Anteriorly**

NOTE that the tongue has been deflected to the (specimen's) right, and the left lingual nerve and vessels and the hypoglossal nerve, sublingual gland and submandibular duct exposed in the floor of the oral cavity. Observe also that the lateral walls of the oral cavity and the oropharynx have been cut in cross section, showing the muscles of mastication laterally, the buccinator muscles medially and the superior pharyngeal constrictor posteriorly.

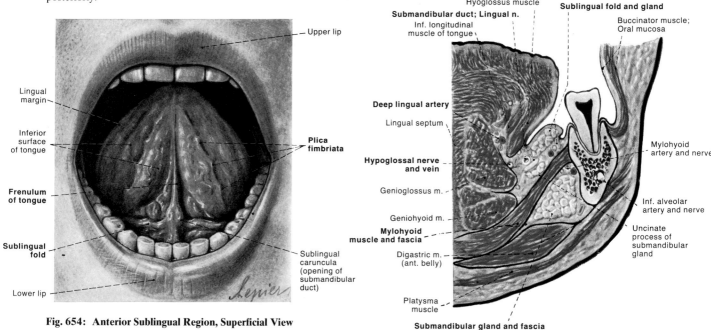

**Fig. 654: Anterior Sublingual Region, Superficial View**

NOTE that the mucous membrane covering the floor of the oral cavity continues over the inferior surface of the tongue, meeting at the midline as an elevated fold called the frenulum of the tongue. Observe the sublingual folds. Along these open the ducts of the sublingual glands, and at their anterior end on each side is an orifice for the submandibular duct called the sublingual caruncula.

**Fig. 655: Frontal Section Through the Tongue, Sublingual and Submandibular Regions**

NOTE the locations of the lingual nerve, submandibular duct and hypoglossal nerve and its accompanying vein. Observe that the mylohyoid muscle separates the sublingual and submandibular regions.

Figs. 653, 654, 655

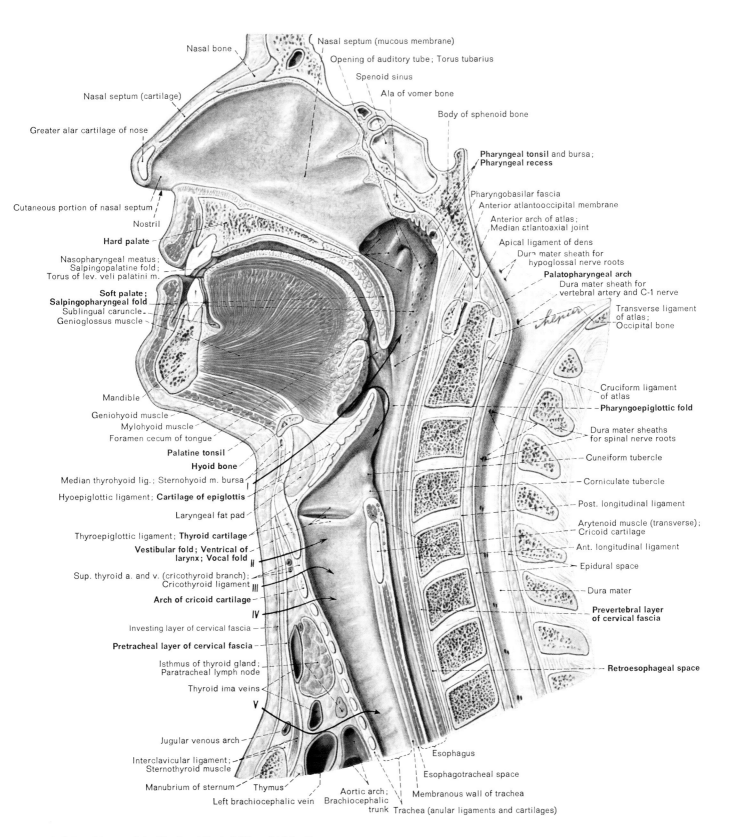

Nasal bone
Nasal septum (mucous membrane)
Opening of auditory tube; Torus tubarius
Spenoid sinus
Ala of vomer bone
Body of sphenoid bone
Nasal septum (cartilage)
Greater alar cartilage of nose

Pharyngeal tonsil and bursa;
Pharyngeal recess

Cutaneous portion of nasal septum
Nostril
Hard palate
Nasopharyngeal meatus;
Salpingopalatine fold;
Torus of lev. veli palatini m.
Soft palate;
Salpingopharyngeal fold
Sublingual caruncle
Genioglossus muscle

Pharyngobasilar fascia
Anterior atlantooccipital membrane
Anterior arch of atlas;
Median atlantoaxial joint
Apical ligament of dens
Dura mater sheath for
hypoglossal nerve roots
Palatopharyngeal arch
Dura mater sheath for
vertebral artery and C-1 nerve
Transverse ligament
of atlas;
Occipital bone

Mandible
Geniohyoid muscle
Mylohyoid muscle
Foramen cecum of tongue
Palatine tonsil
Hyoid bone
Median thyrohyoid lig.; Sternohyoid m. bursa
Hyoepiglottic ligament; Cartilage of epiglottis
Laryngeal fat pad
Thyroepiglottic ligament; Thyroid cartilage
Vestibular fold; Ventrical of
larynx; Vocal fold
Sup. thyroid a. and v. (cricothyroid branch);
Cricothyroid ligament
Arch of cricoid cartilage

Cruciform ligament
of atlas
Pharyngoepiglottic fold
Dura mater sheaths
for spinal nerve roots
Cuneiform tubercle
Corniculate tubercle
Post. longitudinal ligament
Arytenoid muscle (transverse);
Cricoid cartilage
Ant. longitudinal ligament
Epidural space
Dura mater
Prevertebral layer
of cervical fascia

Investing layer of cervical fascia
Pretracheal layer of cervical fascia
Isthmus of thyroid gland;
Paratracheal lymph node
Thyroid ima veins

Retroesophageal space

Jugular venous arch
Interclavicular ligament;
Sternothyroid muscle
Manubrium of sternum    Thymus
Left brachiocephalic vein
Aortic arch;
Brachiocephalic
trunk
Esophagus
Esophagotracheal space
Membranous wall of trachea
Trachea (anular ligaments and cartilages)

**Fig. 656: The Viscera of the Head and Neck: Mid-sagittal Section**

NOTE: 1) the closed oral cavity is occupied principally by the tongue. Observe that the posterior aspect of the oral cavity opens into the oropharanyx. Superiorly, the posterior nasal cavities are continuous with the nasopharynx, whereas inferiorly the laryngeal portion of the pharynx (between the levels of the epiglottis and cricoid cartilages) opens into the larynx.

2) the pharynx continues inferiorly as the esophagus, while the larynx becomes the trachea below the level of the cricoid cartilage.

3) during the act of swallowing (deglutition), as food is directed toward the posterior part of the oral cavity, the soft palate is both elevated and tensed (by the levator and tensor veli palatini muscles) and directed toward the posterior wall of the pharynx, thereby closing off the nasopharynx. Simultaneously the larynx is drawn superiorly toward the epiglottis to the level of the hyoid bone, and the pharynx also ascends. This action closes the laryngeal orifice, thereby preventing food from entering the larynx.

4) arrows I to V: surgical approaches to pharynx, larynx and trachea.

Fig. 656    VII

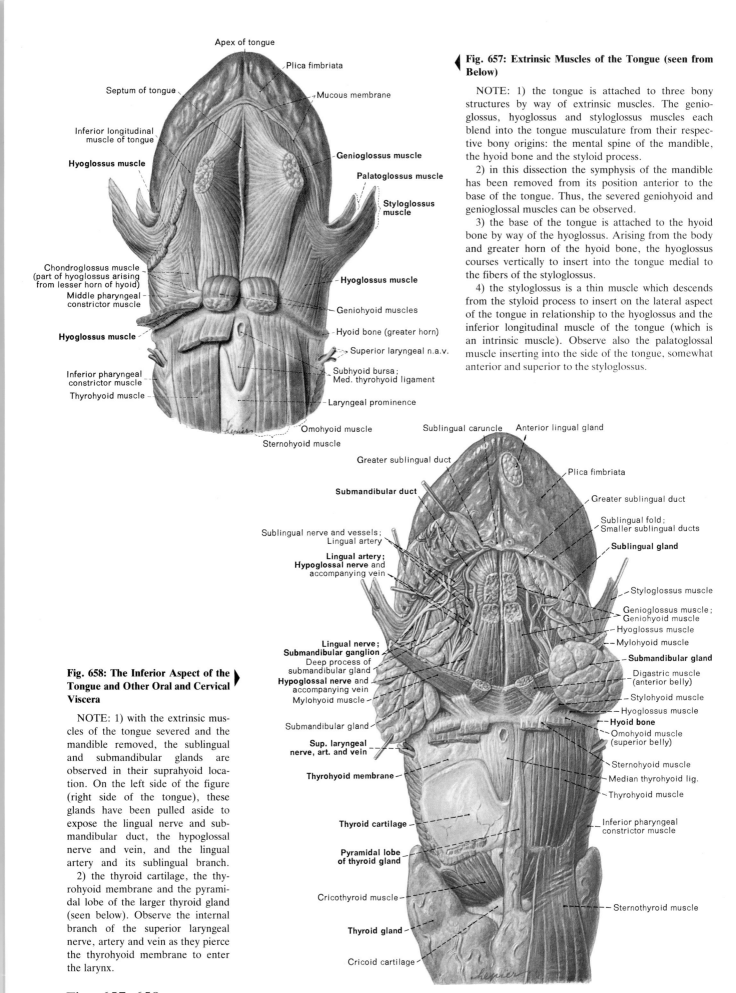

Apex of tongue

Plica fimbriata

Septum of tongue

Mucous membrane

Inferior longitudinal
muscle of tongue

**Genioglossus muscle**

**Hyoglossus muscle**

**Palatoglossus muscle**

**Styloglossus
muscle**

Chondroglossus muscle
(part of hyoglossus arising
from lesser horn of hyoid)

Middle pharyngeal
constrictor muscle

**Hyoglossus muscle**

**Hyoglossus muscle**

Geniohyoid muscles

Hyoid bone (greater horn)

Superior laryngeal n.a.v.

Inferior pharyngeal
constrictor muscle

Thyrohyoid muscle

Subhyoid bursa;
Med. thyrohyoid ligament

Laryngeal prominence

Omohyoid muscle

Sternohyoid muscle

## Fig. 657: Extrinsic Muscles of the Tongue (seen from Below)

NOTE: 1) the tongue is attached to three bony structures by way of extrinsic muscles. The genioglossus, hyoglossus and styloglossus muscles each blend into the tongue musculature from their respective bony origins: the mental spine of the mandible, the hyoid bone and the styloid process.

2) in this dissection the symphysis of the mandible has been removed from its position anterior to the base of the tongue. Thus, the severed geniohyoid and genioglossal muscles can be observed.

3) the base of the tongue is attached to the hyoid bone by way of the hyoglossus. Arising from the body and greater horn of the hyoid bone, the hyoglossus courses vertically to insert into the tongue medial to the fibers of the styloglossus.

4) the styloglossus is a thin muscle which descends from the styloid process to insert on the lateral aspect of the tongue in relationship to the hyoglossus and the inferior longitudinal muscle of the tongue (which is an intrinsic muscle). Observe also the palatoglossal muscle inserting into the side of the tongue, somewhat anterior and superior to the styloglossus.

Sublingual caruncle

Anterior lingual gland

Greater sublingual duct

Plica fimbriata

**Submandibular duct**

Greater sublingual duct

Sublingual fold;
Smaller sublingual ducts

Sublingual nerve and vessels;
Lingual artery

**Sublingual gland**

**Lingual artery;
Hypoglossal nerve and**
accompanying vein

Styloglossus muscle

Genioglossus muscle;
Geniohyoid muscle

Hyoglossus muscle

Mylohyoid muscle

**Lingual nerve;
Submandibular ganglion**
Deep process of
submandibular gland

**Submandibular gland**

Digastric muscle
(anterior belly)

**Hypoglossal nerve and**
accompanying vein

Mylohyoid muscle

Stylohyoid muscle

Hyoglossus muscle

Submandibular gland

**Hyoid bone**

Omohyoid muscle
(superior belly)

**Sup. laryngeal
nerve, art. and vein**

Sternohyoid muscle

Median thyrohyoid lig.

**Thyrohyoid membrane**

Thyrohyoid muscle

Inferior pharyngeal
constrictor muscle

**Thyroid cartilage**

**Pyramidal lobe
of thyroid gland**

Cricothyroid muscle

Sternothyroid muscle

**Thyroid gland**

Cricoid cartilage

## Fig. 658: The Inferior Aspect of the Tongue and Other Oral and Cervical Viscera

NOTE: 1) with the extrinsic muscles of the tongue severed and the mandible removed, the sublingual and submandibular glands are observed in their suprahyoid location. On the left side of the figure (right side of the tongue), these glands have been pulled aside to expose the lingual nerve and submandibular duct, the hypoglossal nerve and vein, and the lingual artery and its sublingual branch.

2) the thyroid cartilage, the thyrohyoid membrane and the pyramidal lobe of the larger thyroid gland (seen below). Observe the internal branch of the superior laryngeal nerve, artery and vein as they pierce the thyrohyoid membrane to enter the larynx.

Figs. 657, 658

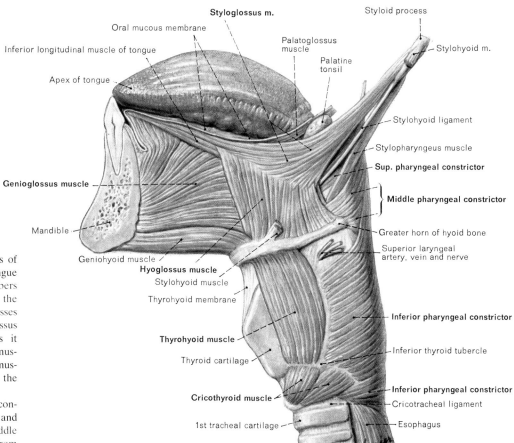

Styloglossus m.

Oral mucous membrane

Inferior longitudinal muscle of tongue

Apex of tongue

Palatoglossus muscle

Palatine tonsil

Styloid process

Stylohyoid m.

Stylohyoid ligament

Stylopharyngeus muscle

**Sup. pharyngeal constrictor**

**Middle pharyngeal constrictor**

Greater horn of hyoid bone

Superior laryngeal artery, vein and nerve

**Genioglossus muscle**

Mandible

Geniohyoid muscle

**Hyoglossus muscle**

Stylohyoid muscle

Thyrohyoid membrane

**Thyrohyoid muscle**

Thyroid cartilage

**Cricothyroid muscle**

1st tracheal cartilage

Trachea

**Inferior pharyngeal constrictor**

Inferior thyroid tubercle

**Inferior pharyngeal constrictor**

Cricotracheal ligament

Esophagus

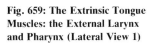

## Fig. 659: The Extrinsic Tongue Muscles: the External Larynx and Pharynx (Lateral View 1)

NOTE: 1) the posterior fibers of the genioglossus draw the tongue forward, while its anterior fibers retract the tongue back into the mouth. The hyoglossus depresses the tongue, while the styloglossus elevates the tongue and pulls it backward. All three of these muscles and the intrinsic tongue muscles as well are innervated by the hypoglossal nerve.

2) the inferior pharyngeal constrictor arises from the cricoid and thyroid cartilages, while the middle pharyngeal constrictor arises from the entire length of the greater horn of the hyoid bone, from the stylohyoid ligament and from the lesser horn (seen in Fig. 660).

3) the thyrohyoid muscle covering the lateral surface of the thyroid cartilage and the two parts of the cricothyroid muscle.

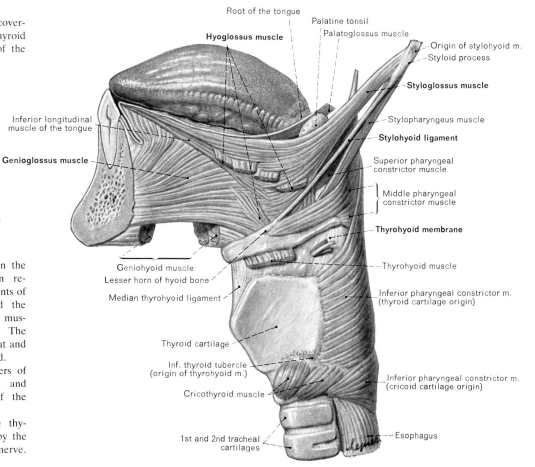

Root of the tongue

Palatine tonsil

Palatoglossus muscle

**Hyoglossus muscle**

Origin of stylohyoid m.

Styloid process

**Styloglossus muscle**

Stylopharyngeus muscle

**Stylohyoid ligament**

Inferior longitudinal muscle of the tongue

**Genioglossus muscle**

Superior pharyngeal constrictor muscle

Middle pharyngeal constrictor muscle

**Thyrohyoid membrane**

Thyrohyoid muscle

Geniohyoid muscle

Lesser horn of hyoid bone

Median thyrohyoid ligament

Thyroid cartilage

Inf. thyroid tubercle (origin of thyrohyoid m.)

Cricothyroid muscle

1st and 2nd tracheal cartilages

Inferior pharyngeal constrictor m. (thyroid cartilage origin)

Inferior pharyngeal constrictor m. (cricoid cartilage origin)

Esophagus

## Fig. 660: The Extrinsic Tongue Muscles: the External Larynx and Pharynx (Lateral View 2)

NOTE: 1) in this dissection the hyoglossus muscle has been removed, revealing the attachments of the stylohyoid ligament and the middle pharyngeal constrictor muscle along the hyoid bone. The geniohyoid muscle has been cut and the thyrohyoid muscle removed.

2) the blending of the fibers of the styloglossus, hyoglossus and genioglossus at the base of the tongue.

3) the penetration of the thyrohyoid membrane laterally by the internal laryngeal vessels and nerve.

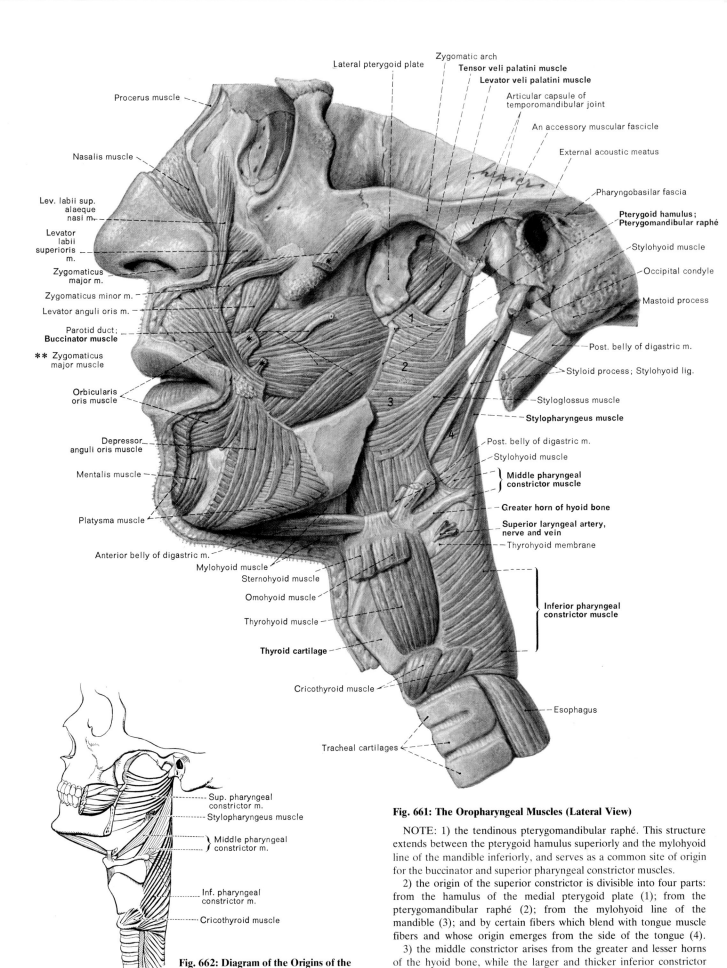

**Procerus muscle**

**Nasalis muscle**

**Lev. labii sup. alaeque nasi m.**

**Levator labii superioris m.**

**Zygomaticus major m.**

**Zygomaticus minor m.**

**Levator anguli oris m.**

**Parotid duct; Buccinator muscle**

**\*\* Zygomaticus major muscle**

**Orbicularis oris muscle**

**Depressor anguli oris muscle**

**Mentalis muscle**

**Platysma muscle**

**Anterior belly of digastric m.**

**Mylohyoid muscle**

**Sternohyoid muscle**

**Omohyoid muscle**

**Thyrohyoid muscle**

**Thyroid cartilage**

**Cricothyroid muscle**

**Tracheal cartilages**

**Lateral pterygoid plate**

**Zygomatic arch**

**Tensor veli palatini muscle**

**Levator veli palatini muscle**

**Articular capsule of temporomandibular joint**

**An accessory muscular fascicle**

**External acoustic meatus**

**Pharyngobasilar fascia**

**Pterygoid hamulus; Pterygomandibular raphé**

**Stylohyoid muscle**

**Occipital condyle**

**Mastoid process**

**Post. belly of digastric m.**

**Styloid process; Stylohyoid lig.**

**Styloglossus muscle**

**Stylopharyngeus muscle**

**Post. belly of digastric m.**

**Stylohyoid muscle**

**Middle pharyngeal constrictor muscle**

**Greater horn of hyoid bone**

**Superior laryngeal artery, nerve and vein**

**Thyrohyoid membrane**

**Inferior pharyngeal constrictor muscle**

**Esophagus**

1  2  3  4

### Fig. 661: The Oropharyngeal Muscles (Lateral View)

NOTE: 1) the tendinous pterygomandibular raphé. This structure extends between the pterygoid hamulus superiorly and the mylohyoid line of the mandible inferiorly, and serves as a common site of origin for the buccinator and superior pharyngeal constrictor muscles.

2) the origin of the superior constrictor is divisible into four parts: from the hamulus of the medial pterygoid plate (1); from the pterygomandibular raphé (2); from the mylohyoid line of the mandible (3); and by certain fibers which blend with tongue muscle fibers and whose origin emerges from the side of the tongue (4).

3) the middle constrictor arises from the greater and lesser horns of the hyoid bone, while the larger and thicker inferior constrictor arises from the thyroid and cricoid cartilages.

**Sup. pharyngeal constrictor m.**

**Stylopharyngeus muscle**

**Middle pharyngeal constrictor m.**

**Inf. pharyngeal constrictor m.**

**Cricothyroid muscle**

### Fig. 662: Diagram of the Origins of the Pharyngeal Constrictor Muscles

Figs. 661, 662

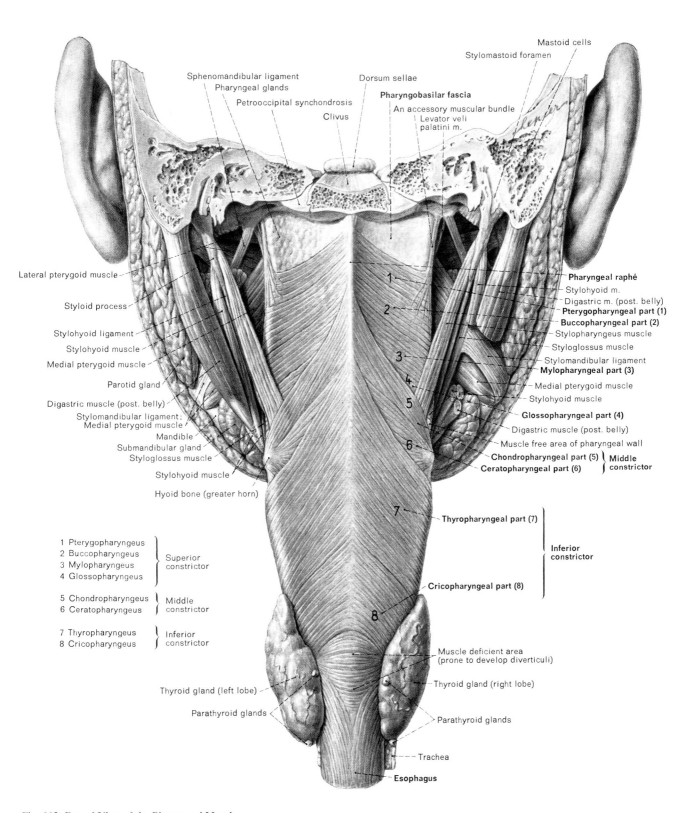

**Fig. 663: Dorsal View of the Pharyngeal Muscles**

NOTE: 1) this posterior view of the pharynx was achieved by making a frontal transection through the petrous and mastoid portions of the temporal bones and through the body of the occipital bone. The styloid processes and their muscular attachments have been left intact.

2) the arrangement of the divisions of the pharyngeal constrictors. Their muscle fibers arise laterally to insert in a posterior median pharyngeal raphé. The superior constrictor is divisible into four parts while the middle and inferior constrictor are each divisible into two. Above the superior constrictor, observe the fibrous pharyngobasilar fascia which attaches to the basal portion of the occipital bone and to the temporal bones. Below the inferior constrictor, the pharynx is continuous with the muscular esophagus.

3) the *superior* and *middle constrictor* muscles and the *thyropharyngeal part of the inferior constrictor* are innervated by the pharyngeal branch of the vagus nerve. These fibers have their cell bodies in the nucleus ambiguus in the brain stem, emerge from the brain with the rootlets of the bulbar part of the accessory nerve and then, by a communicating branch, join the vagus. The cricopharyngeal part of the inferior constrictor is supplied by the recurrent laryngeal branch of the vagus nerve.

Fig. 663     VII

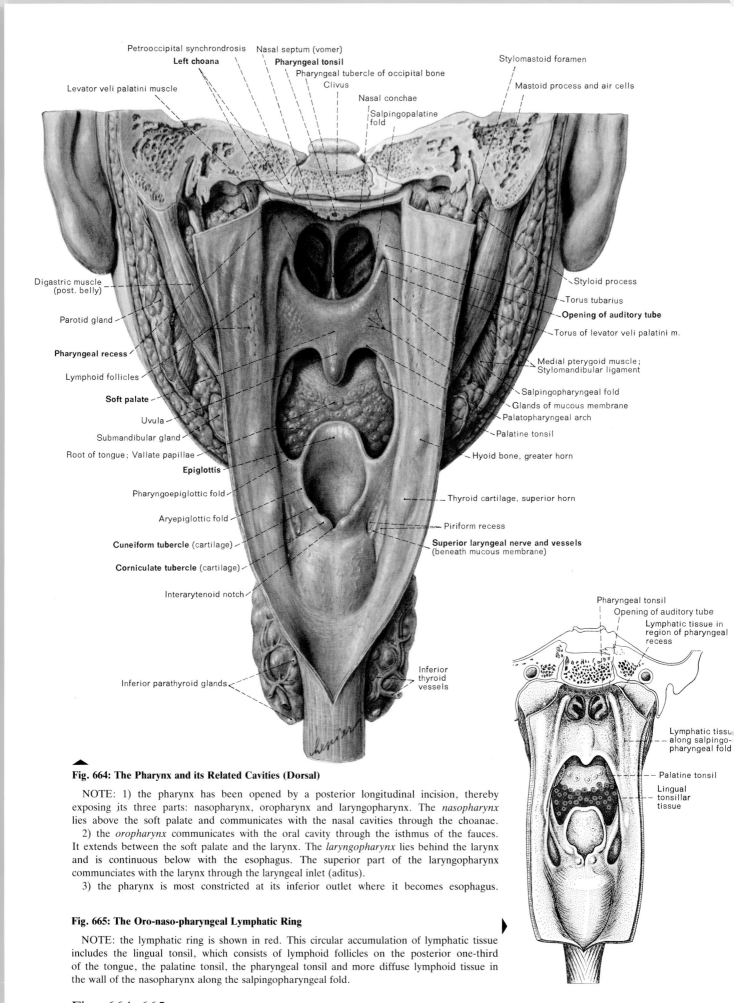

Petrooccipital synchrondrosis
Left choana
Nasal septum (vomer)
**Pharyngeal tonsil**
Pharyngeal tubercle of occipital bone
Clivus
Stylomastoid foramen
Levator veli palatini muscle
Nasal conchae
Salpingopalatine fold
Mastoid process and air cells

Digastric muscle (post. belly)
Parotid gland
**Pharyngeal recess**
Lymphoid follicles
**Soft palate**
Uvula
Submandibular gland
Root of tongue; Vallate papillae
**Epiglottis**
Pharyngoepiglottic fold
Aryepiglottic fold
**Cuneiform tubercle** (cartilage)
**Corniculate tubercle** (cartilage)
Interarytenoid notch
Inferior parathyroid glands

Styloid process
Torus tubarius
**Opening of auditory tube**
Torus of levator veli palatini m.
Medial pterygoid muscle; Stylomandibular ligament
Salpingopharyngeal fold
Glands of mucous membrane
Palatopharyngeal arch
Palatine tonsil
Hyoid bone, greater horn
Thyroid cartilage, superior horn
Piriform recess
**Superior laryngeal nerve and vessels** (beneath mucous membrane)
Inferior thyroid vessels

Pharyngeal tonsil
Opening of auditory tube
Lymphatic tissue in region of pharyngeal recess
Lymphatic tissue along salpingo-pharyngeal fold
Palatine tonsil
Lingual tonsillar tissue

**Fig. 664: The Pharynx and its Related Cavities (Dorsal)**

NOTE: 1) the pharynx has been opened by a posterior longitudinal incision, thereby exposing its three parts: nasopharynx, oropharynx and laryngopharynx. The *nasopharynx* lies above the soft palate and communicates with the nasal cavities through the choanae.

2) the *oropharynx* communicates with the oral cavity through the isthmus of the fauces. It extends between the soft palate and the larynx. The *laryngopharynx* lies behind the larynx and is continuous below with the esophagus. The superior part of the laryngopharynx communicates with the larynx through the laryngeal inlet (aditus).

3) the pharynx is most constricted at its inferior outlet where it becomes esophagus.

**Fig. 665: The Oro-naso-pharyngeal Lymphatic Ring**

NOTE: the lymphatic ring is shown in red. This circular accumulation of lymphatic tissue includes the lingual tonsil, which consists of lymphoid follicles on the posterior one-third of the tongue, the palatine tonsil, the pharyngeal tonsil and more diffuse lymphoid tissue in the wall of the nasopharynx along the salpingopharyngeal fold.

Figs. 664, 665

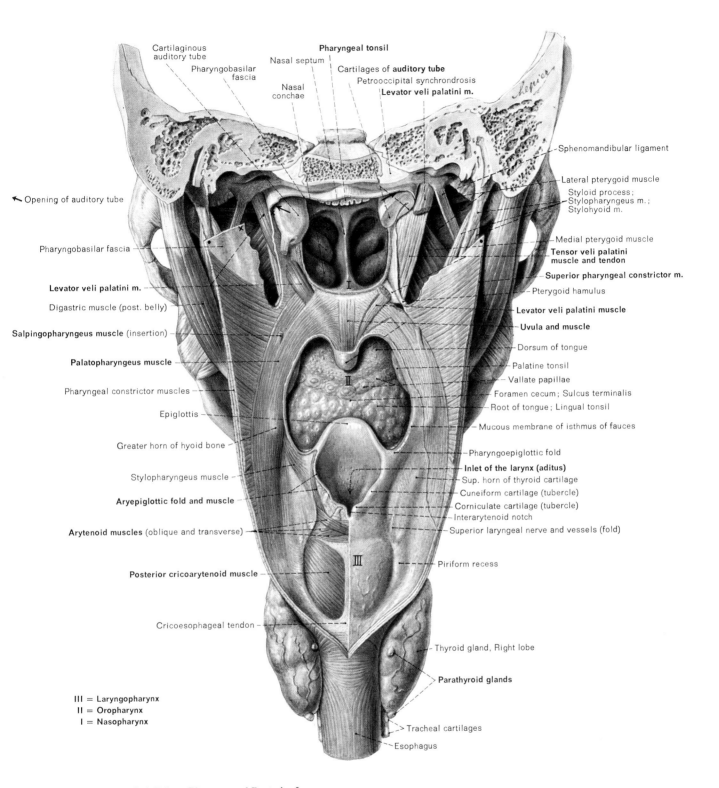

Cartilaginous auditory tube
Pharyngobasilar fascia
Nasal septum
Nasal conchae
**Pharyngeal tonsil**
Cartilages of **auditory tube**
Petrooccipital synchrondrosis
**Levator veli palatini m.**

Opening of auditory tube

Sphenomandibular ligament
Lateral pterygoid muscle
Styloid process;
Stylopharyngeus m.;
Stylohyoid m.

Pharyngobasilar fascia
Medial pterygoid muscle
**Tensor veli palatini muscle and tendon**
**Superior pharyngeal constrictor m.**
Pterygoid hamulus
**Levator veli palatini m.**
Digastric muscle (post. belly)
**Salpingopharyngeus muscle (insertion)**
**Palatopharyngeus muscle**
Pharyngeal constrictor muscles
Epiglottis
Greater horn of hyoid bone
Stylopharyngeus muscle
**Aryepiglottic fold and muscle**
**Arytenoid muscles (oblique and transverse)**
**Posterior cricoarytenoid muscle**
Cricoesophageal tendon

**Levator veli palatini muscle**
**Uvula and muscle**
Dorsum of tongue
Palatine tonsil
Vallate papillae
Foramen cecum; Sulcus terminalis
Root of tongue; Lingual tonsil
Mucous membrane of isthmus of fauces
Pharyngoepiglottic fold
**Inlet of the larynx (aditus)**
Sup. horn of thyroid cartilage
Cuneiform cartilage (tubercle)
Corniculate cartilage (tubercle)
Interarytenoid notch
Superior laryngeal nerve and vessels (fold)
Piriform recess
Thyroid gland, Right lobe
**Parathyroid glands**
Tracheal cartilages
Esophagus

III = Laryngopharynx
II = Oropharynx
I = Nasopharynx

**Fig. 666: Muscles of the Soft Palate, Pharynx, and Posterior Larynx**

NOTE: 1) the dissection in this figure is similar to that in Figure 664. The pharynx has been opened dorsally by a midline incision and the mucous membrane has been removed from the soft palate, pharynx and the left posterior larynx. On the right side, a portion of the levator veli palatini muscle has been removed in order to expose the adjacent belly and tendon of the tensor veli palatini muscle.

2) the muscles of the soft palate. Both the muscle of the uvula and the levator veli palatini muscle are innervated by the vagus and accessory nerve contributions to the pharyngeal plexus, whereas the tensor veli palatini muscle is innervated by the mandibular division of the trigeminal nerve.

3) the palatopharyngeus muscle arising by two fascicles from the soft palate. The muscle fibers of these two fascicles arise posterior and anterior to the insertion of the levator veli palatini muscle. The fascicles descend and merge and then insert into the posterior border of the thyroid cartilage and onto the adjacent pharyngeal wall.

Fig. 666    VII

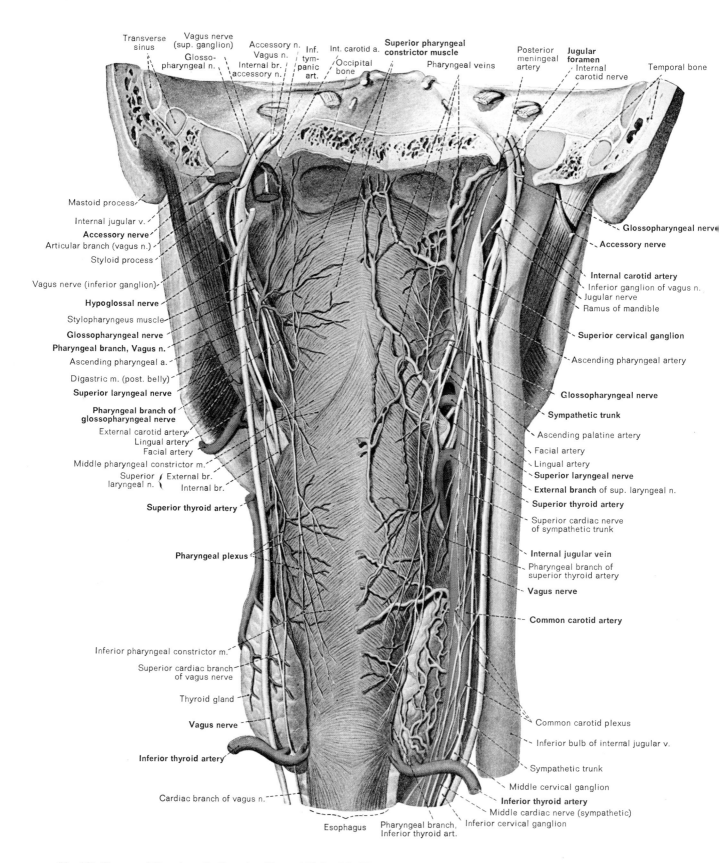

**Fig. 667: Nerves and Vessels on the Dorsal and Lateral Walls of the Pharynx**

NOTE: 1) the head has been split longitudinally. The pharynx, larynx and facial structures were separated from the vertebral column and its associated muscles. This posterior view of the pharynx also shows the large nerves and blood vessels which course through the neck. On the right side, observe the carotid artery, internal jugular vein, vagus nerve and sympathetic trunk.

2) on the left side, the glossopharyngeal and hypoglossal nerves were exposed by the removal of the carotid arteries and internal jugular vein. Along with the jugular vein, the jugular foramen transmits the 9th, 10th and 11th cranial nerves.

3) the thyroid gland and its superior and inferior thyroid arteries. The superior and middle thyroid veins drain into the internal jugular vein, while the inferior thyroid veins (not shown) usually drain into the left brachiocephalic vein.

Fig. 667

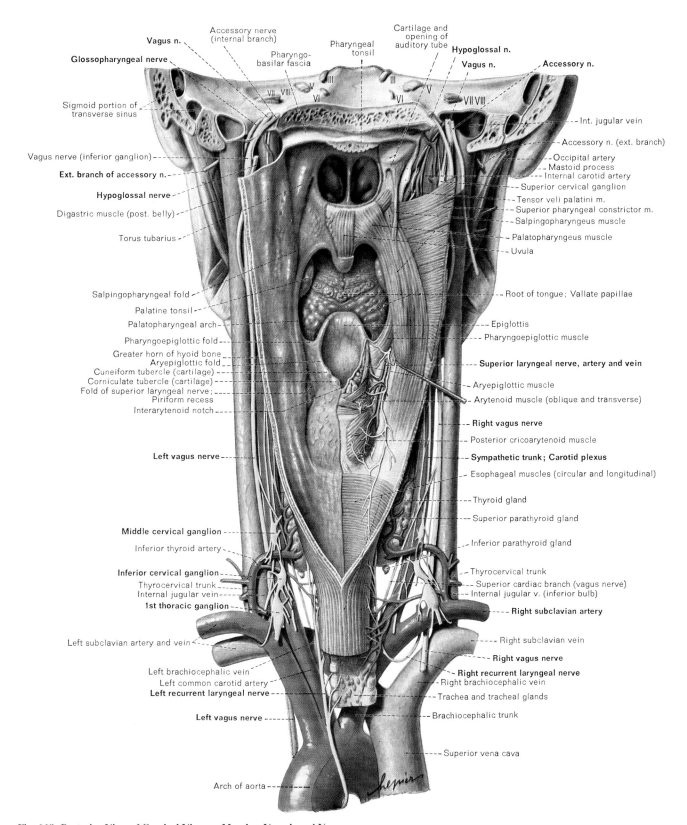

**Fig. 668: Posterior View of Cervical Viscera: Muscles, Vessels and Nerves**

NOTE: 1) in this posterior view of the vessels and nerves of the neck, the dorsal wall of the pharynx has been opened longitudinally, revealing the nasal, oral and laryngeal orifices which communicate with the pharynx. Observe the superior laryngeal artery, vein and nerve entering the larynx from above.

2) the recurrent laryngeal nerves ascending from the thorax to the larynx in the tracheoesophageal groove. On the left side, the recurrent laryngeal nerve courses around the arch of the aorta to reach this groove, while on the right side the recurrent laryngeal nerve curves around the subclavian artery.

3) the inferior cervical ganglion (at the level of 7th cervical vertebra). This ganglion is fused with the 1st thoracic sympathetic ganglion in about 80% of cases. The fused 1st thoracic and inferior cervical ganglion is called the stellate ganglion.

Fig. 668   VII

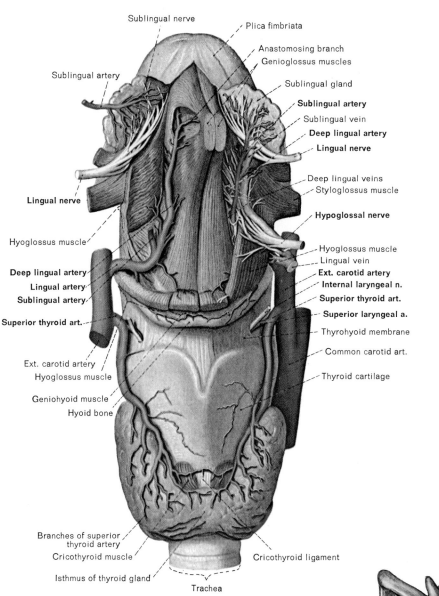

Sublingual nerve
Plica fimbriata
Anastomosing branch
Genioglossus muscles
Sublingual artery
Sublingual gland
Sublingual artery
Sublingual vein
Deep lingual artery
Lingual nerve
Deep lingual veins
Styloglossus muscle
Lingual nerve
Hypoglossal nerve
Hyoglossus muscle
Hyoglossus muscle
Lingual vein
Deep lingual artery
Ext. carotid artery
Lingual artery
Internal laryngeal n.
Sublingual artery
Superior thyroid art.
Superior laryngeal a.
Superior thyroid art.
Thyrohyoid membrane
Common carotid art.
Ext. carotid artery
Hyoglossus muscle
Thyroid cartilage
Geniohyoid muscle
Hyoid bone
Branches of superior thyroid artery
Cricothyroid muscle
Cricothyroid ligament
Isthmus of thyroid gland
Trachea

## Fig. 669: Ventral View of Larynx, Tongue and Thyroid Gland: Vessels and Nerves

NOTE: 1) the superior thyroid arteries descending to the thyroid gland. In their course they give off the superior laryngeal arteries, which penetrate the thyrohyoid membrane to gain entrance to the interior of the larynx, accompanied by the internal laryngeal branch of the superior laryngeal nerve. Observe also the cranial and medial course of the lingual artery deep to the hyoglossus muscle and its suprahyoid, sublingual and deep lingual branches.

2) the lingual nerves as they enter the tongue to supply its anterior two-thirds with general sensation. The motor nerve to the tongue is the hypoglossal, and it is seen coursing along with accompanying veins (venae comitantes). The hypoglossal nerve enters the base of the tongue just above the hyoid bone, passing anteriorly across the external carotid and lingual arteries.

3) that the common carotid artery bifurcates at about the level of the upper border of the thyroid cartilage. Observe also that the lingual artery branches from the external carotid above the hyoid bone, while the superior laryngeal artery arises at the level of the thyrohyoid membrane.

## Fig. 670: The Cartilages and Ligaments of the Larynx (Ventral View)

NOTE: 1) the laryngeal cartilages comprise the skeletal framework of the larynx and they are interconnected by ligaments and membranes. There are *three larger unpaired* cartilages, the cricoid, thyroid and epiglottis and *three sets of paired* cartilages, the arytenoid, cuneiform and corniculate. In this anterior view the unpaired cricoid, thyroid and epiglottis cartilages are all visible.

2) the thyrohyoid membrane and the centrally located thyrohyoid ligament. Attached at the cranial border of the thyroid cartilage, this membrane stretches across the posterior surfaces of the greater horns of the hyoid bone. The medial thyrohyoid ligament extends from the thyroid notch to the body of the hyoid bone. The membrane is pierced by the superior laryngeal vessels and the internal laryngeal nerve.

3) the cricothyroid ligament attaching the contiguous margins of the cricoid and thyroid cartilages. This is a strong ligament and its lateral portions underlie the cricothyroid muscles. Below, the cricotracheal ligament connects the inferior margin of the cricoid cartilage with the first tracheal ring.

Figs. 669, 670

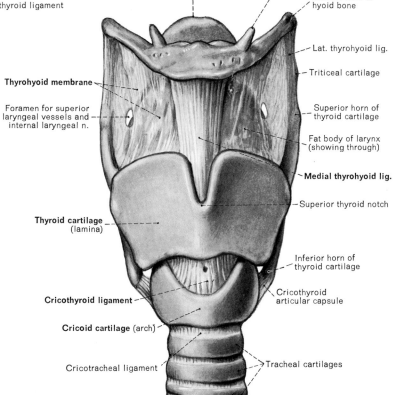

Epiglottis
Lesser horn of hyoid bone
Greater horn of hyoid bone
Lat. thyrohyoid lig.
Thyrohyoid membrane
Triticeal cartilage
Foramen for superior laryngeal vessels and internal laryngeal n.
Superior horn of thyroid cartilage
Fat body of larynx (showing through)
Medial thyrohyoid lig.
Superior thyroid notch
Thyroid cartilage (lamina)
Inferior horn of thyroid cartilage
Cricothyroid articular capsule
Cricothyroid ligament
Cricoid cartilage (arch)
Cricotracheal ligament
Tracheal cartilages

## Fig. 671: Dorsal View of Larynx, Tongue and Thyroid Gland: Vessels and Nerves

NOTE: 1) the glossopharyngeal nerves (IX) as they enter the root or pharyngeal part of the tongue in order to supply the posterior one-third of the surface of the tongue with both general sensation and the special sense of taste. Observe the relationship of the tonsillar branch of the ascending palatine artery with the glossopharyngeal nerve.

2) the courses of the internal branch of the superior laryngeal nerve and the recurrent laryngeal nerve. The internal branch of the superior laryngeal nerve is sensory to the laryngeal mucous membrane as far down as the level of the vocal folds. The recurrent laryngeal nerve is the principal motor nerve of the larynx and supplies all laryngeal muscles except the cricothyroid (which is supplied by the external branch of the superior laryngeal nerve). Additionally, the recurrent nerve supplies sensory innervation to the mucous membrane of the larynx below the level of the vocal folds.

3) the relationships of recurrent laryngeal nerves to the inferior thyroid artery and its inferior laryngeal branches. Observe also the proximity of the recurrent laryngeal nerves to the posterior aspect of the thyroid glands.

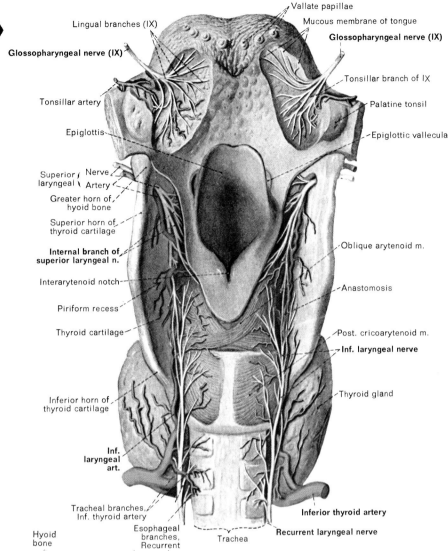

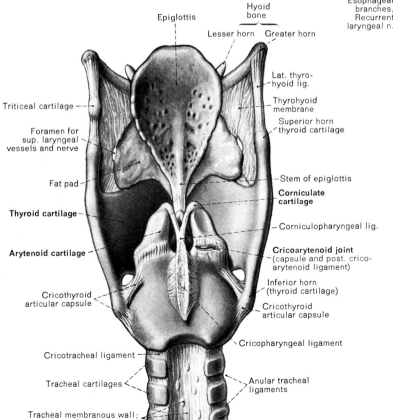

### Fig. 672: The Cartilages and Ligaments of the Larynx

NOTE: 1) the articulation of the paired arytenoid cartilages with the cricoid cartilage below. These synovial cricoarytenoid joints are surrounded by articular capsules and strengthened by the posterior cricoarytenoid ligaments.

2) the cricoarytenoid joints allow for a) *rotation of the arytenoid cartilage* on an axis which is nearly vertical and b) *the horizontal gliding movement* of the arytenoid cartilages.

3) rotation of the arytenoid cartilages results in medial or lateral displacement of the vocal folds, thereby increasing or decreasing the size of the opening between the folds, the rima glottidis. The horizontal gliding action of the arytenoid cartilages permits the bases of these cartilages to be approximated or moved apart. Medial rotation and medial gliding of the arytenoid cartilages occur simultaneously as do the two lateral movements.

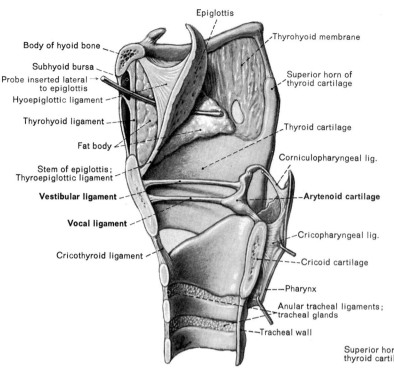

Epiglottis

Thyrohyoid membrane

Body of hyoid bone

Subhyoid bursa

Probe inserted lateral → to epiglottis

Superior horn of thyroid cartilage

Hyoepiglottic ligament

Thyrohyoid ligament

Fat body

Thyroid cartilage

Stem of epiglottis; Thyroepiglottic ligament

Corniculopharyngeal lig.

**Vestibular ligament**

**Arytenoid cartilage**

**Vocal ligament**

Cricopharyngeal lig.

Cricothyroid ligament

Cricoid cartilage

Pharynx

Anular tracheal ligaments; tracheal glands

Tracheal wall

## Fig. 673: The Right Half of the Larynx Showing the Cartilages and the Vestibular and Vocal Ligaments

NOTE: 1) the vestibular ligament is a compact band of fibrous tissue attached anteriorly to the thyroid cartilage and posteriorly to the anterior and lateral surface of the arytenoid cartilage. It is enclosed by mucous membrane to form the vestibular fold (or false vocal fold).

2) the vocal ligament consists of elastic tissue which is attached anteriorly to the thyroid cartilage and posteriorly to the vocal process of the arytenoid cartilage. It, too, is surrounded by mucous membrane which, along with the vocalis muscle, forms the vocal fold. Laryngeal sound waves are produced by oscillations of the vocal folds initiated by puffs of air.

## Fig. 674: The Vocal Ligaments and Conus Elasticus from Above

NOTE that the conus elasticus is a membrane consisting principally of yellow elastic fibers which interconnects the thyroid, cricoid and arytenoid cartilages. It underlies the mucous membrane below the vocal folds and is overlain to some extent by the circothyroid muscle on the exterior of the larynx. Observe the symmetry of the arytenoid cartilages and their related vocal ligaments.

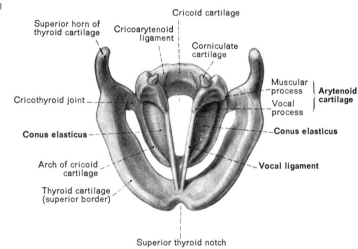

Cricoid cartilage

Superior horn of thyroid cartilage

Cricoarytenoid ligament

Corniculate cartilage

Muscular process

Vocal process

Arytenoid cartilage

Cricothyroid joint

**Conus elasticus**

**Conus elasticus**

Arch of cricoid cartilage

**Vocal ligament**

Thyroid cartilage (superior border)

Superior thyroid notch

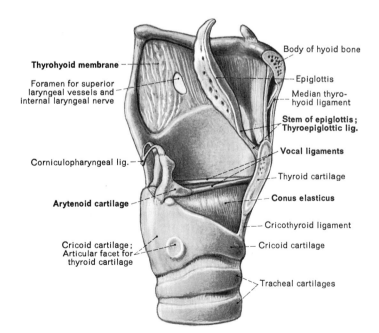

**Thyrohyoid membrane**

Body of hyoid bone

Foramen for superior laryngeal vessels and internal laryngeal nerve

Epiglottis

Median thyro-hyoid ligament

**Stem of epiglottis; Thyroepiglottic lig.**

**Vocal ligaments**

Corniculopharyngeal lig.

Thyroid cartilage

**Conus elasticus**

**Arytenoid cartilage**

Cricothyroid ligament

Cricoid cartilage; Articular facet for thyroid cartilage

Cricoid cartilage

Tracheal cartilages

## Fig. 675: The Upper Left Part of the Larynx

NOTE: 1) the right halves of the hyoid bone, epiglottis and thyroid cartilage have been removed to reveal the interior of the upper left portion of the larynx. The two vocal ligaments, the arytenoid cartilages and the conus elasticus are also displayed.

2) the broad thyrohyoid membrane and its foramen. Observe the attachment of the stem of the epiglottis to the thyroid cartilage by means of the thyroepiglottic ligament.

3) the conus elasticus as it attaches to the vocal fold and the arytenoid, thyroid and cricoid cartilages.

4) although laryngeal sounds are initiated at the vocal folds, the pitch, quality, volume, range, tone and overtone characteristics of the human voice incorporate not only the vocal folds but also the structures in the mouth (tongue, teeth, and palate), the nasal cavities (sinuses), the pharynx, the rest of the larynx, the lungs, diaphragm and abdominal musculature.

Figs. 673, 674, 675

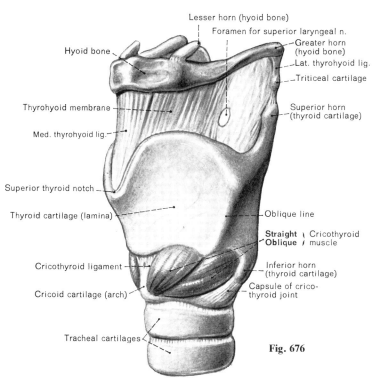

Lesser horn (hyoid bone)
Foramen for superior laryngeal n.
Greater horn (hyoid bone)
Lat. thyrohyoid lig.
Triticeal cartilage
Hyoid bone
Superior horn (thyroid cartilage)
Thyrohyoid membrane
Med. thyrohyoid lig.
Superior thyroid notch
Thyroid cartilage (lamina)
Oblique line
**Straight** \ Cricothyroid
**Oblique** / muscle
Cricothyroid ligament
Inferior horn (thyroid cartilage)
Cricoid cartilage (arch)
Capsule of crico-thyroid joint
Tracheal cartilages

Fig. 676

**Fig. 676: Ventrolateral View of the Exterior Larynx and the Cricothyroid Muscle**

NOTE: 1) the cricothyroid muscle consists of straight and oblique heads. The *straight head* is more vertical and inserts into the lower border of the lamina of the thyroid cartilage, while the *oblique head is* more horizontal and inserts onto the inferior horn of the thyroid cartilage.

2) the circothyroid muscle tilts the anterior part of the cricoid cartilage superiorly. In so doing, the arytenoid cartilages which are attached to the cricoid are pulled dorsally. In addition, the thyroid cartilage is pulled forward and downward. These actions increase the distance between the arytenoid and thyroid cartilages, thereby increasing the tension of and elongating the vocal folds.

**Fig. 677: Laryngeal Muscles (Dorsal)**

NOTE: 1) the *arytenoid muscle* consisting of a *transverse portion* which spans the zone between the two arytenoid cartilages horizontally, and an *oblique portion* which consists of two muscular fascicles that cross one another. Thus, each of the two fascicles of the oblique portion extends from the base of one arytenoid cartilage to the apex of the other cartilage. Some oblique arytenoid fibers continue to the epiglottis along the aryepiglottic fold. These constitute the *aryepiglottis muscle.*

2) the *transverse arytenoid* approximates the arytenoid cartilages, and, therefore, closes the posterior part of the rima glottis. The *oblique arytenoid and aryepiglottic muscles* tend to close the inlet into the larynx by pulling the aryepiglottic folds together and approximating the arytenoid cartilages and the epiglottis.

3) the *posterior cricoarytenoid* muscle extends from the lamina of the cricoid cartilage to the muscular process of the arytenoid cartilage while the *lateral cricoarytenoid* muscle arises laterally from the arch of the cricoid cartilage to insert with the posterior cricoarytenoid muscle onto the arytenoid cartilage.

4) the *posterior cricoarytenoids* are the only abductors of the vocal folds, while the *lateral cricoarytenoids* act as antagonists, and adduct the vocal folds. The posterior muscle abducts by pulling the base of the arytenoid cartilages medially and posteriorly, while the lateral muscle adducts by pulling these same cartilages anteriorly and laterally.

5) the *thyroarytenoid muscle* (Fig. 678) is a thin sheet of muscle radiating from the thyroid cartilage principally backward toward the arytenoid cartilage. Its upper fibers continue to the epiglottis and, joining the aryepiglottic fibers, become the *thyroepiglottic muscle.* Its deepest (and most medial) fibers form the *vocalis muscle* which is attached to the lateral aspect of the vocal fold.

6) the thyroarytenoid muscles draw the arytenoid cartilages toward the thyroid cartilage and, thus, shorten (relax) the vocal folds.

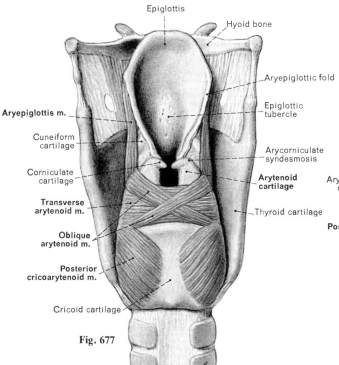

Epiglottis
Hyoid bone
Aryepiglottic fold
Epiglottic tubercle
**Aryepiglottis m.**
Cuneiform cartilage
Arycorniculate syndesmosis
Corniculate cartilage
**Arytenoid cartilage**
**Transverse arytenoid m.**
Thyroid cartilage
**Oblique arytenoid m.**
**Posterior cricoarytenoid m.**
Cricoid cartilage

Fig. 677

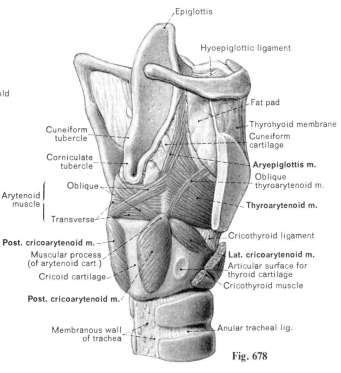

Epiglottis
Hyoepiglottic ligament
Fat pad
Thyrohyoid membrane
Cuneiform tubercle
Cuneiform cartilage
Corniculate tubercle
**Aryepiglottis m.**
Oblique
Oblique thyroarytenoid m.
Arytenoid muscle {
**Thyroarytenoid m.**
Transverse
Cricothyroid ligament
**Post. cricoarytenoid m.**
**Lat. cricoarytenoid m.**
Muscular process (of arytenoid cart.)
Articular surface for thyroid cartilage
Cricoid cartilage
Cricothyroid muscle
**Post. cricoarytenoid m.**
Membranous wall of trachea
Anular tracheal lig.

Fig. 678

**Fig. 678: Laryngeal Muscles (Lateral)**

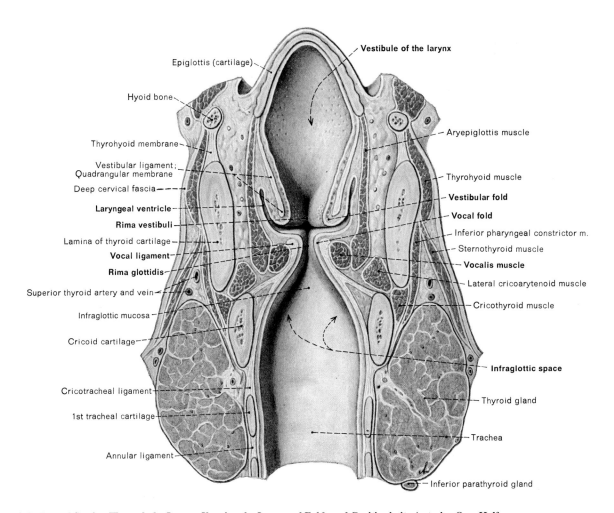

Epiglottis (cartilage)

Vestibule of the larynx

Hyoid bone

Thyrohyoid membrane

Vestibular ligament; Quadrangular membrane

Deep cervical fascia

**Laryngeal ventricle**

**Rima vestibuli**

Lamina of thyroid cartilage

**Vocal ligament**

**Rima glottidis**

Superior thyroid artery and vein

Infraglottic mucosa

Cricoid cartilage

Cricotracheal ligament

1st tracheal cartilage

Annular ligament

Aryepiglottis muscle

Thyrohyoid muscle

**Vestibular fold**

**Vocal fold**

Inferior pharyngeal constrictor m.

Sternothyroid muscle

**Vocalis muscle**

Lateral cricoarytenoid muscle

Cricothyroid muscle

**Infraglottic space**

Thyroid gland

Trachea

Inferior parathyroid gland

**Fig. 679: Frontal Section Through the Larynx Showing the Laryngeal Folds and Cavities in its Anterior One-Half**

NOTE: 1) the paired vocal folds consisting of mucous membrane overlying the vocal ligaments and vocalis muscles. Just superior to the vocal folds observe the vestibular folds. On each side, the vestibular fold is separated from the vocal folds by a recess called the laryngeal ventricle (or sinus).

2) that above the vestibular folds is the vestibule of the larynx which lies just below the laryngeal inlet. Below the vocal folds observe the infraglottic space. This space communicates with the trachea below and is limited by the rima glottidis between the vocal folds above.

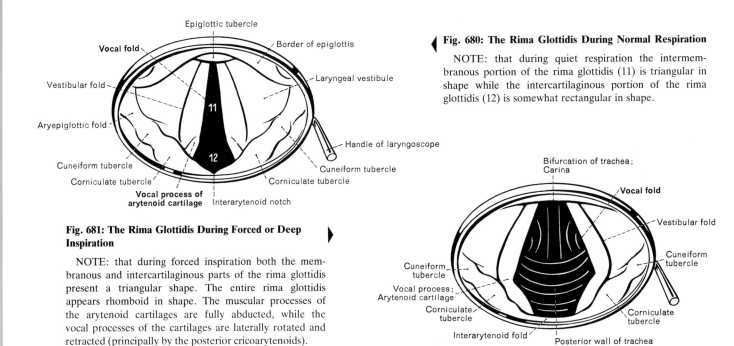

Epiglottic tubercle

**Vocal fold**

Border of epiglottis

Vestibular fold

Laryngeal vestibule

Aryepiglottic fold

Cuneiform tubercle

Corniculate tubercle

Handle of laryngoscope

Cuneiform tubercle

Corniculate tubercle

**Vocal process of arytenoid cartilage**   Interarytenoid notch

11

12

**Fig. 680: The Rima Glottidis During Normal Respiration**

NOTE: that during quiet respiration the intermembranous portion of the rima glottidis (11) is triangular in shape while the intercartilaginous portion of the rima glottidis (12) is somewhat rectangular in shape.

**Fig. 681: The Rima Glottidis During Forced or Deep Inspiration**

NOTE: that during forced inspiration both the membranous and intercartilaginous parts of the rima glottidis present a triangular shape. The entire rima glottidis appears rhomboid in shape. The muscular processes of the arytenoid cartilages are fully abducted, while the vocal processes of the cartilages are laterally rotated and retracted (principally by the posterior cricoarytenoids).

Bifurcation of trachea; Carina

**Vocal fold**

Vestibular fold

Cuneiform tubercle

Cuneiform tubercle

Vocal process; Arytenoid cartilage

Corniculate tubercle

Corniculate tubercle

Interarytenoid fold

Posterior wall of trachea

Figs. 679, 680, 681

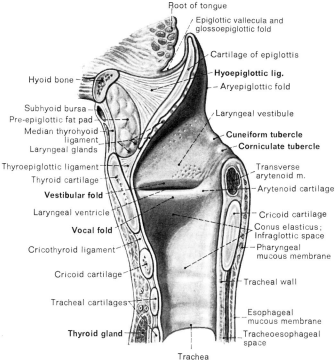

Root of tongue
Epiglottic vallecula and glossoepiglottic fold
Cartilage of epiglottis
**Hyoepiglottic lig.**
Hyoid bone
Aryepiglottic fold
Subhyoid bursa
Pre-epiglottic fat pad
Laryngeal vestibule
Median thyrohyoid ligament
Laryngeal glands
**Cuneiform tubercle**
**Corniculate tubercle**
Thyroepiglottic ligament
Transverse arytenoid m.
Thyroid cartilage
Arytenoid cartilage
**Vestibular fold**
Laryngeal ventricle
Cricoid cartilage
Conus elasticus; Infraglottic space
**Vocal fold**
Pharyngeal mucous membrane
Cricothyroid ligament
Cricoid cartilage
Tracheal wall
Tracheal cartilages
Esophageal mucous membrane
**Thyroid gland**
Tracheoesophageal space
Trachea

## Fig. 682: Midsagittal Section of Larynx

NOTE: 1) the laryngeal inlet through which the larynx communicates with the pharynx. This aperture leads to the laryngeal vestibule, the anterior border of which is the epiglottis. On each side the aryepiglottic folds define the borders of the inlet, which are marked by oval elevations, the cuneiform and corniculate cartilages.

2) the space between the vestibular folds and the vocal folds is known as the ventricle or laryngeal sinus. Below the vocal fold observe how the conus elasticus bounds the infraglottic space laterally, and the communication of this space with the trachea.

3) the attachments of the epiglottis. Superiorly, its hyoepiglottic ligament stretches to the hyoid bone; inferiorly, the thyroepiglottic ligament connects the stem of the epiglottis to the thyroid cartilage; laterally, the aryepiglottic folds extend between the epiglottis and the arytenoid cartilages.

## Fig. 683: Cross Section of Larynx at the Vocal Folds

I = intermembranous portion of rima glottidis

II = intercartilaginous portion of rima glottidis

NOTE: the orientation of the arytenoid cartilages and their articulations with the cricoid cartilage. The vocal folds consist of mucous membrane overlying the vocal ligaments, lateral to which extend the deeper vocalis portions of the thyroarytenoid muscle. By drawing the arytenoid cartilages forward, the thyroarytenoids shorten and relax the vocal folds. Simultaneously, they medially rotate the arytenoid cartilages and, thus, approximate the vocal folds.

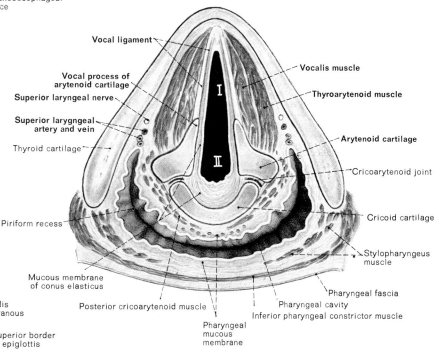

Vocal ligament
Vocal process of arytenoid cartilage
Superior laryngeal nerve
Superior laryngeal artery and vein
Thyroid cartilage
**Vocalis muscle**
**Thyroarytenoid muscle**
**Arytenoid cartilage**
Cricoarytenoid joint
Cricoid cartilage
Piriform recess
Stylopharyngeus muscle
Pharyngeal fascia
Mucous membrane of conus elasticus
Posterior cricoarytenoid muscle
Pharyngeal mucous membrane
Pharyngeal cavity
Inferior pharyngeal constrictor muscle

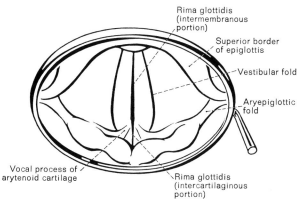

Rima glottidis (intermembranous portion)
Superior border of epiglottis
Vestibular fold
Aryepiglottic fold
Vocal process of arytenoid cartilage
Rima glottidis (intercartilaginous portion)

## Fig. 684: The Rima Glottidis During Whispering

NOTE: that during the production of whispering sounds the intermembranous portion of the vocal folds are approximated, while the intercartilaginous portion of the folds are kept separated. The anterior part of the rima glottidis is narrow and slit-like and the posterior, intercartilaginous portion remains open.

## Fig. 685: The Rima Glottidis During Phonation (Shrill Tones)

NOTE: that during the emission of shrill tones, the vocal folds are approximated and the vocal ligaments tensed resulting in a narrowing of the rima glottidis to a thin slit.

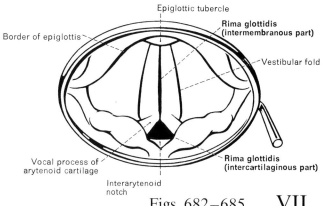

Epiglottic tubercle
Border of epiglottis
**Rima glottidis (intermembranous part)**
Vestibular fold
Vocal process of arytenoid cartilage
Interarytenoid notch
**Rima glottidis (intercartilaginous part)**

Figs. 682–685    VII

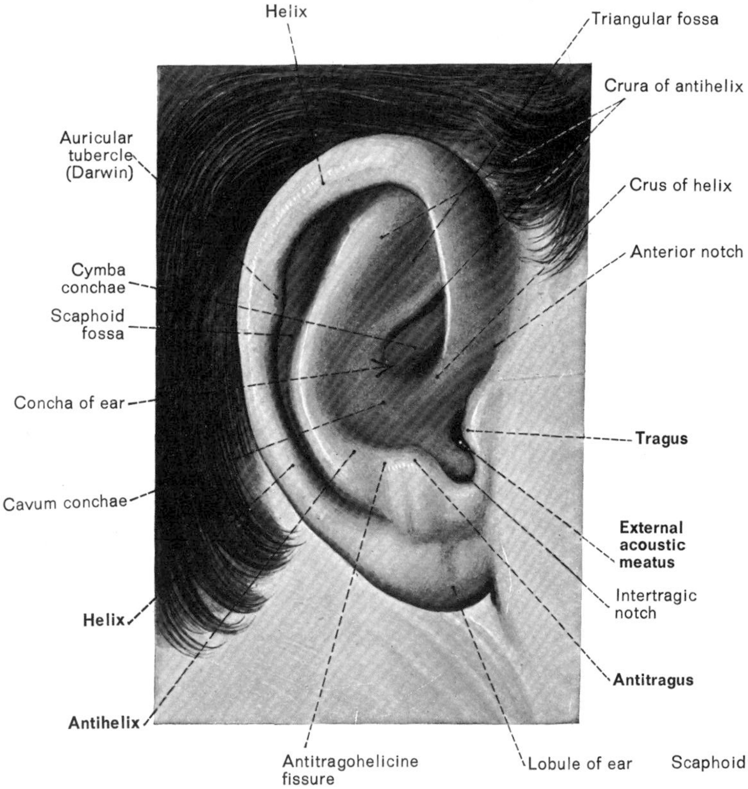

Helix

Triangular fossa

Crura of antihelix

Crus of helix

Auricular
tubercle
(Darwin)

Anterior notch

Cymba
conchae

Scaphoid
fossa

Concha of ear

Tragus

Cavum conchae

External
acoustic
meatus

Helix

Intertragic
notch

Antihelix

Antitragus

Antitragohelicine
fissure

Lobule of ear

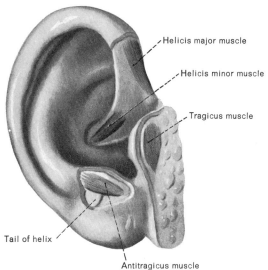

**Fig. 687: The Cartilage of the Right External Ear (seen from Front)**

NOTE: 1) with the skin of the external ear removed, the contours of the single cartilage conform generally with those of the intact auricle. The cartilage is seen to be absent inferiorly at the site of the ear lobe.

2) the attachment of the auricular cartilage to the temporal bone. This attachment is strengthened by the anterior and posterior ligaments (not shown in this figure) which articulate the tragus and spine of the helix to the temporal bone anteriorly, and the concha to the mastoid process posteriorly. The continuous overlying skin completes the attachment.

**Fig. 686: The Right External Ear (Lateral View)**

NOTE: 1) the external ear (or auricle) consists of skin overlying elastic fibrocartilage. It is irregularly shaped and the external acoustic meatus courses through the external ear to the tympanic membrane.

2) the external rim of the auricle is called the helix. Another curved prominence anterior to the helix is the antihelix. Inferiorly, a notch in the cartilage (the intertragic incisure) separates the tragus anteriorly from the antitragus posteriorly.

3) the ear lobe or lobule does not contain cartilage. Instead, it is soft and contains connective tissue and fat.

4) the external acoustic meatus is an oval canal which extends for about 2.5 cm in a S-shaped curve from the concha to the tympanic membrane. It consists of an outer cartilaginous part (1 cm) and a narrower more medial osseous part (1.5 cm).

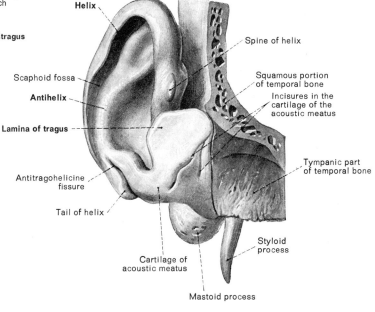

Helix

Spine of helix

Squamous portion
of temporal bone

Incisures in the
cartilage of the
acoustic meatus

Scaphoid fossa

Antihelix

Lamina of tragus

Tympanic part
of temporal bone

Antitragohelicine
fissure

Tail of helix

Cartilage of
acoustic meatus

Styloid
process

Mastoid process

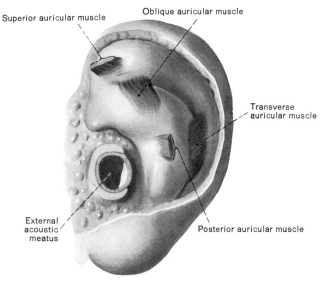

Helicis major muscle

Helicis minor muscle

Tragicus muscle

Tail of helix

Antitragicus muscle

Superior auricular muscle

Oblique auricular muscle

Transverse
auricular muscle

External
acoustic
meatus

Posterior auricular muscle

**Fig. 688: Intrinsic Muscles of External Ear (Lateral Surface)**

**Fig. 689: Muscles Attaching to the Medial Surface of External Ear**

Figs. 686–689

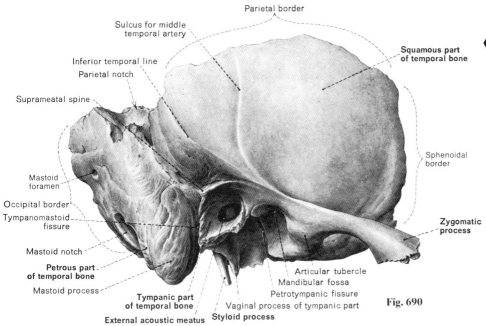

Parietal border

Sulcus for middle
temporal artery

Inferior temporal line
Parietal notch

Suprameatal spine

Mastoid
foramen

Occipital border

Tympanomastoid
fissure

Mastoid notch

**Petrous part**
**of temporal bone**

Mastoid process

**Tympanic part**
**of temporal bone**

**External acoustic meatus**  Styloid process

Vaginal process of tympanic part

Petrotympanic fissure

Mandibular fossa

Articular tubercle

**Zygomatic**
**process**

Sphenoidal
border

**Squamous part**
**of temporal bone**

Fig. 690

**Fig. 690: The Right Temporal Bone**
**(Lateral View)**

NOTE: 1) the temporal bone
which forms the osseous encasement
for the middle and internal ear, consists of three parts: *squamous, tympanic* and *petrous.*

2) the *squamous part* is broad in
shape, thin and flat. From it extends
the zygomatic process. The *tympanic
part* is interposed below the squamous,
and anterior to the petrous parts. The
external acoustic meatus, which leads
to the tympanic membrane, is surrounded by the tympanic part of the
temporal bone.

3) the hard *petrous part* contains
the organ of hearing and the vestibular canals. Its mastoid process is
not solid but contains many air cells,
and its external surface affords
attachment to several muscles.

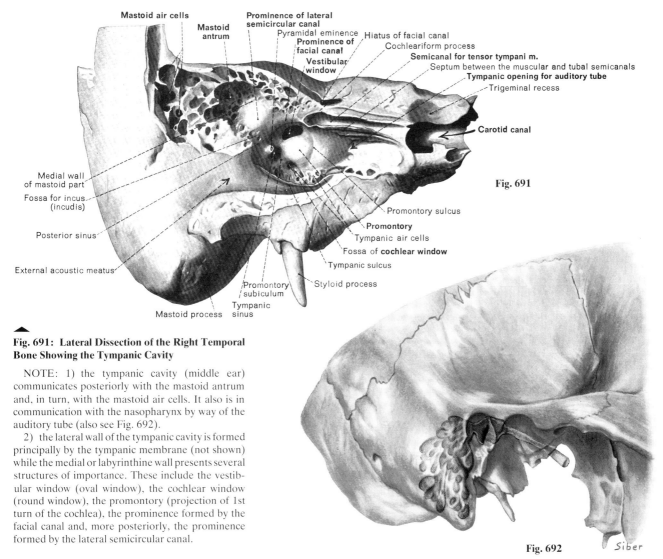

Mastoid air cells

**Mastoid**
**antrum**

**Prominence of lateral**
**semicircular canal**

Pyramidal eminence  Hiatus of facial canal

**Prominence of**
**facial canal**

Cochleariform process

**Semicanal for tensor tympani m.**

**Vestibular**
**window**

Septum between the muscular and tubal semicanals

**Tympanic opening for auditory tube**

Trigeminal recess

**Carotid canal**

Medial wall
of mastoid part

Fossa for incus
(incudis)

Posterior sinus

External acoustic meatus

Promontory sulcus

**Promontory**

Tympanic air cells

Fossa of **cochlear window**

Tympanic sulcus

Promontory
subiculum

Styloid process

Tympanic
sinus

Mastoid process

Fig. 691

**Fig. 691: Lateral Dissection of the Right Temporal**
**Bone Showing the Tympanic Cavity**

NOTE: 1) the tympanic cavity (middle ear)
communicates posteriorly with the mastoid antrum
and, in turn, with the mastoid air cells. It also is in
communication with the nasopharynx by way of the
auditory tube (also see Fig. 692).

2) the lateral wall of the tympanic cavity is formed
principally by the tympanic membrane (not shown)
while the medial or labyrinthine wall presents several
structures of importance. These include the vestibular window (oval window), the cochlear window
(round window), the promontory (projection of 1st
turn of the cochlea), the prominence formed by the
facial canal and, more posteriorly, the prominence
formed by the lateral semicircular canal.

Fig. 692

Siber

**Fig. 692: A Projection of the Middle Ear Air Spaces on the Lateral Surface of the Skull**

NOTE that the mastoid air cells within the mastoid process of the temporal bone (shown in red) communicate with the tympanic cavity (blue).
Coursing between the middle ear and the nasopharynx is the auditory tube (yellow). This communication allows the air pressure in the tympanic
cavity to be the same as external atmospheric pressure and, thus, equivalent on both sides of the tympanic membrane.

## Fig. 693: Frontal Section Through Left External, Middle and Internal Ear

NOTE: 1) the external acoustic meatus commences at the auricle and leads to the external surface of the tympanic membrane. Through the meatus course the sound waves which cause vibration of the tympanum.

2) the middle ear (or tympanic cavity) contains three ossicles (malleus, incus and stapes) and two muscles (tensor tympani and stapedius [not shown]). The cavity of the middle ear communicates with the mastoid antrum and mastoid air cells posteriorly, and the nasopharynx by way of the auditory tube. From the middle ear this tube courses downward, forward and medially. The ossicles interconnect the tympanic membrane with the inner ear.

3) the inner ear contains the coiled cochlea (or organ of hearing) and the three semicircular canals (the vestibular organ) and their associated structures and nerves.

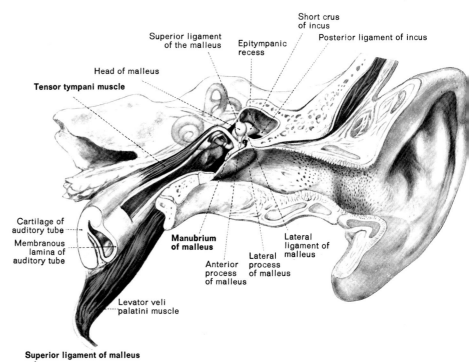

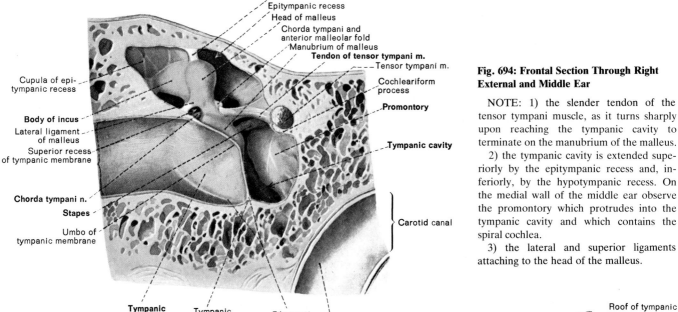

## Fig. 694: Frontal Section Through Right External and Middle Ear

NOTE: 1) the slender tendon of the tensor tympani muscle, as it turns sharply upon reaching the tympanic cavity to terminate on the manubrium of the malleus.

2) the tympanic cavity is extended superiorly by the epitympanic recess and, inferiorly, by the hypotympanic recess. On the medial wall of the middle ear observe the promontory which protrudes into the tympanic cavity and which contains the spiral cochlea.

3) the lateral and superior ligaments attaching to the head of the malleus.

## Fig. 695: Frontal Section of Left Ear Through the Middle Ear Bones

NOTE: 1) when sound waves are received at the tympanic membrane, they cause medial displacements of the manubrium of the malleus. The head of the malleus is tilted laterally, pulling with it the body of the incus. At the same time the long process of the incus is displaced medially, as is the articulation between the incus and the stapes.

2) the base of the stapes rocks as though it were on a fulcrum at the vestibular window, thereby establishing waves in the perilymph. These waves stimulate the auditory receptors and become dissipated at the secondary tympanic membrane covering the cochlear window.

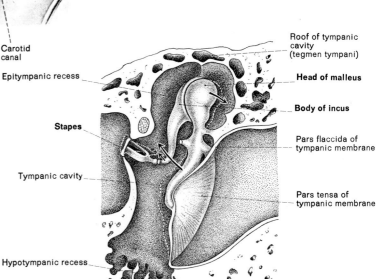

Figs. 693, 694, 695

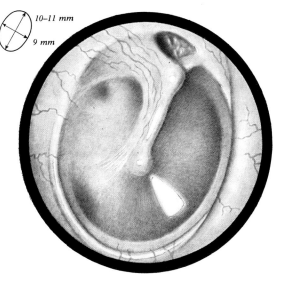

10–11 mm
9 mm

## Fig. 697: Labeled Diagram of Fig. 696

NOTE: 1) the tympanic membrane has been divided into quadrants. The most depressed point is the umbo and is found at the rounded extremity of the handle of the malleus.

2) the anterior and posterior malleolar folds. The more lax part (pars flaccida) of the tympanic membrane lies above and between these folds, while the rest is more tightly stretched (pars tensa).

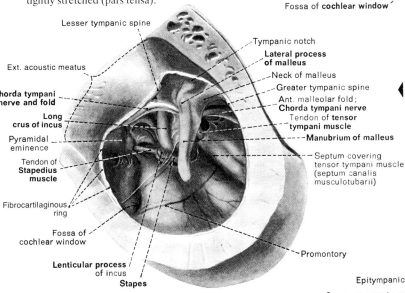

Lesser tympanic spine
Ext. acoustic meatus
Chorda tympani nerve and fold
Long crus of incus
Pyramidal eminence
Tendon of **Stapedius muscle**
Fibrocartilaginous ring
Fossa of cochlear window
**Lenticular process** of incus
**Stapes**

Tympanic notch
**Lateral process of malleus**
Neck of malleus
Greater tympanic spine
Ant. malleolar fold; **Chorda tympani nerve**
Tendon of **tensor tympani muscle**
**Manubrium of malleus**
Septum covering tensor tympani muscle (septum canalis musculotubarii)
Promontory

## Fig. 699: Lateral Wall of the Right Middle Ear (Tympanic Membrane Viewed from within the Tympanic Cavity)

NOTE: 1) the manubrium of the malleus has been severed from the remainder of the ossicle and left attached to the tympanic membrane. The fibrocartilaginous tympanic ring is deficient superiorly, forming the tympanic notch (of Rivinus). The looser portion of the tympanic membrane (pars flaccida) covers this zone.

2) the tympanic membrane below the malleolar folds is the pars tensa. This portion is made taut by the tensor tympani muscle which attaches to the manubrium of the malleus.

3) the innervation of external surface of the tympanic membrane comes from the auriculotemporal branch of the mandibular nerve (V) and the auricular branch of the vagus (X). The inner surface of the membrane receives innervation from the tympanic branch of the glossopharyngeal nerve (IX).

## Fig. 696: Right Tympanic Membrane as seen with an Otoscope in a Living Person

NOTE: that the tympanic membrane is oval in shape and measures about 9 mm across and from 10 to 11 mm vertically (upper inset, actual size). Its blood supply is derived from the deep auricular and anterior tympanic branches of the maxillary artery, and the stylomastoid branch of the posterior auricular artery.

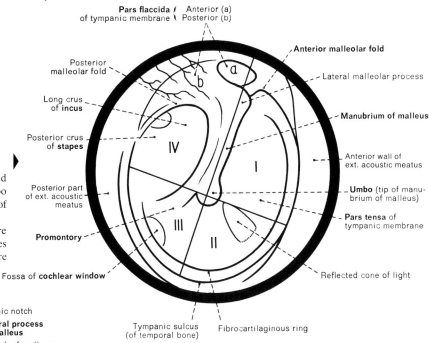

Pars flaccida / Anterior (a)
of tympanic membrane \ Posterior (b)
Posterior malleolar fold
Long crus of **incus**
Posterior crus of **stapes**
Posterior part of ext. acoustic meatus
**Promontory**
Fossa of **cochlear window**
**Anterior malleolar fold**
Lateral malleolar process
**Manubrium of malleus**
Anterior wall of ext. acoustic meatus
**Umbo** (tip of manubrium of malleus)
**Pars tensa** of tympanic membrane
Reflected cone of light
Tympanic sulcus (of temporal bone)
Fibrocartilaginous ring

## Fig. 698: Right Tympanic Cavity seen After Removal of Tympanic Membrane

NOTE: that from this lateral view, the lateral process and manubrium of the malleus, the lenticular process and long crus of the incus, as well as the stapes can be observed upon the removal of the tympanic membrane. Note also the chorda tympani nerve and the tendons of the stapedius and tensor tympani muscles.

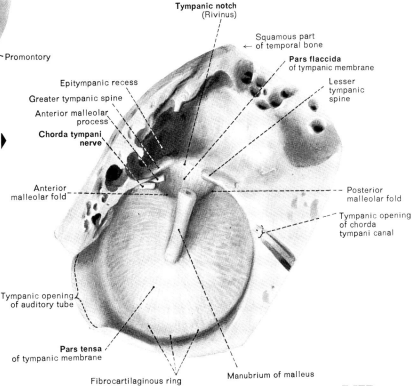

**Tympanic notch** (Rivinus)
Squamous part of temporal bone
**Pars flaccida** of tympanic membrane
Lesser tympanic spine
Epitympanic recess
Greater tympanic spine
Anterior malleolar process
**Chorda tympani nerve**
Anterior malleolar fold
Posterior malleolar fold
Tympanic opening of chorda tympani canal
Tympanic opening of auditory tube
**Pars tensa** of tympanic membrane
Fibrocartilaginous ring
Manubrium of malleus

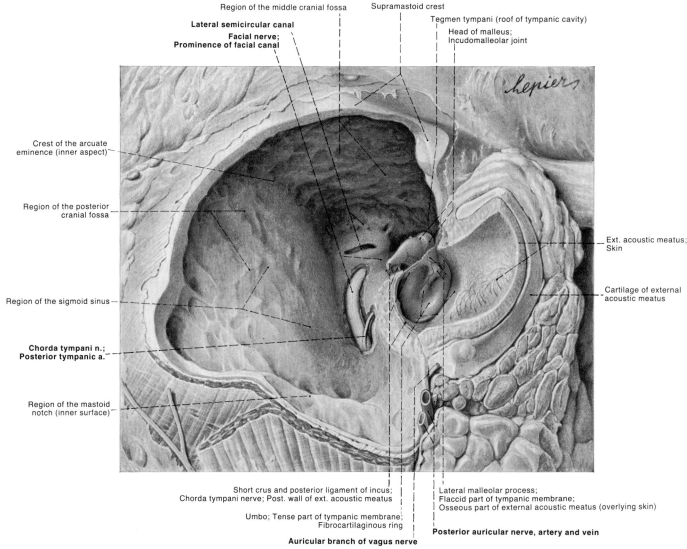

Region of the middle cranial fossa

**Lateral semicircular canal**
**Facial nerve;**
**Prominence of facial canal**

Supramastoid crest

Tegmen tympani (roof of tympanic cavity)

Head of malleus;
Incudomalleolar joint

Crest of the arcuate
eminence (inner aspect)

Region of the posterior
cranial fossa

Region of the sigmoid sinus

**Chorda tympani n.;**
**Posterior tympanic a.**

Region of the mastoid
notch (inner surface)

Ext. acoustic meatus;
Skin

Cartilage of external
acoustic meatus

Short crus and posterior ligament of incus;
Chorda tympani nerve; Post. wall of ext. acoustic meatus

Umbo; Tense part of tympanic membrane;
Fibrocartilaginous ring

**Auricular branch of vagus nerve**

Lateral malleolar process;
Flaccid part of tympanic membrane;
Osseous part of external acoustic meatus (overlying skin)

**Posterior auricular nerve, artery and vein**

**Fig. 700: Lateral Dissection of the Right Temporal Bone: The Tympanic Membrane, Middle Ear, and Facial Canal**

NOTE: 1) that this dissection has proceeded through the mastoid region of the temporal bone, much of which has been removed, as has the posterior wall of the external acoustic meatus. The descending part of the facial canal and the lateral semicircular canal have been opened.

2) the lateral or outer surface of the tympanic membrane. Observe the manubrium of the malleus on the inner surface of the membrane, and the head of the malleus, the incus and the incudomalleolar joint within the tympanic cavity.

3) the junction of the chorda tympani nerve with the facial nerve.

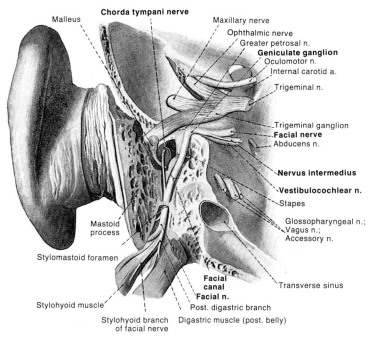

Malleus

**Chorda tympani nerve**

Maxillary nerve

Ophthalmic nerve

Greater petrosal n.

**Geniculate ganglion**

Oculomotor n.

Internal carotid a.

Trigeminal n.

Trigeminal ganglion

**Facial nerve**

Abducens n.

**Nervus intermedius**

**Vestibulocochlear n.**

Stapes

Glossopharyngeal n.;
Vagus n.;
Accessory n.

Mastoid
process

Stylomastoid foramen

Transverse sinus

**Facial**
**canal**
**Facial n.**

Stylohyoid muscle

Post. digastric branch

Stylohyoid branch
of facial nerve

Digastric muscle (post. belly)

**Fig. 701: The Intracranial Course of the Facial Nerve,
View from Behind**

NOTE: 1) that a frontal section has been made through the temporal bone at an angle which opens the facial canal and tympanic cavity from behind. Observe the chorda tympani nerve coursing anteroposteriorly across the middle ear cavity to its junction with the facial nerve.

2) that the internal acoustic meatus in the floor of the cranial cavity can be seen transmitting the facial nerve with its nervous intermedius, as well as the vestibulocochlear nerve. Peripheral to the geniculate ganglion (which serves as the sensory ganglion of VII), the facial nerve enters the facial canal. Within the canal, the facial nerve initially courses laterally and then turns sharply backward and inferiorly (see Figs. 700, 701 and 703).

3) that beyond its junction with the chorda tympani nerve, the main trunk of the facial nerve continues its descent in the temporal bone to emerge on the lateral aspect of the face through the stylomastoid foramen.

Figs. 700, 701

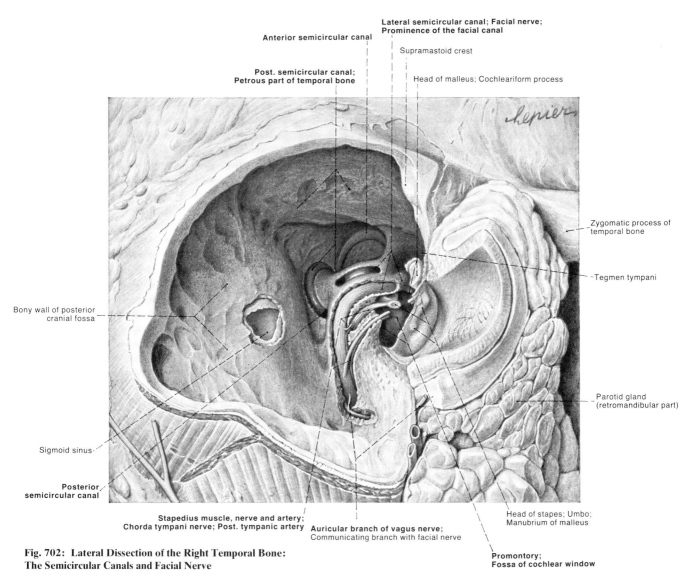

Anterior semicircular canal

Lateral semicircular canal; Facial nerve;
Prominence of the facial canal

Supramastoid crest

Post. semicircular canal;
Petrous part of temporal bone

Head of malleus; Cochleariform process

Zygomatic process of
temporal bone

Tegmen tympani

Bony wall of posterior
cranial fossa

Parotid gland
(retromandibular part)

Sigmoid sinus

Posterior
semicircular canal

Stapedius muscle, nerve and artery;
Chorda tympani nerve; Post. tympanic artery

Auricular branch of vagus nerve;
Communicating branch with facial nerve

Head of stapes; Umbo;
Manubrium of malleus

Promontory;
Fossa of cochlear window

**Fig. 702: Lateral Dissection of the Right Temporal Bone:
The Semicircular Canals and Facial Nerve**

NOTE: 1) that the facial canal has been opened more extensively than in Figure 698, exposing further the chorda tympani nerve and the posterior tympanic artery. This vessel branches from the stylomastoid artery and helps to supply the internal surface of the tympanic membrane. Observe the nerve to the stapedius muscle which arises from the facial nerve near the pyramidal eminence on the posterior wall of the tympanic cavity. Coursing with the nerve is the stapedial artery, and more inferiorly is found the auricular branch of the vagus nerve.

2) that the incus has been removed, thereby revealing the head of the stapes, which is directed laterally. The stapedius muscle inserts onto the posterior surface of the head of the stapes.

3) the anterior, posterior and lateral semicircular canals. These become exposed after removal of the bony prominence over the lateral canal, and additional bone above and behind that prominence.

**Fig. 703: The Facial, Glossopharyngeal and
Vagus Nerves Projected Onto the Temporal Bone,
Lateral View**

NOTE: 1) the tympanic branch of the glossopharyngeal nerve which, along with sympathetic fibers from the caroticotympanic nerve, contributes to the formation of the tympanic plexus (see Figure 710). From this plexus emerges the lesser petrosal nerve which courses to the otic ganglion.

2) the greater petrosal nerve joining with sympathetic branches of the internal carotid plexus (actually the deep petrosal nerve) to form the nerve of the pterygoid canal.

3) the auricular branch of the vagus nerve which is distributed to the upper surface of the external auricle, to the posterior wall and floor of the external acoustic meatus and part of the lateral (outer) surface of the tympanic membrane.

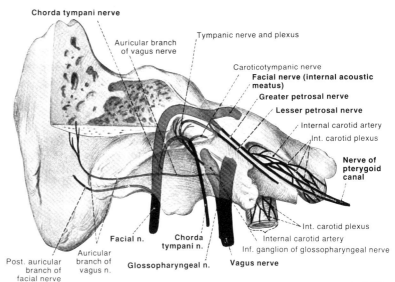

Chorda tympani nerve

Auricular branch
of vagus nerve

Tympanic nerve and plexus

Caroticotympanic nerve
**Facial nerve (internal acoustic
meatus)**
**Greater petrosal nerve**
**Lesser petrosal nerve**
Internal carotid artery
Int. carotid plexus
**Nerve of
pterygoid
canal**

Int. carotid plexus
Internal carotid artery
Inf. ganglion of glossopharyngeal nerve

Post. auricular
branch of
facial nerve

Auricular
branch of
vagus n.

**Facial n.**

**Chorda
tympani n.**

**Glossopharyngeal n.**

**Vagus nerve**

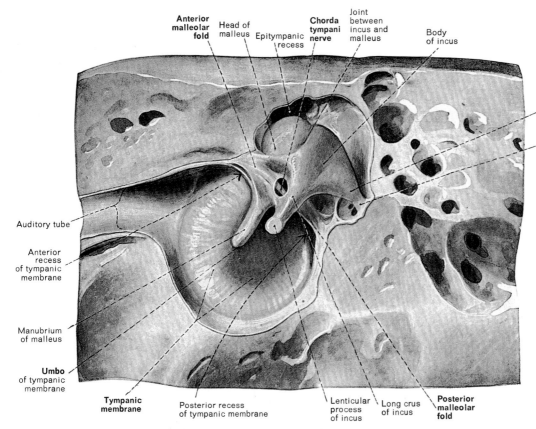

**Anterior malleolar fold** — Head of malleus — Epitympanic recess — **Chorda tympani nerve** — Joint between incus and malleus — Body of incus

Short crus of incus

Posterior ligament of incus

Auditory tube

Anterior recess of tympanic membrane

Manubrium of malleus

**Umbo** of tympanic membrane

**Tympanic membrane** — Posterior recess of tympanic membrane — Lenticular process of incus — Long crus of incus — **Posterior malleolar fold**

**Fig. 704: Lateral Wall of the Right Tympanic Cavity (Viewed from the Medial Aspect)**

NOTE: 1) the tympanic cavity is lined completely with a mucous membrane which attaches onto the surface of all the structures of the middle ear. This tympanic mucosa is continuous with that lining the mastoid air cells posteriorly, and the auditory tube anteriorly.

2) reflections of the tympanic mucous membrane form the anterior and posterior malleolar folds. These are also reflected around the chorda tympani nerve, as it curves along the medial side of the manubrium of the malleus.

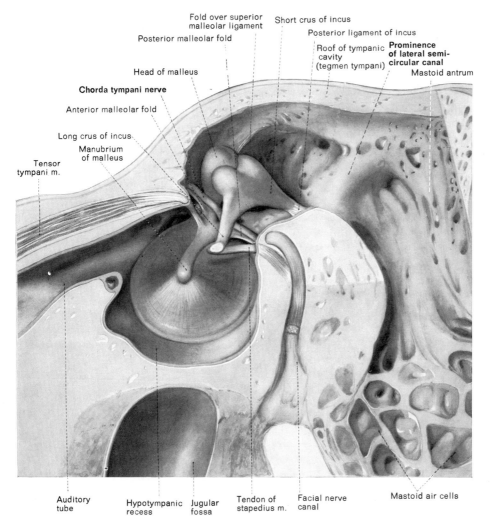

Fold over superior malleolar ligament — Short crus of incus

Posterior malleolar fold — Posterior ligament of incus

Roof of tympanic cavity (tegmen tympani) — **Prominence of lateral semicircular canal**

Head of malleus — Mastoid antrum

**Chorda tympani nerve**

Anterior malleolar fold

Long crus of incus

Manubrium of malleus

Tensor tympani m.

Auditory tube — Hypotympanic recess — Jugular fossa — Tendon of stapedius m. — Facial nerve canal — Mastoid air cells

**Fig. 705: The Muscles, Chorda Tympani Nerve, and Ossicles of the Right Middle Ear**

NOTE: 1) the tendon of the tensor tympani muscle inserting on the manubrium of the malleus and the short tendon of the stapedius as it inserts onto the neck of the stapes close to its articulation with the incus. The tensor tympani draws the manubrium medially, thereby making the tympanic membrane taut. It is innervated by the mandibular division of the trigeminal nerve.

2) the stapedius is the smallest of the skeletal muscles in the body and it is supplied by the facial nerve. It pulls the head of the stapes posteriorly, thereby tilting the base of the stapes in the vestibular window.

3) the direct communication between the nasopharynx, tympanic cavity and mastoid air cells has important clinical meaning, since oro-respiratory tract infections reach the middle ear readily by way of the auditory tube.

Figs. 704, 705

## Fig. 706: Medial Wall of the Right Tympanic Cavity (Viewed from Lateral Aspect)

NOTE: 1) the tympanic membrane has been removed along with the bony roof of the tympanic cavity. The malleus and incus have also been removed and the tendon of the tensor tympani severed. Observe the stapes with its base directed toward the vestibular window and the stapedius muscle still attached to its neck.

2) several bony markings: a) the prominence containing the lateral semicircular canal, b) the curved prominence of the facial canal with its facial nerve, c) the rounded promontory, which is the thin bony covering over the cochlea and d) the hollow pyramidal eminence from which arises the stapedius muscle.

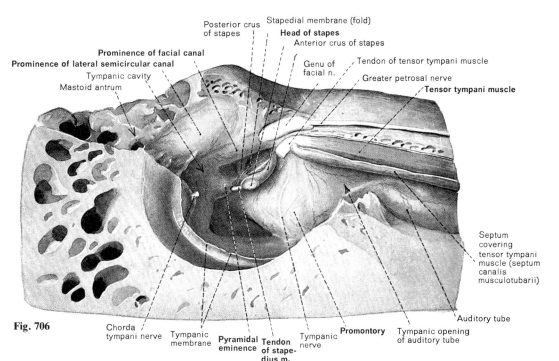

Posterior crus of stapes — Stapedial membrane (fold) — **Head of stapes** — Anterior crus of stapes
Prominence of facial canal — Genu of facial n. — Tendon of tensor tympani muscle — Greater petrosal nerve — **Tensor tympani muscle**
Prominence of lateral semicircular canal — Tympanic cavity — Mastoid antrum
Septum covering tensor tympani muscle (septum canalis musculotubarii)
Chorda tympani nerve — Tympanic membrane — **Pyramidal eminence** — **Tendon of stapedius m.** — Tympanic nerve — **Promontory** — Tympanic opening of auditory tube — Auditory tube

**Fig. 706**

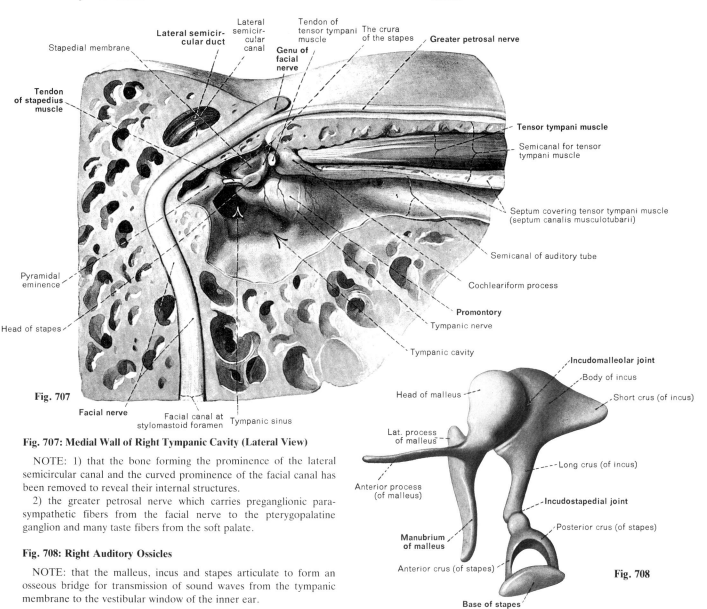

Lateral semicircular duct — Lateral semicircular canal — Tendon of tensor tympani muscle — The crura of the stapes — **Greater petrosal nerve**
Stapedial membrane — **Genu of facial nerve**
**Tendon of stapedius muscle**
— **Tensor tympani muscle**
— Semicanal for tensor tympani muscle
— Septum covering tensor tympani muscle (septum canalis musculotubarii)
— Semicanal of auditory tube
— Cochleariform process
Pyramidal eminence
Head of stapes
— **Promontory**
— Tympanic nerve
— Tympanic cavity
**Fig. 707**
**Facial nerve** — Facial canal at stylomastoid foramen — Tympanic sinus

## Fig. 707: Medial Wall of Right Tympanic Cavity (Lateral View)

NOTE: 1) that the bone forming the prominence of the lateral semicircular canal and the curved prominence of the facial canal has been removed to reveal their internal structures.

2) the greater petrosal nerve which carries preganglionic parasympathetic fibers from the facial nerve to the pterygopalatine ganglion and many taste fibers from the soft palate.

## Fig. 708: Right Auditory Ossicles

NOTE: that the malleus, incus and stapes articulate to form an osseous bridge for transmission of sound waves from the tympanic membrane to the vestibular window of the inner ear.

**Incudomalleolar joint**
Body of incus
Head of malleus — Short crus (of incus)
Lat. process of malleus
Long crus (of incus)
Anterior process (of malleus)
**Incudostapedial joint**
Posterior crus (of stapes)
**Manubrium of malleus**
Anterior crus (of stapes)
Base of stapes
**Fig. 708**

## Fig. 709: Medial Wall of the Right Tympanic Cavity Showing the Stapedius Muscle (Lateral View)

NOTE: 1) the lateral aspect of the pyramidal eminence was removed in order to demonstrate the stapedius muscle. Its tendon emerges through the apex of the eminence and inserts on the neck of the stapes. This muscle measures about 4 mm. in length and its action on the base of the stapes (pulling it laterally) protects the inner ear from damage caused by loud sounds.

2) the tympanic branch of the glossopharyngeal nerve (IX) coursing along the promontory. This nerve is sensory to the mucous membrane of the middle ear and is also known as the nerve of Jacobson. Its fibers are joined by sympathetic fibers and by branches from the facial nerve to form the tympanic plexus.

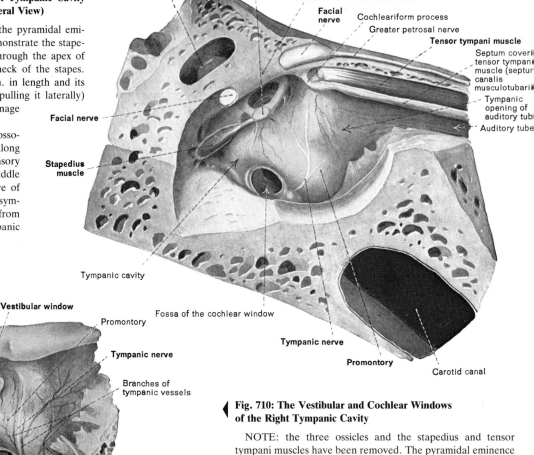

## Fig. 711: The Right Membranous Labyrinth Partially Exposed within the Temporal Bone

NOTE: 1) the membranous labyrinth is in blue, while the roots of the vestibulocochlear nerve are in yellow. The membranous labyrinth lies within the bony labyrinth and generally conforms to it in shape. Between them is found the perilymphatic fluid.

2) within the bony cochlea lie the coils of the cochlear duct. The bony labyrinth consists of the cochlea and the semicircular canals interconnected by the vestibule. In the lateral wall of the vestibule is situated the vestibular window where the stapes has access to the perilymph.

3) the basal end of the cochlear duct communicates with the saccule through the ductus reuniens. The saccule communicates with the utricle and the semicircular canals through the utriculo-saccular duct.

## Fig. 710: The Vestibular and Cochlear Windows of the Right Tympanic Cavity

NOTE: the three ossicles and the stapedius and tensor tympani muscles have been removed. The pyramidal eminence has been opened. On the medial wall of the tympanic cavity observe the oval vestibular window and the round cochlear window which communicate with the internal ear. Coursing along the surface of the promontory can be seen the tympanic vessels and nerve.

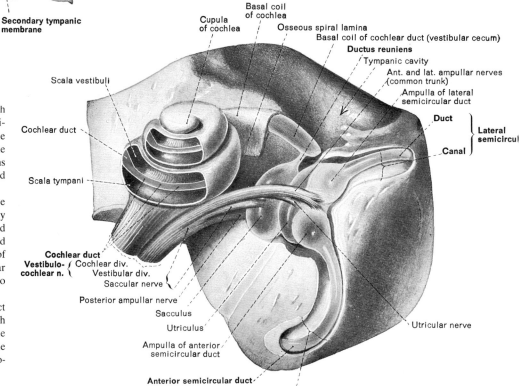

Figs. 709, 710, 711

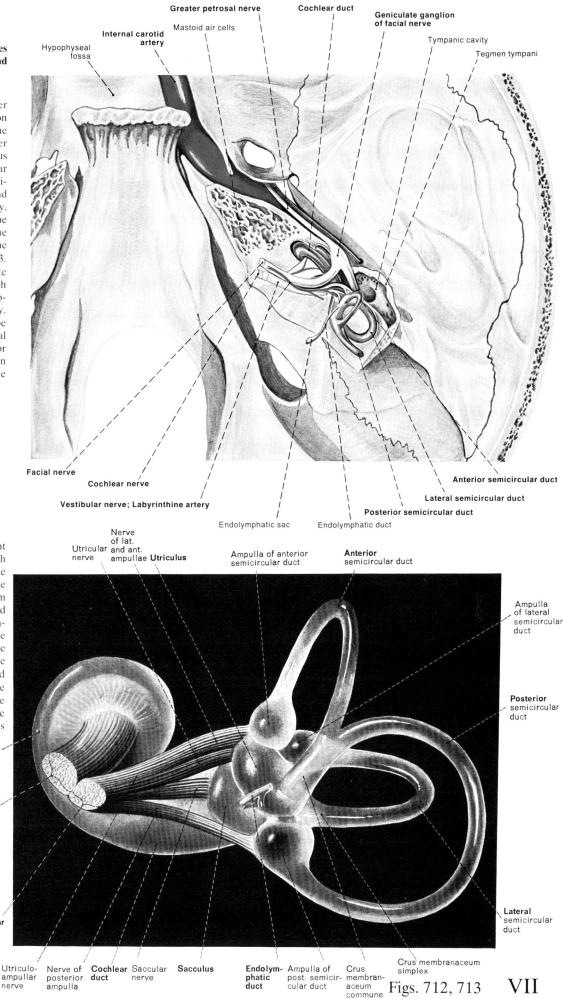

**Fig. 712: The Structures of the Right Inner Ear and the Facial Nerve, Dissected from Above**

NOTE that the upper part of the petrous portion of the right temporal bone has been removed in order to expose the membranous labyrinth, the cochlear duct, the facial and vestibulocochlear nerves and the labyrinthine artery. The orientation of the semicircular ducts and the cochlear duct is nearly the same as that in Figure 713. Observe the geniculate ganglion from which extends the greater petrosal nerve inferomedially. The facial nerve can be seen entering the facial canal lateral and posterior to the ganglion and in relationship to the tympanic cavity.

Hypophyseal fossa
Internal carotid artery
Greater petrosal nerve
Mastoid air cells
Cochlear duct
Geniculate ganglion of facial nerve
Tympanic cavity
Tegmen tympani

Facial nerve
Cochlear nerve
Vestibular nerve; Labyrinthine artery
Endolymphatic sac
Endolymphatic duct
Posterior semicircular duct
Lateral semicircular duct
Anterior semicircular duct

**Fig. 713: The Right Membranous Labyrinth (Medial View)**

NOTE: that the right membranous labyrinth and the branches of the vestibulocochlear nerve have been isolated from the bony labyrinth and shown somewhat diagrammatically. Observe the ampullae of the three semicircular ducts, the sacculus, the utriculus and the cochlear duct. The sites of connection of the endolymphatic duct to the utriculus and sacculus is also indicated.

Utricular nerve
Nerve of lat. and ant. ampullae
**Utriculus**
Ampulla of anterior semicircular duct
**Anterior** semicircular duct
Ampulla of lateral semicircular duct
**Posterior** semicircular duct

**Cochlear duct**

**Cochlear nerve**

**Vestibular nerve**

Lateral semicircular duct

Utriculo-ampullar nerve
Nerve of posterior ampulla
**Cochlear duct**
Saccular nerve
**Sacculus**
**Endolymphatic duct**
Ampulla of post. semicircular duct
Crus membranaceum commune
Crus membranaceum simplex

Figs. 712, 713     VII

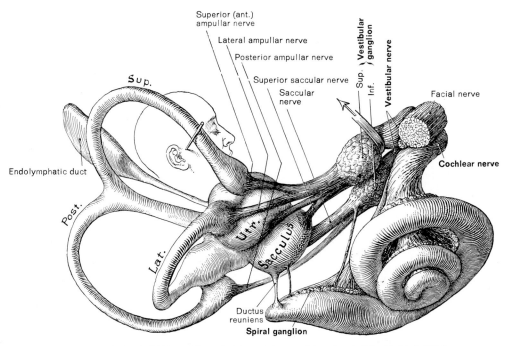

**Fig. 714: The Right Membranous Labyrinth Viewed from the Lateral Aspect (Drawing by Max Brödel, 1934)**

NOTE: 1) nerve branches from each of the ampullae of the semicircular ducts and from the utriculus and sacculus join to form the vestibular division of the vestibulocochlear nerve. The ganglion containing the sensory nerve cell bodies for this division is the vestibular (Scarpa's) ganglion and it has two parts, superior and inferior.

2) the cochlear division of the vestibulocochlear nerve serves the cochlear duct. Its ganglion, the spiral ganglion, is long and coiled. Observe the close relationship between the facial nerve and the vestibulocochlear nerve within the internal acoustic meatus. (Note that the superior semicircular duct is synonymous with the anterior semicircular duct.)

**Fig. 715: Diagram of the Membranous Labyrinth Showing the Stapes**

NOTE: 1) the bony structures are shown as cross hatched, while the perilymphatic spaces are diagrammed as white. The membranous labyrinthine duct system (endolymphatic spaces) which contains the receptors is shown as black.

2) the stapes at the vestibular window. The cochlear window, shown close by, in life is covered by the second tympanic membrane.

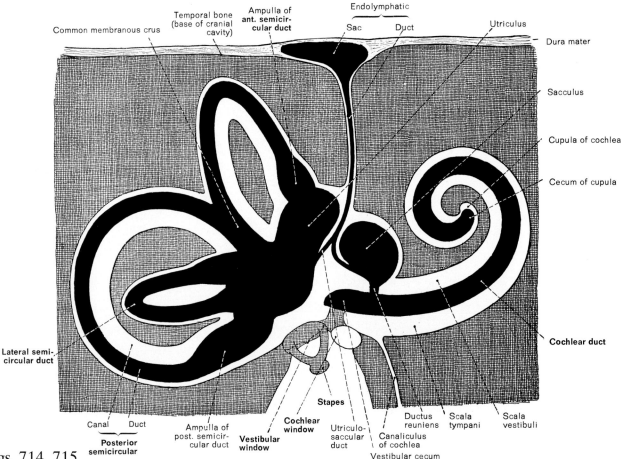

Figs. 714, 715

# Index

Numbers refer to figures in this *Atlas*.